Family Medicine: Prevention, Diagnosis and Treatment

Family Medicine: Prevention, Diagnosis and Treatment

Edited by **Felix Rohmer**

Callisto Reference
New York

Published by Callisto Reference,
106 Park Avenue, Suite 200,
New York, NY 10016, USA
www.callistoreference.com

Family Medicine: Prevention, Diagnosis and Treatment
Edited by Felix Rohmer

International Standard Book Number: 978-1-63239-753-9 (Hardback)

Printed in China.

Contents

	Preface	**IX**
Chapter 1	**Community participation in malaria control strategy of intersect oral collaboration in Ghana: Myth or reality?** Nicodemus O. Owusu	**1**
Chapter 2	**Emergency contraception amongst female college students - knowledge, attitude and practice** Wendwosen T. Nibabe and Tennyson Mgutshini	**9**
Chapter 3	**Service delivery and coverage in primary healthcare in a community-health project in Ibadan, Nigeria** Kabiru K. Salami and William R. Brieger	**16**
Chapter 4	**Missed opportunities in child healthcare** Linda Jonker and Ethelwynn L. Stellenberg	**23**
Chapter 5	**Attitudes toward condom education amongst educators for Deaf and hard-of-hearing adolescents in South Africa** Sumaya Mall and Leslie Swartz	**30**
Chapter 6	**Factors associated with patients' understanding of their management plan in Tshwane clinics** Leticia Fernandez, Theresa Rossouw, Tessa Marcus, Angelika Reinbrech-Schutte, Nicoleen Smit, Hans F. Kinkel, Shehla Memon and Jannie Hugo	**34**
Chapter 7	**The practices of isolating tuberculosis infectious patients at hospitals of Vhembe district, Limpopo Province** Takalani G. Tshitangano	**43**
Chapter 8	**Where there is no morphine: The challenge and hope of palliative care delivery in Tanzania** Kristopher Hartwig, Mervyn Dean, Kari Hartwig, Paul Z. Mmbando, Abduraoof Sayed and Elma de Vries	**50**
Chapter 9	**Sociodemographic characteristics of persons committing suicide in Durban, South Africa: 2006–2007** Soornarain S. Naidoo and Lourens Schlebusch	**58**
Chapter 10	**Implementation of the principles of primary health care in a rural area of South Africa** Surona Visagie and Marguerite Schneider	**65**

Chapter 11 **Overweight and obesity profiles in Niger Delta Region, Nigeria** 75
Alphonsus U. Idung, Festus Abasiubong, Sunday B. Udoh and Uwemedimbuk S. Ekanem

Chapter 12 **The characteristics of HIV and AIDS patients with deep vein thrombosis at Dr. George Mukhari Academic Hospital** 80
Indiran Govender, Honey L. Mabuza and Gboyega A. Ogunbanjo

Chapter 13 **Midwifery workforce profile in Limpopo Province referral hospitals** 83
Sam T. Ntuli and Gboyega A. Ogunbanjo

Chapter 14 **Blood pressure control amongst patients living with hypertension presenting to an urban district hospital outpatient clinic in Kwazulu-Natal** 87
Folafolu A. Adebolu and Mergan Naidoo

Chapter 15 **Injustice to transsexual women in a hetero-normative healthcare system** 93
Douglas Newman-Valentine and Sinegugu Duma

Chapter 16 **Patient knowledge of HIV and its treatment in South Africa** 98
Lauren M. Terblanche and Ethelwynn L. Stellenberg

Chapter 17 **What keeps health professionals working in rural district hospitals in South Africa?** 105
Louis S. Jenkins, Colette Gunst, Julia Blitz and Johan F. Coetzee

Chapter 18 **Profile and correlates of functional status in elderly patients presenting at a primary care clinic in Nigeria** 110
Samuel A. Ajayi, Lawrence A. Adebusoye, Adetola M. Ogunbode, Joshua O. Akinyemi and Ayodeji M. Adebayo

Chapter 19 **Pain management in patients with long-bone fractures in a district hospital in KwaZulu-Natal, South Africa** 117
Adeleye M. Awolola, Laura Campbell and Andrew Ross

Chapter 20 **Medicines availability at a Swaziland hospital and impact on patients** 122
Kholiwe Shabangu and Fatima Suleman

Chapter 21 **A theoretical alternative intraosseous infusion site in severely hypovolemic children** 128
Nkhensani Mogale, Albert-Neels van Schoor and Marius C. Bosman

Chapter 22 **Quality of care for patients with non-communicable diseases in the Dedza District, Malawi** 133
Rachel Wood, Vanessa Viljoen, Lisa Van Der Merwe and Robert Mash

Chapter 23 **Causes of mortality and associated modifiable health care factors for children (< 5-years) admitted at Onandjokwe Hospital, Namibia** 141
Johnface F. Mdala and Robert Mash

Chapter 24 **Risks associated with communication delays in infants from underserved South African communities** 149
Jeannie van der Linde, De Wet Swanepoel, Frances P. Glascoe, E.M. Louw, Jannie F.M. Hugo and Bart Vinck

Chapter 25 **Nurses' compliance with prevention of mother-to-child transmission national guidelines in selected sites in Kinshasa, Democratic Republic of Congo** 156
Augustin R.M. Amboko and Petra Brysiewicz

Chapter 26 **Prevalence and associated risk factors of hypertension amongst adults in a rural community of Limpopo Province, South Africa** 163
Sam T. Ntuli, Eric Maimela, Mariannes Alberts, Solly Choma and Sekgothe Dikotope

Chapter 27 **Prevalence of and factors influencing postnatal depression in a rural community in South Africa** 168
Ethelwynn L. Stellenberg and Johanna M. Abrahams

Chapter 28 **Hypertension in rural communities in Delta State, Nigeria: Prevalence, risk factors and barriers to health care** 176
Mary I. Ofili, Busisiwe P. Ncama and Benn Sartorius

Chapter 29 **Experiences of general practitioners in the Ga-Rankuwa and Mabopane areas in dealing with patients who have sexual problems** 183
Benjamin Mills, Indiran Govender and Jannie Hugo

Chapter 30 **Trends in task shifting in HIV treatment in Africa: Effectiveness, challenges and acceptability to the health professions** 191
Talitha Crowley and Pat Mayers

Chapter 31 **Why are babies born before arrival at health facilities in King Sabata Dalindyebo Local Municipality, Eastern Cape, South Africa? A qualitative study** 200
Adeyinka A. Alabi, Don O'Mahony, Graham Wright and Mohlomi J. Ntsaba

Chapter 32 **HIV and/or AIDS-related deaths and modifiable risk factors: A descriptive study of medical admissions at Oshakati Intermediate Hospital in Northern Namibia** 209
N.K. Mgori and Robert Mash

Chapter 33 **Glass injuries seen in the emergency department of a South African district hospital** 216
Doudou Nzaumvila, Indiran Govender and Efraim B. Kramer

Chapter 34 **Knowledge and perceptions of risk for cardiovascular disease: Findings of a qualitative investigation from a low-income peri-urban community in the Western Cape, South Africa** 224
Sam Surka, Krisela Steyn, Katherine Everett-Murphy, Thomas A. Gaziano and Naomi Levitt

Chapter 35 **Knowledge of community care workers about key family practices in a rural community in South Africa** 232
Ethelwynn Stellenberg, Marjorie van Zyl and Johanna Eygelaar

Chapter 36 **Exploring the meaning of caring amongst student midwives, professional midwives and educators in Tshwane, South Africa** 239
Mmajapi E.T. Masala-Chokwe and Tendani S. Ramukumba

Chapter 37 **Two-year longitudinal health-related fitness, anthropometry and body composition status amongst adolescents in Tlokwe Municipality: The PAHL Study** 247
Oluwatoyi O. Toriola, Makama A. Monyeki and Abel L. Toriola

Chapter 38 **Understanding the organisational culture of district health services: Mahalapye and Ngamiland health districts of Botswana** **254**
Oathokwa Nkomazana, Robert Mash and Nthabiseng Phaladze

Chapter 39 **Intestinal helminth infections amongst HIV-infected adults in Mthatha General Hospital, South Africa** **263**
Olukayode A. Adeleke, Parimalaranie Yogeswaran and Graham Wright

Chapter 40 **The expected and actual communication of health care workers during the management of intrapartum: An interpretive multiple case study** **270**
Doreen K.M. M'Rithaa, Sue Fawcus, Mikko Korpela and Retha De la Harpe

Permissions

List of Contributors

Preface

Family medicine covers prevention, diagnosis and cure of diseases for people of all ages constituting a family or a community. Due to its integrated approach, family medicine is capable of treating almost all the ailments. From theories to research to practical applications, case studies related to all contemporary topics of relevance to this field have been included in this book. The topics covered herein deal with the core areas of family medicine. The progress of this field along with the key concepts have been thoroughly discussed in this text. It aims to serve as a resource guide for students and experts alike and contribute to the growth of the discipline.

All of the data presented henceforth, was collaborated in the wake of recent advancements in the field. The aim of this book is to present the diversified developments from across the globe in a comprehensible manner. The opinions expressed in each chapter belong solely to the contributing authors. Their interpretations of the topics are the integral part of this book, which I have carefully compiled for a better understanding of the readers.

At the end, I would like to thank all those who dedicated their time and efforts for the successful completion of this book. I also wish to convey my gratitude towards my friends and family who supported me at every step.

Editor

1

Community participation in malaria control strategy of intersect oral collaboration in Ghana: Myth or reality?

Author:
Nicodemus O. Owusu[1]

Affiliation:
[1]Faculty of Human and Social Sciences, University of Southampton, United Kingdom

Correspondence to:
Nicodemus Owusu

Email:
kowusosei@yahoo.com

Postal address:
School of Business, Department of Management Studies, University of Cape Coast, Ghana

Background: For many years, malaria has been one of the main health concerns of the government of Ghana. The government has recently implemented a control strategy which will ensure the inclusion of the community members who were previously excluded from the process. Until now, however, scientific study on this strategy has been scanty.

Objectives: The objectives were to investigate the level at which communities have been allowed to participate and to understand whether the idea of community participation in malaria control strategy is a myth or a reality.

Methods: Data were collected in the rural district of Ahafo-Ano South in the Ashanti region of Ghana. An exploratory qualitative approach was employed in order to ascertain the opinions of the local health officials and community members. The level of participation was measured using the framework of Arnstein's 'ladder' of participation, as developed in 1969.

Results: Evidence showed that the level of community participation was only tokenistic. Communities were only informed and/or consulted after decisions had been made, but the real engagement and negotiations were absent. Communities thus had limited opportunities to air their views in the planning process.

Conclusion: This article has revealed that the government's vision of ensuring community participation in the malaria control policy-making process can be said to be a myth rather than a reality.

La participation communautaire dans la stratégie de lutte antipaludique de collaboration orale au Ghana: mythe ou réalité?

Contexte: Le paludisme a été, pendant de nombreuses années, l'une des principales préoccupations du gouvernement du Ghana en matière de santé. Le gouvernement a récemment mis en œuvre une stratégie de contrôle qui assurera l'inclusion des membres de la communauté qui étaient jusqu'ici exclus du processus. Cependant, les études scientifiques sur cette stratégie ont été rares jusqu'ici.

Objectifs: Les objectifs étaient d'étudier le taux de participation des communautés et de déterminer si l'idée de participation de celles-ci à la stratégie de contrôle du paludisme était un mythe ou une réalité.

Méthodes: Les données ont été collectées dans le district rural d'Ahafo-Ano-Sud dans la région Ashanti du Ghana. Une approche exploratoire qualitative a été employée pour déterminer les opinions des responsables de la santé et des membres de la communauté. Le taux de participation a été mesuré à l'aide de «l'échelle» de participation d'Arnstein, développée en 1969.

Résultats: Les résultats ont montré que le niveau de participation de la communauté n'était que symbolique. Les communautés n'avaient été informées et/ou consultées qu'après la prise des décisions, et il n'y avait pas eu d'engagement ni de négociations véritables. Les communautés n'avaient eu que peu d'opportunités d'exprimer leurs points de vue dans le processus de planification.

Conclusion: Cet article montre que la vision du gouvernement de faire participer la communauté au processus d'élaboration d'une politique de contrôle du paludisme est un mythe plutôt qu'une réalité.

Introduction

Setting

For more than a century now, malaria has been one of the key health issues confronting the government of Ghana. The disease has become one of the country's sources of underdevelopment as a result of economic losses and a high rate of morbidity and mortality.[1,2,3] Available evidence shows that about 44% of all outpatient illnesses caused by malaria are treated annually in the government hospitals.[3,4] In addition, it is estimated that 36% of all those admitted at the hospitals and more than 22% of all children under five years of age who die every year can be attributed to malaria.[4,5] With regard to pregnant women, it has been noted that over 13.8% are infected with malaria, with 9.4% of all maternal deaths being caused by the disease.[4,5] Many commentators have argued that these figures are merely the tip of the iceberg since most cases are not reported because they are dealt with at home.[6,7] In terms of economic losses, malaria poses a great financial burden on both households and the economy.[1,8,9] For example, a study has shown that a single episode of malaria in a household can result in an estimated average cost of almost 13.4 new Ghana Cedis ($15.79)[1,8], whilst nationally, just a 1% increase in the malaria morbidity rate might reduce the rate of real gross domestic product (GDP) growth by 0.41%.[8,9]

Faced with these problems, the last 10 years have seen a commitment from the government to address the problem by establishing an intersectoral collaboration strategy (ISC) that will allow grassroots members to be included in the malaria control policy-making process.[6,10,11] Central to the thinking behind this strategy is that by allowing the communities to participate, members would be empowered to have ownership of programme activities, could accept the challenges associated with the control of the disease and, above all, could contribute more effectively to the success of the policy goal of minimising the persistence of malaria in the country.[12,13,14] However, until now, very little has been known about the level of community participation in the ISC strategy for the control of malaria in Ghana. This makes it difficult to know whether this noble collaborative initiative in the country is rhetoric or a reality. This article therefore aims to assess how far communities have really been allowed to participate in control policy-making process in the rural district of Ahafo-Ano South (AAS) in the Ashanti region of Ghana.

The article begins with an explanation of the concept of community participation followed by Arnstein's famous 'ladder' framework.[15] It then tries to analyse which position the study site will occupy on the participation ladder. The article concludes by arguing that simply having communities play a role in the implementation process is not enough – it is more about allowing them to have the necessary influence on the planning process.

Significance of the study

Whilst participation in Ghana has been promoted in the health sector for more than a decade, most studies on the subject, until now, have mostly centred on political issues. There is therefore a paucity of information regarding community participation in the health sector. This makes this study important, when taking into account the timing, the sector and the place where the study was conducted. With respect to the timing, the study was conducted after Ghana had not only signed up to the Roll Back Malaria Agenda and become the recipient of Global Health Funds, but had also received international recognition of being one of the most democratic countries in sub-Saharan Africa. In terms of the sector, from the background readings, it is noted that this study is one of the first empirical studies to have been done with regard to community participation in the health sector in the country. Geographically, the study area is one of the newest and is also the poorest district, both within the Ashanti region and the country as whole. It is also one of the districts that still struggles with the prevention and control of the disease as a result of lack of resources. In essence, the outcomes of this study could help the malaria planning unit and all of the other stakeholders involved in the control programme activities, to enhance their intervention strategies relating to the extent of the community's involvement in programme activities.

The definition of community participation

Although the notion of community participation has been known to be significant in health programme activities, there is still a dispute over its actual meaning and the way it should be assessed.[16,17] It has, however, generally been accepted that community participation is not only the means by which communities become aware of the challenges facing them but also a better instrument for empowering and facilitating better living conditions for those who are underprivileged within the society.[18,19,20] The above characterisation highlights the importance of the power associated with participation,[21] which helps community members to be able to identify what they need, make decisions and develop the means of attaining such desires.[22,23] In so doing, they can take control of their own health and wellbeing. This eventually helps them to build their own capacity to sustain local development rather than having to rely on external agents.[22,23,24]

In addition, it has also been argued that engaging communities provides two contrasting but useful definitions of community participation, namely, 'participation as a means' and 'participation as an end'.[25]

Participation as a means implies that the way people take part in programme activities is characterised by a situation where the goal or objective (not known to all the members) has already been set for them by those in higher positions.[26] Under these circumstances, participation becomes a tool through which the available resources of the community are used in order to attain the desired goal. This kind of participation often appears to be short lived and usually fails to make use of the results of the strenuous efforts put in by the various community members.[22,24] In this way, participation is seen as something imposed by a higher authority as it does not reflect the original ideas of the local community. Rather, it becomes a device employed by powerful organisations, such as governments, looking for involvement as *a means* of utilising community resources such as local knowledge in order to ensure programme effectiveness.[23,27,28]

Participation as an end, however, has the tendency to be a long-term process, contributing toward building and fortifying the self-capabilities of the community members and enabling them to become more involved in health programmes. Participation in this sense helps to achieve goals such as social justice, equity and democracy.[29] In this situation, the source, the form of participation and the process are understood and initiated by the community members' themselves, which enhances integration and empowerment.[30] The underlying idea is that not only are the community members' independence and management skills enhanced, but their capacity to make decisions that have a direct impact on their lives is also nurtured.[31,32,33]

In effect, it can be argued that, through participation, communities can either be led by others to recognise their local health challenges and develop a method of solving them, or they can be empowered to address their own problems and to realise the basic healthcare needs for all of the members (*an end*).[34,35,36.]

Community participation and Arnstein's 'ladder' framework

The main focus of Arnstein's argument on the issue of community participation is on power. According to Arnstein, citizen participation is a process which demonstrates not only the way in which power is shared but also how those that are marginalised in society are allowed to be involved in the decisions that affect them. It is, therefore, a mechanism to allow for the underprivileged to take part in the necessary reforms that can bring about change in their society and to allow them to have a share in the wealth of their community.[15]

In measuring community participation, the various degrees to which a community has connections to power was compared to a ladder.[15,27,32] Based on this analogy, Arnstein suggested a framework with three main levels, as depicted in Figure 1.

8	Citizen control	*Degree of Citizen Power*
7	Delegated power	
6	Partnership	
5	Placation	*Degree of Citizen Tokenism*
4	Consultation	
3	Informing	
2	Therapy	*Non-participation*
1	Manipulation	

Source: Arnstein 1969[15]

FIGURE 1: Arnstein's ladder of participation.

The lowest of all the levels represents a position where no participation takes place at all.[37] After this level, the next levels are characterised by situations wherein those who are marginalised in the society are informed and consulted.[16] Next to these levels are superior degrees which allow community members to be able to influence decisions in various ways through, for example, collaboration with those at a higher level of authority. The final level represents the highest position, where the members have power over the decision-making process.[25,32,36]

In essence, the framework demonstrates the way in which power is redistributed and its significance lies in the standard that is employed in order to make a distinction between those who are at a higher position and the ordinary people found at the lower level of society. At the lower levels, Arnstein[15] argues that there are certain types of participation that provide an opportunity to the community members to either support or be informed about decisions which, by and large, have already been made. Under such circumstances, community participation becomes temporal and is sometimes only ceremonial. In addition, communities are allowed to participate, for example, in developed health programme plans and activities, so as to ensure legitimacy, gain support and prevent future criticism or sabotage. However, at the more advanced (ultimate) levels, the kind of participation that takes place can often be seen as potentially empowering. Participation at these levels allows the community the ability to mobilise and transform themselves and ensures that access to resources and services become relatively more easy.[27,38,39]

Research methods and design

The method for the study was a qualitative exploratory approach involving in-depth interviews and focus group discussions (FGDs) with local health officials and community members at the district, subdistrict and village levels. The data were collected from October 2009 to February 2010 in the AAS district in the Ashanti region. The district occupies a total land area of 124 km^2 and its capital is Mankranso. It has a total population of 174 612, with an adult population of approximately 100 000.[37] The adult literacy rate is 41.1% and, to put it into the national context, the district literacy rate of 41.1% is below the national literacy average rate of 57.9%.[11] In terms of occupation, about 80% are farmers as against the national average of almost 60% of the labour force who are engaged mostly in cocoa, vegetables, plantain and maize farming. However, it is worth mentioning that the choice of this district was for a practical purpose. In fact, whilst all of the districts in Ghana are malaria-endemic districts and therefore any of them could have been chosen, the selection of Ashanti and the AAS district was based on two main reasons: firstly, it was, because of practical considerations (such as availability of background information and familiarity with the local language), an available research network; and secondly, the opportunities for cooperation from the policy actors and the communities were assured.

In total, 80 individual in-depth interviews, including four FGDs (involving 46 participants with approximately 12 participants per group), were conducted. Two groups of interviewees were identified. The first group selected was from the local public health staff (20 interviewees), whilst the second was from within the communities. The latter group included community residents and a number of village health volunteers in malaria control programme activities. The sample size included both genders whose ages ranged from

18 to 70 years. Individual interviews lasted for approximately 45 minutes, whereas the FGDs took about two hours.

Data analysis

In analysing the data, all the audio-taped interviews were first transcribed from the local language (Ashanti) to English and this was done with care so as to maintain the original meaning of the dialogue that took place.[40,41] In achieving this, three main guiding principles were used, in line with other qualitative research enquiries. Firstly, the full interviews were read through with the aim of identifying the common themes. Secondly, each sentence was examined for the purpose of identifying the main idea behind the sentence and to give it a name or concept, that is to say, there were certain statements that could be understood only in a Ghanaian or local context and these thus needed to be interpreted for the researcher. In this way, by asking for the local explanations of certain concepts, the researcher's subjectivity was controlled during this creation process. Finally, concepts that were alike were put together to form categories which were more specific and could be generalised.[42,43] Overall, two major categories were identified and these included the local health officials' and the community members' perspectives on the extent to which they participate in the control policy process.

Ethical considerations

Permission to undertake this research was approved by the University of Southampton Ethics Board and, subsequently, by the Ministry of Health in Ghana. All participants were assured of confidentiality and the whole project was explained to them verbally, often in their own local language. Consent forms were also given to participants who agreed to take part.

Results

Characteristics of study population – The socio-demographic characteristics of the participants

Of the 80 participants who took part in the interviews, 44 (55%) were women and 36 (45%) were men. The overall mean age was 39.5 ± 1.5 years (ranging between 18 and 70 years) with the highest number of participants found in the 30–49 year age group (45%). Seventy percent (*n* = 56) of the participants were married and in terms of education, only 11% (*n* = 5) of the women and 15% (*n* = 5) of the men had education equal to senior secondary school or above. All of the rest of the women had education either up to junior secondary school (*n* = 30; 69%) or no education at all (*n* = 9; 20%), whilst 75% (*n* = 27) of the men had education up to junior secondary school and 10% (*n* = 4) had no education at all. With regard to occupation, more than two-thirds of the interviewees were farmers (74%), whilst just over one-quarter (*n* = 21; 26%), including government officials, were either salaried workers or local people who owned their own business (e.g. a shop). In essence, most of the interviewees were poor rural farmers.

The opinions from local health officials on community participation

In using Arnstein's framework, the results of this study demonstrated that there was no real community participation in the NMCP (National Malaria Control Programme) policy-making process in the study site. Evidence in the study, so far, has shown that the mechanism used for public participation in the NMCP policy-making process could be described, in the words of Arnstein, as being 'tokenistic' with 'informing' and 'consultation' (p. 217)[15] being the types of participation.

This description was the result of the opinions expressed by the most of the local health staff who were interviewed. During the interview, it was found that although some of the officers (*n* = 5; 25%) believed that there had been participation, the majority of the interviewed officers (*n* = 15; 75%) expressed their doubts regarding the extent of community participation during the planning process. According to the views shared by the majority of interviewees, despite the fact that the local health representatives were often informed about the planning process, they had no power to influence any decision that would be made during meetings, as was reflected in most of the arguments made by some of the participants during the interviews:

> 'We consult them when it is necessary and it is not always the case that their decisions are acted upon in the process.' (P3, Male, 38, District malaria control officer)

> 'Although community members are those closer to the problem especially malaria, we can take decision without them, or we usually call on them but in the end, their views do not count very much.' (P5, Female, 26, Community health nurse)

> 'I am not surprised that the community members are side-lined when it comes to the final decision on priorities because it is the government who has the resources. It is a pity but that is the reality of the situation.' (P11, Male, 35, Non-governmental organisation [NGO] worker)

Firstly, these arguments confirm that the final outcome of the malaria control programme activities do not represent the views of all those involved. This indicates that the use of ISC as a mechanism to enhance community participation in (e.g. NMCP) policy-making process is not effective. Secondly, the general picture that one can get from these arguments is that when it comes to the planning process, the inclusion of community members' priorities, as well as the chances to explore the cultural significance of their views, is lacking. Such limited participation by the communities' can lead to the neglect of important sources of lay knowledge particularly top local decisions' (p. 79).[44] This raises a question as to whether community participation in NMCP at the local level is a means or an end. From the above analysis, it is fair to say that the community participation in the malaria control policy-making process may be described aptly as a tool for the attainment of the needed goal of the health authorities through the use of the community's own resources (*a means*). This is in contrast with having communities themselves becoming more involved in developing their own capabilities in order to achieve the desired goals (*an end*) without being dictated to by the health officials.[45,46,47]

However, the few officials who believed that participation *had* taken place argued that, faced with the constraints within the various districts, all of the institutional mechanisms that had been put in place at the community level were the ideal way to consult the community members. Arguments made in support of this claim reflected the views that the complex nature of the concept 'participation' had made the issue more difficult to handle. This can be seen from the following statements:

> 'Participation is a "subtle concept" and it can be interpreted by different people in various ways, so it all depends upon how one views it.' (P2, Female, 41, District health manager)

> '[*I*]f we do not communicate to [*sic*] them, how can we even get their views? They have representatives and all of them are invited to attend some of the general meetings.' (P12, Male, 29, District health worker)

> 'We expect their representatives to consult their local people before they come and we believe that whatever they present here reflect [*sic*] the views of the community.' (P18, Female, 33, Local health education officer)

> 'We have selected community health committee members who are frequently consulted. These committee members act as the voices for the community. So, yes, they are part of the process although we make the final decision.' (P10, Female, 28, District clinical nurse)

The above arguments suggest that through decentralisation, provision has been made for the community members to participate in the planning process, of which authorities at the higher level are aware. To these officials, with this decentralisation policy, there is an opportunity given to the community members to participate in the health (e.g. NMCP) decision-making process through their local representatives.

Local residents' views on the extent of their participation

Similar to the majority of health officials, almost all of the community members (n = 46; 76%) also held the view that despite the fact that members have been participating in the process in various forums (e.g. general meetings, workshops, interviews and, indirectly, through their local health committees), the level of participation leaves much to be desired. For most of the members (n = 46; 76%), the participation of the community has been a reaction to what the health planners would like them to do. This was reflected in most of the arguments put forward by the majority of those who voiced their opinions during the FGDs. For example, one participant made the following statement:

> '[*T*]hey always come here to tell us what they intend to do but how they arrived at such decision is not something we have any means to know.' (P57, Male, 55, Local chief)

Others added:

> '[*I*]t is all good for them to contact us after they have taken a decision and come to seek our support but what I would have liked is to have us during the time of decision taking [*sic*].' (P77, Male, 23, Local youth organiser)

> 'Although we have our community health committees, they only bring us into the discussion when they have made a decision on how they want us to give our support. I find it wrong.' (P81, Female, 35, Head of women's traders association)

> '[*W*]e are only to obey what they tell us to do but nobody comes to say, this date or that date we want you to come so we can all decide on what is best for you.' (P55, Female, 33, Zonal health committee member)

> 'Often when the health officials who come here … I think they purposely come here to make us know what they intend to do which is not the same as asking for our opinions.' (P60, Male, 44, Elected zonal assemblyman)

However, from the perspective of a minority group within the interviewees (n = 14; 24%), it was noted that although they did admit that there was only consultation, they were satisfied with the type of participatory approach that was adopted. During the interview, various assertions were made by the interviewees. For example, one of the farmers said:

> 'Definitely, we are not considered at the initial stages of the planning process, but when it comes to health, it is good that doctors, nurses do the planning.' (P62, Male, 61, Local chief cocoa farmer)

In addition, a local taxi driver also expressed his concern, saying:

> 'I think we do need these experts to decide for us, especially health complex issues that affect our lives like malaria. I think it will be wrong to let us decide on our own.' (P75, Male, 31, Local taxi driver)

Finally, at the time of the FGDs, another participant said:

> 'They are trained to do that job and we are only to support them. So consulting us alone for me is okay.' (P59, Male, 40, Local shop owner)

The views expressed above by the community members reflect two divergent but important fundamental views regarding how the concept of community participation is defined in the literature. Firstly, there were those (n = 14; 24%, i.e. minority views) who acknowledged that community participation had been minimal, but nonetheless accepted it to be a step in the right direction. For them, if there was any participation at all, it should be as a reaction to the wishes of the health experts. This perception of participation agrees with the narrowest level of Rifkin's[24] idea of health which is considered to be a condition where there is no existence of illness (the medical approach). In this context, community participation is described as being a process whereby community members perform certain tasks, such as providing a healthy environment within a community, under the directives of health experts.[24] What this means is that community members are only service users and must therefore follow the orders provided by the professionals without taking part actively in policy issues that affect them.[46,47]

Thus, with regard to malaria, some members within the community wanted to be passive when it comes to decisions that affect their own health. They preferred, instead, to leave such a task in the hands of the health experts whilst following their orders.

In contrast, the second group, (*n* = 46; 76%, i.e. majority views) saw community participation in a wider context and perceived community participation to be the community members' involvement in NMCP policy decisions without necessarily resorting to the dictates of the health experts. This way of seeing community participation is consistent with the second approach of Rifkin,[24] which is called the *health service approach*. With this approach, community participation is viewed in the wider context as 'the mobilisation of community people to take an active part in the delivery of health services' (p. 241).[24]

To this group of people, decision-making regarding malaria should not be left solely in the hands of health professionals; instead, the community members should also be involved. This is in contrast to the minority group who argued that because of the complex nature of health and, for that matter, malaria, decisions should not be left to anyone other than the health professionals. This seems to suggest that the second group's majority opinion exemplifies the belief that the definition of health should not be merely the absence of disease (the medical approach), but should rather have the broader meaning of the word, which involves 'the physical, mental and social wellbeing of the individual'.[48]

Discussion

This study finding reflects the extent to which community members are given the chance to voice their concerns regarding NMCP activities in the AAS district of the Ashanti region in Ghana. There have been underlying variations in the definitions of community participation by those involved in malaria control programme activities which have given rise to both convergent and divergent perceptions.

On the one hand, the perspective of the local officials is there *has* been community participation. To them, as long as community representatives from the district health sector are invited to attend meetings, the community members are participating in the NMCP process. It is felt that these representatives represent the interests of the community and therefore have the opportunity to bring their communities' concerns to the discussion table.

On the other hand, there are those who think that there has been *limited* involvement of communities in the planning process. Some interviewed local officers agreed with the idea that when community groups are invited to participate, the ultimate real decisions are still in the hands of the state officials. There is therefore none of the empowerment and effective participation which the health policy of decentralisation purports to achieve.[49,50]

This raises a question as to whether community participation in NMCP at the local level is employed as a *means* or an *end*. From the above analysis, it is fair to say that the concept of community participation offers no opportunity to community members to attain real power at the local level policy-making processes. Instead, the community members, including their representatives, only play, in the words of Arnstein, a ritual role.[15] They are not permitted to have control over their own health situation but rather are coopted into direct forms of participation which are in essence inactive, passive and, eventually, a convenient way of controlling participation[44] – the participation is not really intended to have any significant input from the community members toward the decision-making process.

From the context of Arnstein's ladder of participation framework,[15] such participation can be regarded as tokenistic and the highest quality of participation is at consultation levels. This only guarantees the provision of information and consultation on issues and it neither leads to community empowerment nor ensures direct incorporation of input from the communities into the policy-making process. This implies that the communities are only used as tools (means) for achieving policy goals rather than being the actual decision makers (an end) regarding their local health problems.

Overall, the findings have demonstrated some key issues which demonstrate that successful implementation of the ISC strategy in the malaria control planning process has not yet taken place. In essence, despite the fact that the process and the right to participate may be devolved to the local level, the community's influence, which could mould and challenge policy development, as well as supervise the outcomes, is still in the hands of the health authorities. This is in contrast to the national health policy statement which is aimed at ensuring the empowerment of the community. However, what the health officials fail to realise is that participation is not merely about having the opportunity to consult or being informed about policy outcomes or attending meetings, but also about having the power to control inputs which would otherwise have been controlled by others who may or may not address the communities' priorities.[23]

This finding also reflects the power relationship between the community (weak) and the health experts (strong). To adopt this kind of 'induced' form of participation means that communities only accept ideas on local development that have been developed for them by health authorities instead of the members developing these ideas by themselves.

Community members thus only participated in the NMCP policy-making process when the health authorities had to inform them about certain activities rather than engaging with them regarding policy plans. Consequently, the community members had no power to influence negotiations and, under this type of participation, Arnstein has argued that community participants seem to be participating in policy process solely to give backing to government's decisions.[15] In addition, the health authorities only consulted the community members by organising general community meetings, but there was no guarantee that their suggestions and input on priorities would be considered or acted upon in the final priority selection. This kind of participation, in the words of Arnstein, is regarded as 'placation'.[15] In effect, participation by the communities could be deemed merely ceremonial, seeing as the policy-making process still bears all the features of a top-down system of decisionmaking.[49,50,51]

This is in contrast to Arnstein's idea that citizen participation involves the exchange of power through a mechanism which could promote the interests of communities in the policy processes. Participation that does not give power to the local community members can be considered to be a fruitless exercise which leads the members nowhere and 'only maintains [*the*] status quo' (p. 219).[15]

On the whole, using Arnstein's ladder of participation, it is fair to say that rather than being a reality, the level of community participation in the NMCP policy-making process could be termed as a myth characterised merely by provision of information and consultation.

Limitations

Although the methods employed in this study were useful, the author acknowledges that this study is not without its limitations. One potential limitation is that the responses to questions were based on individuals' own perceptions and could therefore be said to be subjective, rather than objective. However, this was addressed through the use of the triangulation method which involves cross-checking with others for further details as well as finding out more from the existing records and literature. Using such a method to establish the validity of the information received helped with a better comprehension of the issue under study.[52]

The second limitation was that the study was confined to only one district in Ghana and, as such, the results could not be generalised since other people in other districts could have their own opinions on the subject.

Conclusion

This article has considered the extent to which communities get involved in malaria control policy issues in the AAS district in Ghana. The study used Arnstein's ladder of participation framework to measure the level of participation. The findings showed that although the community members were allowed to take part at the district level policy-making process of malaria control, there was no power offered to the local residents. Indeed, their participation has been limited purely to information, consultation and placation throughout the process. As such, whilst the idea of participation is rooted in both international and national health policy documents, there is little explicit practical operation thereof in terms of power sharing.

This study's results, therefore, raise concerns over the effectiveness of the ISC policy strategy of national control programme to enhance community participation. Whilst it can be argued that the government is committed to controlling malaria, the same cannot be said about its commitment in promoting community participation through the ISC strategy. Having no clear and effective mechanisms for the empowerment of community members seems to put the achievement of the ideals of Alma Ata of 1978[48] and the Millennium Development Goals[53] beyond the reach of the Ghanaian government at present.

Acknowledgements

The author gratefully acknowledges the community leaders and Malaria Control Programme staff in the Ahafo-Ano South district of the Ashanti region in Ghana, for all their logistical support.

Competing interests

The author declares that he has no financial or personal relationship(s) which may have inappropriately influenced him in writing this article.

References

1. Asante FA, Asenso-Okyere K. Economic burden of malaria in Ghana. Technical report submitted to the World Health Organization (WHO), Africa Regional Office (AFRO). Legon: University of Ghana; 2003.
2. Dugbartey AT, Dugbartey MT, Apedo MY. Delayed neuropsychiatric effects of malaria in Ghana. J Nerv Ment Dis. 1998;186(3):183–186. http://dx.doi.org/10.1097/00005053-199803000-00007
3. Owusu-Agyei S, Awini E, Anto F, et al. Assessing malaria control in the Kassena-Nankana district of northern Ghana through repeated surveys using the RBM tools. Malaria J. 2007;6:103. http://dx.doi.org/10.1186/1475-2875-6-103
4. Ministry of Health. The Annual Report on National Malaria Control Programme. Accra, Ghana; 2008.
5. The Global Fund to Fight AIDS, TB and Malaria. Global Fund Results Report, 2012. Accra, Ghana; 2102.
6. USAID President's Malaria Initiative (PMI). Malaria Operational Plan – FY08 Final Version. A reflection on collaborative discussions with the national malaria control programmes and partners in country, Ghana. USAID; 2012.
7. Breman JG, Alilio MS, Mills A. Conquering the intolerable burden of malaria: what's new, what's needed. Am J Trop Med Hyg. 2004;64(Suppl.2):1–15.
8. Asenso-Okyere WK, Dzator JA. Household cost of seeking malaria care: a retrospective study of two districts in Ghana. Soc Sci Med. 1997;45(5):659–667. http://dx.doi.org/10.1016/S0277-9536(96)00383-8
9. Asante FA, Asenso-Okyere K, d'Almeida S, et al. Economic burden of malaria in the African region: evidence from Ghana. Survey Report 2(4); 2004.
10. Ministry of Health. Health sector programme of work – 2007. Independent review. Accra, Ghana; 2008.
11. Ministry of Health. Health sector programme of work – 2010. Independent review. Accra, Ghana; 2011.
12. World Bank. Rolling back malaria: the World Bank Global Strategy & Booster Programme. Washington, DC: World Bank; 2007.
13. WHO/RBM. The Roll Back Malaria strategy for improving access to treatment through home management of malaria. Geneva: WHO/HTM/MAL/1101; 2005.
14. Atkinson JA, Vallely A, Fitzgerald L, et al. The architecture and effect of participation: a systematic review of community participation for communicable disease control and elimination. Implications for malaria elimination. Malaria J. 2011;10:225. http://dx.doi.org/10.1186/1475-2875-10-225
15. Arnstein S. A ladder of citizen participation. JAIP. 1969;35(4):216–224.
16. Jewkes R, Murcott A. Meanings of community. Soc Sci Med. 1996;43(4):555–563. http://dx.doi.org/10.1016/0277-9536(95)00439-4
17. Lupton C, Peckham S, Taylor P. Managing public involvement in health care purchasing. Buckingham, UK: Open University Press; 1998.
18. Zakus JDL, Lysack CL. Revisiting community participation. Health Policy Plann. 1998;13:1–12. http://dx.doi.org/10.1093/heapol/13.1.1
19. Boyce WF. Disadvantaged persons' participation in health promotion projects: some structural dimensions. Soc Sci Med. 2001;52(10):1551–1564. http://dx.doi.org/10.1016/S0277-9536(00)00268-9
20. World Health Organization. Community involvement in health development: challenging health services. A report of a WHO study group: WHO Technical Report Series 1989;89. Geneva: WHO; 1989.
21. Boyce W, Lysack C. Understanding the community in Canadian CBR: critical lessons from abroad. Can J Rehabil. 1997;10(4):261–271.

22. Ndekha A, Hansen EH, Mølgaard P, et al. Community participation as an interactive learning process: experiences from a schistosomiasis control project in Zimbabwe. Acta Trop. 2003;85:325–338. http://dx.doi.org/10.1016/S0001-706X(02)00256-5
23. Bandesha G, Litva A. Perceptions of community participation and health gain in a community project for the South Asian population: a qualitative study. J Public Health (Oxf). 2005;27(3):241–245. http://dx.doi.org/10.1093/pubmed/fdi044
24. Rifkin SB. Lessons from community participation in health programmes. Health Policy Plann. 1986;1:240–249. http://dx.doi.org/10.1093/heapol/1.3.240
25. Nelson N, Wright S. Power and participatory development: theory and practice. London: Intermediate Technology Publications; 1995.
26. Oakley P. Projects with people: the practice of participation in rural development. Geneva: International Labour Office; 1991.
27. Morgan L. Community participation in health: perpetual allures, persistent challenge. Health Policy Plann. 2001;16(3):221–230. http://dx.doi.org/10.1093/heapol/16.3.221
28. Hayward C, Simpson L, Wood L. Still left out in the cold: problematising participatory research and development. Sociol Ruralis. 2004;44(1):95–108. http://dx.doi.org/10.1111/j.1467-9523.2004.00264.x
29. Woelk GB. Cultural and structural influences in the creation of and participation in community health programmes. Soc Sci Med. 1992;35:419–424. http://dx.doi.org/10.1016/0277-9536(92)90334-M
30. Rifkin SB, Muller F, Bichmann W. Primary health care: on measuring participation. Soc Sci Med. 1988; 26(9):931–940. http://dx.doi.org/10.1016/0277-9536(88)90413-3
31. Kaseje DC, Sempebwa EK. An integrated rural health project in Saradidi, Kenya. Soc Sci Med. 1989;28:1063–1071. http://dx.doi.org/10.1016/0277-9536(89)90389-4
32. Eyre R, Gauld R. Community participation in a rural community health trust: the case of Lawrence New Zealand. Health Promot Int. 2003;18(3):189–197. http://dx.doi.org/10.1093/heapro/dag014
33. Everatt D, Marais H, Dube N. Analysing the depth and quality of public participation in the integrated development planning process in Gauteng. Politikon. 2010;37:2–3, 223–249.
34. Cohen JM, Uphoff NT. Participation's place in rural development: seeking clarity through specificity. World Dev. 1980;8(3):213–235. http://dx.doi.org/10.1016/0305-750X(80)90011-X
35. Simovska V. The changing meanings of participation in school based health education and health promotion. Health EducRes. 2007;22(6):864–878. http://dx.doi.org/10.1093/her/cym023
36. Abers RN. Reflections on what makes empowered participatory governance happen. In: Fung A, Wright EO, editors. Deepening democracy: institutional innovations in empowered participatory governance. London: Verso, 2003; p. 200–207.
37. Ministry of Health. District Annual Report,Ahafo-Ano South, 2008.Mankraso, Ghana; 2008.
38. Espino F, Koops V, Manderson L. Community participation and tropical disease control in resources-poor settings. WHO Special Programme for Research and Training in Tropical Disease; 2004.
39. World Health Organization. Community involvement in health indicators: report on a WHO Study. WHO Regional Office for Europe; 1991.
40. Kvåle S. Interviews: an introduction to qualitative research interviewing. Thousand Oaks, CA: Sage Publications; 1999.
41. Yin RK. Case study research: design and methods.5th ed. Applied Social Research Methods Series. Newbury Park, CA: Sage Publications Inc.; 1994.
42. Strauss A, Corbin J. Basics of qualitative research: techniques and procedures for developing grounded theory. Thousand Oaks, CA: Sage Publications; 1996.
43. Denzin NK, Lincoln YS. Handbook of qualitative research. Thousand Oaks, CA: Sage Publications; 1994.
44. Anderson RB, Barnett C. The indigenous land claims in New Zealand and Canada: from grievance to enterprise. The Saskatchewan Institute of Public Policy 2006, Paper No 39. Regina, SA: University of Regina; 2006.
45. Nikkhah HA, Redzuan M. Participation as a medium of empowerment in community development. Eur J Soc Sci. 2009;11(1):170–176.
46. Oakley P. Community involvement in health development: an examination of critical issues. Geneva: World Health Organization; 1989.
47. La Bonte R. Power, participation and partnerships for health promotion. Australia, Victoria: Victorian Health Promotion Foundation; 1997.
48. World Health Organization. Declaration of Alma-Ata. USSR: International Conference on Primary Health Care, Alma-Ata, USSR. 6–12 September; 1978.
49. Blair H. Participation and accountability at the periphery: democratic local governance in six countries. World Dev. 2001;28(1):21–39. http://dx.doi.org/10.1016/S0305-750X(99)00109-6
50. Brinkerhoff D, Crosby B. Managing policy reform: concepts and tools for decision makers in developing and transitioning countries. Bloomfield, CT: Kumarian Press; 2002.
51. Laverack G, Wallerstein N. Measuring community empowerment: a fresh look at organizational domains. Health Promot Int. 2001;16:179–185. http://dx.doi.org/10.1093/heapro/16.2.179
52. Jick TD. Mixing qualitative and quantitative methods: triangulation in action. AdminSciQuart.1979;24(4):602–611.
53. United Nations Development Programme/Government of Ghana. 2010 Ghana Millennium Development Goals Report. Accra, Ghana; 2012

2

Emergency contraception amongst female college students – knowledge, attitude and practice

Authors:
Wendwosen T. Nibabe[1]
Tennyson Mgutshini[2]

Affiliations:
[1]Ethiopian Society of Obstetricians and Gynaecologists, Addis Ababa

[2]College of Human Sciences, University of South Africa, South Africa

Correspondence to:
Tennyson Mgutshini

Email:
mgutst@unisa.ac.za

Postal address:
The University of South Africa, Preller Street, Pretoria, UNISA, 0003, South Africa

Background: Unwanted teenage pregnancies have a notable detrimental impact on the learners' trajectory and have been associated with jeopardising the students' educational progress and future career prospects. These pregnancies are mostly unplanned and unintended and many are terminated, either legally or illegally.

Aim: The aim of this study was to explore the contributory role played by the knowledge, attitude and practices of female college students with respect to the utilisation of emergency contraceptives.

Setting: Three tertiary institutions in Dessie, Ethiopia.

Methods: Quantitative self-administered questionnaires were used to collect descriptive data from 352 female college students.

Results: The study revealed that there was a high percentage (78.3%) of unwanted pregnancies amongst those engaging in sex. Significantly, nearly half (43.3%) of these unwanted pregnancies resulted in abortion. Only 10% of the students sampled admitted to ever having used emergency contraception. Even though more than half (69.9%) of the students knew about emergency contraception, only 27% of them felt confident that they understood when it was most effective.

Conclusion: These and other observed findings confirm the need for improvement of female college students' knowledge and timely utilisation of emergency contraception.

La contraception d'urgence chez les étudiantes inscrites dans l'enseignement supérieur – connaissances, attitudes et pratiques

Présentation: Les grossesses non désirées des adolescentes ont un impact négatif notoire sur les parcours des apprenantes et ont été associées à la mise en péril des progrès des étudiantes en termes d'études et de perspectives professionnelles. Ces grossesses sont, pour l'essentiel, non planifiées et non désirées, et nombre sont interrompues, que ce soit légalement ou illégalement.

Objectif: L'objectif de l'étude était d'étudier le rôle joué par les connaissances, les attitudes et les pratiques des étudiantes inscrites dans l'enseignement supérieur quant à l'utilisation des contraceptifs d'urgence.

Cadre: Trois établissements d'enseignement supérieur à Dessie, en Éthiopie.

Méthodes: Des questionnaires quantitatifs auto-administrés ont été utilisés afin de recueillir des données descriptives auprès de 352 étudiantes suivant des études supérieures.

Résultats: L'étude a révélé qu'il existait un fort pourcentage (78.3%) de grossesses non désirées parmi les jeunes filles prenant part à des activités sexuelles. Il convient de noter que près de la moitié (43.3%) de ces grossesses non désirées se soldait par un avortement. Seules 10% des étudiantes interrogées ont déclaré avoir utilisé une contraception d'urgence. Bien que plus de la moitié (69.9%) des étudiantes savait que la contraception d'urgence existait, 2% d'entre elles seulement étaient certaines de bien comprendre à quel moment celle-ci était la plus efficace.

Conclusion: Ces conclusions, auxquelles viennent s'ajouter celles d'autres études, confirment la nécessité d'améliorer les connaissances des étudiantes inscrites dans l'enseignement supérieur sur la contraception d'urgence et son utilisation en temps opportun.

Introduction

Emergency contraception is a method of preventing unwanted pregnancy resulting from unintended sexual activity, contraceptive failure or sexual assault,[1] as well as from a lack of knowledge about or access to contraception. Its primary use is in reducing the need for abortions and the negative maternal health consequences associated therewith.[2] Related literary sources suggest that, for most of the youth, tertiary education represents a shift toward greater independence from home – an opportunity to form new friendships and, for some, an opportunity to experience romantic and/or sexual relationships. Higher education students' unwanted pregnancies pose a major public health problem globally. This problem also presents in Ethiopia, where there are added challenges resulting from the fact that some parts of society adhere to strict cultural and religious practices that forbid premarital sex. Unwanted pregnancies have a notable detrimental impact on the learners' trajectory and have been associated with jeopardising the students' educational progress and future career prospects. These pregnancies are mostly unplanned and unintended and many are terminated, either legally or illegally.[3]

Predecessor research suggests that 'emergency contraception (EC) can substantially reduce a woman's chance of becoming pregnant when taken soon after sex'.[4,5,6] By inference, this offers protection from the negative consequences of unplanned pregnancies as described above. When used within 72 hours after sexual contact, emergency contraceptive tablets have the capacity to prevent pregnancy by 75% - 58% and, when combined with the use of intra-uterine contraceptive devices (IUCDs), as many as 99% of unwanted pregnancies can be prevented.[7] Although options for and information about emergency contraception have increased, further efforts are needed in order to improve women's access to this important backup method of birth control.[2] In global terms, an estimated 46 million induced abortions are performed annually with 78 000 maternal deaths each year.[8] In Ethiopia, unsafe abortions account for nearly 60% of all gynaecological admissions and almost 30.0% of all obstetric admissions.[9] Approximately 22% – 54% of direct obstetric deaths are as a result of unsafe abortion. Emergency contraception is increasingly regarded as the primary means to reduce abortion rates.[10] In Ethiopia, women who undergo induced abortions are more likely statistically to be below the age of 30 years and literate, often having studied beyond the level of secondary education.[11]

Some, including Ambaw,[12] Tilahun,[3] Mengist[13] and Tamire and Enqueselassie,[11] have conducted research in different universities in Ethiopia and all concur that the number of students who have a positive attitude toward sexual practice and the number of those who are experiencing penetrative sex and induced abortion are increasing. Despite this, their awareness with regard to preventing unintended pregnancy after incidental sex is relatively limited. It is this consensus that sets the backdrop for the acknowledgement that making emergency contraceptive pills (ECPs) accessible to college students is a crucial first step in helping to curb the growing rates of unintended pregnancy and unsafe abortion.[14] Imbedded within this is the need for a clearer understanding of the factors that promote or limit students' use of emergency contraceptives.

Statement of the research problem

In spite of the high rate of unwanted pregnancies, the uptake of emergency contraception to prevent such an occurrence amongst college students at different colleges in Ethiopia is disproportionately low. The factors that influence utilisation patterns are as yet poorly understood. This poses a range of major public health problems – including an increased risk of complications associated with illegal abortions in the country – and may be associated with dropout and non-completion of education amongst students due to unintended pregnancies. This area of research has not been given much attention within the Ethiopian context and, to date, only a few non-research-based reports exist, with much of the discourse being conducted within mass media outlets. This background dictates a need for primary research to offer empirical insights into the reasons for low uptake of emergency contraception as a first step toward the reduction of pregnancy in college students. In keeping with this imperative, the current study looks specifically at the role by played by attitudes, knowledge and practice in determining the usage of emergency contraceptives. For the study, 'attitude' will be conceptualised as being a hypothetical construct that represent an individual's degree of like or dislike for something. This is often referred to as the attitude object. People can also be conflicted about or ambivalent toward an object, meaning that they possess both positive and negative attitudes simultaneously toward the item in question. Attitudes are judgements.[15]

Objectives

In attempting to achieve the aim of the study, a number of key objectives were identified and include: (1) to assess the students' pre-existing knowledge with regard to emergency contraception; (2) to assess students' pre-existing attitudes about sex and how can these affect their use of emergency contraception; (3) to assess the utilisation level of emergency contraceptives amongst students; and (4) to utilise the findings to develop practical recommendations for service providers.

Research method and design

Study design and setting

There are six colleges in Dessie, Ethiopia, of which three were selected by a simple random sampling method. A quantitative descriptive cross-sectional study was conducted at these three colleges. Primary data were collected via self-administered structured questionnaires to assess female college students' *Knowledge*, *Attitude* and *Practice* toward sex and emergency contraception.

Study population and sampling

In this study, all female students in the selected colleges (N = 2554) were considered as a source population and the required sample size was drawn from this population. Multi-stage sampling was used to guide the selection process. To start, three colleges out of the total six colleges in the city were selected using simple random sampling. The selected colleges were Dessie Teacher's Education College (6 departments, 40 classes and 1110 female students), Admas University College (6 departments, 8 classes and 248 female students) and ALKAN University College (2 departments, 15 classes and 451 female students).

Sample size calculation

The sample size was calculated using a one-sample population proportion formula. Assuming the proportion of students who are aware of emergency contraception to be 50% and assuming a non-response rate of 10%, the required sample was calculated using the following formula:

$$n = [(z\acute{a}/2)^{2}*p(1-p)*(D)]/d^2 = [(1.96)^2(0.5)(0.5)]/(0.05)^2 = 384.16$$

Adding a 10% non-response rate, 384.16 +10% = 423 study subjects. But since the total population is less than 10 000 or $n/N > 10\%$ it was essential to use population correction. Therefore, nf = ni/[1 + ni/N] = 423/[1+423/2554]=363.

Where:
n = the desired sample size
p = proportion of students who have knowledge about emergency contraceptives = 50% (used to obtain a maximum sample size as there was no previous study conducted in this regard in Dessie) $(z\acute{a}/2)^2$ = critical value at 95% confidence level of certainty (1.96)
d^2 = the margin of error between the sample and the population = 5%
D = design effect (one stage)
nf = final sample size after correction
ni = initial sample size before correction

The required sample size was thus 363.

Based on proportional allocation, 223 students from Dessie Teacher's Education College, 50 students from Admas University College and 90 students from ALKAN University College were included in the study.

Data collection

Data were collected using a structured self-administered questionnaire. To assess whether the instrument covered all dimensions of the construct, relevant literature and experts in the field were consulted, with due consideration to the research problem. In addition, the instrument items were adapted in part from a standardised questionnaire used in the nationwide survey conducted by the Ethiopian Family Guidance Association and others from instruments of similar studies conducted and published in different journals.[16] The questionnaires were pre-tested with students in two departments at Dessie Teacher's Education College. Based on pre-test feedback and suggestions, some questions were rephrased or amended and the final questionnaire was then prepared. Of the total questionnaires distributed to the respondents, five were incomplete and six were returned blank, resulting in a response rate of 97%.

Data collection process

The questionnaire was administered at the three colleges over a number of days. There were three data collectors in total with each collecting data from one college. Randomly-selected students from different departments and different classes were divided into groups of 10 and distributed into different groups.

The students were briefed about the purpose of the initial meeting and very detailed information about the study was presented when they gathered in the lecture halls. They were then informed about the survey – its objectives and procedures – and were assured that the information collected would be treated as confidential and used only for research purposes. This approach was chosen so as to aid the dissemination of information in the most convenient manner. The interactive presentation of the study overview allowed potential participants opportunities to seek clarification. The purpose of this was to reduce the non-response rate. After these initial information sessions, prospective respondents were given a week-long cooling-off period to consider their decision about giving consent. In addition to this, the students were reassured throughout all stages of the study about their right to opt out of the study without repercussions. Students who gave consent were provided with the questionnaire and were given access to an area where they could complete their questionnaire in private.

Validity and reliability

To promote validity and reliability within the study, a number of measures were introduced, including ensuring homogeneity in the ages of the students surveyed. For example, the study focused primarily on students at the same level of study. The students also had to meet pre-identified criteria, such as being 18 years or older and being a fulltime student, which helped to eliminate any bias resulting from differential selection of study subjects. There were, however, elements within the study which introduced some heterogeneity, for example, the participants were from different cultures and religions and included members from both rural and urban areas.

Data management and analysis

A total of 352 female college students at the three chosen institutions completed the questionnaire. The data from the questionnaires were analysed by a statistician using SPSS for Windows, version 16.0. Descriptive statistics were elicited for each of the questions.

Ethical issues

Multi-site ethical clearance was obtained from the higher degrees committee of the Department of Health Studies at the University of South Africa as well as from each of the three colleges that were included in the study. Written permission was provided by each of these entities with the express proviso that participating students would be guaranteed the freedom to refuse participation without fear of prejudice. In keeping with this, prospective participants were invited to take part in the study by letter initially and this was then followed up verbally on their arrival at the research site. Privacy and confidentiality were maintained both during and after the administration of the questionnaire by ensuring that the students in the lecture halls were separated out adequately and by posting individual questionnaires using registered post. At the beginning and at the completion of each questionnaire, data collectors thanked the study subjects for their willingness and for giving their time to participate in the study.

Results

Demographic data

All respondents were aged between 18 and 25 years. Of this group, 29.8% (*n* = 105) participants were between 18 and 19 years old; 34.1% (*n* = 120) were between 20 and 21 years old; 18.5% (*n* = 65) were between 22 and 23 years old; and 17.6% (*n* = 62) were between the ages of 24 and 25. For the religious breakdown of the respondents, 67.3% (*n* = 237) were Orthodox Christians; 30.1% (*n* = 106) were Muslim; 2% (*n* = 7) were Protestant; 0.3% (*n* = 1) were Catholic; and 0.3% (*n* = 1) had other affiliations. The educational level of the respondents ranged from first year (25%; *n* = 88) to third year (40.62%; *n* = 143), as indicated in Table 1.

Of the respondents, 83.24% (*n* = 293) were unmarried and 16.76% (*n* = 59) married. The majority of the respondents (37.5%; *n* = 132) lived with their friends; 34.1% (*n* = 120) lived alone; and 28.4% (*n* = 100) lived with their family.

Identified independent variables were fit into five separate binary logistic-regression models (models 1–5) to examine the association between each of the predictor and outcome variables (emergency contraception awareness; attitude toward sex and emergency contraception; and sexual practice and utilisation of emergency contraception). In model 1, the dependent variable was dichotomised and coded as 1 (aware of emergency contraception) and as 0 (never heard about emergency contraception). In a similar fashion, the dependent variables (attitude toward sex and attitude toward emergency contraception) in model 2 and 3 were dichotomised and coded as 1 (favourable attitude) and 0 (unfavourable attitude). The fourth and fifth independent variables were dichotomised and coded as 1 (ever practised) and 0 (never practised). Categorical independent variables were categorised meaningfully and then grouped.

Students' knowledge of emergency contraceptives

One hundred and eighty-seven (53.3%) of the students knew about at least one regular modern contraceptive method and 79 (22.4%) knew about two or more modern methods, which is lower than a similar study conducted in the Oromia regional state of Ethiopia (85.6%).[13] Amongst the modern methods known of by the respondents, injectable contraceptives were the most commonly-known method (22.7%), followed by pills (12.5%). On the other hand, 22.7% (*n* = 80) of the students did not know about any of the commonly-used contraceptive methods.

Of the 352 respondents, 69.9% (*n* = 246) had heard about emergency contraception. Of those who knew about emergency contraception, 8.9% (*n* = 22) had obtained their information from reading leaflets, 38.6% (*n* = 95) from radio and TV, 30.9% (*n* = 76) from health education at different health facilities and 21.5% (*n* = 53) from college during different lectures and peer discussion. Regarding the type of contraceptives used as emergency, 53.7% (*n* = 132) said pills, 11.4% (*n* = 28) said IUCD and 19.1% (*n* = 47) cited both pills and IUCD. Of these students, 15.9% (*n* = 39) did not know which particular contraceptive is used as emergency contraception. With respect to the type of drug used as emergency contraception, 46.3% (*n* = 114) replied that it is the same as the drug found in ordinary contraceptives and 41.9% (*n* = 103) answered that it is the same one, but stronger than the ordinary contraceptives. Concerning the time limit for taking pills and the insertion of an IUCD as emergency contraception, only 32.1% (*n* = 79) indicated correctly that emergency contraceptive pills should be taken within 72 hours, whilst only 6.5% (*n* = 16) replied that an IUCD should be inserted within 5 days.

To assess the level of actual knowledge, a series of eight knowledge questions (on method identification; drug composition; time frame for effective use; time interval between doses; effectiveness of the drug; appropriate situations for use; and places where emergency contraception can be found) were posed to those students who had heard of emergency contraception. To generate the summarised level of knowledge, the response on each question was first scored and tallied and then the total of each respondent was scored ranging from 0–8 (0% – 100%). A cumulative/total score was calculated and then the respondents were classified as poor, fair or good with respect to their level of knowledge about emergency contraception. Hence, respondents who scored zero were considered as *'not having the knowledge'*; those who scored 12.5% – 50% as *'fair knowledge'*; and those who scored more than 50% as *'good knowledge'*.

TABLE 1: Age distribution of female college students.

Age of respondents in years	Frequency	Percent	Valid Percent	Cumulative Percent
18–19	105	29.8	29.8	29.8
20–21	120	34.1	34.1	63.9
22–23	65	18.5	18.5	82.4
24–25	62	17.6	17.6	36.9
Total	**352**	**100.0**	**100.0**	**100.0**

Attitude of students toward sex

Students were questioned extensively about their attitudes toward sexual relationships. A set of nine statements pertaining to relationships and sex were included in the questionnaire. Six positive and three negative items were included in order to maintain the balance of responses. The nine items were answered as either 'agreed strongly', 'agreed slightly', 'had no opinion about the statement under consideration', 'disagreed slightly', or 'disagreed strongly' (a five-point Likert scale). For positively-worded statements, those who selected 'agree' were regarded as having a positive attitude and those who chose 'disagree' were considered to have a negative attitude. Conversely, for negatively-worded statements, those who selected 'agreed' were clustered as having a negative outlook, whereas those who said 'disagree' were categorised as having a positive attitude. The responses on each attitudinal items were scored and tallied, then the total of each respondent's score was ranged from 0–9 (0% – 100%). A score of 50% and above was considered to be a *'favourable attitude'* whereas those scoring below 50% were thought of as having an *'unfavourable attitude'*. The summarised attitudinal index indicates that 84.4% of the total respondents had a favourable attitude toward sexual relationships.

Attitude toward emergency contraceptives

Respondents were again questioned about their attitudes toward emergency contraception. The five items were answered as either 'agree strongly', 'agree slightly', 'neutral', 'disagree slightly' or 'disagree strongly'. For positively-worded statements, those who selected 'agree' were regarded as having a positive attitude and those who chose 'disagree' were considered to have a negative attitude. Conversely, for negatively-worded statements, those who selected 'disagree' were clustered as having a positive outlook whereas those who said 'agree' were categorised as having a negative attitude. The responses on each attitudinal item were scored and tallied, then the total of each respondent's score was ranged between 0 and 5 (0% – 100%). A score of 50% and above was considered as being a *'favourable attitude'*, whereas those scoring below 50% were thought of as having an *'unfavourable attitude'*.

Respondents' sexual practice

Respondents were asked whether they had ever had sexual intercourse and, if so, whether they had a history of pregnancy and at what age they became pregnant. Amongst the respondents, 36.6% (n = 129) had experienced sexual intercourse. Of the total 129 students that had sexual experience, 46.5% (n = 60) had a history of pregnancy. The majority (76.7%; n = 45) of these students had fallen pregnant between 15 and 19 years of age. Of these pregnancies, 78.3% (n = 47) were not planned. Of the total pregnancies, 43.3% (n = 26) resulted in an unsafe abortion.

Respondents' utilisation of emergency contraception

Of the 246 students who had heard about emergency contraception, only 15.4% (n = 38) of the students made use of it, which is still higher than a study conducted in Adama University and Jimma University of Ethiopia (4.7% and 6.8%, respectively).[3,10] The higher use of emergency contraception in this study could be because of the fact that a higher proportion of them (36.6%; n = 129) had a history of sexual intercourse when compared with those at Adama University[3] (29%; n = 194).

With regard to regularity of use, 71.1% (n = 27) of the students had used emergency contraception only once and 28.9% (n = 11) of them had used it twice. Of the students who had ever used emergency contraception, 68.4% (n = 26) obtained it from nurses and the rest (31.6%; n = 12) directly from pharmacists. The majority of them (63.2%; n = 24) used it because of miscalculation of their safe sexual time. Most of the sexually-active respondents who had a history of sexual practice (56.6%; n = 73) complained that the main challenge with regard to utilisation of emergency contraceptives was their unavailability in pharmacies at the time of need. The second challenge mentioned by 23.3% (n = 30) of the respondents was fear of stigma. A diagrammatic overview is presented in Table 2.

Discussion

Knowledge of students about emergency contraceptives

Similar procedures were followed by Ayana[16] and Desta and Regassa.[17] Based on the summary index, about 66.1% fell into the range of 'fair knowledge' and only 33.9% had good knowledge of emergency contraception. The level of knowledge here is comparable to that conducted in Bahirdar University (34.8%)[18] and slightly higher than a study

TABLE 2: Practice with regard to emergency contraception amongst female college students at Dessie Teacher's Education College, ALKAN University College and Admas University College in Dessie, Ethiopia (2012).

Practice indicators	Number	Percent
Have you ever used emergency contraceptive pills? (n = 246)		
Yes	38	15.4
No/Others	208	84.6
How many times have you used this method during the last year? (n = 38)		
Once	27	71.1
Twice/Others	11	28.9
Who recommend use of emergency contraception? (n = 38)		
A friend	4	10.5
Partner (male)	9	23.7
Health professional/Others	25	65.8
Who provided you with emergency contraception? (n = 38)		
Nurses	26	68.4
Pharmacists/	12	31.6
Why did you use emergency contraception? (n = 38)		
Time was miscalculated	24	63.2
Condom broke	3	7.9
Pills missed	6	15.8
Withdrawal failed/Others	5	13.2
What were the challenges you faced to get emergency contraception? (n = 129)		
Price	6	4.7
Not available in pharmacies	73	56.6
Fear of stigma	30	23.3
Lack of knowledge/Others	20	15.5

conducted in Jimma University (22.8%),[19] but lower than a study conducted in Addis Ababa University (43.5%).[11]

Binary logistic-regression analysis showed that students aged 18–19 and 20–21 are respectively 86.5% and 74.5% less knowledgeable than their reference age (24–25), with $p < 0.001$, adjusted odds ratio (AOR) 0.135, 95% confidence interval (CI) 0.056–0.323 for the students aged 18–19; and $p < 0.005$, AOR 0.255, 95% CI 0.106–0.610 for students aged 20–21. In the case of level of education, as years of study increased there was a relative increase in the knowledge about emergency contraception, making third-year students a reference ($p < 0.001$, AOR = 0.077, (95% CI 0.035–0.170) for first-year students and for second-year students ($p < 0.001$, AOR 0.141, 95% CI 0.066–0.301), which means they were respectively 92% and 86% less knowledgeable than third-year students. There is also a statistically-significant association between marital status and knowledge about emergency contraception. Married respondents had more knowledge than unmarried respondents (AOR 2.094, 95%CI 1.040–4.213).

Attitude of students toward sex

In model 2, level of education had a significant association with attitude toward sex, where those in first year were 0.258 times less likely to have a favourable attitude toward sex than respondents at the third-year level.

Attitude toward emergency contraceptives

A similar procedure was followed by previous researchers.[18,20] The summarised attitudinal index indicates that 63.6% of the respondents who had ever heard of emergency contraception had a favourable attitude toward it. This figure is better than studies conducted in Addis Ababa University (53%)[11], Bahirdar University (56.7%)[18] and Hawassa post-secondary school female students (65.6%),[16] but less than a study conducted amongst female students at Haramaya University.[17]

In this study, there is also a statistically-significant association between age and educational level of the respondents and their attitude toward emergency contraception. Students aged 18–19 showed 86.5% less-positive attitudes towards emergency contraception ($p < 0.001$, 95% CI 0.056–0.323) compared with students aged 24–25. Similarly, students aged 20–21 were 74.5% less positive toward emergency contraception compared with their 24–25 year-old counterparts ($p < 0.005$, 95% CI.0.106–0.610). Again, first- and second-year students reported less-positive attitudes toward emergency contraception than third-year students ($p < 0.001$, AOR 0.077, 95% CI 0.035–0.170; and $p < 0.0.001$, AOR 0.141, 95% CI 0.066–0.301, respectively).

Respondents' sexual practice

There are no independent variables having a statistically-significant association with model 4 (sexual practice), except the marital status of the respondents – unmarried students are less likely to indulge in sexual practice ($p < 0.001$, AOR 0.0.370 and 95% CI 0.124–0.535). A similar study in Addis Ababa showed a lower rate of unwanted pregnancy (73.5%; $n = 36$),[2] an equivalent rate of induced abortion (71.7%; $n = 38$) and a lower rate of unsafe abortion (29%; $n = 11$). The possible explanation for the low rate of safe abortion, high rate of unsafe abortion and high rate of unwanted pregnancy and delivery in this study could be due to a lack of health facilities with sufficiently-trained staff; a lack of awareness about where to get safe preventive methods; and financial problems that made the respondents take measures that threatened their life or their future.

Respondents' utilisation of emergency contraception

Of the variables that were studied, only two independent variables emerged as being statistically significant in terms of their association with utilisation of emergency contraception, namely, (1) age of the respondents and (2) marital status. Students aged from 22–23 years old were 2.9 times more likely to utilise emergency contraception than younger fellow students ($p < 0.05$, 95% CI 1.007–8.368) and married students were 0.359 times less likely to utilise emergency contraception than unmarried students ($p < 0.005$, 95% CI 0.169–0.760).

Limitations of the study

There were a number of limitations with regard to this study. Firstly, the data were collected only from female students in colleges. In the rural areas, where only a small proportion of individuals get an opportunity to attend college, the result from the current study has limited statistical power and cannot be generalised to all youth in the study area, thus possibly overestimating the result. Secondly, self-reported information is subjected to reporting errors, missed values and bias. Since the study touches on sensitive issues, the possibility of underestimation cannot be excluded, even though the study was anonymous. Thirdly, the young females were extremely impatient during the collection, which was expected for this age. They were impatient with regard to the questions presented, as well as the time required. Many felt shy with respect to some issues, especially those related to sex, and there were 11 non-responses. Lastly, the current study offers a quantitative exploration and future researchers could offer clarifying insights through the use of qualitative methodologies.

Conclusion

The study findings revealed that whilst overall awareness of emergency contraception was within the expected norms, specific knowledge of is very low (33.9%) amongst the female students of Dessie Teacher's Education College, Admas University College and ALKAN University College. Of those who had ever heard of emergency contraception, 63.6% reported favourable attitudes toward emergency contraception. The present study has also documented that the knowledge and attitude of female college students toward emergency contraception was affected by a range of personal characteristics including age and level of education, whilst marital status, attitude towards sex and utilisation of emergency contraception are affected by level of education and marital status. Finally, a high rate of sexual activity and unwanted pregnancies have been reported. This prompts a need for sexual health services to initiate important measures, such as provision of continuous sex education, guidance and counselling services – especially during the first year of university – and increasing accessibility of emergency contraception and other preventive methods to the users. It is worth noting that the campus health workers can play an important role by spreading the knowledge of emergency contraception widely throughout the student community through individual counselling when female students visit the clinic.

Recommendations

Strengthening information education and communication in colleges on sexual reproductive health, with special emphasis on different family-planning methods – including emergency contraception – will be a problem-solving procedure for female college students. Contraception information sessions should cover all details of how the emergency contraceptives work and how they should be taken.

Clinics guided by special policies should be available to provide reproductive health services for adolescence and young female students, in particular over weekends and during the evenings.

A collaborative effort between service providers, health institutes and colleges is of paramount importance. It would be a good idea to make emergency contraceptives, especially emergency contraceptive pills, available at all drug-dispensing institutes including private and government institutions, non-governmental organisations, pharmacies, clinics and community-based distribution agents. Facilitating conditions to distribute or sell without prescription, after sufficient training and information sessions for both dispensers and clients, could be helpful.

There is also a need to empower young people to discuss sexual and reproductive health issues with their parents, friends and others.

The majority of the female college students did not have any actual knowledge about emergency contraceptives. It is thus recommended that emergency contraceptives be advertised in clinics, in colleges, at schools and also during radio and television broadcasts.

Strengthening of sexual health clubs starting from the lower levels of education is also important. Educators should provide moments to reflect, to think about the responsibilities involved in sexual practices and to discuss gender relations in terms of relationships because this aspect is linked directly to pregnancy in female college students. Emergency contraception should also be included in the curriculum of the students along with other family planning methods.

Acknowledgements

The authors would like to acknowledge the Dean of the College of Humans Sciences at UNISA, Professor Moeketsi, for her support of this study.

Competing interests

The authors declare that they have no financial or personal relationship(s) which may have inappropriately influenced them in writing this article.

Authors' contributions

WTN (Ethiopian Society of Obstetricians and Gynaecologists) and TM (University of South Africa) were the sole contributors to the conception and preparation of the manuscript. WTN was the primary researcher.

References

1. Gebeyohanis E. Assessment of knowledge, attitude and utilization of emergency contraception among Mekelle University female undergraduate students. Master's thesis. Addis Ababa: School of Public Health, Addis Ababa University Medical Faculty; 2009.
2. Lemma DA. Emergency contraception in Addis Ababa: practice of service providers. Master's thesis. Pretoria: University of South Africa; 2009.
3. Tilahun D, Assefa T, Belachew T. Knowledge, attitude and practice of emergency contraceptives among Adama University female students. Ethiop J Health Sci. 2010;20(3):195–202. PMid:22434979, PMCid:PMC3275848
4. NARAL Pro-choice America. Emergency contraception (EC): an important and underutilized contraceptive option. [document on the Internet]. c2011 [cited 2013 October 21]. Available from http://www.prochoiceamerica.org/media/fact-sheets/birth-contol-emergency-contraception.pdf
5. Association of Reproductive Health Professionals. Update on emergency contraception. [page on Internet]. c2011 [cited 2013 Nov 10]. Available from http://www.arhp.org/Publications-and-Resources/Clinical-Proceedings/EC/Introduction
6. Guttmacher Institute. Emergency contraception. [document on the Internet]. c2012 [cited 2012 September 26]. Available from www.guttmacher.org/statecenter/spibs/spib_EC.pdf
7. International Consortium for Emergency Contraception. Emergency contraceptive pills. Medical and service delivery guidelines. Washington DC. 2nd edition; 2004.
8. Pavin L. Emergency Contraception. CMAJ. 2003;169(6):230–244.
9. Federal Ministry of Health. Technical and procedural guidelines for safe abortion services in Ethiopia. Addis Ababa: Ethiopia; 2006.
10. Abera H, Tebeje B. Knowledge, attitudes, and practices towards emergency contraception among female Jimma University students, Jimma, Southwest Ethiopia. Ethiopian Journal of Reproductive Health.2009;3(1):37–43.
11. Tamire W, Enqueselassie F. Knowledge, attitude, and practice on emergency contraceptives among female university students in Addis Ababa, Ethiopia. Ethiop J Health Dev. 2007;21(2):111–116. http://dx.doi.org/10.4314/ejhd.v21i2.10037
12. Ambaw F. Predictors of sexual value systems among Jimma University students, Southwest Ethiopia. Ethiop J Health Sci.2008;18(3):109–116.
13. Mengistu S. Assessment of level of awareness and utilization of emergency contraception, among college female students in Oromia Regional state, Arsi Zone, Asella town, South-East Ethiopia. Master's thesis. Addis Ababa: School of Public Health, Addis Ababa University; 2007.
14. Parker C. Adolescents and emergency contraceptive pills in developing countries. Family Health International Working Paper Series WP05-01, 2005; p. 1–18.
15. Nolen-Hoeksema S. Atkinson and Hilgard's introduction to psychology. 15th ed. Kentucky: Wadsworth Inc; 2009.
16. Ayana WB. Emergency contraceptive: Post-secondary school female students' and service providers' perspective (the case of Awassa Town). Master's thesis. Addis Ababa: Addis Ababa University School of Graduate Studies; 2008.
17. Desta B, Regassa N. On emergency contraception among female students of Haramaya University, Ethiopia: surveying the level of knowledge and attitude. Master's thesis. Addis Ababa: Institute of Population Studies, Addis Ababa University; 2011.
18. Atsede D. Emergency contraceptive: knowledge, attitudes, and practices (KAP) among Bahir Dar University female students [unpublished thesis]. Addis Ababa; 2007.
19. Nasir T. Knowledge, attitude and practice of emergency contraception among graduating female students of Jimma University, Southwest Ethiopia. Ethiop J Health Sci. 2010;20(2):91–97.
20. Tajure N, Pharm B. Knowledge, attitude and practice of emergency contraception among graduating female students of Jimma University, Southwest Ethiopia. Ethiop J Health Sci. 2010;20(2):91–97. PMid:22434966, PMCid:PMC3275837

Service delivery and coverage in primary healthcare in a community-health project in Ibadan, Nigeria

Authors:
Kabiru K. Salami[1]
William R. Brieger[2]

Affiliations:
[1]Department of Sociology, University of Ibadan, Nigeria

[2]Department of International Health, Bloomberg School of Public Health, Johns Hopkins University, USA

Correspondence to:
Kabiru Salami

Email:
kabsalami@yahoo.co.uk

Postal address:
Department of Sociology, University of Ibadan, Ibadan Nigeria

Background: Standard health-service delivery aimed toward improving maternal and child health status remains elusive in Nigeria because of inaccuracies in data documentation leading to a lack of relatively stable evidence.

Objectives: Through a community-health project, this study tested the accuracy of record keeping in primary healthcare services in nine clinics run in Ibadan, Nigeria.

Methods: A validation exercise was performed through a sample of the 10 most recent names extracted from three registers maintained by each clinic.

Results: A review of the register covering a period of four years showed a steady increase in: fully-immunised children, registration for antenatal care during the first trimester of pregnancy, the number of women who attended antenatal care at least three times, the overall number of women who booked for antenatal care and women who delivered in Eniosa Community-Health Project facilities over the four-year period. It was possible to trace 86% of those selected from the antenatal care register, 88.9% of those from the birth register and 81.1% of those from the immunisation register. Four women who should have been included for antenatal care, seven who had delivered (but were not in the register) and 13 who reportedly received immunisation but were not listed were found during the validation exercise.

Conclusion: This study concludes that the names appearing in the register are likely to represent valid events, but that the registers did not capture all such events in the community.

Validation de la fourniture de service et de la couverture en soins de santé primaires: l'expérience tirée d'un projet de santé communautaire à Ibadan, au Nigeria

Contexte: La fourniture de services de santé normaux visant à améliorer les conditions de santé de la mère et de l'enfant reste rare au Nigeria en raison d'imprécisions dans les données documentées, qui entraînent un manque de preuves suffisamment solides.

Objectifs: Au moyen d'un projet de santé communautaire, cette étude a testé la précision des traces écrites laissées par les services de soins de santé primaires dans neuf cliniques d'Idaban, au Nigeria.

Méthodes: Un exercice de validation a été effectué sur un échantillon des 10 noms les plus récents tirés de trois registres tenus par chaque clinique.

Résultats: Un examen du registre couvrant une période de quatre ans a montré une augmentation régulière du nombre d'enfants totalement vaccinés, de l'inscription aux soins prénatals pendant le premier trimestre de la grossesse, le nombre de femmes venues au moins trois fois pour des soins prénataux, le nombre total de femmes qui se sont inscrites aux soins prénatals et les femmes ayant accouché dans les locaux du Projet de santé communautaire Eniosa sur la période de quatre ans. Il était possible de retrouver 86% de celles choisies dans le registre de soins prénatals, 88.9% de ceux du registre de naissance et 81.1% de ceux du registre des vaccinations. Quatre femmes qui auraient dû être incluses aux soins prénataux, sept qui avaient accouché (mais n'étaient pas dans le registre) et 13 qu'on disait avoir été vaccinées mais n'étaient pas sur la liste furent trouvées lors de l'exercice de validation.

Conclusion: Cette étude conclut qu'il est probable que les noms apparaissant dans le registre reflètent des événements valides, mais que les registres n'avaient pas enregistré tous ces événements dans la communauté.

Introduction

Background

Despite the declaration and commitment asserted by the Nigerian national health policy (NHP) that 'Primary health care (PHC) shall remain the basic philosophy and strategy for national health development'[1] and that 'PHC is the key to attaining the goal for all people of Nigeria', studies on evaluation of health indices have shown slow progress toward agreed health goals[2] and steady deteriorating conditions have been shown during every health system evaluation carried out in Nigeria.[3] Lack of a standard healthcare system is one major factor in sub-Saharan Africa,[2] with Nigeria ranking 187th for its health systems performance out of 191 member States.[4,5] Access to healthcare is restricted by geographic-, socioeconomic- and/or financial- and sociocultural factors.[6,7] In many countries in sub-Saharan Africa a substantial proportion of all health services are provided by the private sector.[8,9,10,11] Even in government facilities where there are qualified personnel[12] and relatively cheaper services, Batega[13] reported shorter opening hours, irregular drug supply or unavailable drugs and the poor attitude of health workers. Other studies have reported on the factors that determine the health behaviour of patients in various contexts, including physical-, socioeconomic-, cultural- and political factors.[14,15,16]

Access to a PHC facility is projected as being a basic social right,[17] but proximity to the nearest facility,[18] socioeconomic status of the individual,[14,19] cultural beliefs and practices[20] and a low level of trust and confidence in the health provider have been a major barrier, particularly in rural areas, thereby hindering the access to services. Both non-use and late use have also been reported in studies, especially amongst mothers of under-five children in Nigeria,[21] as being responsible for the high rate of maternal mortality in Africa. Several studies have reported various factors, including place of residence, breastfeeding status, place of delivery, access to postnatal care and maternal age and education, as influencing child health and survival.[22,23,24] The consequences of maternal-health challenges in Africa have undermined social- and economic development and are more devastating in resource-poor settings.[25] The overall implication is that the highest infant- and maternal mortality in the world has been reported in sub-Saharan Africa, with the region accounting for half of the 8.8 million under-five year mortality globally in 2008.[17] In addition, an estimated 1000 deaths per 100 000 live births occurred in Africa, with one in 20 women dying as a result of pregnancy-related conditions in Africa compared with one in 4000 deaths amongst European women.[26] A recent report by a consortium of United Nations agencies attested to a sharp drop in maternal mortality in East Asia, but a slow one in Africa in the last two decades, with maternal deaths falling to about 287 000 in 2010.[27] The very quick drop in the maternal mortality in East Asia, as opposed to the slow drop in Africa, was attributed to an increase in contraception and antiretroviral drugs for mothers with HIV and to a greater numbers of births attended by specialists.[27] Although there is ample evidence of success stories worldwide, there is a need to validate the hospital-based reporting in Nigeria in order to arrive at reliable and valid data. The Eniosa Community-Health Project (ECHP) in Lagelu local government area (LGA) validated the major services and coverage in the project registers from the end users at the end of four years of the existence of the project. The ECHP was the first non-profit, private charitable organisation to run PHC services in Nigeria and aims to achieve a sustainable healthcare system in rural Nigerian communities. This study was part of the performance assessment of a community-health project in Nigeria.

Eniosa Community-Health Project

The Eniosa Community-Health Project is one of several health and development activities in Nigeria. This community-health project was supported in Nigeria by the Tulsi Chanrai Foundation, a charitable, philanthropic and non-profit private voluntary organisation. The Chanrai family has been in business in Nigeria since 1891 – well over a century. The Foundation provided PHC services in the rural areas of Oyo, Osun and Kaduna States at the time of this assessment. The first such PHC system was called the ECHP, established in September 1997 and situated in the Lagelu and Akinyele Local Government Areas of Oyo State. It was designed to address the health needs of the community at an affordable cost and made healthcare available to people on their doorstep.

The ECHP was started as a pilot PHC project of the Tulsi Chanrai Foundation with the objective being to develop a sustainable and replicable model PHC system in Eniosa. Another objective was to reduce morbidity and mortality amongst mothers and children and to prevent early childhood diseases. The ECHP area covers 11 larger villages with clinics and numerous surrounding hamlets. The project covers an area of approximately 25 km^2 with an estimated population of 20 500 people. This article was derived from the larger assessment study and focuses on activities at nine of the clinics, excluding the base at Eniosa and the clinic at Atapa which was newly-established at the time of the study.

Indigenously-trained health workers, supervised by a doctor and a nurse-midwife based at Eniosa Base Clinic, set up and run the centres. The clinics are staffed by locally-selected 'health workers' who have finished their school certificate and have received a three-month pre-service training session and subsequent in-service training on a weekly basis. The main services provided by the clinics include quality pre- and post-natal care, clean and safe delivery, immunisation and growth monitoring of infants, nutrition interventions for malnourished children and general health promotion. The validation exercise was part of the 2002 evaluation exercise for the Foundation and the aim of this study was to test the accuracy of record keeping in PHC services in the nine clinics run by the ECHP in Ibadan, Nigeria.

Research method and design

Eniosa community is located in the western part of Lagelu LGA, 15 km northeast of Ibadan, the Oyo State capital. The LGA is primarily rural and agricultural and has an estimated population of 69 000 based on the 1991 census. This assessment began with a review of clinic records. All the clinics started to offer full treatment in 1998 and the project was planned to expand to other States in Nigeria in 2001. The Eniosa project maintained records for each of the following: antenatal care (ANC) register, drug register, immunisation register, family visit diary, outpatient department (OPD) register, data summary sheets and an obstetric activities register. For example, from the ANC register, the total number of pregnant mothers who booked, attended ANC and delivered at the clinic was recorded on a tally sheet. From the drug register, the evaluation team made note of the actual number of drugs available, the number of drugs given out free-of-charge (mainly to small children under the age of one year) and the number sold to adults. The immunisation register provided the opportunity to identify how much of each antigen given out; this included the total number of children who started with the immunisation process and the actual number who were fully immunised. Being a retrospective descriptive analysis of the clinic records, a unique model in this assessment is the testing of the accuracy of the record keeping in the clinic. This was carried out by validating some of the activities carried out in each clinic. The validation exercise was performed by taking a sample of names from three of the registers, namely the ANC booking register, delivery register and immunisation register. The 10 most recent client names were extracted from each of the three registers. The clients' villages were located with the assistance of the health worker in each clinic. Care was taken not to allow the health worker to influence the responses, so once the team got to the target village they excused the health worker and the researchers tried to locate the client (or parent of the client, in the case of immunisation) by asking for directions from co-villagers. Validation questions consisted of simply asking whether the client had utilised the particular service and asking for the time of utilisation. Accuracy of the dates reported by clients was also confirmed with physical evidence such as birth certificates or immunisation cards. All villages were visited at least once, but in those villages where the clients either traveled or were not available for the interview, two more attempts were made to visit them.

The validation exercise also consisted of trying to locate persons who should have been in the register during the period between the date of the tenth client's register entry and the current date. For example, if the 10 names on the birth register extended between November 2001 and April 2002, then the team would ask village leaders and members whether any other person had delivered a baby during that period. If a non-recorded event had happened, the person was located and information was obtained with regard to the place and date of booking, delivery or immunisation, as appropriate. On returning from the field, all questionnaires were checked and edited on a daily basis by the evaluation team. The data were coded and entered into the computer using the EPI INFO package version 6.04 for analysis. The data gathered were analysed and descriptive statistics was used in order to report the findings of the study.

Results

Results of review of records

Treatment was provided free for infants in the Eniosa system. Figure 1a reflects the treatment register and shows that whilst the number of patients paying for treatment was similar over the four-year period, the number of those receiving free treatment increased steadily. It should be noted that three of the clinics were not yet providing treatment in 1998. There were 5622 treatments recorded for 1998, of which 1865 (33%) were free. By 2001, this had increased to 11 376 treatments, of which 6420 (56%) were free. Figure 1b shows a steady increase in fully-immunised children (as found in the Eniosa registers) from 126 in 1998 to 337 in 2001. As can be seen, recording of BCG vaccinations increased through 2000, but dipped slightly in 2001. On the other hand, Measles vaccinations increased over the four-year period, from 116 to 337. The register reported DPT3 and Polio3 jointly, showing that they increased from 117 contacts in 1998 to 398 contacts in 2001. Details on DPT drop-out obtained from the coverage survey showed that whilst 86.1% children were administered with DPT1 and 71.9% children with DPT3, it appeared that 14.2% of children who started with their DPT immunisation did not complete third contact.

Antenatal Care and Safe Delivery are two of the major services provided by the ECHP. Figure 1c was drawn from the ANC and delivery registers in the Eniosa clinics. Ogunremi clinic was not yet functioning in 1998. The chart shows an increase in registration for all four indicators. Registration during the first trimester of pregnancy increased from 68 in 1998 to 161 in 2001. Likewise, the number of women who attended ANC at least three times rose from 174 in 1998 to 322 in 2001. Overall, 250 women booked for ANC services in 1998, whilst 380 did so in 2001. Finally, 206 women delivered in Eniosa facilities in 1998 and the number increased to 379 in 2001.

Eniosa clinics started offering Family Planning Services in 2000. The register shows that there were six condom packs distributed in 2000 and 101 in 2001. Twelve IUCD insertions were performed in 2000 and 19 in 2001. Six women received injectable contraception in 2000 versus 30 in 2001.

Family and/or village visits are a daily activity of the health worker. They check each house to find out if anyone has been sick, to update the birth register and to encourage the use of services. A register was also kept on family and/or village visits. Figure 1d shows that the number of families visited increased from 7544 in 1998 to 15 248 in 2000. The total number of visits that involved health education increased from 787 in 1998 to 1183 in 2001, with the overall percentage of visits devoted to health education being 6.6% in 1998 and 10.4% in 2000. Growth monitoring occurred during home visits and showed a steady increase from 1890 to 6050 over the period.

Eniosa Health Care has a supplemental nutrition programme for malnourished children under the age of five. These are identified through regular growth monitoring and village visits. Each mother receives four packets, the contents of which include dried cowpeas, cowpea flour for making *akara* (bean cakes), soybean flour for making soya milk and maize flour fortified with ingredients such as dried fish for making pap. This is expected to last for approximately one week and the mothers are encouraged to return to collect more until the child improves. A total of 172 children have benefited from this programme over the four-year period, as can be seen in Figure 1e.

Other registers were also reviewed. Table 1 highlights referrals made from 1998–2001. Two general types of referrals were made: those for complicated delivery and those for other medical or surgical reasons. Village-based clinics made their referrals to the Eniosa Base Clinic, whilst the Eniosa clinic made its referrals to appropriate specialist clinics and hospitals in Ibadan. Over the four-year period the number of referrals for delivery from village clinic to the base decreased from 23 to 12. Referrals for other reasons increased from 17 to 45 from 1998–2000 and then dropped to 29 in 2001. There were, on average, four referrals outside the Eniosa system over the four-year period.

Results from service utilisation

Table 2 shows the results of the register validation exercise. It was possible to trace 86% of those patients selected from the ANC register, 88.9% of those from the birth register and 81.1% of those from the immunisation register. All of these confirmed that they had in fact used the service specified. After asking in each village visited whether any additional people should have been registered within the dates selected for those found in the register, the interviewers found four people who should have been included for ANC, seven who had delivered, but were not in the register, and 13 who reported receiving immunisation but were not listed. Three of the unregistered ANC clients claimed to have registered, whilst one had not yet sought care. The birth register is filled out based on information obtained during home visits, since it includes all places of delivery, not only those occurring at Eniosa clinics. Of the 13 who were not included in the immunisation register, nine said that their child was vaccinated at an ECHP clinic, one went to a private clinic and three could not remember. Table 3 shows that most births occurred at home (45.3%), followed by Eniosa clinics (37.2%). Of the seven who had delivered but were not registered, only two (14.3% each) reported an assisted birth (traditional birth attendant [TBA] or ECHP staff).

This study documented the number of assisted deliveries in all places where the 86 registered- and unregistered births that are described in Table 3 occurred. Assisted delivery comprised those births where an ECHP health worker, a trained TBA or a health staff member of another clinic attended the birth. Overall, 58.1% of the births were attended by a trained attendant. All births in a clinic were delivered by a trained person, whilst only 28.0% of deliveries outside a clinic received the attention of a trained attendant. Both trained TBAs and ECHP staff visited homes for deliveries if necessary.

Multiple reasons were obtained from the women (41.9%) who delivered without trained assistance. Ten claimed they delivered unassisted because they went into labour after

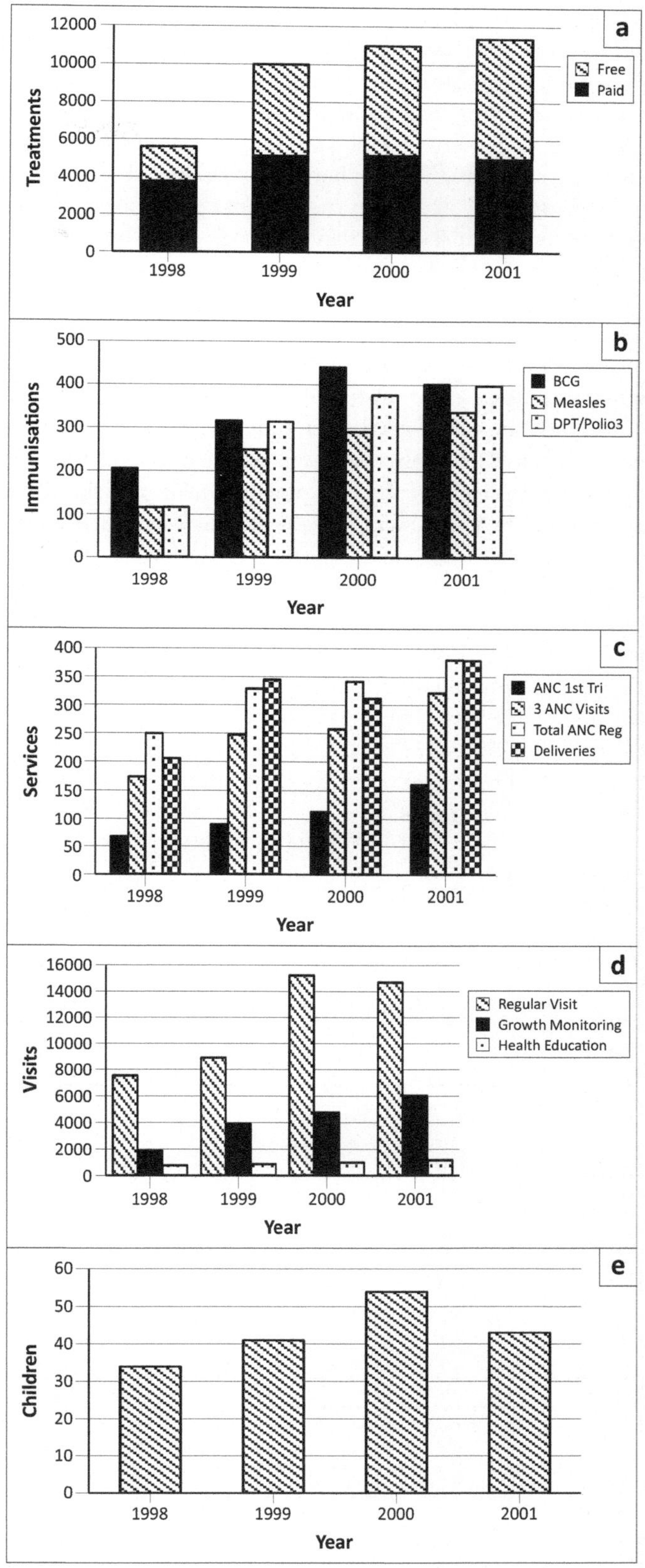

FIGURE 1: Review of records and utilisation thereof. (a) Treatments given; (b) Immunisations given; (c) Maternity services; (d) Family and village visits; (e) Malnourished children receiving food supplements.

TABLE 1: Patients referred from various village clinics to Eniosa community-health project base and from base to Ibadan hospitals (1998–2001).

Names of clinics	1998		1999		2000		2001	
	Delivery	Others	Delivery	Others	Delivery	Others	Delivery	Others
Village clinics	23	17	19	29	14	45	12	29
ECHP base	0	0	3	3	2	4	1	3
Total	**23**	**17**	**22**	**32**	**16**	**49**	**13**	**32**

ECHP, Eniosa Community-Health Project.

clinic hours or late at night. Six claimed that the health worker was not around. Five complained about distance or lack of transport. Three said it was because they delivered on a weekend or holiday, whilst two said that labour came on suddenly. Two more said they preferred to deliver at church. One each said that it was not her first experience, that she had not registered for ANC, that she did not tell anyone she was in labour and that she had delivered on the road on the way to the clinic. Five did not provide any explanation.

The registers also included a record of adverse events such as miscarriage, still births and deaths, as seen in Table 4. As with other register reviews, the year 1998 does not reflect those clinics that were yet to open fully. In absolute terms it is hoped that the 2001 figures reflect access to improved quality maternity services, as all child outcome measures for 2001 are lower than 1999. It was possible to make a calculation of infant mortality rate from the birth and death data available in the registers. Table 4 shows the proportion of recorded births that were delivered by a trained attendant and the infant mortality rate for the years 1998–2001. It should be recalled that the validation of the birth register identified that approximately 8% of births may not have been recorded. Due to their sensitive nature, child deaths were not validated, meaning that the infant mortality calculations in the table can only be called estimates.

TABLE 2: Register validation.

Registration status	ANC		Birth		Immunisation	
	n	%	*n*	%	*n*	%
Names selected	90	–	90	–	90	–
People traced	74	86.0	80	88.9	73	81.1
Traced and confirmed	74	100.0	80	100.0	73	100.0
Total found	78	–	87	–	86	–
Not registered	4	5.1	7	8.0	13	15.1

ANC, Antenatal care.

TABLE 3: Place of delivery.

Place delivered	In birth register		Not in register		Total	
	n	%	*n*	%	*N*	%
Home	34	43.0	5	71.4	39	45.3
ECHP	32	40.5	0	0	32	37.2
Church	8	10.1	1	14.3	9	10.5
Other clinics	5	6.3	0	0	5	5.8
On the road	0	0	1	14.3	1	1.2
Total	**79**	**91.9**	**7**	**8.1**	**86**	**100**

ECHP, Eniosa Community-Health Project.

Ethical considerations

On getting to the village, field staff sought the consents of the participants. As a normal practice in traditional society, the head of the village was met initially and the purpose of the visit was explained to him. The field staff proceeded to interview the respondents after the approval of the village heads. Field staff also explained to the respondents the purpose of the study, the duration of the interview and the benefit to be derived as a result of their participation. Participation was voluntary and respondents were made to know that they were free to withdraw from the interview at any time they wanted. The study involved little or no harm; however, the base clinic of ECHP had been prepared to take care of prospective participants whose participation, in any case, had had an adverse effect. All the questionnaires used to gather the data in this study were locked in a safe and kept in a place that is accessible only by the researchers.

Trustworthiness

The instrument used for the study was pretested for standardisation and to ascertain its validity and reliability. The pretest took place amongst women of a similar or almost similar sociodemographic structure in a nearby community where ECHP was not in operation. At the end of the pretesting, responses gathered were considered in order to validate the content and to improve its standard. All these processes were put in place to ensure the trustworthiness of the study through validity and reliability.

Discussion

This validation exercise of the ECHP employed a variety of methods to gather information and it should be stated that the detailed record keeping at both the facility- and central level was a most valuable resource for the current exercise. These records allowed a vision of programme activities and results over a four-year span. Previous assessments had also relied on these well-kept records. What was different about the ECHP assessment was the sampling of names and tracing them to their different villages for interviews regarding their use of the facility.

A review of the health-facility records showed a general increase in service utilisation between 1998 and 2001. Some of the increase between 1998 and 1999 was due to the opening

TABLE 4: Birth records, Mortality estimates and Adverse events (1998–2001).

Activities	1998	1999	2000	2001	Total
Review of Register of Adverse Events					
Miscarriage	5 (12.5%)	14 (35.0%)	12 (30.0%)	9 (22.5%)	40
Stillbirth	2 (28.6%)	3 (42.8%)	1 (14.3%)	1 (14.3%)	7
Death at birth	3 (60.0%)	2 (40.0%)	0	0	5
Infant death	2 (5.7%)	11 (31.4%)	13 (37.1%)	9 (25.8%)	35
Maternal death	1 (50.0%)	0	0	1 (50.0%)	2
Births and Infant Mortality Estimates					
Births by trained attendant	135 (54.4%)	211 (64.5%)	186 (61.6%)	307 (81.0%)	839
Births by untrained attendant	113 (45.6%)	116 (35.5%)	116 (38.4%)	72 (19.0%)	417
Infant mortality estimates per 1000 live births	5 (20.2%)	13 (39.8%)	13 (43.0%)	9 (23.7%)	40
Total births recorded	**248**	**327**	**302**	**379**	**1256**

of a new clinic, but overall the trend was still positive. The exception was a drop in BCG immunisations in 2001. As is evident from the immunisation programme, as reported in the Nigeria Demographic and Health Survey (NDHS) 1999,[28] measles vaccinations occur less than other immunisations. Whilst this implies room for improvement in follow up, one should be encouraged by the survey findings that show a significantly lower drop-out rate amongst children in the ECHP area.

Home visits showed a slight drop in 2001. It is worth noting that throughout the years, few home visits were recorded as being for the purpose of health education. Clearly, many of the visits were 'educational' in general in that they encouraged utilisation of services, but these records show that the visits, which are generally well received by the villagers, could have a more specific educational agenda. A monthly plan for educational outreach could be developed for the programme.

A unique aspect of the assessment of ECHP was the register validation exercise. Basically, the records as they stand are accurate in that names listed as having utilised a service did in fact do so. This lack of 'false positive' service statistics is a testimony to the honesty of the health staff. What was discovered in the process of tracing the listed clients was that a few people who had obtained a service were not recorded. This ranged from 5.1% of ANC clients traced to 15.1% of children who had reportedly received immunisation. One can thus conclude that the names appearing in the register are likely to represent valid events, but that the registers did not actually capture all such events in the community.

Eight per cent of births that had occurred in the record-review period had not been recorded and, as expected, none had taken place at an ECHP facility. In general, the health workers during their home visits were able to keep track of non-facility-based births, but these had slipped through and affected the calculations of infant mortality, contributed to an underestimation of the births in the area and child-health needs and resulted in an over-estimation of maternity service utilisation, particularly the proportion who were delivered by a trained attendant. As it stands, two-fifths of births were delivered by an untrained attendant, which is slightly higher than NDHS (1999)[28] reported for the southwestern zone of the country. The proportion delivered by a trained attendant showed a general increase over the period, whilst the estimated infant mortality using the register information shows a decrease.

It is suggested that even though immunisation completion rates and ANC utilisation are high, there is always room for improvement. Village health committees should be involved in tracing defaulters and in other outreach activities. Training of TBAs should continue with an effort at reducing the somewhat large proportion of births that are delivered by untrained attendants. Village visits should also be used as an opportunity to validate and update clinics records. It is ascertained that the high rate of positive validated data in the field was based on the high and total commitment of the Tulsi Chanrai Foundation staff; but yet further commitment is necessary in order to cultivate loyalty, improve performance and optimise cooperation amongst the community people. Finally, record-validation exercise should become an annual event and an in-service learning experience for the staff.

Conclusion

This study concludes that the names appearing in the register are likely to represent valid events, but that the registers did not capture all such events in the community.

Acknowledgements

The efforts of Dr Paul Kadansamy, the Director of PHC for the Chanrai Foundation are appreciated with regard to the provision of adequate logistics during the survey. All the interviewers in this study have performed well and their commitment in accuracy in documentation is acknowledged. The entire community and the respondents gave us their attention over the period of the study and we acknowledge them here.

Competing interest

The authors declare that they have no financial or personal relationship(s) which may have inappropriately influenced them in writing this article.

Authors' contributions

K.K.S (University of Ibadan) and W.R.B (Johns Hopkins University) both made substantive intellectual contributions to various stages that led to this article, including the conception, design and implementation of the study from whence this article is generated. Analysis of data in this study was carried out by K.K.S and supervised by W.R.B. The draft copy of the article was prepared by K.K.S., with input from W.R.B. and both authors read the draft and agreed with the content of the article.

References

1. Federal Ministry of Health, Nigeria. The national health policy and strategy to achieve health for all Nigerians. Lagos; 1988.
2. Travis P, Bennett S, Haines A, et al. Overcoming health-systems constraints to achieve the Millennium Development Goals. Lancet. 2004;364(9437):900–906. Erratum in Lancet. 2005;365(9456):294.
3. Reid M. Nigeria still searching for right formula. Bull World Health Org. 2008;86(9): 663–665.
4. Asuzu MC. The necessity for a health systems reform in Nigeria. Journal of Community Medicine & Primary Health Care. 2004;16(1):1–3. http://dx.doi.org/10.2471/BLT.08.020908, PMid:18797638, PMCid:PMC2649488
5. National Strategic Health Development Plan. The National Strategic Health Development Plan Framework (2009–2015). [document on internet]. [c2009] [cited 2013 Aug. 26]. Available from: http://www.internationalhealthpartnership.net/fileadmin/uploads/ihp/Documents/Country_Pages/Nigeria/Nigeria%20National%20Strategic%20Health%20Development%20Plan%20Framework%202009-2015.pdf
6. Gilson L, Schneider H (editors). Understanding health service access: concepts and experience. Global Forum Update on Research for Health. 2007;4:28–32.
7. Hausmann-Muela S, Ribera JM, Nyamongo I. Health-seeking behaviour and the health system response. DCPP Working Paper No. 14. Washington, DC: Disease Control Priorities Project. 2003; p. 1–37.
8. Economic Commission for Africa. Mainstreaming health equity in the development agenda of African countries. African Centre for Gender and Social Development (ACGS); 2008.

9. WHO, UNAIDS. Guidelines on provider-initiated HIV testing and counselling in health facilities. Geneva, Switzerland; 2007.
10. Majumder A. Utilisation of health care in North Bengal: A study of health seeking patterns in an interdisciplinary framework. J Soc Sci. 2006;13(1):43–51.
11. Doctor HV, Findley SE, Ager A, et al. Using community-based research to shape the design and delivery of maternal health services in Northern Nigeria. Reprod Health Matters. 2012;20(39):104–112. http://dx.doi.org/10.1016/S0968-8080(12)39615-8
12. Kimani JK,Ettarh RR. Determinant of pathways to HIV testing in rural and urban Kenya: Evidence from the 2008 Kenya Demographic and Health Survey. Journal of Rural and Tropical Public Health. 2012;11:1–7.
13. Batega DW. Knowledge, attitudes and practices about malaria treatment and prevention in Uganda: A literature review. USAID; 2004.
14. Ettarh RR, Kimani J. Determinants of under-five mortality in rural and urban Kenya. Rural Remote Health. 2012;12:1812.
15. Babalola S, Fatusi A. Determinants of use of maternal health services in Nigeria – looking beyond individual and household factors. BMC Pregnancy and Childbirth. 2009;9:43. http://dx.doi.org/10.1186/1471-2393-9-43, PMid:19754941, PMCid:PMC2754433
16. Kroeger A. Anthropological and socio-medical health care research in developing countries. Soc Sci Med. 1983;17(3):147–161. http://dx.doi.org/10.1016/0277-9536(83)90248-4
17. United Nations. The Millennium Development Goals Report. New York: UN; 2010.
18. Oti SO, Odimegwu C. Perinatal mortality in Nigeria: do place of delivery and delivery assistants matter? The Open Demography Journal. 2011;4:1–10.
19. Uchudi JM. Covariates of child mortality in Mali: Does the health-seeking behavior of the mother matter? J Biosoc Sci. 2001;33(1):33–54. http://dx.doi.org/10.1017/S0021932001000335, PMid:11316394
20. Katung PY. Socio-economic factors responsible for poor utilisation of the primary health care services in a rural community in Nigeria. Niger J Med. 2001;10(1):28–29.
21. McTavish S, Moore S, Harper S, et al. National female literacy, individual socio-economic status, and maternal health care use in sub-Saharan Africa. Soc Sci Med. 2010; 71(11):1958–1963. http://dx.doi.org/10.1016/j.socscimed.2010.09.007, PMid:20980089
22. Doctor HV. Does living in a female-headed household lower child mortality? The case of rural Nigeria. Rural Remote Health. 2011;11(2):1635.
23. Jones G, Steketee RW, Black RE, et al. How many child deaths can we prevent this year? Lancet. 2003;362(9377):65–71. http://dx.doi.org/10.1016/S0140-6736(03)13811-1
24. Black RE, Morris SS, Bryce J. Where and why are 10 million children dying every year? Lancet. 2003;361(9376):2226–2234. http://dx.doi.org/10.1016/S0140-6736(03)13779-8
25. Asante FA, Asenso-Okyere K. Economic burden of malaria in Ghana. WHO-AFRO; 2008.
26. World Health Organization. Health strategies: Health for all policy in the 21st century in the African region: Agenda 2020. WHO-AFRO; 2008.
27. McNeil DG Jr. Maternal deaths plunged over 2 decades to about 287,000 in 2010, U.N. Reports. The New York Times – Health; May 16, 2012.
28. National Population Commission. Nigeria Demographic and Health Survey 1999. Calverton, Maryland: National Population Commission, Abuja Nigeria; 2000.

4

Missed opportunities in child healthcare

Authors:
Linda Jonker[1]
Ethelwynn L. Stellenberg[1]

Affiliations:
[1]Faculty of Health Sciences, Department of Nursing, Stellenbosch University, South Africa

Correspondence to:
Ethelwynn Stellenberg

Email:
elstel@sun.ac.za

Postal address:
PO Box 19063, Francie van Zijl Drive, Tygerberg 7500, South Africa

Background: Various policies in health, such as Integrated Management of Childhood Illnesses, were introduced to enhance integrated service delivery in child healthcare. During clinical practice the researcher observed that integrated services may not be rendered.

Objectives: This article describes the experiences of mothers that utilised comprehensive child health services in the Cape Metropolitan area of South Africa. Services included treatment for diseases; preventative interventions such as immunisation; and promotive interventions, such as improvement in nutrition and promotion of breastfeeding.

Method: A qualitative, descriptive phenomenological approach was applied to explore the experiences and perceptions of mothers and/or carers utilising child healthcare services. Thirty percent of the clinics were selected purposively from the total population. A convenience purposive non-probability sampling method was applied to select 17 mothers who met the criteria and gave written consent. Interviews were conducted and recorded digitally using an interview guide. The data analysis was done using Tesch's eight step model.

Results: Findings of the study indicated varied experiences. Not all mothers received information about the *Road to Health* book or card. According to the mothers, integrated child healthcare services were not practised. The consequences were missed opportunities in immunisation, provision of vitamin A, absence of growth monitoring, feeding assessment and provision of nutritional advice.

Conclusion: There is a need for simple interventions such as oral rehydration, early recognition and treatment of diseases, immunisation, growth monitoring and appropriate nutrition advice. These services were not offered diligently. Such interventions could contribute to reducing the incidence of child morbidity and mortality.

Opportunités manquées dans le domaine des soins de santé aux enfants.

Contexte: Différentes politiques, telles que la Gestion intégrée des maladies enfantines, ont été mises en place pour améliorer la prestation de services intégrés dans le domaine des soins de santé aux enfants. Au cours de la pratique clinique le chercheur a remarqué que les services intégrés ne sont pas toujours assurés.

Objectifs: Cet article décrit les expériences des mères qui ont utilisé les services de santé généralisés aux enfants dans la zone métropolitaine du Cap en Afrique du Sud. Ces services comprenaient le traitement des maladies; les interventions préventives telles que la vaccination; et les interventions incitatives, telles que l'amélioration de la nutrition et la promotion de l'allaitement.

Méthode: Une approche phénoménologique, qualitative et descriptive a été appliquée pour étudier les expériences et perceptions des mères/personnes en charge qui utilisent les services de santé aux enfants. Trente pour cent des cliniques ont été sélectionnées à dessein parmi toute la population. On a appliqué une méthode pratique d'échantillonnage aléatoire et raisonnée pour sélectionner les 17 mères qui répondaient aux critères et ont donné leur consentement par écrit. On a effectué des entrevues et des enregistrements numériques à l'aide d'un guide d'entrevue. Pour l'analyse des données on a utilisé le modèle en huit étapes de Tesch.

Résultats: Les résultats de l'étude ont montré des expériences variées. Les mères n'ont pas toutes reçu les renseignements sur le livret ou la carte « le Chemin de la Santé ». Selon les mères, il n'y avait pas de services de santé intégrés aux enfants. Les conséquences sont les opportunités manquées de vaccination, de fourniture de vitamines A, l'absence de contrôle de la croissance, d'évaluation de l'alimentation et de conseils nutritionnels.

Conclusion: Il faut donc des interventions simples, comme la réhydratation orale, le dépistage précoce et le traitement des maladies, la vaccination, le contrôle de la croissance, et des conseils pour une nutrition appropriée. Ces services ne sont pas offerts assidûment. Ces interventions pourraient permettre de réduire le taux de morbidité et de mortalité chez les enfants.

Introduction

Diligent provision of simple health interventions could reduce child mortality and morbidity. Examples of these interventions could include oral rehydration, early recognition and treatment of diseases, immunisation, growth monitoring and appropriate nutrition advice. However, despite improvements in healthcare delivery, implementation of appropriate programmes and having policies and legislation based upon best practices, South Africa has failed to reduce the maternal and under-five child mortality rate[1]. In fact, South Africa is one of 12 countries where the incidence of mortality in children younger than five years increased during the period 1990–2008.[2] Missed opportunities may have contributed toward the incidence of mortality. However, important underlying conditions may be missed if the integrated approach to child healthcare is not practised.

Setting

The research was conducted in the eastern side of the Cape Metropole in South Africa, which contains 10 clinics. The clinics included in the study are managed jointly by both the Provincial Government of the Western Cape and the Metro Municipal Health Services. Clinics from both authorities were selected in order to prevent prejudice and bias in the sampling process. The area was selected intentionally because children were referred to a hospital rendering primary-, secondary- and tertiary-level services. This provided the opportunity to obtain information about the child health services in the continuum of child healthcare services.

The researcher observed that policies and guidelines for rendering child health services may be disregarded in some clinical areas. It appeared as if integration of healthcare services was not practised in some places. Against this background, the researcher embarked upon a scientific study to determine if the observations made were a true reflection of services rendered.

Key focus area

Mothers with children younger than two years of age and who utilised the healthcare offered at clinics, private general practitioners and hospitals were interviewed in order to obtain their actual experiences in the utilisation of these services.

Contribution to the field

The findings of this research paper could create awareness for healthcare providers, policy makers in health and Nursing and Medical Education Institutions about the clients' perception of services. By identifying experiences of those utilising the services, insight could be provided to practitioners and policy makers regarding the challenges faced by the users. Healthcare providers could use the information to reflect on their own practice measured against policy guidelines. Integrated comprehensive healthcare delivery could contribute toward minimising missed opportunities and, ultimately, toward helping to decrease morbidity and mortality in children younger than five years of age.

Background

Many of the deaths in the under- five population have been avoidable and could be attributed to the incorrect implementation of health programmes.[3] For example, separating the provision of curative and preventive paediatric care has resulted in many missed opportunities for immunisation.[4] Fewer opportunities are missed if immunisation and nutrition services are available all day, rather than for limited periods of the week. Human Rights Watch cautions that the health system's inability to ensure accountability, oversight and effective response contributes to morbidity and mortality.[5] Countries that made the most progress in reduction of child mortality were those that had higher coverage of integrated primary healthcare. The strongest predictor of changes in the under-five mortality rates were improvements in access to and provision of all the clinical services.

The healthcare of children is a parental responsibility, but society and the government have a moral responsibility to ensure that the rights of children according to the Constitution are protected. Child mortality is a basic reflection of the health status of children and an alternative marker of the quality of healthcare.[6]

Changes in society have influenced healthcare delivery to children. Prior to 1994, the plight of women and children was caused by a variety of social problems which included poverty, lack of nutrition and sanitation, unemployment, lack of immunisation programmes and unsafe water. Improvements after 1994 can (amongst others) be ascribed to the implementation of free services, the Expanded Programme on Immunization and Integrated Management of Childhood Illnesses programme.[7] South Africa declared Primary Health Care (PHC) as the centrepiece of all its health policies since 1994.[8] Key health promotion activities include: immunisation, the Integrated Management of Childhood Illness (IMCI) strategy, childhood infection prevention, neonatal health and developmental screening, growth monitoring and nutrition.[9]

The availability of programmes and policies does not imply that services are rendered as envisaged. An important way of evaluating the implementation of a programme is by obtaining detailed information on the clients' experiences. Information on the experiences of the persons affected by the programme gives a more meaningful evaluation of what takes place during implementation.

Problems with the implementation of programmes within the healthcare package for children influence the quality of services rendered. Despite the fact that integrated PHC was adopted as a vehicle for service delivery, a lack of integration of services still exists. There is a need for high quality healthcare that will minimise the inequalities in society (wealth and social privileges) that impact on child health.[10] Concerns regarding the rendering of child services could also be related to the quality of the data collected, which influences healthcare planning. The geographical access to services does not influence mortality but rather, the quality of care plays a significant role in the child mortality rates. This may be significant as there is a tendency to regard services in metropolitan areas as good, because of accessibility to primary healthcare.[11]

Policies direct or indicate the context and mode of implementation. Deviating from the intended methodology could result in unintended consequences. An example of this is where separating the provision of curative and preventive paediatric care could result in many missed opportunities for immunisation. Fewer opportunities are missed if immunisation and nutrition services are available all day, every day, rather than for a limited period each week.[4] A survey in Ghana revealed that logistical challenges at hospitals, a shortage of nurses and a lack of knowledge were responsible for missed opportunities.[12]

Another aspect that may influence the implementation of policy directions could be monetary in nature. Sustainable funding for integrated programmes could be a problem, as funders tend to fund individual programmes. These programmes may then be implemented as a vertical service and related healthcare aspects may not be attended to.[13] South Africa spends healthcare funds on quaternary (highly-specialised tertiary) and curative healthcare which should preferably be spent at a PHC level, where more people can be helped.[14] Despite the fact that South Africa spends 8.7% of its Gross Domestic Product (GDP) on health, its healthcare outcomes are not as good as countries that are poorer and spend much less on health. Contributing factors are, amongst others, poor training of nurses and midwives; a curative rather than preventive approach; a lack of services providing education to schools and communities on nutrition; and a lack of infrastructure, equipment and consumables.[15] Consequently, the integration of services may be compromised.

Ethical considerations

The proposal was submitted to the Health Research Ethics Committee for Human Research at University of Stellenbosch for ethics clearance (N10/11/392), as well as the Metro Municipal Health Services (ID 10230) and the Provincial Department of Health of the Western Cape (RP 29/2011).

Informed consent was obtained to both conduct and make a digital recording of the interview. Respondents were provided with the ability to contact the researcher for feedback. Privacy and confidentiality, as well as limited access to research documents, were explained.

Research methods and design

A qualitative, descriptive phenomenological approach was applied in order to explore the experiences and perceptions of mothers utilising child health services for children younger than two years. This design was appropriate as the researcher focused on actual services rendered. Phenomenologists conduct research in natural settings and consider it the best place to observe, ask questions and do interviews.[16] In the experience of the researcher, service providers could rationalise omissions in adhering to guidelines to poor record keeping rather than poor compliance with policies.

A field diary was kept. Observations made by researcher were recorded and information obtained from the child's handheld *Road to Health* book.

For the purposes of this study and to improve understanding and ensure rigour in the study, the meaning of 'mother' is conceptualised as being the biological mother, adoptive mother, grandmother, foster mother, sibling or father who brings the child to the clinic (this terminology was adopted in order to incorporate the different caregivers who bring children for child healthcare services).

Population and sampling

The target population was the mothers and/or carers of children younger than 24 months old who used the services at the clinics in a section of the eastern side of the metropolitan area in Cape Town, South Africa. A purposive sample of n = 3 (30%) of the clinics was selected from the total population. A convenience purposive non-probability sampling method was applied with regard to interviewing 17 mothers who met the criteria and gave written informed consent. According to De Vos et al.,[17] a sample of n = 10 is adequate in qualitative research or until data saturation is met.

Data collection

The researcher (an independent nurse practitioner) conducted and digitally recorded the interviews with each participant using an interview guide. In-depth, open-ended questions were developed by considering the literature, objectives, expert opinion and own experience in the field. Questions explored the experiences of the mothers about the services received. Observations and information from the child's *Road to Health* book were documented in the field diary. Participants' responses were explored for interrelatedness during the course of the interview. An interview guide was used, as can be seen in Box 1.

Data analysis

The data analysis was done using Tesch's eight step model,[18] supported by the guidelines supplied by Burns and Grove.[19] The analysis involved the transcription of digitally-recorded interviews according to the coding of the data, the generating of themes and subthemes, interpretation and organisation of data and the drawing of conclusions.

BOX 1: Interview guide.

- Tell me about the *Road to Health* book of your child.
- Tell me for what services do you bring your child to the clinic.
- Tell me what happens when you bring your child to the clinic.
- Tell me what happens when you take your child to the doctor.
- Tell me what happens when you take your child to the hospital.
- Tell me what they told you about your child's weight.
- Tell me what they told you about your child's diet/food.
- Is there anything you want to share with me regarding the services at the clinics?
- Is there any suggestion you want to share regarding how the services can be improved?

Ensuring quality

A pre-test was conducted at one clinic, where two respondents were interviewed. The value of the pre-test was that it elicited shortfalls in the methodology and ensured rigour in the process.

Dependability was ensured by the careful description of each step of the data collection and analyses processes. The researcher completed the data analysis and coding processes. A colleague assisted by doing a similar process of assigning codes to the transcribed data. An expert in qualitative research and nursing reviewed the data analyses and the data coding processes. The expert evaluated the dependability of data analysis.

Conformability was maintained by keeping field notes during the interviews and data analysis processes; any preconceived ideas and observations were noted and bracketed. The Modelling Role-Modelling Nursing theory of Erickson, Tomlin and Swain, as mentioned by George's work on nursing theories,[26] was utilised as the conceptual theoretical framework to facilitate its application to the broad population. Detailed records of the coding and analysis process were kept. The reflective memos, marginal remarks and the record of the data trail will assist if the processes should be replicated.

Results

Interviews were conducted at three clinics. At clinic A, six participants were interviewed, four at clinic B and seven at clinic C, making it a total of 17 participants interviewed. Findings relate to participant characteristics and services utilised and their experiences at service delivery points.

Participant characteristics and services utilised

Sixteen children were accompanied by their biological mother and one child by the grandmother. Eight mothers had only one child; eight had two children and one had five children. The age of the children ranged between three weeks and 18 months. The group appeared to consist of mothers who normally visited clinics and could provide information on their experiences.

All mothers used the clinic as a service provider. Eleven mothers also used private medical practitioners and eight mothers used the hospitals for the healthcare of their children. The hospital was used by choice and also after hours, if no clinic was open.

The mothers were interviewed about services received at all service providers as they form part of the continuum of care.

Experiences of participants at service delivery points

The participants' experiences were highlighted and discussed according to the classification of Binkin et al.,[6] who found in a meta-analysis of studies that the interventions by health workers to reduce the under-five mortality rate can be grouped into three broad groups, namely: treatment for diseases; preventive interventions, such as immunisation; and promotive interventions, such as improvement in nutrition and promotion of breastfeeding. The missed opportunities could then be highlighted.

Treatment for diseases

Children with life-threatening conditions require immediate action from mothers, as well as their healthcare providers. Various methods of educating mothers can be utilised, such as posters, pamphlets, peer education and health information messages in the *Road to Health* book. The mothers knew about these conditions and knew not to wait in queues if the child is very sick:

> 'You tell them and after 10 minutes they say you must come this side – five minutes. So if very sick they help you quickly ...' (Participant B1, Female)

The information was depicted on the walls of the facilities and photographs assisted mothers in the recognition of sick children. Only one facility had no rehydration corner and the participants verbalised their confusion in this regard:

> 'I sat as normal I went to the place indicated, place was locked. Said someone will see to you. I left after 90 minutes.' (Participant A6, Female)

Underlying illnesses should be managed according to the IMCI protocol that requires that growth, nutrition and immunisations should be assessed at each visit. The findings reflected that mothers could not recall if integrated or holistic management was rendered when the child was ill. Missed opportunities regarding the dispensing of vitamin A indicated that an integrated service was not practised:

> 'Look at everything ... Do not discuss weight and feeds. Will ask if child is still on the breast.' (Participant A1, Female)

Preventive interventions

Immunisation services should be offered every day at all facilities. The mothers' experiences with immunisation services indicate that the concept of 'seamless health services' does not exist as far as immunisation was concerned. One of the mothers at clinic C related that this was the second time that the child was not immunised as a result of staffing problems. Immunisation services were not offered at the hospitals and private practitioners:

> 'Take child to doctor if in hurry. Clinic takes too long. Mostly doctors do not weigh or check immunisation. Examine and finish. Do not look at Road to Health card.' (Participant A4, Female)

Mothers explained that the card might be checked, but they were then referred back to the clinics. The successes of the Expanded Programme on Immunization were seen in obtaining polio-free status; reduction in incidence of measles morbidity and mortality; and the decrease in neonatal tetanus incidence.[3] The measles outbreak of 2009–2010 in South Africa is a direct consequence of low herd cover. The higher the immunisation coverage, the better the herd immunity appears to be.[20] It was also found that children were not immunised because of the unavailability of vaccines:

> '…[s]upposed to come for her injections last week but they did not have any in stock.' (Participant A5, Female)

The guidelines are clear on the level of child care to be offered. Healthcare guidelines and policies such as the Expanded Programme on Immunization (South Africa) require immunisation services to be available at all service delivery points such as clinics, community health centres and hospitals. The Department of Health supports the participation of the private sector.[21] Information available on 10 November 2011 on the website of the Department of Health actually motivates parents to visit their clinic or medical practitioner to obtain immunisations. The public is assured that the nursing sister will take the child's weight, length and head circumference in order to determine if the child is growing at the expected rate.[22]

Vitamin A and deworming should be offered at six-monthly intervals. In this study it appeared as if the provision of vitamin A was overlooked as only one child received all the required dosages. In a survey on missed opportunities in a Cape Town clinic, it was found that separating the provision of curative and preventive paediatric care resulted in many missed opportunities for immunisation. One of the findings is applicable to the provision of vitamin A.[4] The recommendations of this study appear not to have been implemented as integrated services were not rendered at some facilities, according to the lived experiences of the mothers. Nurses attend to queues, not to children, according to one participant:

> '… [*T*]hey have to do all the queues …' (Participant B2, Female)

Health promotion activities

The *Road to Health* book should be provided at the birth of the child. Postnatal care of the participants took place at private and public healthcare facilities. In public facilities, children were born at primary, secondary and tertiary levels of care. The mothers' experiences indicated that information on the *Road to Health* book or card was not offered to every mother:

> 'No, I asked, but they said it is my child's card ...' (Participant C3, Female)

> '… [*N*]othing, only said it is the clinic card. It must be used when I take the child to the clinic …' (Participant C5, Female)

Mothers should receive information on aspects that will enable them to care for their children. The *Road to Health* book or card is an excellent source of information for mothers. However, it was found that this opportunity could be better utilised. The omission to explain the card could imply that mothers were not enabled to assess the health of the child or to practise preventive healthcare in order to improve their child's health and prevent unnecessary healthcare costs.[23] Health information messages in the book provide valuable information about feeding, oral rehydration, play and stimulation and safety of the child. There are drawings of children with danger signs that prompt the mother when to take the child to a healthcare service provider:

> 'Everything about her is in it; also messages if she is sick that I can read; her birth weight and stuff. Everything is in it ...' (Participant A3, Female)

Nutrition advice should be offered diligently. Weight and growth of children younger than 24 months should be assessed at each contact session, at least once a month. Mothers received information about the weight gain of the child, but feeding assessments and nutritional advice were not offered:

> 'They did explain that every time I come to the clinic the nurse will weigh the baby and the baby must pick up weight and if it goes down it is bad ...' (Participant A5, Female)

> 'No, I was actually planning to ask them if she had picked up …' (Participant B4, Female)

The mothers revealed incorrect feeding practices but received no advice regarding how to correct the practices. Grandmothers and family members seem to be a frequent source or provider of nutrition information:

> 'My mother told me to give him water …' (Participant C7, Female)

Inadequate knowledge about appropriate foods and feeding practices are often a greater determinant of malnutrition than actual lack of food.[24] Participants related in this study that although they had access to the services, the nutrition services were not provided. Therefore, the concern was that the mothers were not able to improve the nutrition status of the child as a result of the possible lack of knowledge.

Monitoring growth requires assessment of weight, length and head circumference. All children were weighed. No mother verbalised that the child's length or head circumference were measured. Mothers knew that the weight was plotted on the growth card, but the curve was not discussed:

> 'Your child is growing well mommy [*mimicking the staff*].' (Participant C1, Female)

Some mothers received no information about the weight gain. Three mothers had children with low weight for their age. The mothers were informed about the concern when the child's growth curved crossed the -2SD line:

'Last time they said she is low weight for her age and then they discussed it …' (Participant B3, Female)

In this specific instance, the curve indicated unsatisfactory weight gain in the preceding months, but no feeding assessments were done during that period. Numerous gaps existed in the implementation of growth monitoring and nutrition promotion within the South African context. These gaps included inaccurate assessment of the weight of the children, a failure to plot weights, the inability of nursing staff to have identified the nutritionally at risk, poor utilisation of the *Road to Health* card and poor communication with caregivers.[1] The national guidelines indicate that growth monitoring is an integral part of the immunisation visit. Another aspect of growth monitoring includes health advice to mothers regarding good nutrition.[6]

Discussion

Missed opportunities

Table 1 summarises the missed opportunities found at the time of the study.

South Africa adopted good policies and guidelines based upon best practices after 1994. Delivering healthcare is regulated by these policies and guidelines. These standards of provision can be confirmed as the minimum desired or acceptable level of healthcare. Two aspects must be taken into account when this is interpreted: firstly, the national norms and standards define what should be offered; and secondly, the local norms and standards define what is offered. This revolves around staff competency.[25] Health managers are responsible to ensure that healthcare workers are competent to deliver healthcare according to minimum standards. The findings of the study indicated that services were not integrated. Applying guidelines to practised integrated services could have prevented these missed opportunities and could also have contributed to lower the morbidity and mortality rates in children. Countries that had made the most progress, as measured by the average annual reduction of mortality, were those which had higher coverage of integrated primary healthcare. They also found that the strongest predictor of changes in the under-five mortality rates were improvements in access to and provision of all the clinical services.[6]

Recommendations

Rendering of child services should be done using an integrated approach. This approach is not entrenched and urgent attention is required to ensure adherence to policies. Every contact visit should be utilised for the checking of growth, nutrition and immunisation status.

Maternal services should be strengthened so as to ensure that health promotion and education activities are offered. This should include explaining the *Road to Health* book to the mother and/or carer.

The private sector, medical officers and hospitals should participate and render child services according to policy objectives as determined for child services. This should be supported by health managers who are responsible for ensuring that quality integrated healthcare is rendered to all children who utilise child health services. This approach is endorsed by the National Department of Health.[22]

Limitations of the study

This research was limited to clinics in the eastern section of the Cape Metropole of the Western Cape Province, South Africa.

Conclusion

Research was conducted in the eastern side of the Cape Metropole in South Africa. Mothers were interviewed in order to determine their experiences regarding the healthcare offered for their children younger than two years old. Despite improvements in healthcare delivery, implementation of appropriate programmes and having policies and legislation based upon best practices, South Africa has failed to reduce the maternal and under-five child mortality rate.[1] Diligent provision of simple health interventions could contribute to a reduction in child mortality and morbidity.

Mothers' experiences revealed that integrated comprehensive services were not practised. Healthcare workers tend to ascribe omissions in service delivery to poor record keeping. However, mothers' experiences suggested that the services not rendered were missed opportunities that could be the result of not applying integrated services.

Each contact visit is an opportunity to ensure that all required services according to age are rendered and omissions are rectified. Clinics can be busy places, with long queues of people waiting for healthcare services. Mothers have to care for families and may find it difficult to spend long hours in queues.

Further research to determine why hospitals, obstetrical services and the private sector do not follow national policies is needed. The underlying reasons why service providers do not seem to adhere to policies should be determined and addressed. Identifying the root causes could assist in addressing the shortfalls in service delivery.

TABLE 1: Missed opportunities.

Child health service	Missed opportunities
Immunisations	12 of 17 child immunisations were not done as required for the child's age
Vitamin A provision	3 of 4 children did not received Vitamin A according to age
Information provided about *Road to Health* book	13 of 17 mothers received no information about the *Road to Health* book
Developmental assessments done	16 of 17 children had no developmental assessments done for the required age
Nutrition information and feeding assessment	7 of 17 could not recall any information given or feeding assessments done

The provision of equipment and manpower at clinics may be a contributing factor and should be investigated.

Providing only one aspect of child healthcare may lead to missed opportunities with regard to providing immunisations, as well as failure to dispense important disease prevention drugs such as vitamin A and deworming tablets. The child's nutritional status and diet may not be assessed and the mother may not receive advice on appropriate nutrition according to the child's age. These missed opportunities contribute to the high incidence in child mortality and morbidity. South African healthcare policies require that integrated healthcare be rendered for children.

Acknowledgements

Dr E.L. Stellenberg from the Faculty of Health Sciences, University of Stellenbosch, is acknowledged for her motivation and continuous support, direction and inspiration throughout my studies and the writing of this article. I am grateful to the Metro Municipal Health Services and Provincial Department of Health of the Western Cape that granted permission to conduct the research in the clinics. Lastly, thanks go to the staff of the three clinics who kindly provided me the opportunity and space to interview the mothers.

Competing interests

The authors declare that they have no financial or personal relationships which may have inappropriately influenced them in writing this article.

Authors' contributions

E.L.S. (Stellenbosch University) was the main study leader and made considerable contributions towards the original research project and thesis. She also made substantial corrections and additions to the article. L.J. (Stellenbosch University) contributed to the study concept, design, analysis and interpretation, as well as the original drafting of the article.

References

1. Barron P, Roma-Reardon J. South African Health Review 2008. Durban: Health Systems Trust; 2008.
2. Chopra M, Daviaud E, Pattinson R, et al. Saving the lives of South Africa's mothers, babies, and children: can the health system deliver? Lancet. 374(9692):835–846. http://dx.doi.org/10.1016/S0140-6736(09)61123-5
3. Day C, Gray A. Health and related indicators In: Barron P, Roma-Reardon J, editors. South African Health Review 2008. Durban: Health Systems Trust, 2008; 239–396.
4. Bachmann MO, Barron P. Missed opportunities for immunisation in curative and preventive services in a community health centre. A follow-up survey. S Afr Med J. 1996;86(8):947–949.
5. Human Rights Watch. 'Stop making excuses': accountability for maternal health care in South Africa. New York: Human Rights Watch; 2011.
6. Binkin N, Chopra M, Simen-Kapeu A, et al. Do improvements in outreach, clinical, and family and community-based services predict improvements in child survival? An analysis of serial cross-sectional national surveys. BMC Public Health. 2011;11:456. http://dx.doi.org/10.1186/1471-2458-11-456
7. McKerrow N, Mulaudzi M. Child mortality in South Africa: using existing data. In: Padarath A, Fonn S, editors. South African Health Review 2010. Durban: Health Systems, 2010; p. 59–72.
8. Mhlanga RE. Maternal, newborn and child health: 30 years on. In: Barron P, Roma-Reardon J, editors. South African Health Review 2008. Durban: Health Systems Trust, 2008; p. 132–138.
9. Hogan B. 2008: In: Barron P, Roma-Reardon J, editors. South African Health Review 2008. Durban: Health Systems Trust, 2008; p. vii–xii.
10. Saloojee H, Bamford L. Key childhood health promotion and disease prevention programmes. In: Ijumba P, Padarath A, editors. South African Health Review 2006. Durban: Health Systems Trust, 2006; p. 181–202.
11. Sartorius BKD, Kahn K, Vounatsou P, et al. Young and vulnerable: Spatial-temporal trends and risk factors for infant mortality in rural South Africa (Agincourt), 1992–2007. BMC Public Health. 2010;10:645. http://dx.doi.org/10.1186/1471-2458-10-645
12. Brugha R, Kevany JP. Maximizing immunization coverage through home visits: a controlled trial in an urban area of Ghana. Bull World Health Organ. 1996;74(5):517–524.
13. Shefer AM, Luman ET, Lyons BH, et al. Vaccination status of children in the Women, Infants, and Children (WIC) program. American Journal of Preventive Medicine. 2001;20(4)(Suppl. 1):47–54. http://dx.doi.org/10.1016/S0749-3797(01)00279-3
14. Mannak M. Child, maternal mortality reaches crisis levels. [blog on the Internet] 2011 [cited 2014 Apr 22]. Available from: http://www.bhfglobal.com/child-maternal-mortality-reach-crisis-levels-250511.
15. Mafubela D. Why South Africa's health record is poor. Mail and Guardian 2011 Mar 28. [Available online from: http://www.mg.co.za/article/2011-03-28-why-south-africas-health-record-is-poor]
16. Munhall PL. Nursing research: a qualitative perspective. 3rd ed. London: Jones & Bartlett Learning; 2001.
17. De Vos AS, Strydom H, Fouche CB, et al. Research at grass roots: for the social sciences and human services professions. 3rd ed. Pretoria: Van Schaik; 2005.
18. Tesch R. Qualitative research: analysis types and software tools. Bristol: Falmer Press; 1990.
19. Burns N, Grove SK. The practice of nursing research: appraisal, synthesis, and generation of evidence. 6th ed. Missouri: Saunders; 2009.
20. Trotter CL, Maiden MC. Meningococcal vaccines and herd immunity: lessons learned from serogroup C conjugate vaccination programs. Expert Rev Vaccines. 2009;8(7):851–861. http://dx.doi.org/10.1586/erv.09.48
21. National Department of Health. Vaccinator's Manual: 'Immunisation that works'. Expanded programme on immunisation in South Africa(EPI-SA). Pretoria: NDOH; 2013.
22. National Department of Health. New EPI vaccines guidelines. Pretoria: NDOH; 2010.
23. National Department of Health. A policy on quality in health care for South Africa. Abbreviated version. Pretoria: NDOH; 2007.
24. Krebs NF, Hambidge KM, Mazariegos M, et al. Complementary feeding: a Global Network cluster randomized controlled trial. BMC Pediatr. 2011;11:4. http://dx.doi.org/10.1186/1471-2431-11-4
25. Department of Health. The primary health care package for South Africa – a set of norms and standards. Pretoria: NDOH.
26. George JB. Nursing theories. The base for professional nursing practice. 6th ed. New Jersey: Prentice Hall; 2010.

Attitudes toward condom education amongst educators for Deaf and hard-of-hearing adolescents in South Africa

Authors:
Sumaya Mall[1]
Leslie Swartz[1]

Affiliations:
[1]Alan J Flisher Centre for Public Mental Health, Department of Psychology, Stellenbosch University, South Africa

Correspondence to:
Sumaya Mall

Email:
sumaya.mall@gmail.com

Postal address:
18 Rhodes Avenue, Mowbray 7700, South Africa

Background: Disabled adolescents are at a critical time in their psychosocial and sexual development.

Aim: This study explores the attitudes of educators working in schools for Deaf and hard-of-hearing pupils in South Africa toward condom education for their pupils.

Methods: We conducted a combination of individual in-depth and joint interviews with a total of 27 participants. The sample comprised educators, school psychologists, school nurses and teaching assistants.

Results: Results showed that educators were aware of the HIV risk for their pupils and reported the risk of sexual abuse or premature sexual activity as being risk factors for HIV infection. None of the schools had a written condom education policy. Whilst some schools were integrating condom education in existing school curricula, others faced moral or religious dilemmas in doing so. There were differences in attitudes, both amongst schools and amongst educators in the same schools.

Conclusions: Given the context of a burgeoning HIV epidemic, it is vital to address adequate condom education in schools.

Attitudes des éducateurs d'adolescents sourds et malentendants en Afrique du Sud, envers l'éducation sur l'usage des préservatifs.

Contexte: Les adolescents handicapés sont à un moment critique de leur développement psychosocial et sexuel.

Objectif: Cette étude examine les attitudes des éducateurs des écoles de Sourds et Malentendants en Afrique du Sud envers l'éducation sur l'usage des préservatifs pour leurs élèves.

Méthodes: Nous avons procédé à une combinaison d'entretiens individuels et en groupe approfondis avec un total de 27 participants. L'échantillon comprenait des éducateurs, des psychologues scolaires, des infirmières scolaires et des maîtres auxiliaires.

Résultats: Les résultats ont montré que les éducateurs étaient au courant des risques de VIH chez leurs élèves et ils ont signalé que le risque d'abus sexuels ou d'activité sexuelle prématurée étaient des facteurs de risque d'infection par le VIH. Aucune des écoles n'avait de politique écrite d'éducation sur l'usage des préservatifs. Bien que certaines écoles aient intégré l'éducation sur l'usage des préservatifs dans leur programme scolaire, d'autres étaient confrontées à des dilemmes moraux ou religieux. On a remarqué qu'il y avait des différences d'attitudes entre les écoles et parmi les éducateurs d'une même école.

Conclusions: Etant donné le contexte d'une épidémie croissante de VIH, il est indispensable d'aborder sérieusement l'éducation sur l'usage des préservatifs dans les écoles.

Introduction

Despite the fact that people with disabilities may be more vulnerable to HIV than the general population, some HIV services are inaccessible to them.[1] Accessibility to services is a particular issue for members of the Deaf[1] community because information is rarely available in accessible formats such as Sign Language.[2] In addition, particularly in lower-income countries, people with hearing loss are more likely than the rest of the population to face literacy challenges because

1.We use the capital letter 'D' to denote that Deafness is a cultural identity that refers to individuals with hearing loss who communicate in Sign Language and are members of a Deaf community

of their reduced access to adequate schooling. Written materials may also be of little use.[3,4] South Africa has the highest number of HIV-positive people of any country, meaning that addressing the issue of prevention is thus a pressing concern for its Deaf community. There is also little information on the needs of this community regarding HIV services.[5,6] As part of a larger study,[6] we report here on data exploring attitudes to sexuality and condom education amongst educators of Deaf and hard-of-hearing pupils in six schools in Gauteng and the Western Cape provinces in South Africa.

Research methods and design

Participants and study sites

Having obtained the required ethical and institutional permission, the first author (SM) interviewed educators at six schools for Deaf and hard-of-hearing students in Cape Town and Johannesburg. All the schools catering for this population in Cape Town were selected, as were the two schools in Johannesburg with the longest history of Deaf education. For practical reasons, the two more recently established schools in Johannesburg were not studied. Within the schools, we employed purposive sampling and recruited 27 participants (of whom six were Deaf or hard-of-hearing) across the six schools. We interviewed 19 high school teachers, two school psychologists, one matron or 'hostel mother', three teaching assistants and two school nurses through a combination of joint interviews (two participants) and individual in-depth interviews. All had worked at their respective schools for between 10 and 20 years. All hearing participants were interviewed in English or Afrikaans (as per their choice) and Deaf participants were assisted by a South African Sign Language (SASL) interpreter. Interviews were recorded and transcribed by an independent transcription service.

Measures

We developed an open-ended interview guide by studying key issues from both Deaf studies and behavioural adolescent literature pertaining to sexual behaviour or HIV. Key domains were: challenges facing Deaf and hard-of-hearing youth regarding HIV; schools' initiatives to address HIV risk and concerns; and schools' policies on condom usage.

Data analysis

We used the framework approach, which consists of three phases:[7] (1) familiarising oneself with the data (i.e. reading the transcriptions, developing codes and assigning data and themes to the codes developed); (2) summarising and synthesising coded data; (3) developing associations or patterns within concepts and themes and ensuring that participants have been presented accurately. Initially, responses were read for emergent themes, which were then coded. Care was taken to ensure the codes captured the respondents' meaning accurately. A second researcher (LS) coded the interviews independently in order to ensure validity of the categories. We used NVivo 7.0 (QSR International 2008), a qualitative software program, for data management.

Ethical considerations

As the first author was based at the University of Cape Town (UCT) at the start of the study, ethical approval to conduct the study was provided by the Human Ethics Research Committee of UCT's Faculty of Health Sciences (REC REF 423 2009). The Faculty of Health Sciences Committee at Stellenbosch University later reviewed the application and also provided ethical approval. The research team adhered to all ethical procedures during the research process, including informed consent for all participants where they were assured their responses would remain confidential. They were also assured that they could discontinue their participation in the study at any time.

Results

Participants' views on their pupils' sexuality

Several participants believed that Deaf children are at risk of sexual abuse. One explained:

> '... people with disabilities, they are at more risk when coming to, to, to sexual activities ... they are at more risk [*of sexual abuse*] ... they [*the perpetrators*] don't regard them as you know, people, normal people you see, so they take advantage of that ...' (High School teacher 1, Life Orientation, Female)

Schools' policies on condom education

None of the schools had a written policy regarding condom usage and educators had different views of the issue. One participant, for example, thought it was important to have condom demonstrations so that Deaf pupils can understand how to use them, but a colleague working in the same school thought that condom demonstrations were problematic and that they could encourage premature sexual activity:

> 'So I almost want to say, the thing that's bad, the motivation from the adults [*to*] use a condom ... actually encourages, to say ... it's all right, ... the message that actually comes through is, you can have go ahead and have sex ... it's actually a bad message ... that is given out to the community ...' (High School teacher 2, Afrikaans, Male)

Another school (although historically Catholic) had a long history of educating pupils about condoms. Two Deaf teachers who had completed their schooling at the school reported that they had received condom education there over 20 years ago:

> 'We don't have any nuns here now, when I was young, they gave us sex education, but it did not start from the nuns, they took somebody from outside to present sexuality to us, 22 years ago, they gave us sex education and showed us on a banana how to use a condom.' (High School teacher 3, Life Orientation, Female)

However, a school nurse mentioned that the school's previous principal (a nun) had not allowed her to distribute condoms to pupils:

> '... [*u*]ntil the end of last year, we had a, a nun that was our principal ... I was given a donation of condoms ... and I wanted to hand them out and she wouldn't allow me to ... we have a volunteer – she's been doing the sex education with the children.

She would hand out condoms in her classroom, so I gave her the box, so the condoms did eventually get to the kids.' (School Nurse 1, Female)

Although the principal at another Catholic school reported that staff were under pressure from the nuns not to have condom demonstrations at school, four participants working at that school said that demonstrations did, in fact, occur. The principal also conceded the reality of early sexual risk behaviour amongst pupils and the necessity of condoms:

'At the very least [*I tell the pupils*] use condoms, which I know as a Catholic I shouldn't promote, but I mean if a child is already sexually active ...' (School Principal 1, Female)

The principal of another historically Catholic school was adamant that condom demonstrations were not allowed at her school:

'It's [*condom usage*] not encouraged and I respect, I am not a Catholic but I am the principal of this school and I had, I have decided to come and work in this school and ... I feel it's right that I uphold their ethos. If I feel, if I can't do that then ... I should terminate my service because I have applied to be in this school.' (School Principal 2, Female)

However, one of her staff members, a teacher, explained that there may be room for adaptation of certain values:

'The owners of the school are Catholic sisters ... but now I've put a poster up there with A, B, C [*abstain, be faithful, condomise*] ... and nobody has taken down you know, take them down ... the only thing they would not allow is the condom dispensers.' (High School teacher 4, Life Orientation, Female)

Discussion

Our findings reveal a mixed picture. Whilst one school had no limitations regarding condom education, religious and moral issues influenced two of the other schools' condom education programmes. One Catholic school had successfully managed to reconcile religious belief with HIV prevention needs. Whilst educators in the other traditionally Catholic schools were making efforts to do the same, they were not always supported by their principals, who believed that a Catholic stance on condom usage should be upheld.

It may be chance (for example, dependant on who a child has as a teacher) that decides what kind of sex education (if any) a child in a school for Deaf and hard-of-hearing pupils receives and whether or not the child learns about condom use. For some educators, there seems to be a clash between their religious values and the threat of an emerging HIV epidemic. This finding resonates with that of Rohleder and Swartz,[8] a study that found that carers feared that providing HIV prevention information to disabled people would place them at risk of sexual abuse. Rohleder[9] found that staff at disability organisations sometimes viewed condom education for disabled people as being immoral; their views were grounded in religious beliefs. Given the vulnerability of Deaf and hard-of-hearing adolescents to HIV infection, this issue is not simply one of values. Providing sexuality education to pupils who are Deaf or hard-of-hearing poses challenges at the best of times, because of the communication barriers, but as far as we are aware, the question of the role of religious beliefs and values has not (until now) been explored sufficiently. As quoted above, one of the participants says, 'I have decided to come and work in this school' and, therefore, out of respect for the school, believes that it is incumbent on her to operate in keeping with the values she sees as being central to the school. This is an admirable stance and resonates with attitudes toward contraception within many religious bodies and organisations.[10]

Conclusion

The parents of the pupils have had no such choice in terms of the values of the school – either the pupils attend this school or they do not receive education. This may well have an impact on their future health. This situation, it is important to recognise, is a product not of the views of the educators themselves (they are entitled to their own beliefs regarding sexuality education) but of the social context in which education for Deaf pupils (and indeed for many other disabled children) continues to be coupled with religious institutions. Many within the schools, as we have shown, are doing all they can to provide sexuality education. A broader engagement, balancing the rights of religious schools (and educators) to their beliefs against the rights of the pupils to have access to sexuality and health promotion, needs to be undertaken.

Acknowledgements

We wish to acknowledge the NRF-SA Norway partnership for funding this study. We would like to acknowledge the role of the late Professor Alan Flisher for his insight during the conceptual stages of this study.

Competing interests

The authors declare that they have no financial or personal relationship(s) which may have inappropriately influenced them in writing this article.

Authors' contributions

S.M. and L.S. (both Stellenbosch University) conceptualised the study questions and designed the interview guide. S.M. collected the data and both S.M. and L.S. analysed the data. S.M. led the writing of the manuscript, whilst L.S. assisted.

References

1. Mall S, Swartz L. Addressing intersections in HIV/AIDS and mental health: The role of organizations for d/Deaf and hard of hearing individuals in South Africa. Am Ann Deaf. 2012;156(5):492–500. http://dx.doi.org/10.1353/aad.2012.1604
2. Bisol CA, Sperb TM, Brewer TH, et al. HIV/AIDS knowledge and health-related attitudes and behaviors among deaf and hearing adolescents in southern Brazil. Am Ann Deaf. 2008;153(4):349–356. http://dx.doi.org/10.1353/aad.0.0055
3. Groce N, Yousafzai A, Dlamini P, et al. HIV/AIDS and disability: A pilot survey of HIV/AIDS knowledge among a deaf population in Swaziland. Int J Rehabil Res. 2006;29(4), 319–324. http://dx.doi.org/10.1097/MRR.0b013e328010c68f

4. Groce NE, Yousafzai AK, van der Maas F. HIV/AIDS and disability: Differences in HIV/AIDS knowledge between deaf and hearing people in Nigeria. Disabil Rehabil. 2007;29(5):367–371. http://dx.doi.org/10.1080/09638280600834567
5. Mall S, Swartz L. Parents' anxieties about the risk of HIV/AIDS for Deaf and hard of hearing adolescents in South Africa: A qualitative study. J Health Psychol. 2012;17(5):764–773. http://dx.doi.org/10.1177/1359105311421051
6. Mall S, Swartz L. Sexuality, disability and human rights: Strengthening healthcare for disabled people. SAMJ. 2012;102(10):792–793.
7. Ritchie J, Lewis J. Qualitative research practice. A guide for social science students and researchers. London, UK: SAGE Publications; 2003.
8. Rohleder P, Swartz L. Providing sex education to persons with learning disabilities in the era of HIV/AIDS: tensions between discourses of human rights and restriction. J Health Psychol. 2009;14(4):601–610. http://dx.doi.org/10.1177/1359105309103579
9. Rohleder P. HIV/AIDS and disability: An exploration of organizations' responses to HIV/AIDS as it affects people with disabilities. [Unpublished doctoral dissertation]. Department of Psychology, Stellenbosch University, South Africa; 2008.
10. Mishtal J, Dannefer R. Reconciling religious identity and reproductive practices: The Church and contraception in Poland. Eur J Contracept Reprod Health Care. 2010;15(4):232–242. http://dx.doi.org/10.3109/13625187.2010.498595

Factors associated with patients' understanding of their management plan in Tshwane clinics

Authors:
Leticia Fernandez[1]
Theresa Rossouw[1]
Tessa Marcus[1]
Angelika Reinbrech-Schutte[1]
Nicoleen Smit[1]
Hans F. Kinkel[1,2]
Shehla Memon[1,2]
Jannie Hugo[1]

Affiliations:
[1]Department of Family Medicine, University of Pretoria, South Africa

[2]Foundation for Professional Development, South Africa

Correspondence to:
Leticia Fernandez

Email:
fernandezlet@gmail.com

Postal address: Department of Family Medicine, University of Pretoria, P/Bag x323, Arcadia, Pretoria 0007, South Africa

Background: This research focused on patients' views regarding healthcare services and identified factors associated with understanding of their management plan.

Aim: To develop a baseline for patient–clinician collaboration and the extent to which patients felt included and understood their treatment plan.

Setting: Tshwane district (South Africa) public health outpatient clinics.

Method: Medical students interviewed 447 patients in 22 clinics in Tshwane district. Agreement was measured by the percentage of cases in which patients and clinicians were in accord about a particular aspect of the consultation.

Results: About one-third of patients incorrectly answered questions on whether changes in lifestyle or diet were prescribed as part of their treatment. The likelihood that patients understood their plan was associated with seeing the same clinician three or more times; having a consultation in their same or a similar language; patient participation in the diagnosis; and feeling that the clinician had explained their health problems to them.

Conclusions: There is need for greater emphasis on continuity of care, the clinicians' ability to speak the patient's language and involving patients in the consultation.

Les facteurs associés à la compréhension par les patients de leurs plans de prise en charge dans des centres médicaux de Tshwane

Présentation: Cette étude se concentrait sur les points de vue des patients concernant les services de santé et les facteurs identifiés associés à la compréhension de leur plan de prise en charge.

Objectif: Développer une référence pour la collaboration entre patients et médecins et déterminer la mesure dans laquelle les patients avaient le sentiment d'être inclus à la préparation de leur plan de prise en charge et de le comprendre.

Cadre: Centres médicaux publics accueillant des patients en consultation externe dans le district de Tshwane (Afrique du Sud).

Méthode: Des étudiants en médecine ont interrogé 447 patients dans 22 centres médicaux dans le district de Tshwane. La concordance était mesurée par le pourcentage de cas dans lesquels les patients et les médecins étaient d'accord sur un aspect particulier de la consultation.

Résultats: Environ un tiers des patients n'a pas su répondre correctement aux questions visant à déterminer si des changements dans leur style de vie ou régime alimentaire avaient été prescrits dans le cadre de leur traitement. La probabilité que les patients comprennent leur plan était associée au fait de consulter le même médecin à trois reprises ou plus, de consulter dans leur langue ou dans une langue similaire, de participer au diagnostic, et au sentiment que le médecin leur avait expliqué le problème de santé dont ils souffraient.

Conclusions: Il est nécessaire de mettre davantage l'accent sur la continuité de la prise en charge, la capacité des médecins à parler la langue de leurs patients, et l'implication des patients dans la consultation.

Introduction

South Africa is a multicultural, multilingual society where there is extreme social inequality and extensive racial inequity that manifest both in health outcomes and access to quality healthcare. For the majority of the population, historically-created racialised endemic poverty and social dislocation have produced substantial health and education deficits over generations.[1,2] The resultant disease burden has been further compounded by the HIV and tuberculosis (TB) epidemics, which threaten to overwhelm an already-stretched public healthcare delivery system.[3]

In the presence of fragmented health systems, low levels of health literacy, severe shortages of staff and medical professionals and poor staff morale, quality of care in public clinics and hospitals has remained low for the most vulnerable groups in South Africa.[1,3,4] A recent study to evaluate the quality of services in 16 HIV clinics in and around Pretoria that offer antiretroviral treatment (ART) found that they underperformed in critical areas when measured against performance standards for ART initiation. Clinician consultations were amongst the weakest areas in terms of quality of service. The study found that psychosocial histories were taken from only 50% of the patients, physical examinations were performed in only 41% of these consultations and only 38% of patients were asked to bring all concurrent medications to their next visit. In the case of female patients, only 56% were asked if they were pregnant and only 39% were referred for a pap smear. Moreover, the authors report that longer consultations were not necessarily associated with higher quality of clinician care.[5]

In the next decades, improving the quality of healthcare and health outcomes may well depend on changes in the delivery of care, such as promoting patient-centred care that will contribute to better relationships and more effective collaboration between patients and clinicians.[4,7,8] Patient-centred care improves outcomes because it is informed by patient understanding of the issues and their treatment preferences, as well as their interest and commitment to managing their own health.[7,8,9] In this sense, the caregiver acts as an interpreter of the patients' symptoms and health needs and engages with them as partners in the quest to improve their long-term health prospects.[10]

The positive impact of patient-centred care has been documented in several previous studies on emotional, mental and functional health, treatment adherence, physiological status (e.g. blood pressure), symptoms resolution and pain control.[11,12] Specific benefits associated with positive patient–clinician communication include a reduction in patient distress and blood pressure when clinicians provide clear information and emotional support, as well as diminished patient anxiety when clinicians encourage questions and share in the decision-making process.[11] Patient participation during consultation and agreement with the clinician about causes and treatment for their symptoms are significantly associated with better medication adherence and clinical outcomes.[8,12]

Amongst the current barriers to effective patient-centred practices in public clinics and hospitals in South Africa are a lack of continuity of care, time constraints, limited resources and language and cultural differences.[13,14,15] Continuity of care is especially important in patient-centred care because it creates the opportunity for developing a therapeutic relationship between patients and clinicians over time.

The concept of continuity of care has evolved with changes in the context of healthcare delivery over time. In the 1950s, when single-physician practices were the prevailing mode, continuity of care referred to having a personal caregiver. As the number of medical partnerships increased, concerns about patient anonymity led to the redefinition of continuity of care as coordination amongst caregivers to ensure uninterrupted patient care. Later on, the restructuring of the healthcare systems of the 1990s resulted in redefining continuity of care to include not only continuity by the same caregiver or group of caregivers, but also coordination of services along the components of the care delivery system.[16]

More recently, the hierarchical model of continuity portrays a continuum of care from informational to longitudinal to interpersonal continuity. At the lowest level, informational continuity refers to a group of clinicians having access to comprehensive knowledge about a patient without necessarily developing a relationship. Longitudinal continuity refers to patients receiving care from a team of clinicians who are responsible for coordinating healthcare services. At the highest level, interpersonal continuity involves a relationship in which the patient develops trust in a clinician, who then assumes responsibility for the patient's overall healthcare.[17]

Throughout the changes in the concept of continuity of care, however, the one constant has been that it represents the patient's perspective. The three major themes have been the importance of a personal caregiver committed to the patient's wellbeing, communication of patient information between caregivers and coordination between caregivers to ensure uninterrupted care.[16] Basically, continuity of care is about the way that individuals experience and practitioners provide healthcare over time.[6] Continuity of care happens when healthcare is connected, coherent and consistent.[18] Continuity of care improves the quality of care with clinicians enjoying greater patient trust. It also contributes to improved health outcomes with, amongst other things, patients being more likely to follow advice, having fewer and shorter hospitalisations and making less use of emergency services.[19,20,21,22,23,24,25,26,27]

Clinician cultural and linguistic competences are also important, especially in patient-centred care, since they aim to bridge cultural and socioeconomic differences, improve communication and develop a meaningful patient–clinician relationship. Clearly, when clinicians are unable to understand their patients' complaints or needs and patients, in turn, do not understand the advice of the clinician, quality of care is compromised.[28,29]

We report findings from a quality-improvement project conducted in Tshwane clinics to develop a baseline for patient–clinician collaboration during consultation. The project is part of the service-learning opportunities designed for medical students by the University of Pretoria's Departments of Family Medicine and Public Health. This study measured the extent to which patients report that clinicians adhere to standards of performance during consultation; the relationship between patient–clinician collaboration on patient understanding of management plans; and whether other factors, such as language and continuity of care, mediate the information exchanged between patient and clinician.

Research methods and design

The authors developed the research objectives, protocols and instruments to establish a baseline for patient-clinician collaboration during consultations in Tshwane's public health clinics. Between one and four Year 5 medical students from the University of Pretoria were assigned to each of the 22 clinics that participated in the study, depending on the facility size and its ability to accommodate students.

The questionnaires for patients and clinicians were developed in English, mirrored each other and contained several statements about the consultation. The language of the interview with patients was expected to be English, but students reported that if they felt it was needed they used Afrikaans or some other African languages they knew. However, a limitation of this study is that we did not record the language or languages of the interview, neither did we measure the language proficiencies of the interviewers and respondents. (See appendix 1 for sample questionnaire)

Statements about the consultation could be answered as 'true', 'partly true', 'partly false' or 'false'. The answer categories for statements about the patient's management plan were 'yes', 'no' or 'not sure'. For example, patients were asked to evaluate the statement, *'The clinician listened to my questions and concerns without interrupting me'*. The patient's answer was compared to the clinician's response to a similar statement, namely, *'I listened to this patient's questions and concerns without interrupting'*. In addition, data were collected about the patient's age, gender, first language, language of consultation and the number of times the patient had seen the same clinician.

Patients were selected as a sample of convenience and their names and other identifying information were not collected or entered in the database. The only link between the patient and clinician was the patient's file number, which students recorded in both the patient and the clinician questionnaires. Each student interviewed 10 patients post-consultation. The clinician was asked to complete the corresponding form on their own immediately after the consultation to ensure that the interaction would refer to the particular patient interviewed. After interviewing a patient, the student collected the completed questionnaire from the clinician and matched them by the patient's file number. Clinicians and patients were blinded to each other's answers, which students were instructed to treat as confidential information. Students entered the matched patient–clinician data into a database prepared by the authors for this study.

In this paper we present the combined findings from all the clinics in the research project. In total, there were 447 paired patient–clinician observations. However, one variable, the number of visits to the same clinician, had 78 missing cases (17.5%), which reduced the usable dataset to 366 pairs of observations. Preliminary analysis showed that the cases with missing data did not differ significantly in terms of patients' age, gender or language from those with no missing data. In order to address the missing values in the dataset and maximise the sample size, we used the imputing function of Stata, using as regressors all other patient variables in the survey to inform the imputation of values for the number of visits. No imputations were done for any other variable. We present our findings using the larger dataset with imputed values. Findings from the analysis with the smaller data set with no imputations are similar, except that the association between number of visits to the same clinician and the dependent variables do not reach statistical significance using the smaller dataset with no imputed values, even though the direction of the coefficients are similar.

Data analysis

The two outcomes of interest are whether patients gave the same answer as their clinician regarding the statements (a) *'My treatment or management plan includes changes in lifestyle'*, and (b) *'My treatment or management plan includes changes in diet'*. We coded each of these variables as 1 if both the patient and the clinician answered the same ('yes', 'no' or 'not sure') and coded 0 otherwise. We hypothesised that patients would be more aware of these details of the management plan when they experienced greater collaboration during consultation, have continuity of care and/or the consultation is in their first or a similar language.

The independent or explanatory variables central to the analysis are:

(1) **Continuity of care:** The number of visits with the same clinician was obtained from patients. This variable is coded 1 if the patient had met the same clinician three or more times and 0 if the patient saw the clinician for the first or second time. The choice of three or more consultations as a cut-off point was based on empirical comparisons. Prior to imputation, the percentage of respondents who matched their clinicians' responses about whether their management plan included changes in lifestyle was 70.6% for those seeing the clinician for the first time ($n = 197$); 71.7% if they had seen the same clinician for the second time ($n = 53$); and 79.4% amongst those seeing the clinician for the third time ($n = 34$). These differences became of statistical significance after the imputation of missing values for the number of times seeing the same clinician.

(2) **Language concordance:** This variable is coded as 1 if the consultation was conducted in the patient's first language or a same or similar language; and coded 0 if the language of consultation is different from the first language of the patient. This variable takes into account that some languages are related, such that speaking one facilitates understanding and communicating in the other. For example, IsiZulu, IsiXhosa and Xitsonga are considered similar languages, as are Sepedi, Sesotho and Setswana.

(3) **Consultation elements:** The statements included in the analysis were selected based on two criteria: significant bivariate correlation with the dependent variables and/or their conceptual relevance to patient-centred care. Each variable is coded as 1 if both the patient and clinician answered 'true' or 'partly true' and 0 otherwise.

The next section presents the sample characteristics, the extent of agreement between patients and clinicians and the results of multivariate analysis. Because of the dichotomous nature of our dependent variables, we use logistic regressions to assess the role of continuity of care, language concordance and selected consultation elements on patients' understanding of their management plan.

Ethical considerations

This study was approved by The University of Pretoria's Faculty of Health Sciences Research Ethics Committee (Protocol #75/2010). Prior to data collection, students received training about the purpose of the study and the use of protocols to recruit and interview patients. Students also attended a second session to address any issues related to the study. There were no anticipated risks associated with participation in the study for either the patients or the clinicians and the potential benefits to the patients included improvement in clinician understanding of patient perspectives regarding medical services. Patients recruited for the study were informed that their participation was voluntary and that their answers would be strictly confidential and anonymous, with no negative consequences in terms of treatment at the clinic based on their answers or if they chose not to participate.

TABLE 1: Sample characteristics: patients interviewed in Tshwane District clinics.

Variables	Patients (n = 443)	%
Gender		
Female	293	66.1
Male	150	33.9
Age group		
< 25	46	10.4
25–44	165	37.2
45–54	101	22.8
55–64	80	18.1
65+	51	11.5
Consultations with clinician		
First time with this clinician	213	48.1
Second time with this clinician	59	13.3
Three or more times with this clinician	171	38.6
Language of consultation and patient's first language		
Patients whose consultation was in a language different from their first language	238	53.7
English	186	42.2
Afrikaans	36	8.1
Sepedi/Sesotho/Setswana	14	2.9
Isizulu	2	0.5
Patients whose consultation was in their same or similar language	205	46.3
Sepedi/Sesotho/Setswana	74	16.7
Afrikaans	68	15.3
English	31	7.0
Isizulu/Isixhosa/Isindebele	26	5.9
Other	6	1.4

Results

The characteristics of patients interviewed in the participating Tshwane district clinics are listed in Table 1. Most of the patients interviewed were female (66%; n = 293) and over half (52%; n = 232) were aged 45 or older, with 12% (n = 51) aged 65 or older. Since patients in the clinics are assigned to the next available clinician, 48% (n = 213) of the patients consulted with a clinician that they were meeting for the first time, 13% (n = 59) had seen their clinician once before and 39% (n = 171) had seen their clinician three or more times.

Table 1 shows that there is a large diversity of languages spoken at the clinics by both patients and clinicians. Fifty-four per cent (n = 238) of the patients who had a consultation in a language other than their first language, had this consultation in English (42%; n = 186) or Afrikaans (8%; n = 36). On the other hand, close to half the patients in the sample (46%; n = 205) had a consultation in their own or a similar language, mostly in the related languages of Sepedi/Sesotho/Setswana (17%; n = 74) and in Afrikaans (15%; n = 68).

Table 2 shows several of the statements that patients and clinicians were asked to evaluate independently after the consultation. Most patients and clinicians answered that these statements were true or partly true about their consultation, resulting in very high agreement.

Table 3 compares answers from clinicians and patients regarding the management plan. The first two statements, whether the patient has the same understanding as her or his clinician regarding the need for changes in lifestyle and changes in diet as part of the management plan, are the

TABLE 2: Agreement in patient–clinician matched items (n = 443).

Questions to patients	Questions to clinicians	Percentage matched answers†
The clinician listened to my questions and concerns without interrupting me.	I listened to this patient's questions and concerns without interrupting.	98.4
The clinician examined me in order to find out what's wrong with me.	I examined this patient in order to find out what's wrong with her or him.	92.1
I participated in the diagnosis of my condition or disease.	This patient participated in the diagnosis of her or his condition or disease.	87.8
The clinician explained to me what's wrong with my health.	I explained to this patient what's wrong with her or his health.	95.5
I had the opportunity to ask questions of the clinician.	I encouraged this patient to ask me questions about her or his condition or disease.	92.8
I feel confident I can explain to someone at home the treatment or management plan for my condition.	This patient will be able to explain to someone at home the management plan for her/his condition.	95.5

†, Matched answers are those where clinician and patient answered that the statement was true or partly true.

outcome variables in this analysis. Approximately 67% (n = 296) of the clinicians said that the management plan of the patient they had just consulted included changes in lifestyle, 32% (n = 142) answered that it did not and 1% (n = 5) said they were not sure. It is noteworthy that the few cases (n = 5; 1%) in which clinicians answered that they were 'not sure' about the changes in their patient's management plan usually referred to seeing a patient for the first time and not finding sufficient information about their management plan on the patient's records. This issue is complex and will not be discussed for now as it is outside the scope of this study.

Patients' answers regarding the need for changes in lifestyle as part of their management plan had a similar distribution: 61% (n = 268) said 'yes', 35% (n = 155) said 'no' and close to 5% (n = 20) were 'not sure'. Matching the answers between clinicians and their patients in the last column shows that approximately 74% (n = 327) gave the same answer, with most agreeing that changes in lifestyle were necessary (52%; n = 229). Table 3 also shows that 77% (n = 339) of the patients matched their clinician's responses regarding changes in diet and 84% (n = 372) matched their clinician's responses about the need to see another doctor, specialist or therapist.

Table 4 shows the odds of patient–clinician agreement regarding whether changes in lifestyle and diet are part of the patient's management plan. The dependent variable is the odds of patients correctly answering whether their management plan includes changes in lifestyle or changes in diet.

The most important findings from the multivariate analysis is that the odds of patients understanding whether their management plan includes changes in lifestyle are about 70% – 80% higher if they had seen the same clinician more than twice or if their consultation was in their first (or a similar) language compared with those whose consultation was in a different language. Similarly, the odds of correctly answering whether the management plan includes changes in diet were 60% higher for patients consulting in their first or a similar language than for those consulting in a different language.

Table 4 shows that, in addition to the impact of language and continuity of care on better patient understanding of their management plan, patients who agreed with their clinicians that they participated in their diagnosis were about twice as likely to answer correctly whether their management plans included changes in lifestyle or diet, respectively, compared with patients who said they did not participate in the diagnosis. Similarly, when patients agreed with their clinician that their health problem had been explained to them, they were substantially more likely to answer correctly whether or not their management plan included changes in diet.

TABLE 4: Odds ratios of patient–clinician agreement about the management plan.

Variables	Patient–clinician agree† as to whether management plan includes changes in: Lifestyle‡	Diet‡
Patient's age	1.00	1.00
Gender		
Male	-	-
Female	0.80	1.27
Times consulting with same clinician		
One or two time	-	-
Three or more times	**1.67****	1.02
Language of consultation		
Different from patient's first language	-	-
Same or similar to patient's first language	**1.83****	**1.60****
Matched statements about the consultation		
The patient participated in the diagnosis of her or his condition		
Patient and clinician disagree	-	-
Patient and clinician agree	**2.40****	**1.78***
The clinician explained the health problem to the patient		
Patient and clinician disagreed	-	-
Patient and clinician agreed	2.06	**2.71****
The patient had opportunity to ask questions		
Patient and clinician disagreed	-	-
Patient and clinician agreed	1.20	0.94
The patient understands what's wrong with her or his health		
Patient and clinician disagreed	-	-
Patient and clinician agreed	2.26	0.53
Number of observations	441	441

†, Clinician and patient answered the same (Yes, No or Not Sure).
‡, Disagree is the omitted category.
*, Coefficients statistically significant at $p <= 0.10$; ** $p <= 0.05$.

TABLE 3: Clinicians' vs. patients' understanding of their management plan.

Statements about the patient's management plan	Clinicians' answers *n*	Clinicians' answers %	Patients' answers *n*	Patients' answers %	Matched clinician-patient agreement † *n*	Matched clinician-patient agreement † %
The treatment or management plan includes changes in lifestyle (*n* = 443)						
Yes	260	58.7	268	60.5	229	51.7
No	142	32.1	155	35.0	97	21.9
Not Sure	5	1.1	20	4.5	1	0.2
Total matching, %	-	-	-	-	-	**73.8**
The treatment or management plan includes changes in diet (*n* = 443)						
Yes	260	58.7	242	54.6	201	45.4
No	183	41.3	189	42.7	138	31.2
Not Sure	0	0.0	12	2.7	0	0.0
Total matching, %	-	-	242	54.6	-	**76.5**
The treatment or management plan includes seeing another doctor, specialist or therapist (*n* = 442)						
Yes	89	20.1	97	21.9	64	14.5
No	348	78.7	335	75.8	308	69.7
Not Sure	5	1.1	10	2.3	0	0.0
Total matching, %	-	-	-	-	-	**84.2**

†, Clinician and patient answered the same (Yes, No or Not Sure). Non-matching responses are not included in the last column.

Discussion

Given the low quality of care in public South African clinics, it was surprising to find that patients consistently gave very positive assessments about their clinician, as is shown in Table 2. The vast majority of patients interviewed agreed that during their consultation the clinician listened to their questions and concerns, conducted a physical examination, gave them a chance to ask questions, gave them an explanation for their health problems and allowed them to participate in the diagnosis. In addition, nearly all patients agreed that they were informed well enough to explain their treatment or management plan to others.

Even with the seemingly small variation in answers, in preliminary analysis we found that three statements had a statistically-significant association with whether or not patients understood their management plan ($p < 0.05$). These statements were (1) whether the patient participated in the diagnosis, (2) whether the clinician explained the health problem to the patient and (3) whether the patient understood what was wrong with his or her health.

However, the clear bias toward positive assessment of clinicians by their patients warrants future research to understand the limitations of these items. Students suggested two possible reasons: (1) that patients may have been concerned about the confidentiality of their answers, even if assured otherwise and (2) that patients may have little background or other experiences that would help them assess whether their consultation was thorough or not.

We found greater disagreement in comparing the answers of patients and clinicians regarding the content of the management plan (Table 3), which may be because these items refer to factual knowledge. Patients in many cases were not sure or did not know whether their management plans included changes in lifestyle or diet, or referrals to other doctors. This suggests that the exchange of information during the consultation was not understood fully in the same way by patients and clinicians.

An issue with potentially-significant consequences for health outcomes is the relatively high proportion of patients who do not know whether their management plan includes changes in lifestyle or diet. Immediately after their consultation, about 26% (n = 116) of the patients were confused about whether or not they needed to modify their lifestyle and 24% (n = 104) did not know if they needed to modify their diets. In fact, one-third of all the patients in the study did not answer correctly one or both items about lifestyle and diet changes prescribed in their management plan.

Our main findings are that patients have a significantly better understanding of their management plan when consultations are conducted in the patient's first or a similar language, with a clinician they have seen several times before. Patients also need to feel involved during the consultation and understand the explanation regarding their condition. This suggests the need for greater emphasis on continuity of care and on addressing obstacles to effective communication, either by improving clinician linguistic competencies or by matching clinician–patient language capabilities to whatever extent possible. These are likely to be cost-effective patient-centred interventions with a potentially large impact on patient health outcomes.

There are three limitations of this study. Firstly, the participants were selected as a sample of convenience and may not be representative of the population presenting to all Tshwane clinics. Secondly, the questionnaires were developed only in English and the English language proficiency of respondents was not measured so that there is no information as to whether statements were understood as intended. Thirdly, we imputed missing values for the variable that measured the number of times that the patient had seen a particular clinician. Although we did not find significant differences between those who answered and the missing cases, our findings should be taken as tentative until further research corroborates them.

Conclusion

This study contributes to patient-centred research that shows how clinicians, through their communication skills and interactions during consultations, have the potential to exert a positive influence with regard to their patients' health behaviours and outcomes.

In this study, about one-third of the patients presenting in public clinics answered questions incorrectly on whether changes in lifestyle or diet were prescribed as part of their treatment, even though they had just left the consulting room. Clinicians may not be aware of the confusion their patients are experiencing about their medical advice or treatment. This may be due to the stresses of treating a high volume of patients or the need to keep a focus on making the correct diagnosis.

Patient-centred care argues that consultation should be tailored to address each individual's needs and preferences. The shift requires that clinicians engage in conversations with their patients in collaborative ways. This collaboration has the potential to empower patients to participate actively in health matters and is likely to result in better clinical outcomes.[30,31]

Clinician linguistic competence appears to be especially important. As in other multi-lingual societies, language in South Africa is a marker for imputed or actual cultural differences. Whereas clinicians invariably speak English and/or Afrikaans, the majority of their patients speak their own and other indigenous languages and only a little English or Afrikaans.[32] In this way, the communication barriers between patients and clinicians that arise from the structure of a healthcare system that anonymises and depersonalises health services are reinforced perversely by language differences. Researchers have reported that medical students doing clinical rotations in health facilities are often frustrated by their inability to connect to and understand the cultural experiences and social constrains that impact the health outcomes of their patients.[32] Currently, language barriers are addressed on an *ad hoc* basis in most clinics and hospitals in South Africa, with translation help from a staff member if needed.[29,32] However, more research is needed in order to understand the extent to which miscommunication due to language barriers reflects on poor health outcomes.

Engaging patients in the consultation and building positive therapeutic relationships are dynamics that are easier to introduce through continuity of care and in the presence of greater patient–clinician language concordance. Admittedly, continuity of care and matching patients to clinicians who are able to speak the same or a similar language may not be possible or cost-effective in large clinic or hospital settings, where it may require investment in staff training and in the development of strategies to address organisational and structural challenges. However, continuity of care may be more easily implemented in primary care at the community level where some innovative transformations are already taking place. Examples of innovative practices include Lusikisiki public clinics in rural South Africa, where HIV services have been integrated into primary healthcare through decentralisation of services and by task shifting within each clinic to distribute workloads more evenly;[33] another successful innovation has been the adoption of new technologies (eg. geographic information systems [GIS]) in Hlabisa subdistrict primary healthcare clinics to study and address the relationship between distance to roads and clinics and various health outcomes, including the prevalence of HIV amongst women attending prenatal clinics.[34,35]

Ultimately, improvements in the health of the most vulnerable segments of South Africa may require systemic commitment to patient-centred practices and making community-level primary care the first and most important part of the healthcare system. It may also require that medical training incorporate curricula enriched by the perspectives that social sciences research and linguistic studies can bring to the understanding of health-impacting behaviours. In this regard, reviews of studies with diverse patient populations find strong evidence that cultural and linguistic competence have positive impacts on health outcomes, including improved adherence to treatment and following recommended changes in lifestyle.[36]

Cultural and linguistic components may include a broad range of practices, from endorsement of influential community members and using materials in the preferred language, to adapting messages to cultural values and having providers or peer educators from the same cultural, ethnic or racial groups. Some components may be more relevant than others, indicating that there is need for further research to identify the specific cultural and linguistic components that may be most effective within particular populations.[37]

Acknowledgements

The authors are indebted to the 2012 class of fifth-year students who took part in this research. We thank them for their commitment to the project as well as their insightful feedback.

Competing interests

The authors declare that they have no financial or personal relationship(s) that may have inappropriately influenced them in writing this article.

Authors' contributions

J.H. (University of Pretoria) was the project leader. J.H., A.R. and T.R. (University of Pretoria) conceptualised and designed the study. L.F., T.R., N.S. (University of Pretoria) and H.K. and S.M. (University of Pretoria and Foundation for Professional Development) were responsible for experimental and questionnaire design. T.M. (University of Pretoria) made significant conceptual contributions to the article. L.F., T.M. and T.R. conducted the analysis and interpretation of the findings and prepared the manuscript. N.S. contributed to data collection and preparation.

References

1. Coovadia H, Jewkes R, Barron P, et al. The health and health system of South Africa: historical roots of current public health challenges. Lancet. 2009;374(9692):817–834. http://dx.doi.org/10.1016/S0140-6736(09)60951-X
2. Ardington C, Case A. Interactions between mental health and socioeconomic status in the South African national income dynamics study. J Stud Econ Econometrics. 2010;34(3):69–85.
3. Chopra M, Lawn JE, Sanders D, et al. Achieving the health Millennium Development Goals for South Africa: challenges and priorities. Lancet. 2009;374(9694):1023–1031. http://dx.doi.org/10.1016/S0140-6736(09)61122-3
4. Hugo JF, Cooper ID, Thigiti J, et al. Equity in health care: does family medicine have a role? Afr J Prm Health Care Fam Med. 2010;2(1). Art.#243, 3 pages.
5. Kinkel H, Adelekan A, Wolvaardt G. Assessment of service quality of public ART clinics in South Africa. Pretoria, South Africa: Foundation for Professional Development; 2011.
6. Marcus TS. Community oriented primary care L2: Primary health. Cape Town, South Africa: Pearson; 2013.
7. Cliff B. The evolution of patient-centered care. J Healthc Manag. 2012;57(2):86-–88.
8. Loh A, Leonhart R, Wills CE, et al. The impact of patient participation on adherence and clinical outcome in primary care of depression. Patient Educ Couns. 2007;65(1):69–78. http://dx.doi.org/10.1016/j.pec.2006.05.007
9. Institute of Medicine. Crossing the quality chasm: a new health system for the 21st century. Washington, DC: National Academy Press; 2001.
10. Travaline JM, Ruchinskas R, D'Alonzo GE Jr. Patient–physician communication: why and how. J Am Osteopath Assoc. Clinical Practice. 2005;105(1):13-18.
11. Stewart MA. Effective physician–patient communication and health outcomes: a review. CMAJ. 1995;152(9):1423–1433.
12. Staiger TO, Jarvik JG, Deyo RA, et al. Brief report: patient–physician agreement as a predictor of outcomes in patients with back pain. J Gen Intern Med. 2005;20(10):935–937. http://dx.doi.org/10.1111/j.1525-1497.2005.0175.x
13. Hu P, Reuben DB. Effects of managed care on the length of time that elderly patients spend with physicians during ambulatory visits: National Ambulatory Medical Care Survey. Med Care. 2002;40(7):606–613. http://dx.doi.org/10.1097/00005650-200207000-00007
14. Betancourt JR, Green AR, Carrillo JE, et al. Defining cultural competence: a practical framework for addressing racial/ethnic disparities in health and health care. Public Health Rep. 2003; 118(4): 293-302.
15. Kundhal KK, Kundhal PS. Cultural diversity: an evolving challenge to physician–patient communication. JAMA. 2003;289(1):94. http://dx.doi.org/10.1001/jama.289.1.94
16. Uijen AA, Schers HJ, Schellevis FG, et al. How unique is continuity of care? A review of continuity and related concepts. Fam Pract. 2012;29(3):264–271. http://dx.doi.org/10.1093/fampra/cmr104
17. Saultz JW. Defining and measuring interpersonal continuity of care. Ann Fam Med. 2003;1(3):134–143. http://dx.doi.org/10.1370/afm.23

18. Haggerty JL, Reid RJ, Freeman GK, et al. Continuity of care: a multidisciplinary review. BMJ. 2003;327(7425):1219–1221. http://dx.doi.org/10.1136/bmj.327.7425.1219

19. Alazri M, Heywood P, Neal RD, et al. Continuity of care: literature review and implications. Sultan Qaboos Univ Med J. 2007;7(3):197–206.

20. Schers H, van den Hoogen H, Bor H, et al. Familiarity with a GP and patients' evaluations of care. A cross-sectional study. Fam Pract. 2005;22(1):15–19. http://dx.doi.org/10.1093/fampra/cmh721

21. Morgan ED, Pasquarella M, Holman JR. Continuity of care and patient satisfaction in a family practice clinic. J Am Board Fam Pract. 2004;17(5):341–346. http://dx.doi.org/10.3122/jabfm.17.5.341

22. Love MM, Mainous AG 3rd, Talbert JC, et al. Continuity of care and the physician–patient relationship: the importance of continuity for adult patients with asthma. J Fam Pract. 2000;49(11):998–1004.

23. Campbell SM, Roland MO, Buetow SA. Defining quality of care. Soc Sci Med. 2000;51(11):1611–1625. http://dx.doi.org/10.1016/S0277-9536(00)00057-5

24. Devroey D, Coigniez P, Vandevoorde J, et al. Prevention and follow-up of cardiovascular disease among patients without a personal GP. Fam Pract. 2003;20(4):420–424. http://dx.doi.org/10.1093/fampra/cmg415

25. Mainous AG III, Koopman RJ, Gill JM, et al. Relationship between continuity of care and diabetes control: Evidence from the third National Health and Nutrition Examination Survey. Am J Public Health. 2004;94(1):66–70. http://dx.doi.org/10.2105/AJPH.94.1.66

26. Lackland DT, Egan BM. Lack of continuous care is associated with higher rates of stroke in hypertensive medicaid beneficiaries. Am J Hypertens. 2002;15:142A. http://dx.doi.org/10.1016/S0895-7061(02)02660-2

27. Hänninen J, Takala J, Keinänen-Kiukaanniemi S. Good continuity of care may improve quality of life in Type 2 diabetes. Diabetes Res Clin Pract. 2001;51(1):21–27. http://dx.doi.org/10.1016/S0168-8227(00)00198-4

28. Hudelson P, Vilpert S. Overcoming language barriers with foreign-language speaking patients: a survey to investigate intra-hospital variation in attitudes and practices. BMC Health Serv Res. 2009;9:187. http://dx.doi.org/10.1186/1472-6963-9-187

29. Schlemmer A, Mash B. The effects of a language barrier in a South African district hospital. S Afr Med J. 2006;96(10):1084–1087.

30. Miles A, Mezzich J. The care of the patient and the soul of the clinic: person-centered medicine as an emergent model of modern clinical practice. Int J Pers Cent Med. 2011;1(2):207–222.

31. Fehrson G, Henbest R. In search of excellence. Expanding the patient-centred clinical method: a three-stage assessment. J Fam Pract. 1993;10(1):49–54. http://dx.doi.org/10.1093/fampra/10.1.49

32. Marcus TS. The place of social science in medical education: a case study of language and culture in experiential learning in a multilingual society. Multicultural Learning and Teaching. 2011;6(2):2161–2412. http://dx.doi.org/10.2202/2161-2412.1077

33. Bedelu M, Ford N, Hilderbrand K, et al. Implementing antiretroviral therapy in rural communities: The Lusikisiki model of decentralized HIV/AIDS care. J Infect Dis. 2007;196(Suppl 3):S464–468. http://dx.doi.org/10.1086/521114

34. Tanser F, le Sueur D, Solarsh G, et al. HIV heterogeneity and proximity of homestead to roads in rural South Africa: an exploration using a geographical information system. Trop Med Int Health. 2000;5(1):40–46. http://dx.doi.org/10.1046/j.1365-3156.2000.00513.x

35. Tanser F. Geographical information systems (GIS) innovations for primary health care in developing countries. Innov: Technol, Govern, Global. 2006;1(2):106–122. http://dx.doi.org/10.1162/itgg.2006.1.2.106

36. Goode TD, Dunne MC, Bronheim SM. The evidence base for cultural and linguistic competency in health care. New York, NY: Commonwealth Fund; 2006.

37. Guerrero EG, Campos M, Urada D, et al. Do cultural and linguistic competence matter in Latinos' completion of mandated substance abuse treatment? Subst Abuse Treat Prev Policy. 2012;7:34. http://dx.doi.org/10.1186/1747-597X-7-34

Appendix 1 starts on next the page →

Appendix 1

UNIVERSITY OF PRETORIA DEPARTMENT OF FAMILY MEDICINE

QI – PATIENT COLLABORATION INDEX **DATE (MM/DD/YYYY) |__|__|_______|** **INTERVIEWER:____________**

DR's NAME: ______________________ CLINIC/HOSPITAL: ____________________ FILE NUMBER: __________________

PATIENT GENDER: _______________ AGE: __________ TOTAL NUMBER OF TIMES PATIENT HAS SEEN THIS CLINICIAN ___________

MAIN LANGUAGE OF CONSULTATION: ___________________ IF OTHER (SPECIFY): ___________________

PATIENT'S FIRST LANGUAGE: _________________________ IF OTHER (SPECIFY): ___________________

I will read you some statements. After I read each statement, please tell me if in your case it is "true," "partly true," "partly false," or "false.

1. The clinician listened to my questions and concerns without interrupting me.	**TRUE** **PARTLY TRUE** **PARTLY FALSE** **FALSE**	2. The clinician examined me in order to find out what's wrong with me.	**TRUE** **PARTLY TRUE** **PARTLY FALSE** **FALSE**
3. I participated in the diagnosis of my condition or disease.	**TRUE** **PARTLY TRUE** **PARTLY FALSE** **FALSE**	4. The clinician explained to me what's wrong with my health.	**TRUE** **PARTLY TRUE** **PARTLY FALSE** **FALSE**
5. I had the opportunity to ask questions to the clinician.	**TRUE** **PARTLY TRUE** **PARTLY FALSE** **FALSE**	6. I understand what is wrong with my health.	**TRUE** **PARTLY TRUE** **PARTLY FALSE** **FALSE**
7. I agree with the medical treatment to manage my condition or disease.	**TRUE** **PARTLY TRUE** **PARTLY FALSE** **FALSE**	8. I feel confident I can explain to someone at home the treatment or management plan for my condition.	**TRUE** **PARTLY TRUE** **PARTLY FALSE** **FALSE**

I just have a few more questions. For the following statements, please answer "yes," "no" or "not sure" if you are not sure or don't know.

9. My treatment or management plan includes changes in lifestyle.	**YES** **NO** **NOT SURE**	10. (IF YES) I know what I am supposed to change regarding my lifestyle.	**YES** **NO** **NOT SURE**
11. My treatment or management plan includes changes in diet.	**YES** **NO** **NOT SURE**	12. (IF YES) I know the changes that I need to make to my diet.	**YES** **NO** **NOT SURE**
13. My treatment or management plan includes medicines.	**YES** **NO** **NOT SURE**	14. (IF YES) I know when and how to take my medicines.	**YES** **NO** **NOT SURE**
15. My management plan includes to see another doctor, specialist or therapist.	**YES** **NO** **NOT SURE**	16. (IF YES) I have a referral form or letter to see the other doctor.	**YES** **NO** **NOT SURE**

THANK YOU FOR YOUR PARTICIPATION!

The practices of isolating tuberculosis infectious patients at hospitals of Vhembe district, Limpopo Province

Author:
Takalani G. Tshitangano[1]

Affiliation:
[1]Department of Public Health, University of Venda, South Africa

Correspondence to:
Takalani Tshitangano

Email:
takalani.tshitangano@univen.ac.za

Postal address:
PO Bag X 5050, Thohoyandou 0950, South Africa

Background: Airborne infections pose a serious threat to susceptible individuals whenever they are together in confined spaces with patients coughing up tuberculosis (TB) bacilli. In healthcare facilities, those with infectious TB should, as far as possible, be isolated from non-infectious patients in order to prevent exposure to the infectious droplet nuclei generated by infected patients.

Aim: This article aims to describe the use of masks and isolation of infectious TB patients at hospitals of Vhembe district, Limpopo Province in order to inform future policy and practices.

Setting: This study was conducted at seven of the eight hospitals in Vhembe district.

Methods: A cross-sectional qualitative design of a descriptive nature was used. Purposive sampling was used to select 57 focus group participants. Necessary approval, permission and clearance were obtained. The participants' rights were respected.

Results: This study confirmed that TB cubicles were not reserved for patients with infectious TB and that many TB inpatients at hospitals of Vhembe district were not isolated; masks were not used consistently or appropriately by patients, staff or visitors. Furthermore, the movement of TB inpatients in isolation was not restricted.

Conclusions: There is an unnecessary risk of becoming infected with TB at the rural hospitals of Vhembe district as a result of incorrect isolation practices. The development and implementation of a quality control programme, as well as ongoing training at the hospital level, would improve the TB infection control measures practised by healthcare workers at hospitals in Vhembe district and reduce the risk of acquiring TB at these hospitals.

L'habitude d'isoler les patients infectés par la tuberculose dans les hôpitaux du district de Vhembe, dans la province du Limpopo.

Contexte: Les infections aéroportées sont une sérieuse menace pour les personnes sensibles quand elles se trouvent ensemble dans un espace confiné avec des patients qui toussent et projettent des bacilles de tuberculose (TB). Dans les établissements de santé, les personnes infectées par la tuberculose devraient, autant que possible, être isolées des patients non-infectieux pour éviter l'exposition aux noyaux de gouttelettes infectieuses produites par les patients infectés.

Objectif: Cet article a pour objet de décrire l'utilisation de masques et l'isolation des patients atteints de tuberculose infectieuse dans les hôpitaux du district de Vhembe, dans la province du Limpopo, afin d'élaborer les politiques et pratiques futures.

Cadre: Cette étude a été menée dans sept des huit hôpitaux du district de Vhembe.

Méthodes: On a utilisé une étude transversale qualitative de nature descriptive. On a utilisé l'échantillonnage au jugé pour choisir 57 participants pour le groupe témoin. On a obtenu l'approbation, la permission et l'autorisation nécessaires. On a respecté les droits des participants.

Résultats: Cette étude a confirmé que les compartiments pour tuberculeux n'était pas réservés aux patients atteints de tuberculeuse infectieuse et que beaucoup de patients tuberculeux hospitalisés dans les hôpitaux du district de Vhembe n'étaient pas isolés; les masques n'étaient pas utilisés systématiquement ou correctement par les patients, le personnel ou les visiteurs. En outre, les mouvements des patients tuberculeux hospitalisés en isolation n'étaient pas limités.

Conclusions: Il y a des risques inutiles d'être infecté par la tuberculose dans les hôpitaux ruraux du district de Vhembe en raison des mauvaises pratiques d'isolation. Le développement et la mise en œuvre du programme de contrôle de qualité, ainsi qu'une formation continue au niveau de l'hôpital, améliorerait les mesures de contrôle de l'infection tuberculeuse pratiquées par le personnel hospitalier dans les hôpitaux du district de Vhembe et réduirait les risques de contagion tuberculeuse à ces hôpitaux.

Introduction

Airborne infections pose a serious threat to susceptible individuals whenever they are placed together with the index case in confined spaces.[1] According to Escombe et al., airborne tuberculosis (TB) transmission occurs particularly in overcrowded settings containing TB infectious patients, such as hospitals, clinics, homeless shelters, and prisons.[1] Therefore, the World Health Organization (WHO) advises that infectious TB patients be isolated from other patients in order to protect these other patients from the infectious droplet nuclei that infectious patients generate.[2]

The US Centers for Disease Control and Prevention (CDC) describes isolation as 'the separation of persons who have a specific infectious illness from those who are healthy and the restriction of their movement to stop the spread of that disease'.[3] Sissolack, Marais and Mehtar see quarantine as another form of isolation.[4] However, quarantine is described by the CDC as the 'separation and restriction of movement of persons who, while not yet ill, have been exposed to an infectious agent and therefore may become infectious to stop the spread of an infectious disease'.[3] The WHO suggests a third less effective way of separating infectious TB patients from non-infectious patients, namely, to establish a separate area within a hospital ward.[2] In this study, isolation refers to separation of individuals having a particular disease or who have been exposed to an infectious agent from those who are healthy; this includes the establishment of a separate area within a hospital ward and the restriction of the movement of the infected patients in order to minimise the spread of disease.

The problem is that, according to the WHO, 'of every 100 hospitalized patients at any given time, 7 in developed and 10 in developing countries will acquire at least one of the infections acquired in health care settings'.[5] Tuberculosis is one of these infections. Authors worldwide warn that the risk of becoming infected with TB in healthcare settings is increasing daily.[2,3,4,5] Lin et al. indicated that infections acquired in healthcare settings represent an important indicator of healthcare quality and patient safety, which makes it an important health issue for research.[6] The WHO acknowledges that infections acquired in healthcare settings are a recognised public health problem and a global public threat for both patients and healthcare professionals.[7] Mixing infectious TB patients with patients who do not have TB, especially those with HIV or other immune-compromised conditions, fuels TB transmission risks.[5]

A comprehensive infection, prevention and control (IPC) programme helps to decrease the spread of TB, including drug-resistant TB. This study was part of a larger study that was conducted in 2012, which examined other IPC interventions with regard to TB, namely, availability of a TB infection control plan at hospitals, existence of health service delay in TB diagnosis and treatment, TB infection control trainings for healthcare workers (HCWs), environmental control practices and sputum collection practices.[8,9] These studies found that IPC interventions were not aligned to the WHO policy on TB infection control in healthcare facilities, households and congregate settings, because of a lack of TB infection control plans in hospitals.[10]

Purpose of the study

This article aims to describe the use of masks and isolation of infectious TB patients at hospitals of Vhembe district, Limpopo Province in order to inform future policy and practice.

Objectives

The objectives of this study were as follows:

- Explore and describe how the movement of an infectious TB patient was handled in the isolation ward.
- Explore and describe the management of visitation in the isolation ward.
- Explore and describe where infectious TB patients were placed in the hospital.
- Explore and describe the use of masks in the TB ward or isolation cubicles at hospitals in Vhembe district.

Research methods and design

Study design

In this study, a cross-sectional qualitative design of a descriptive nature was used.[11] Vhembe district has eight public hospitals. One hospital, however, is a psychiatric hospital and does not admit TB patients. This study was thus conducted in 2012 at only seven of the eight hospitals of Vhembe district. The target population of this study was all the HCWs at these hospitals. The HCWs in this study were professionals involved in the care of TB patients, namely, laboratory staff members, surgical ward nurses, antiretroviral (ARV) clinic nurses, TB focal point staff, paediatric ward nurses, outpatient department (OPD)/casualty nurses, X-ray staff members, TB ward nurses, medical ward nurses, infection control nurses, occupational health and safety (OHS) nurses, pharmacy staff members, sub-acute ward nurses, maternity ward nurses, psychiatric ward nurses and doctors. This target population was chosen because HCWs are in direct contact with infectious patients and are more at risk of acquiring infectious conditions such as TB.[6]

Study population and sampling strategy

Purposive sampling of a maximum variation type[12] was used to select a variety of representative focus group participants believed to have the necessary TB control knowledge needed in this study. The participants in the focus group discussions varied, comprising the deputy manager of nursing, laboratory staff members, surgical ward nurses, ARV clinic nurses, TB focal point staff, paediatric ward nurses, OPD/casualty nurses, X-ray staff members, TB ward nurses, medical ward nurses, infection control nurses, OHS nurses, pharmacy staff members, sub-acute ward nurses, maternity ward nurses and psychiatric ward nurses. Although doctors were amongst the population targeted for this study, they did not consent to participation and thus did not take part in the study.

The sample size for the focus group discussions was one focus group per participating hospital, making up 7 focus groups. Each focus group comprised five to 10 members, making a total sample size of 57 participants.

The central question for the focus group discussions was: 'How would you describe the practices of isolating an infectious TB patient in this hospital?' In response to the answers given by the focus group members, follow-up probing questions were asked, as prepared for in the unstructured focus group discussion guide. The content and construct validity of the focus group discussion guide and checklist were ensured through consultation with the Vhembe district TB coordinator as well as the WHO TB infection control policy.[10]

Data collection

The pilot study at the first hospital afforded the researcher the opportunity to pre-test the focus group discussion guide as well as the checklist in order to check the reliability of the checklist by using a test–re-test and an inter-rater test, in order to determine whether the wording and constructs were clear and to evaluate the feasibility of the entire study. The data collection tools and processes were then readjusted accordingly. The data collected from the pilot study formed part of the empirical data for this study so as not to lose important information.

A checklist was developed to record participants' responses to the central question that asked: 'Is there a TB ward away from non-infectious wards in this hospital'. This checklist had 3 columns, two for answers of 'Yes' and 'No' and a further column that allowed the participants to describe the availability of TB wards that are kept separate from the non-infectious wards.

Data analysis

Mixed methods were used to analyse the data. Qualitative data collected through focus group discussions were analysed using the open coding method following Tesch's[13] 8-step criteria as described by Creswell,[14] whereas data collected through the checklist were analysed using quasi-statistics, where the number of hospitals with or without a separate TB ward were counted.[11,12] The results from quasi-statistics as well as those from open coding analysis were combined, giving rise to the conclusions of the study. Lincoln and Guba's[15] model comprising four criteria or measures to ensure trustworthiness of the study findings, namely, truth value (credibility), applicability (transferability), consistency (dependability) and neutrality (confirmability), was adopted.

Trustworthiness

In order to ensure credibility of the study findings, three data-collection instruments (focus group discussions; document study; and observation) presented methodological triangulation, whilst the use of both quantitative and qualitative data analysis methods demonstrated data analysis triangulation. The researcher also took photographs of what was observed for further reference. Member checks afforded participants an opportunity to verify whether the researcher had captured exactly what they had said. Prolonged engagement of participants during focus group discussions, which lasted one to one-and-a-half hours, enabled the researcher to collect all the information regarding TB infection control practices until data saturation was achieved.[15] Persistent observations which lasted from one-and-a-half to two hours per hospital, helped the researcher to gather information regarding all environmental TB control measures practised in the study hospitals.

In order to ensure transferability of the study findings, a thick description was documented in clear simple language regarding how themes were identified, how code books were built, how subcategories were induced and how categories emerged, so as to afford readers a chance to decide for themselves if the results are transferable to their own contexts.

In order to ensure dependability of the study findings, the auditor (who happened to be a neutral colleague from the same university) examined the running account of the process of inquiry as well as the findings and recommendations, attesting to the fact that the findings are supported by the data and that the study is internally coherent. An extensive and detailed record of the study process was documented for others to replicate.[11] The proposal for this study was presented to a panel of experts (comprising professors and doctors) serving on the Higher Degrees Ethics Committee of the University of Venda; and a certificate of ethical clearance was issued by the university as a way of showing its belief in the methodology's ability to yield dependable results. The proposal was also evaluated by the Private Research Ethics Committee of the University of Limpopo, who issued approval to conduct the study, again as a way of showing a belief in the ability of the methodology to yield dependable results. The proposal for this study was presented at the International Nurses' Conference held from 27 June to 4 July 2009 in Durban, South Africa for peer-review and the inputs from this conference were taken into consideration. The researcher is an experienced healthcare professional in the field of TB management. The researcher's TB management knowledge and expertise added value to the process of data collection, coding, formulation and naming of subcategories, establishment of relationships and model development, which attest to the dependability of the findings.

In order to ensure confirmability of the study findings, the researcher has thus far published 11 papers in Department of Higher Education and Training-accredited peer-reviewed journals. Three of the published papers have been presented at national conferences for peer-review purposes.

Ethical considerations

Approval for the study was obtained from both the University of Venda (UNIVEN) Higher Degree Committees and the Limpopo Provincial Department of Health. Ethical clearance was obtained from the UNIVEN Ethics Committee (project number SHS/10/PDC/02) and the Limpopo Provincial Department of Health provided a letter that gave permission for data collection at each of the seven hospitals.

Ethical clearance obtained from UNIVEN Ethics Committee, together with the permission letter from the province, were used to negotiate entrance to each hospital where data were collected. Informed written consent was obtained from each participant. Ethical principles such as the principle of justice, beneficence and self-determination were observed when dealing with participants. In addition, hospitals where data was collected were allocated codes A–G to ensure that the participants' rights to privacy, anonymity and confidentiality were respected.

Results

This study confirmed that TB cubicles were not reserved for patients with infectious TB and that many TB inpatients at hospitals of Vhembe district were not isolated; masks were not used consistently or appropriately by patients or staff or visitors. Furthermore, the movement of TB inpatients in isolation was not restricted. These findings were arranged into categories, which are discussed in detail hereunder. Table 1 provides details of the participants whose views have been quoted in the text.

Tuberculosis inpatients were not isolated; cubicles were not reserved

The probing question was: 'Is there a TB ward away from the non-infectious wards in this hospital?' Four hospitals did not have dedicated TB wards, but had TB cubicles established within the medical ward. Only two of the hospitals had TB wards established a distance away from the other wards, but these wards were used in different ways depending on the hospital. One hospital used the TB ward to isolate only TB inpatients who were on streptomycin. The other hospital had divided its TB ward into cubicles, one for multi-drug-resistant (MDR)-TB inpatients; one for non-pulmonary TB inpatients; one for sputum-negative TB inpatients; one for sputum positive inpatients; and the other one for TB suspect inpatients. One hospital did not have an area or ward dedicated for either TB suspects or confirmed TB inpatients. In this hospital, infectious and non-infectious inpatients were mixed together in a medical ward (see Table 2).

TABLE 1: Participants' demographics.

Participant number	Position	Hospital	Gender	Age
1	Medical ward nurse	D	F	48
2	General ward nurse	G	F	33
3	Medical ward nurse	B	F	37
4	TB ward nurse	C	M	52
5	Male medical ward nurse	C	M	46
6	Female medical ward nurse	C	F	43
7	Female medical ward nurse	F	F	46
8	Male medical ward nurse	F	F	43
9	TB ward nurse	A	F	47

TB, tuberculosis.

The movement of tuberculosis inpatients in isolation was not restricted

When participants were asked how the movement of infectious TB patients was handled in the isolation ward at each hospital, participants from the majority of the hospitals ($n = 6$) indicated that TB inpatient movement was not restricted.

According to one participant from hospital D: 'Patients' movement [*sic*] are not restricted' (P1).

The general ward nurse from hospital G confirmed this, saying: 'TB patients' movements are not restricted' (P2).

A medical ward nurse from hospital B added: 'TB patients are allowed to go wherever they want' (P3).

The TB ward nurse, Male medical ward nurse and Female medical ward nurse from hospital C further said that movements of TB patients are not restricted in the hospital 'because it is difficult to control the movement of a patient who can walk' (P4, 5, 6).

Only one participating hospital restricted its TB patients' movements. According to participants 7 and 8 from hospital F, there is a fence around the TB ward which restricts the movement of TB patients. Patients are only allowed to go out when it is necessary and then the appropriate precautionary measures are put in place.

Masks were not used consistently or appropriately

When a probing question was asked, namely: 'How would you describe the use of masks in TB ward or isolation cubicles in this hospital?', participants' responses included mask use by TB inpatients, visitors and HCWs.

Mask use by inpatients

With regard to the use of masks by TB inpatients, the study revealed a variation of mask use, with only two hospitals

TABLE 2: Availability of tuberculosis wards away from non-infectious wards: Quantitative data.

Hospital	Is there a tuberculosis ward away from non-infectious wards in this hospital?
A	**Yes:** There is a cubicle for TB suspects in the TB ward; TB ward is for all confirmed TB cases.
B	**No:** TB patients are nursed in medical wards
C	**No:** Separate areas for TB suspects for now. TB patients are nursed in a medical ward. TB ward is for patients on streptomycin only.
D	**Yes:** TB suspects are nursed in TB ward in a suspect cubicle. Confirmed cases are nursed in TB wards in their own cubicles.
E	**No:** TB patients are admitted in their isolation ward, which isolates all infectious cases, even when non-TB.
F	**No:** There is no TB ward. TB patients are nursed in a medical ward, but there are cubicles for TB suspects, one for sputum-positive TB and one for MDR-TB.
G	**No:** There is no TB ward. All TB patients are nursed in medical ward amongst other non-infectious patients.
Conclusion:	Four hospitals do not have separate TB wards. Of the three that do have TB wards, one utilises this ward only to care for patients on streptomycin.

TB, tuberculosis; MDR, multi-drug resistant.

giving patients surgical masks. One participant, a medical ward nurse from hospital D said: 'All patients in the TB cubicle put on surgical masks' (P1).

One hospital was giving patients N95 respirators. Three participants from hospital C said: 'TB suspects are given N95 mask [*sic*]' (P4, 5, 6).

That being said, the majority (n = 5) of the hospitals did not give patients masks at all. According to the general ward nurse from hospital G: '[*I*]solated TB patients are not given disposable masks to put on' (P2).

This claim was confirmed by participants 7 and 8 from hospital F. Additional confirmation was made by the medical ward nurse from hospital B, who said: '[*I*]solated TB patients are not given masks to put on' (P3).

The researcher further observed that neither patients nor HCWs had masks on in a TB cubicle which is within one of the medical wards in hospital B.

Mask use by visitors

With regard to the use of masks by visitors at TB cubicles and wards, participants from the majority of the hospitals (n = 6) indicated that visitors are given masks and allowed to see their patients in bed. Out of these six, five gave surgical masks and one gave N95 respirators. One hospital did not give masks at all and yet allowed visitors to see their patients in bed. According to one of the participants from hospital F: 'Visitors are also given a mask N95. There is a courtesy nurse who supplies visitors with masks and educates them on proper use and disposal' (P7).

A participants from hospital B said: 'Visitors see their TB patients in beds. There is no visitor restriction. Masks are sometimes used by visitors' (P3).

Participants 4, 5 and 6 from hospital C confirmed this by saying that visitors are not restricted and are allowed to see their TB suspect patient without a mask. At the female medical ward, visitors of MDR-TB patients are given masks and are restricted. In the TB ward, visitors are given masks if they are available and are not allowed to see their patients in bed, but rather see them outside in the open air.

A participant from hospital A added:

> 'Visitors see their TB suspect or confirmed TB patients in bed. There is no visitor restriction. Visitors get into the ward with paper disposable mask on they take from a container mounted on the wall at the entrance of the TB ward. These masks are disposed into the dirty bin upon leaving the TB wards.' (P9)

Mask use by healthcare workers

With regard to the use of masks by HCWs at TB cubicles and wards, the same confusion regarding which mask to use was revealed by the fact that HCWs at two hospitals put on N95 masks in TB cubicles and wards. According to participants 7 and 8 from hospital F, 'whenever a nurse enters one of the TB cubicles' he or she puts on an N95 mask.

Three participants from hospital C said: 'Nurses put on surgical masks in TB cubicles' (P4, 5 & 6).

However, HCWs at the majority of the hospitals (n = 4) did not put on masks at all in TB cubicles. According to a participants from hospital B: 'Nurses do not put on masks in TB cubicles' (P3).

Discussion

This study discovered that TB inpatients were not isolated and that the TB cubicles were not reserved for patients with infectious TB. Furthermore, the movement of TB inpatients in isolation was not restricted and masks were not used either consistently or appropriately by patients, staff or visitors in wards that cared for infectious TB patients.

These findings concur with those of Basu, Andrew and Poolman, who assert that the 'capacity for safe airborne isolation does not exist in South African hospitals'.[16] According to Basu et al., non-XDR (extensively drug resistant)-TB patients are frequently admitted to the wards with other patients who have a TB disease and risk super infection and/or nosocomial infection.[16] Similarly, Sissolak et al. discovered a total lack of isolation facilities in South Africa.[4] Knirsch et al. also found that practices and facilities in South Africa were inadequate for both the recognition and isolation of potential TB patients.[17] Scablon et al. warn that hospitals can be breeding grounds for drug-resistant TB.[18] Hussey, director of the Institute of Infectious Diseases and Molecular Medicine at the University of Cape Town confirmed that 'hospitals could be dangerous environments, especially for patients with HIV-compromised immune systems'.[19] To substantiate that fact, the Church of Scotland hospital study in 2006 discovered that the majority of drug-resistant TB cases were associated with nosocomial infections.[19] To make matters worse, Port Elizabeth's Joseph Pearson TB hospital nurses reported that 'MDR-TB patients were contracting XDR-TB strains at an intense rate in a situation where XDR-TB patients were in a different ward from MDR-TB patients'.[4]

Siegel et al. believe that minimising the spread of tuberculosis pathogens in hospitals requires the use of TB isolation wards.[20] Amon, Girard and Keshavjee concur, stating that 'under South African law, authorities may detain an individual suffering from an infectious disease until the disease ceases to present a public health risk',[21] and state further that the draft government policy guideline[22] calls for the isolation of all MDR- and XDR-TB patients in a specialist facility for a minimum of six months. In its implementation of the guideline, the South African isolation wards where patients are quarantined in South Africa are described as prison-like by the Southern African AIDS Information Dissemination Service.[19] To substantiate this fact, Amon et al. highlight that:

> [*i*]n March 2009, the AIDS Law Project reported that approximately 1,700 people, including children were detained in TB isolation facilities, many of them in substandard conditions that violated South African constitutional rights and national health legislation.[21]

Eric Goemaere, cited in Amon et al., contends that 'incarcerating the sick in substandard isolation facilities discourages diagnosis'.[21] Furthermore, public health experts cited in Amon et al. noted that 'holding MDR- and XDR-TB patients in overcrowded hospitals with inadequate ventilation increases the risk of nosocomial TB transmissions'.[21]

Furthermore, Doctors without Borders in Cape Town found that more patients would be diagnosed and treated successfully if they were followed treatment in their own homes, rather than being isolated in specialised hospitals.[19]

On the contrary, the WHO recommends that facilities should establish isolation wards,[10] believing that if these isolation wards are located away from other wards with non-TB patients in a separate building, TB transmission would be prevented.[2] According to the WHO, 'two wards housed in separate buildings should be established, namely a medical ward with TB suspects and a TB ward with only patients on TB therapy'.[2]

The WHO further prescribes the following isolation practices that should be enforced strictly during isolation of inpatients:[2]

- 'Inpatients should not be allowed to leave their rooms or wander the hospital grounds, except for when infectious TB patients must undergo essential diagnostic procedures outside their rooms. Thus, a designated area outside for confirmed infectious TB patients can be used for fresh air'.[2]
- 'Whenever inpatients leave the isolation areas for medically essential procedures or diagnostic examination, a disposable surgical mask should be given'.[2]
- 'If possible, visitation hours should be held in a designated area outdoors'.[2]
- Isolation should be continued for a minimum of two weeks except for MDR-TB, which is said to remain infectious for a prolonged period.

The WHO also stipulates that both HCWs and patients must adhere to the airborne precautions in isolation rooms and/or areas.[10] In addition, settings where isolation facilities do not exist require sophisticated and expensive environmental controls for the reduction of nosocomial transmission. Furthermore, the WHO warns that:

> [*t*]he difficulty of ensuring effective separation of patients necessitates the need to avoid hospital admission, or rapidly discharging patients with suspected or confirmed TB, which is sometimes difficult as it is dependent on the seriousness of the patient's condition.[2]

In the light of the possibility that in certain instances it is difficult to discharge patients rapidly or avoid hospitalisation, it is imperative that enough isolation rooms be made available in each hospital.[2]

According to the CDC, 'the classification of the risk assessment of the health-care setting is used to determine how many isolation rooms each setting needs, depending on the number of TB patients examined'.[23] The CDC states that:

> [*a*]t least one isolation room is needed for settings in which TB patients stay while they are being treated, and additional rooms might be needed depending on the magnitude of patient-days of persons with suspected or confirmed TB disease. Additional rooms might be considered if options are limited for transferring patients with suspected or confirmed TB disease to other settings with isolation rooms.[23]

Furthermore, settings that plan to manage patients with TB disease should have at least one isolation room or enclosure. According to the CDC:

> [*i*]solation rooms should be single-patient rooms in which environmental factors and entry of visitors and HCWs are controlled to minimize the transmission of M. tuberculosis. [*Furthermore*], all HCWs who enter an isolation room should wear at least N95 disposable respirators. Visitors may be offered respiratory protection (i.e., N95) and should be instructed by HCWs on the use of the respirator before entering an isolation room.[3]

In addition, isolation rooms should have specific requirements for controlled ventilation, negative pressure, and air filtration. Each patient in the isolation room should have a private bathroom. According to the CDC:

> [*p*]ersons with suspected or confirmed TB disease who are in-patients should remain in isolation rooms until they are determined to be non-infectious and have demonstrated a clinical response to a standard multidrug anti-tuberculosis treatment regimen or until an alternative diagnosis is made. Therefore, if the alternative diagnosis cannot be clearly established, even with three negative sputum smear results, empiric treatment of TB disease should strongly be considered.[23]

HCWs should ensure that doors to isolation rooms are kept closed except in cases where patients, HCWs or others need to enter or exit the room.[3]

In addition, respiratory protection with an N95 or higher-level respirator is recommended for personnel entering the TB isolation wards in order to prevent droplet infection of *Mycobacterium tuberculosis*.[20] Masks must also be placed on coughing patients (cough etiquette/respiratory hygiene) so as to limit potential dissemination of infectious respiratory secretions from the infectious TB patients to others.[20]

Recommendations

The following simple recommendations were made:

> Hospitals should 'demonstrate a commitment to preventing transmission of infectious agents by incorporating infection control into the objectives of the organization's patient and occupational

safety programs'.[21] Policies and procedures explaining how these measures should be applied, including systems used for the identification and communication of information about patients with potentially transmissible infectious TB, are essential for ensuring the success of these measures.[21] A key administrative measure that could be taken is the provision of both fiscal and human resources for the maintenance of infection control and occupational health programmes that are responsive to emerging needs. Specific components that could be addressed include facility construction and design decisions,[19] as well as adequate supplies and equipment, including effective facility ventilation systems.[11] The involvement of the healthcare administrators in infection control processes would ensure an improvement of their awareness regarding the rationale and resource requirements for the efficient and effective following of recommended infection control practices.

Several administrative factors may affect adherence to isolation practices in healthcare settings namely institutional culture, individual worker behavior, and the work environment.

In their 2005 *Guidelines for preventing the transmission of Mycobacterium tuberculosis in health-care settings*, the CDC state that:

> [s]afety culture (or safety climate) refers to a work environment where a shared commitment to safety on the part of management and the workforce is understood and followed. A safety culture is created through (1) the actions management takes to improve patient and worker safety; (2) worker participation in safety planning; (3) the availability of appropriate protective equipment; (4) influence of group norms regarding acceptable safety practices; and (5) the organization's socialization process for new personnel. [*Each of these factors was found to have*] a direct bearing on adherence to transmission prevention recommendations.[24]

Education regarding improvements to adherence is one of the IPC interventions that has been studied in detail. It is interesting to note that self-reported adherence is much higher in groups that have received some level of educational intervention.[24] Educational interventions incorporating video-taped and performance feedback are said to be more successful with regard to improving adherence.[25]

Conclusion

Isolation practices suggested by the national as well as international legislative frameworks regarding infectious TB patients were not being adhered to in rural hospitals of Vhembe district.

Acknowledgements

The author thanks the authorities for granting permission to enter the hospitals to collect data; and all participants for active participations in sharing information for this study.

Competing interests

The author declares that she has no financial or personal relationship(s) that may have inappropriately influenced her in writing this article.

References

1. Escombe AR, Moore DAJ, Gilman RH, et al. Upper-room ultraviolet light and negative air ionization to prevent tuberculosis transmission. PloS Med. 2009;6(3):e1000043. http://dx.doi.org/10.1371/journal.pmed.1000043
2. World Health Organization. Guidelines for the prevention of tuberculosis in health care facilities in resource-limited settings [document on the Internet]. c1999 [cited 2014 Sep 14]. Available from: http://www.who.int/tb/publications/who_tb_99_269/en/
3. US Centers for Disease Control and Prevention. Guidelines for preventing the transmission of Mycobacterium tuberculosis in health-care facilities, 1994. MMWR. 1994;43(RR-13):1–141.
4. Sissolak D, Marais F, Mehtar S. TB infection control prevention and control experiences of South African nurses – a phenomenological study. 2011;11:262.
5. World Health Organization. Health care-associated infections fact sheet [document on the Internet]. 2013 [cited 2013 May 14]. Available from: http://www.who.int/gpsc/country-work/gpsc_ccisc_fact_sheet_en.pdf
6. Lin CF, Yang CY, Lu MS, et al. Effectiveness of a nosocomial infection control training in improving knowledge in patient-hired attendants and outsourced workers in Taiwan. J Nurs Res. 2006;16(3):187–194. http://dx.doi.org/10.1097/01.JNR.0000387305.96622.5b
7. World Health Organization. Global tuberculosis control 2010 [document on the Internet]. c2010 [cited 2014 Sep 14]. Available from: http://www.who.int/tb/publications/global_report/2010/en/
8. Tshitangano, TG, Maputle MS, Netshikweta ML. Practices of tuberculosis sputum specimen collection at resource-limited hospitals in Vhembe district, Limpopo Province, South Africa. Afr J Phys Health Educ Recr Dance. 2013;19(Suppl 1):116–125.
9. Tshitangano, TG, Maputle MS, Netshikweta ML. Environmental tuberculosis control measures at resource-limited hospitals in Vhembe district, Limpopo Province, South Africa. Afr J Phys Health Educ Recr Dance. 2013;19(Suppl 1):107–115.
10. World Health Organization. WHO policy on TB infection control in health-care facilities, congregate settings and households [document on the Internet]. c2009 [cited 2014 Sep 14]. Available from: http://whqlibdoc.who.int/publications/2009/9789241598323_eng.pdf
11. Kumar D. Research methodology: A step-by-step guide for beginners. 3rd ed. Washington, DC: SAGE Publications Ltd; 2011.
12. O'Leary Z. The essential guide to doing research. London: SAGE Publications Ltd; 2004.
13. Tesch R. Qualitative research: analysis types and software tools. New York: Routledge; 1990.
14. Creswell JW. Research design: qualitative, quantitative, and mixed methods approaches. 3rd ed.London: SAGE Publications Ltd; 2009.
15. Lincoln Y, Guba E. Naturalistic inquiry. London: SAGE Publications Ltd; 1985.
16. Basu S, Andrew J, Poolman EM. Prevention of nosocomial transmission of extensively drug-resistant tuberculosis in rural South African district hospitals: an epidemiological modelling study. Lancet. 2007;370(9597):1500–1507. http://dx.doi.org/10.1016/S0140-6736(07)61636-5
17. Knirsch CA, Jain N, Pablos-Mendez A, et al. Respiratory isolation of tuberculosis patients using clinical guidelines and an automated clinical decision support system. Infect Control Hosp Epidemiol. 2008;19(2):94–100. http://dx.doi.org/10.2307/30141996
18. US Centers for Disease Control and Prevention. Tuberculosis control laws and policies: a handbook for public health and legal practitioners [document on the Internet]. c2009 [cited 2014 Sep 14]. Available from: http://www.cdc.gov/tb/programs/TBLawPolicyHandbook.pdf
19. Schablon A, Beckmann G, Harling M, et al. Prevalence of latent tuberculosis infection among health care workers in a hospital for pulmonary diseases. J Occup Med Toxicol. 2009;4:1. http://dx.doi.org/10.1186/1745-6673-4-1
20. Siegel JD, Rhinehart E, Jackson M, et al. Guideline for isolation precautions: preventing transmission of infectious agents in healthcare settings [document on the Internet]. c2007 [cited 2014 Sep 14]. Available from: http://www.cdc.gov/hicpac/ pdf/isolation/isolation2007.pdf
21. Amon JJ, Girard F, Keshavjee S. Limitations on human rights in the context of drug-resistant tuberculosis: A reply to Boggio et al. Health and Human Rights. 2009;11(1):1–10.
22. Republic of South Africa: Department of Health. The national infection prevention and control policy & strategy [document on the Internet]. c2007 [cited 2014 Sep 23]. Available from: http://www0.sun.ac.za/ruralhealth/ukwandahome/rudasaresources2009/DOH/5%20-%20ipc-policy.pdf
23. US Centers for Disease Control and Prevention. Guidelines for environmental infection control in health-care facilities. Recommendations of CDC and the Healthcare Infection Control Practices Advisory Committee (HICPAC). MMWR. 2003;52(RR-10):1–48.
24. US Centers for Disease Control and Prevention. Guidelines for preventing the transmission of Mycobacterium tuberculosis in health-care settings, 2005. MMWR. 2005;54(RR-17):1–141.
25. US Centers for Disease Control and Prevention. Tuberculosis transmission in a homeless shelter population – New York, 2000–2003. MMWR. 2005;54(6):149–152.

8

Where there is no morphine: The challenge and hope of palliative care delivery in Tanzania

Authors:
Kristopher Hartwig[1]
Mervyn Dean[2]
Kari Hartwig[3]
Paul Z. Mmbando[1]
Abduraoof Sayed[4]
Elma de Vries[5]

Affiliations:
[1]Evangelical Lutheran Church in Tanzania, Tanzania

[2]Consulting Palliative Care Physician, Tanzania

[3]College of Health Sciences, Walden University, United States

[4]Department of Community Health, University of Cape Town, South Africa

[5]Division of Family Medicine, University of Cape Town, South Africa

Correspondence to:
Kristopher Hartwig

Email:
kristopher.hartwig@gmail.com

Postal address:
PO Box 3033, Arusha, Tanzania

Background: In Tanzania, a country of 42 million, access to oral morphine is rare.

Aim: To demonstrate the effectiveness of palliative care teams in reducing patients' pain and in increasing other positive life qualities in the absence of morphine; and to document the psychological burden experienced by their clinical providers, trained in morphine delivery, as they observed their patients suffering and in extreme pain.

Setting: One hundred and forty-five cancer patients were included from 13 rural hospitals spread across Tanzania.

Method: A mixed method study beginning with a retrospective quantitative analysis of cancer patients who were administered the APCA African POS tool four times. Bivariate analyses of the scores at time one and four were compared across the domains. The qualitative arm included an analysis of interviews with six nurses, each with more than five years' palliative care experience and no access to strong opioids.

Results: Patients and their family caregivers identified statistically significant ($p < 0.001$) improvements in all of the domains. Thematic analysis of nurse interviews described the patient and family benefits from palliative care but also their great distress when 'bad cases' arose who would likely benefit only from oral morphine.

Conclusion: People living with chronic cancer-related pain who receive palliative care experience profound physical, spiritual and emotional benefits even without oral morphine. These results demonstrate the need for continued advocacy to increase the availability of oral morphine in these settings in addition to palliative care services.

Là où il n'y a pas de morphine: les défis et espoirs de la fourniture de soins palliatifs en Tanzanie.

Contexte: En Tanzanie, un pays de 42 millions d'habitants, l'accès à la morphine par voie orale est rare.

But: Montrer l'efficacité des équipes de soins palliatifs dans la réduction de la douleur des patients et l'amélioration d'autres qualités de vie en l'absence de morphine; et documenter la charge psychologique vécue par les prestataires cliniques formés à l'utilisation de la morphine lorsqu'ils observaient chez leurs patients une souffrance et une douleur extrême.

Cadre: Cent quarante-cinq patients atteints du cancer venant de 13 hôpitaux ruraux répartis dans toute la Tanzanie ont été étudiés.

Méthode: Une étude à méthode mixte commençant par une analyse quantitative rétrospective des patients atteints du cancer à qui l'outil Afrique POS APCA avait été administré à quatre reprises. Des analyses bivariées des résultats au moment un et quatre ont été comparées pour tous les domaines. Le volet qualitatif comprenait une analyse d'entretiens avec six infirmiers/-ières ayant chacun plus de cinq ans d'expérience en soins palliatifs et sans accès à des opioïdes puissants.

Résultats: Les patients et leurs soignants familiaux ont identifié des améliorations statistiquement positives ($p < 0{,}001$) dans tous les domaines. L'analyse thématique des entretiens auprès des infirmiers/-ières a décrit les bienfaits des soins palliatifs pour le patient et sa famille, mais aussi leur grande détresse lorsque des « mauvais cas » surviennent pour qui seule la morphine par voie orale pourrait probablement apporter un soulagement.

Conclusion: Les personnes vivant avec une douleur chronique liée au cancer qui reçoivent des soins palliatifs sont physiquement, spirituellement et émotionnellement profondément soulagées, même sans morphine par voie orale. Ces résultats montrent le besoin de plaidoyer permanent en faveur de l'accroissement de la disponibilité de morphine par voie orale dans ces contextes en plus des services de soins palliatifs.

Introduction

In rural Tanzania, as in much of the developing world, diagnosis of cancer occurs late in the clinical course of disease, with the result that palliative care is often the best and only option for care.[1,2] Yet, in low- and middle-income countries, few palliative care services are available as a result of a shortage of trained professionals, a lack of opioids for pain treatment and limited integration into standard medical care.[3,4]

The World Health Organization (WHO) defines palliative care as being a holistic approach for patients and their families who are living with life-threatening diseases, particularly emphasising the treatment of pain.[5] Oral morphine is widely accepted as being the first-line drug for treatment of moderate- to severe cancer pain,[6] but it is of limited availability in much of the world despite ongoing advocacy for recognition of pain relief as a basic human right.[7,8] The result is that many people living with cancer are left to die at home, or in hospital, with no effective way to relieve their physical suffering. Efforts to provide palliative care without access to oral morphine have lacked credibility. Anne Merriman, a pioneer in African palliative care, observed that 'palliative care without morphine is only supportive care… and lack of access to morphine is torture.'[9]

In 2010, the WHO estimated that over 14 000 of Tanzania's population of over 40 million will die of cancer each year.[10] Due to the vast distances involved, the immobility of the very sick and limited training of clinical staff, very few patients will have access to a palliative care service.

Tanzania's Pharmaceutical Board requires individual hospitals to apply for a licence to administer morphine; few hospitals currently have this licence and even when such a service is available the supply of oral morphine may be limited as a result of stringent reporting and access regulations. Overall consumption of morphine at the national level remains very low,[11] presumably because of low availability (in 2010, only four hospitals had licences to dispense morphine) and limited prescription, even when available.

Palliative care is relatively new to Tanzania. Initial efforts began in the early 1990s at the Ocean Road Cancer Institute in Dar es Salaam, but it was not until this century that other organisations began concerted efforts with regard to provision of palliative care. By 2002 there were three further sites: PASADA (Pastoral Activities and Services for people with AIDS, Dar es Salaam Archdiocese), Muheza Hospice (Tanga Region) and Selian Hospice (Arusha Region).[12] What is the experience of the few palliative care patients and their providers in settings with no morphine? There is little available in the literature to document the value and limitations of palliative care in these settings. Through a retrospective study of data gathered from 2009 to 2010, we aim to address this gap.

Background to the study

In 2004, the Evangelical Lutheran Church in Tanzania (ELCT) began a programme in palliative care, emulating the growth of Selian's service. Using a hospital-based approach, trained palliative care teams were developed through 18 rural ELCT hospitals, scattered widely throughout the country (Figure 1). In 2007, the ELCT programme, in collaboration with the Foundation for Hospices in Sub-Saharan Africa (FHSSA) and the African Palliative Care Association (APCA), received funding from the US government's President's Emergency Program for AIDS Relief (PEPFAR) in order to initiate the CHAT program (Continuum of care for people living with HIV/AIDS in Tanzania)[13,14,15,16] in 13 of the ELCT hospitals, which varied in size from 60 to 400 beds and served catchment areas of between 100 000 and 400 000 people.

CHAT ran from 2007 to 2010 and comprised a supervising palliative care team and mobile hospital-based teams with vehicle transport that provided home-based care (HBC) and monitored pain and the quality of care systematically with a validated assessment tool, the APCA African Palliative Outcome Scale (POS). CHAT funders allowed all patients with terminal illness, including cancer, admission to the programme.

The palliative care teams had been trained to treat moderate to severe pain using the WHO Analgesic Ladder[17] within the limits of the drugs they had at their disposal. At the time of the study oral morphine was not accessible in most of rural Tanzania, including the 13 sites that were part of CHAT. As a result, the practice of pain management faced significant challenges requiring each palliative care team clinician and nurse to become proficient in the systematic use of the available analgesics, of which tramadol was the most potent.

Studies have very clearly shown the benefit of HBC programmes for people living with HIV,[18] but there is little information about such care for cancer patients where oral morphine is lacking. While it might be intuitive that the general well-being of any patient would be enhanced by attention from a palliative care team, is the team's efficacy compromised by the absence of morphine? Although tramadol has been studied in the treatment of cancer pain, it has been in the context of more potent options.[19,20,21,22] The teams administered tramadol to a maximum dose of 400 mg/d to all patients with moderate to severe pain and combined it according to patient response and tolerance with ibuprofen, paracetamol and/or amitriptyline.

The aim of this paper is twofold. First is to document, using the POS indicators, the value of palliative care for patients living with cancer but without access to morphine. Second is to document the psychological burden experienced by their clinical providers, who are trained in morphine delivery but have no access to the drug, as they observe their patients suffer in pain.

Research methods and design

The study was conducted from January 2009 to December 2010, employing a combination of quantitative and qualitative

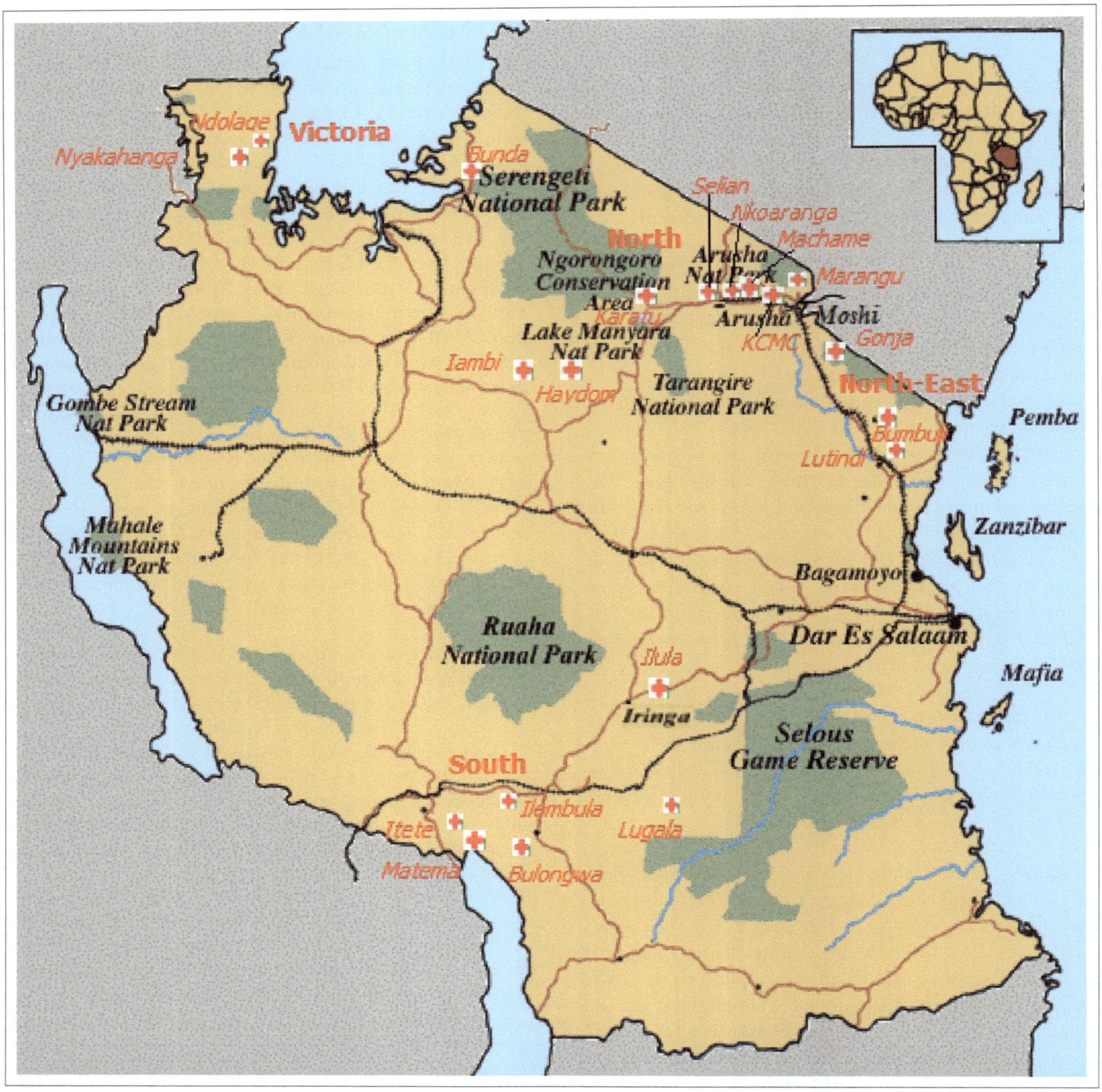

Note: Each cross represents an Evangelical Lutheran Church in Tanzania hospital. Four additional hospitals have opened or are in the process of opening, three located in the northeast and one in the far northwest.

FIGURE 1: Location of Evangelical Lutheran Church in Tanzania hospitals on map of Tanzania.

methods. The quantitative component comprised a retrospective cohort analysis of 145 cancer patients across the 13 hospital sites that did not have access to oral morphine. The qualitative arm involved face-to-face interviews with nurses from the hospital sites.

Retrospective cohort analysis

The POS, designed to be administered four times over two to four weeks, has been validated in several of the African languages for people over the age of 18 years and for a variety of disease conditions.[23,24] For our study a Swahili version of the POS – Swahili is the official language of Tanzania – was used by the attending nurse with translation into the local dialect or language where necessary. The POS contains seven questions for the patient and three questions for family caregivers. Patients identify physical symptoms, including pain and psychological status, on a scale of zero to five. (See Table 1 for the English version of the APCA African POS).

Inclusion criteria for the study were people over 18 years of age living with cancer for whom three or four POS assessments had been performed between January 2009 and December 2010. The data were taken from the reports which were submitted monthly to the central ELCT office as part of the routine data collected by the CHAT project. Each hospital assigned patient numbers and all POS files used

TABLE 1: African Palliative Care Association Palliative Outcome Scale (APCA POS).

Questions	Rating
Ask the patient	
Q1. Please rate your pain (from) = no pain to 5 = worst/overwhelming pain) during the last 3 days	0 (no pain) – 5 (worst/overwhelming pain)
Q2. Have any other symptoms (e.g. nausea, coughing or constipation) been affecting how you feel in the last 3 days?	0 (not at all) – 5 (overwhelmingly)
Q3. Have you been feeling worried about your illness in the past 3 days?	0 (not at all) – 5 (overwhelming worry)
Q4. Over the past 3 days, have you been able to share how you are feeling with your family or friends?	0 (not at all) – 5 (yes, I've talked freely)
Q5. Over the past 3 days, have you felt that life was worthwhile?	0 (no, not at all) – 5 (yes, all the time)
Q6. Over the past 3 days, have you felt at peace?	0 (no, not at all) – 5 (yes, all the time)
Q7. Have you had enough help and advice for your family to plan for the future?	0 (not at all) – 5 (as much as wanted)
Ask the family carer	
Q8. How much information have you and your family been given?	0 (none) – 5 (as much as wanted) N/A
Q9. How confident does the family feel caring for ________________?	0 (not at all) – 5 (very confident) N/A
Q10. Has the family been feeling worried about the Client over the last 3 days?	0 (not at all) – 5 (severe worry) N/A

this numbering system to protect patient confidentiality. All records were kept in a locked file with patient identifiers in a separate file.

The APCA POS data were entered into Microsoft Excel and analysed using Stata version 11 (StataCorp. 2009. Stata Statistical Software Release 11. College Station, TX: StataCorp LP). Prior to data analysis, low-scoring positive scores, such as a '2' for minimal worry were reversed numerically so that all negative scores were skewed toward the higher numbers and could be compared with ease. To assess statistical significance over time, scores from the first and last visits were compared for each question. The Shapiro-Wilk test indicated that the key outcome variables, pain and other domains as measured by the POS were not distributed normally, thus the non-parametric Wilcoxon-signed rank test was applied. The statistical level of significance was set at $p < 0.05$.

Qualitative analysis

In order to assess clinical providers' perspectives on quality of pain management for cancer patients in settings without morphine, the first author conducted face-to-face interviews with six nurses from six of the CHAT hospitals. We selected nurses using criterion sampling,[25] specifically, years of experience and palliative care training. Three of the nurses held diplomas in palliative care whilst the other three each had at least seven years of experience working in palliative care. All six nurses had received training from APCA, Nairobi Hospice or Hospice Uganda, each being a well-established programme in East Africa.

We used a semi-structured interview guide to conduct each interview and tape-recorded all sessions. The core questions asked the nurse to (1) describe in detail the case of a patient with cancer who, whilst under their team's care, had poor pain control; (2) describe the case of a patient with cancer with very good pain control; and (3) reflect on the value of palliative care in the setting of no access to oral morphine for chronic pain control.

The first author conducted all the interviews; five in Swahili and one in English. The same author transcribed all of the interviews and translated the Swahili interviews into English prior to data analysis. Two authors (K.H. and M.D.) conducted a thematic analysis of the interview transcripts with particular attention to the nurses' perspectives on their patients' pain control and quality of life and their own experience in coping as professionals with no access to morphine. The two analysts used an iterative process of independently identifying themes and quotes within the interviews and then comparing results. The final set of themes emerged after discussion and further iterative analysis of the transcripts.

Ethical considerations

The University of Cape Town (UCT) and the National Institute of Medical Research (NIMR) of Tanzania gave ethical approval for the study (UCT: HREC REF 319/210, IRB Number IRB00001938; NIMR: NIMR/HQ/R.8a/Vol. 1X/1025). Each nurse provided written voluntary consent to be interviewed.

Results

Of the 153 satisfactorily-completed POS records, eight patients had died before the third visit, leaving 145 records for inclusion in the study. Women made up 87 (60%) of the patients and had an average age of 57 compared with men at 56. Given the limited diagnostic procedures and treatments available in rural areas precise diagnoses, including co-morbidities, are rarely available so we did not attempt to collect such data.

The results for each domain of the POS showed a statistically-significant change from first to last visit ($p < 0.001$). The worst problem at each visit was pain, with the average first visit pain score being 3.8 (slightly higher for men), which compared with the next worst score of 3.4 for patient anxiety. By the last visit the average pain score for both men and women was 2.3, similar to that of several other symptoms (Table 2). Table 3 illustrates improvement over time in every domain for both patients and family members.

Multiple themes and subthemes arose from the nurse interviews, including the challenge of pain management without access to morphine; the psychological burden on the caregivers; advocacy for oral morphine; the value of holistic care for patients and family; and improved pain management for most patients. The nurses all provided examples of observing patients' pain being eased and emotional and spiritual well-being improving, even if pain was not completely relieved over time. In the interests of complete confidentiality, no demographic data were recorded for the nurses, who were given study numbers for reference purposes.

TABLE 2: Gender comparisons.

Gender	Number	Average Age	Visit 1 Average Pain	Visit 4 Average Pain	*p*-value
Female	87 (60%)	57	3.71	2.31	< 0.001
Male	58 (40%)	56	4.02	2.31	< 0.001
Total	145	–	–	–	–
Average	–	57	3.83	2.31	< 0.001

TABLE 3: Summary statistics of Palliative Outcome Scale scores at each visit (1 to 4).

Questions	Visit	*N*	Mean	SD	Median	Min	Max	*p*-value
Q1. Please rate your pain (from 0 = no pain to 5 = worst/ overwhelming pain) during the last 3 days	1	145	3.8	1.0	4	1	5	< 0.001
	2	145	3.1	1.0	3	1	5	
	3	145	2.7	1.0	3	0	5	
	4	145	2.3	1.2	2	0	5	
Q2. Have any other symptoms (e.g. nausea, coughing or constipation) been affecting how you feel in the last 3 days?	1	145	2.6	1.5	3	0	5	< 0.001
	2	145	2.0	1.4	2	0	5	
	3	145	1.7	1.3	2	0	5	
	4	144	1.5	1.3	2	0	5	
Q3. Have you been feeling worried about your illness in the past 3 days?	1	145	3.4	1.6	4	0	5	< 0.001
	2	144	2.7	1.4	3	0	5	
	3	144	2.3	1.3	2	0	5	
	4	143	2.1	1.4	2	0	5	
Q4. Over the past 3 days, have you been able to share how you are feeling with your family or friends?	1	145	3.5	1.7	4	0	5	< 0.001
	2	144	3.8	1.3	4	0	5	
	3	145	4.1	1.1	4	1	5	
	4	145	4.2	1.1	5	1	5	
Q5. Over the past 3 days have you felt that life was worthwhile?	1	145	2.0	1.7	1	0	5	< 0.001
	2	145	2.5	1.6	2	0	5	
	3	145	2.9	1.5	3	0	5	
	4	145	3.0	1.6	3	0	5	
Q6. Over the past 3 days, have you felt at peace?	1	145	1.8	1.5	2	0	5	< 0.001
	2	145	2.4	1.5	2	0	5	
	3	145	2.7	1.5	3	0	5	
	4	145	2.8	1.5	3	0	5	
Q7. Have you had enough help and advice for your family to plan for the future?	1	144	2.9	1.9	3	0	5	< 0.001
	2	144	3.7	1.3	4	0	5	
	3	142	4.0	1.2	4	0	5	
	4	143	4.1	1.2	5	0	5	
Q8. How much information have you and your family been given?	1	142	3.3	1.6	3	0	5	< 0.001
	2	141	4.0	1.1	4	1	5	
	3	142	4.4	0.8	5	1	5	
	4	143	4.6	0.7	5	2	5	
Q9. How confident does the family feel caring for ____?	1	141	4.1	1.2	5	0	5	< 0.001
	2	140	4.3	1.0	5	1	5	
	3	141	4.5	0.9	5	1	5	
	4	142	4.5	0.9	5	1	5	
Q10. Has the family been feeling worried about the patient over the last 3 days?	1	142	3.1	1.6	3	0	5	< 0.001
	2	141	2.6	1.5	3	0	5	
	3	141	2.2	1.4	2	0	5	
	4	143	2.1	1.6	2	0	5	

At a funeral for a patient attended by the palliative care team, families shared their appreciation:

> 'They felt that the medications for pain made a real difference. They did not see that the pain was as bad as when she had been hospitalised, even when her condition was worsening.' (Nurse 2)

Nurse 1 added:

> 'Many are so happy to be visited and listened to, because we really try hard to address all of their problems, and comfort them even when they are in pain.'

Although pain reduction is a primary service, the emotional and psychological support provided to patients and their families can be seen in these quotes as well as the POS scores.

The value of the holistic nature of a palliative care approach in a context of limited resources was best summarised by this quote:

> 'With our African setup you cannot simply say that now I managed the physical pain and everything is OK. There are other aspects of pain like the social pain, the spiritual pain and so on. They contribute a lot to pain and so if you are able to manage these other pains like the social pain and the spiritual pain and psychosocial pain then you will find that to some extent a lot of these pains are associated with the physical. For example, there might be family conflicts, or poverty, the child is not going to school, the breadwinner is unable to work; so you find some of these elements are adding pain into the physical pain.' (Nurse 3)

All six nurses however, felt that their pain management would be improved by having access to oral morphine. Four of the six nurses trained to use morphine for severe, chronic pain expressed concern over not having access to potent pain relievers. Each nurse could easily tell the story of one or more patients who had suffered considerable unrelieved pain before death. Table 4 provides quotes from the nurses which exemplify some of these challenges of patient care and the psychological burden on the nurses.

The nurses' collective frustration with the limited access to oral morphine also proved to be an incentive for advocacy. Each of them spoke of lobbying within their own hospital with doctors and pharmacists. In addition, they spoke of the need to reduce government bureaucracy so that more hospitals could provide morphine. Nurse 5 spoke passionately:

> 'My thoughts and advice is that the relevant ministries and government leaders should make the process of getting pain medications to be fair and easy. After all it is a basic human right for patients to get that service.' (Nurse 5)

Discussion

Our results indicate that even in the absence of morphine there is a benefit in providing palliative care to cancer patients. Overall pain scores improved from an average of 3.8 out of 5 (moderately severe pain) to 2.3 out of 5 (moderate pain) and non-pain symptoms and other indicators – psychological, spiritual and family issues – improved significantly as well. Both women and men experienced similar decreases in pain and positive changes in the other domains over the period of the four visits. However, the average last visit POS score still indicates a moderate degree of pain and is higher than that reported by facilities using morphine.[26,27] For example, in South Africa average APCA African POS scores went from 4 to 1 over six visits with morphine compared with our results of 4 to 2 with no morphine.[27] This suggests the value of holistic palliative care to patients without access to morphine. However, without a breakdown by disease process it is difficult to assess how comparable the two populations are. The nurses, despite their frustration at not having access to oral morphine, nonetheless affirm the value of palliative care in the absence of morphine. In this rural Tanzanian setting palliative care is valuable and offers a significant degree of pain control in the absence of oral morphine, but not to the degree that could be achieved if morphine was available. Given that much of the world currently lacks access to a strong opioid for treating cancer pain,[28] this finding has significance. Recent availability of the APCA African POS as a validated tool makes such assessment feasible. There are few examples of results in the peer-reviewed literature using the APCA African POS.[26,27] This study contributes to a nascent body of literature on this tool in different African settings.

From the nurse interviews there is, as a result of their training, a clear belief that pain control would be even better with oral morphine. All recalled difficult pain cases which might have been better managed had they only been able to access morphine. There is a burden to the team in having knowledge of optimal treatment without being able to deliver it. The psychological hardship for palliative and other community teams in resource-constrained environments is an area that has been under-researched.

There are a number of limitations to this study. We did not have access to a comparison hospital site with access to morphine and using POS – such direct comparison would have been very useful. Having only one investigator doing interviews and translations raises the possibility of bias and error. For the language of the POS, whilst Swahili is the dominant language in Tanzania there are more than 120 distinct languages in the country, some of which are in use amongst the 13 rural sites of this study. Translations from Swahili into the local language were occasionally done on the spot by the health professional administering the POS, or through a family interpreter.

Nonetheless, our results are in line with data from other palliative care providers in Africa. Loy et al.'s work[29] shows the positive impact of palliative care for HIV clients and

TABLE 4: Nurse interview quotes.

Theme	Quote
Caregiver stress	'It is a challenge [*not having morphine*], actually a very big one. You get there and you have nothing with which to help the pain. Sometimes the person needs help, and when you fail to deliver that help, it is as if you have done nothing. They may even wonder why you bothered to visit.' (Nurse 5)
	'As a PC [*palliative care*] professional you can only be satisfied when you feel you are doing the right thing, although you are not curing you are doing the right thing. But if you are not doing the right thing [*giving oral morphine*] you feel as if you are mismanaging the patient.' (Nurse 3)
Unrelieved pain	'For this case, it was very difficult to control her pain using tramadol and ibuprofen. There was not much improvement. It became necessary for me to go to KCMC [*regional hospital*] where we were able to get oral morphine. She was so happy to get that medication! She continued with it ... but near the end she was unable to get it again, as we were unable to refill the medication. So we used tramadol and others as we had done before. It did not give her relief like when she had the morphine. The challenge was, if only in our institutions morphine would be available, in order that for patients like her with strong pain they might get some relief...Truly, I felt very badly; terrible. I kept thinking that there was medicine just there at KCMC. But the restrictions of the pharmacy, that they cannot just give it to anybody, it really hurt me. If only this woman had lived somewhere like Arusha, being near a place like Selian, where oral morphine is available without severe restriction.' (Nurse 6)
	'... a patient who was 70 years old or so, who had been found to have cancer of the prostate ... We worked with him with the pain. We started Diclopar [*diclofenac plus paracetamol*] four times daily and tramadol 50 mg four times daily. It did not help much ... Still the pain continued ... We had to increase pain medications, the tramadol to 100 mg four times daily. But 3 days later we found the pain to still be so much. More medications were added... amitriptyline and diazepam at night. From then pain reduced slightly but not a great deal. He continued until he was called by God... These patients are here. They do not respond satisfactorily to our pain medications and are not satisfied with our care.' (Nurse 5)
	37 y.o. female with advanced ovarian cancer taking tramadol orally. 'She reported to us with very advanced disease and very advanced pain; it was too late to really help her ... But all along her pain was not responding ... When she recognised what was going on, she didn't want to see us ... We had to gradually convince them that our services would help; it took time. Then when we did the pain did not improve. It began as overwhelming and was helped only slightly by our medications. Eventually she was unable to swallow and she died... That last time when she could not swallow tramadol, perhaps morphine in the mouth might have been absorbed and she could have had the chance of relief.' (Nurse 4)

the nurse interviews in this study point out that clients have a great appreciation and sense of improvement when receiving palliative care. In South Africa, with access to oral morphine and where the POS is used regularly, average pain scores improved from 4 to 1 over time.[27] Detailed data comparison from South Africa and APCA would be an area for further study, with the hypothesis that pain control is improved significantly with the availability of oral morphine.

Pursuit of oral morphine is an ongoing challenge for many palliative care advocates around the world. The mention of advocacy by several of the nurses suggests that there appears to be little danger of palliative care teams abandoning their pursuit of oral morphine access. This study, and indeed the CHAT project with its associated emphasis on quality measurement, is an important advocacy tool for accessing oral morphine and for palliative care in general. The availability of client-centred data is valuable in care provision, particularly in areas such as rural Tanzania where information is limited. In this regard the POS is an invaluable tool.[30,31,32]

The information in this and similar studies can be used to lobby government decisions regarding health policy. As Mmbando described in the APCA newsletter of April 2011,[33] and as was written up in the FHSSA newsletter,[34] it is as a result of this very emphasis on quality and advocacy that 12 out of 13 CHAT sites (including all sites from which the nurse interviewees came) had, as of February 2011, been granted approval for oral morphine usage by the Tanzania Food and Drug Authority. A year later (January 2012), continued advocacy and training brought morphine access to a total of 19 ELCT facilities, including all of the CHAT sites. With other programmes such as Muheza in Tanga Region and Tearfund in the Lake Zone[35] having gained access to oral morphine, the prospects for pain management in rural Tanzania are much improved. By the end of 2012, there were 50 facilities – a mix of public and private – which had gained approval for oral morphine use through the Tanzania Food and Drug Authority (Paul Mmbando, personal communication, August 16, 2013). Although no funding is available at this time, future research in these same hospitals with similar patient populations to this study would be desirable in order to observe if there are differences in POS results now that morphine is more widely available.

Conclusion

This study shows that palliative care without morphine is beneficial to cancer patients, but comparison with other studies suggests that pain control would be even better with access to oral morphine. A degree of pain relief for most cancer patients can be accomplished without strong opioids in the context of palliative care. A trained palliative care team, equipped with education and medications, can be a powerful advocate for people at the end of life, whether the disease be cancer, HIV, or any other. Effectiveness of the care, whether for pain or other domains of palliative care, can be measured and shown to be of value for clients and their families, but there is a psychological burden for nurses trained in palliative care and the use of morphine when they are asked to deliver palliative care without access to the world's most available strong analgesic.

Whilst palliative care team leaders can become excellent advocates for accessing oral morphine, more research is warranted in the area of supporting such teams that often operate without the full range of tools necessary to meet all of their patients' needs.

Acknowledgements

Dr Geoffrey Sigalla of ELCT, Shelley Smith of FHSSA and Richard Kaye and Tony Powell of APCA all provided key teamwork and input in the development of the infrastructure and monitoring that allowed this care and research to be possible. The USAID office in Dar es Salaam was critical in facilitating the significant PEPFAR funds and guidance necessary in order to provide continuous staffing and outreach over 3 years.

Competing interests

The authors declare that they have no financial or personal relationship(s) which may have inappropriately influenced them in writing this article.

Authors' contributions

K.H. (Evangelical Lutheran Church, Tanzania) was lead author and researcher. P.M. (Evangelical Lutheran Church, Tanzania) provided conceptual contributions, as did E.V. (University of Cape Town). A.S. (University of Cape Town) provided analysis for the quantitative data, K.H. (Walden University) assisted with qualitative analysis and concepts and M.D. (Consulting Palliative Care Physician, Tanzania) provided conceptual, analytical and editorial assistance.

References

1. Pampallona S, Bollini P. Palliative care in developing countries: Why research is needed. J Pain Palliat Care Pharmacother. 2004;17(3–4):171–182.
2. Krakauer EL. Just palliative care: responding responsibly to the suffering of the poor. J Pain Symptom Manage. 2008;36(5):505–512. http://dx.doi.org/10.1016/j.jpainsymman.2007.11.015, PMid:18971074
3. Stjernswärd J. Instituting palliative care in developing countries – an urgently needed and achievable goal. J Pain Palliat Care Pharmacother. 2003;17(3–4):xxix–xxxvi. PMid:15022945
4. Logie D. Africans die in pain because of fears of opiate addiction. BMJ. 2007;335(7622):685. http://dx.doi.org/10.1136/bmj.39353.715359.DB, PMid:17916825, PMCid:PMC2001053
5. World Health Organization. Definition of palliative care. [page on internet] nd [cited 2010 Jun. 04]. Available from: http://www.who.int/cancer/palliative/definition/en/
6. World Health Organization. WHO Model List of Essential Medicines. 17th list (March 2011). [document on internet] c2011 [cited 2012 Nov. 05]. Available from: http://whqlibdoc.who.int/hq/2011/a95053_eng.pdf
7. Human Rights Watch. 'Please, do not make us suffer any more...'. [page on internet] c2009 [cited 2010 Oct. 02]. Available from: http://www.hrw.org/en/reports/2009/03/02/please-do-not-make-us-suffer-any-more
8. Gwyther L, Brennan F, Harding R. Advancing palliative care as a human right. J Pain Symptom Manage. 2009;38(5):767–774. http://dx.doi.org/10.1016/j.jpainsymman.2009.03.003, PMid:19783399
9. Smith R. A way to provide palliative care globally. [blog on online journal]. c2012 [cited 2012 Sep. 29]. Available from: http://blogs.bmj.com/bmj/2012/06/25/richard-smith-a-way-to-provide-palliative-care-globally/
10. World Health Organization. Noncommunicable diseases: United Republic of Tanzania. [document on internet]. c2011 [cited 2013 Sep. 16]. Available from: http://www.who.int/nmh/countries/tza_en.pdf

11. Pain and Policy Studies Group. United Republic of Tanzania: Consumption data at-a-glance. [page on internet]. c2012 [cited 2012 Jan. 31]. Available from: http://www.painpolicy.wisc.edu/country/profile/united-republic-tanzania

12. International Observatory on End of Life Care. Country reports in alphabetical order. [page on internet]. nd [cited 2010 Jun. 04]. Available from: http://www.eolc-observatory.net/global_analysis/country_by_country.php

13. Hartwig K. The development of hospice care in Arusha, Tanzania: Lessons from the neighbouring states of Kenya and Uganda J Palliat Care. 2001;17(2):121–125.

14. Mmbando P, Hartwig KA, Hofgren B, et al. Care for the most vulnerable children in Tanzania: A faith-based model of care and support for children affected by HIV. J Health Care Poor Underserved. 2009;20(4 Suppl):13–21. http://dx.doi.org/10.1353/hpu.0.0195, PMid:20168028

15. Hartwig KN, Hartwig KA, DiSorbo P, et al. Scaling up a community-based palliative care program among faith-based hospitals in Tanzania. J Palliat Care, 2010;26(3):194–201. PMid:21047042

16. Nanney E, Smith S, Hartwig K, et al. Scaling up palliative care services in rural Tanzania. J Pain Symptom Manage. 2010;40(1):15–18. http://dx.doi.org/10.1016/j.jpainsymman.2010.04.002, PMid:20619207

17. World Health Organization. Cancer Pain Relief. Geneva, Switzerland: World Health Organization; 1986.

18. Mermin J, Were W, Ekwaru JP, et al. Mortality in HIV-infected Ugandan adults receiving antiretroviral treatment and survival of their HIV-uninfected children: A prospective cohort study. Lancet. 2008;371(9614):752–759. http://dx.doi.org/10.1016/S0140-6736(08)60345-1

19. Leppert W, Luczak J. The role of tramadol in cancer pain treatment – a review. Support Care Cancer. 2005;13(1):5–17. http://dx.doi.org/10.1007/s00520-004-0720-4, PMid:15668743

20. Grond S, Sablotzki A. Clinical pharmacology of tramadol. Clin Pharmacokinet. 2004;43(13):879–923. http://dx.doi.org/10.2165/00003088-200443130-00004

21. Grond S, Radbruch L, Meuser T, et al. High-dose tramadol in comparison to low-dose morphine for cancer pain relief. J Pain Symptom Manage. 1999;18(3):174–179. http://dx.doi.org/10.1016/S0885-3924(99)00060-3

22. Wilder-Smith CH, Schimke J, Osterwalder B, et al. Oral tramadol, a mu-opioid agonist and monoamine reuptake-blocker, and morphine for strong cancer-related pain. Ann Oncol. 1994;5(2):141–146. PMid:8186157

23. Powell RA, Downing J, Harding R, et al. Development of the APCA African Palliative Outcome Scale. J Pain Symptom Manage. 2007;33(2):229–232. http://dx.doi.org/10.1016/j.jpainsymman.2006.10.008, PMid:17280929

24. Harding R, Selman L, Agupio G, et al. Validation of a core outcome measure for palliative care in Africa: the APCA African Palliative Outcome Scale. Health Qual Life Out. 2010;8:10. http://dx.doi.org/10.1186/1477-7525-8-10, PMid:20100332, PMCid:PMC2825183

25. Patton, M.Q. Qualitative Research & Evaluation Methods. 3rd ed. Thousand Oaks: Sage Publications; 2002.

26. Tapsfield JB, Bates MJ. Hospital based palliative care in sub-Saharan Africa; A six month review from Malawi. BMC Palliat Care. 2011;10:12. http://dx.doi.org/10.1186/1472-684X-10-12, PMid:21740584, PMCid:PMC3146929

27. African Palliative Care Association. Example of the use of the APCA African POS at the Hospice and Palliative Care Association of South Africa. [page on internet]. nd [cited 2013 Sep 13]. Available from: http://www.africanpalliativecare.org/index.php?option=com_content&view=article&id=51%3Aexample-of-the-use-of-the-apca-african-pos-at-thehospice-and-palliative-care-association-of-south-africa&catid=8%3Afrank&Itemid=50

28. The Board of Regents of the University of Wisconsin System. Opioid consumption motion chart. [chart on internet]. nd [cited 2011 May 5]. Available from: http://ppsg-production.heroku.com/chart

29. Loy G, Harding R, Collins K, et al. Multidimensional outcomes for HIV outpatients receiving integrated palliative care: a prospective longitudinal natural experiment. Presented at AIDSImpact Santa Fe 2011. [page on internet]. c2011 [cited 2012 Nov. 12]. Available from: www.aidsimpact.com/2011/Academics/Programme/abstract/?id=333

30. Harding R, Gwyther L, Mwangi-Powell F, et al. How can we improve palliative care patient outcomes in low- and middle-income countries? Successful outcomes research in sub-Saharan Africa. J Pain Symptom Manage. 2010;40(1):23–26. http://dx.doi.org/10.1016/j.jpainsymman.2010.04.007, PMid:20619209

31. Harding R, Selman L, Agupio G, et al. The prevalence and burden of symptoms amongst cancer patients attending palliative care in two African countries. Eur J Cancer. 2011;47(1):51–56. http://dx.doi.org/10.1016/j.ejca.2010.08.003, PMid:20822896

32. Dix O. Impact of the APCA African Palliative Outcome Scale (POS) on care and practice. [document on internet]. c2012 [cited 2013 Aug. 01]. Available from: http://www.csi.kcl.ac.uk/files/Impact_of_APCA_POS.pdf

33. African Palliative Care Association UK. Newsletter. [document on internet]. [c2011 [cited 2011 May 15]. Available from: http://www.apca.org.uk/newsletter.php?issue=7#32 with APCA membership

34. Foundation for Hospices in Sub-Saharan Africa. Newsletter. [document on internet]. [c2011 [cited 2012 Mar. 17]. Available from: http://www.fhssa.org/files/public/Quarterly/Focus_on_Comp_Qtr2_2011.pdf

35. Palliative Care Works. [Example of other efforts outside of Evangelical Lutheran Church in Tanzania successfully promoting palliative care in Tanzania]. [page on internet]. nd [cited 2012 Mar. 17]. Available from: http://www.palliativecareworks.org/news.html

9

Sociodemographic characteristics of persons committing suicide in Durban, South Africa: 2006–2007

Authors:
Soornarain S. Naidoo[1]
Lourens Schlebusch[2]

Affiliations:
[1]Department of Family Medicine, University of KwaZulu-Natal, South Africa

[2]Department of Behavioural Medicine, University of KwaZulu-Natal, South Africa

Correspondence to:
Soornarain Naidoo

Email:
naidoos79@ukzn.ac.za

Postal address:
Department of Family Medicine, University of KwaZulu-Natal, Private Bag X7, Congella, Durban, 4013

Background: Suicidal behaviour is a leading contributor to the burden of disease worldwide and varies widely between countries. South African figures are amongst the highest in the world, with recent trends indicating a disturbing rise, especially amongst the younger age groups, across all races.

Aim: This study analysed sociodemographic characteristics and trends relating to suicides committed in Durban, South Africa during the period of 2006–2007.

Method: A retrospective analysis of suicidal deaths (during 2006–2007), extracted from autopsy registers at all three government-run mortuaries in Durban, was conducted.

Results: The total number of suicides in Durban increased by 6.68% from 2006 to 2007. Suicide accounted for an average of 8.8% of all non-natural deaths per year of the study. The overall suicide rates of 14.53 (2006) and 15.53 (2007) per 100 000 population are comparable with national and global figures. The majority of suicides occurred in single unemployed persons, men and younger age groups. The largest number of suicides per year was recorded in black people, followed by Indian, white and mixed-race people. Hanging was the preferred method in the majority of victims, followed by self-poisoning, shooting and jumping.

Conclusions: The findings indicate a disturbingly high suicide rate amongst the various population and age groups in Durban. The dominant methods used may be influenced by ease of access. The reported trends may worsen unless there is a swift and decisive public health response and cohesive community-based programmes which include a supportive multidisciplinary network.

Caractéristiques sociodémographiques des personnes qui se sont suicidées à Durban, en Afrique du Sud: 2006–2007

Présentation: Le comportement suicidaire est l'un des principaux facteurs contribuant à la charge mondiale de morbidité et varie dans une large mesure d'un pays à l'autre. L'Afrique du Sud enregistre l'un des taux de suicide les plus élevés du monde, les tendances récentes révélant une hausse dérangeante, notamment chez les plus jeunes, toutes races confondues.

Objectif: Cette étude a consisté en l'analyse des caractéristiques sociodémographiques et des tendances associées aux suicides enregistrés à Durban, en Afrique du Sud, au cours de la période 2006-2007.

Méthode: Une analyse rétrospective des décès par suicide (en 2006-2007), recensés par le biais des rapports d'autopsie dans les trois morgues publiques de Durban, a été réalisée.

Résultats: Le nombre total de suicides à Durban a augmenté de 6.68 % entre 2006 et 2007. Le suicide était en moyenne la cause de 8.8 % des décès de causes non naturelle au cours de l'année concernée par l'étude. Les taux de suicide généraux de 14.53 (2006) et 15.53 (2007) pour 100 000 personnes sont comparables avec les chiffres enregistrés dans le pays et dans le monde. Les personnes qui s'étaient suicidées étaient célibataires et sans emploi, de sexe masculin et appartenaient à la tranche d'âge des plus jeunes. Le plus grand nombre de suicides par an a été enregistré chez des individus d'origine africaine, suivi par des individus d'origine indienne, européenne et métisse. La mort par pendaison était la méthode privilégiée par la majorité des victimes, suivie par l'ingestion de substances toxiques, les armes à feu et les sauts.

Conclusions: Les conclusions révèlent un taux de suicide particulièrement élevé chez les jeunes des différents groupes de population à Durban. Les principales méthodes utilisées pourraient être justifiées par leur facilité d'accès. Les tendances révélées par ce rapport pourraient s'aggraver en l'absence d'intervention de santé publique rapide et décisive et de programme communautaire cohésif accompagné d'un réseau d'entraide pluridisciplinaire.

Introduction

Suicidal behaviour (comprising suicidal ideation, planning, attempts and completed or fatal episodes) has increased globally over the last decade and has been identified as being one of the major contributors to the high disease and healthcare burden in many low- to middle-income countries.[1] According to the World Health Organization (WHO), approximately 1.53 million people will die annually from suicide by 2020, compared with the 0.88 million suicides that occurred in 2002.[2] Suicide rates are higher amongst men (with male to female ratios up to 3:1) throughout the world except in China, where female rates are consistently higher than those for men, particularly in rural areas.[3,4] Globally, the majority of suicides occur in people aged 35–44 years in both sexes and the ratio of suicide attempts to suicide varies from 20–40:1.[2]

In South Africa, it was reported in 2008 that approximately 6500 suicides and 130 000 suicide attempts occurred annually.[5] It is widely believed that these figures have since increased.[1] Non-fatal suicidal behaviour in South Africa outnumbers suicides, with the ratio varying between 8:1 and 20:1, depending on the geographical area and the racial group of the study sample.[6] The average age for suicide nationally is 34 years and the highest number of suicides occur in the 15–19 year age group, followed by the 10–14 year group.[7] Suicide rates have been increasing steadily in all population groups in the country over the last decade, although the prevalence varies considerably across age and race groups. Suicide has been labelled as the third major cause of death in Indian, black and mixed-race people after homicide and natural deaths and it is the second major cause of deaths in white people.[8,9,10]

A wide range of methods is used by persons committing suicide.[1] These depend on a number of factors such as the mental state of the suicidal person; intention to die (high or low); intensity of the trigger factor or stressor and the ensuing crisis; threshold or tolerance to trigger factors; personal or popular choices in terms of knowledge of prior effectiveness of the method; access to the agent or instrument to be used; and the environment where the act is planned to take place. At a global level, shooting, hanging and self-poisoning have remained the leading agents of choice.[4,6,11,12] Figures released for South Africa in the last decade have shown that hanging and shooting were the most preferred methods, followed by other methods such as self-poisoning with agents such as pesticides and poisons, drug overdoses, self-gassing and self-immolation.[13,14,15,16,17] An analysis of the autopsy register in the Eastern Cape Province in South Africa (previously called Transkei) for the period 1993–2003 showed an increasing trend of hangings from 5.2 per 100 000 in 1993 to 16.2 per 100 000 in 2003, particularly in the younger (20–29 year) age group.[13] This is consistent with other studies on choice of method in South Africa.[6]

Homicide-suicide and extended suicide, especially involving adult men, intimate partners, and/or family members, have increased notably in South Africa, attracting much publicity, mainly because of their associated physical trauma and psychosocial impact. Several case study reports have been published highlighting characteristics of the perpetrator (usually male and often employed in the security or police services, or unemployed); the victim (usually female); the location of the event (usually the home); and the method generally used (firearms).[6,18,19,20]

Durban is the third-largest city in South Africa and the largest in KwaZulu-Natal Province. It accounts for 1.4% of the geographical area of the KwaZulu-Natal Province but, according to the 2001 national population census, was home to 3.2 million (34%) of the province's population.[21] Sixty percent of the province's economic activity takes place in this port city, with 68% of its inhabitants being of a working age (15–65 years) and 27.9% being unemployed, 88.6% of whom are black South Africans. A demographic analysis of the city in 2001 showed that 68.3% of the residents were black, 2.9% mixed-race, 19.9% Indian and 8.9% white, with 51.94% being women and 48.06% men. The reported age profile of the city's inhabitants in 2001 is reflected in Table 1.[21]

This study was part of a larger study carried out by the lead researcher during the period 2007–2011,[1] and was intended to analyse the existing suicide trends amongst the different population groups in Durban, South Africa, as well as sociodemographic characteristics of persons who committed suicide in Durban during the period 2006–2007.

Research method and design

Medico-legal autopsies of all unnatural deaths occurring in the Durban municipality are routinely carried out in three state mortuaries (Phoenix, Gale Street and Pinetown). Final cause of death is entered into the autopsy record following the routine inquest procedure. This process, including finalisation of the inquest docket prepared for each case and authentication of the exact cause of death, can sometimes take as long as two years.

This epidemiological study was conducted in 2010–2011. A retrospective analysis of the autopsy registers at the three government-run mortuaries in the Durban Municipality was conducted for the period 2006–2007. All suicidal deaths were further extracted from these registers and analysed. The rationale for choosing the above study period was to ensure that only authentic suicide cases finalised via the inquest methodology employed in South Africa were included for

TABLE 1: Durban population age groupings.

Age	0–14	15–24	25–44	45–64	65+
Residents (%)	27.7	21.2	32.5	14.5	4.2

Source: Statistics South Africa[21]

analysis in the study. Cases that were classified as 'deaths due to other causes' or those that could not be finalised via the inquest process were excluded from this study.

Ethical considerations

Ethical approval to conduct the study was granted by the University of KwaZulu-Natal's Biomedical Research Ethics Committee (Reference number HSS/0181/06D) and the KwaZulu-Natal Provincial Department of Health.

Data analysis

All data were captured and analysed using the Statistical Software Package for Social Sciences® (SPSS) version 19 (IBM Corp, Armonk, NY, 2010) and SAS/STAT software version 8.2 (Cary, NC, SAS Institute, 2010).

Results

Prevalence of suicide in Durban

During the two-year study period, 6046 and 5550 non-natural deaths were recorded for 2006 and 2007 respectively. Suicide accounted for 7.7% (n = 465) of these non-natural deaths (N = 6046) in 2006 and 9.0% (n = 497) of non-natural deaths (N = 5550) in 2007. The suicide incidence rate for Durban in 2006 was 14.53/100 000 population and that for 2007 was 15.53/100 000 population. These calculations were based on the 2001 national census figures.[21]

Suicide victim characteristics

Male suicides outnumbered female suicides (Table 2) in both 2006 (ratio 3.2: 1) and 2007 (3.6: 1).This was also reflected in the monthly mean calculations for both years. The monthly mean for male suicides was 27.54 (SD = 10.2) in 2006 and 32.17 (SD = 7.3) in 2007, whereas that for females was 9.33 (SD = 3.8) in 2006 and 8.83 (SD = 2.4) in 2007. In both years, the largest number of suicides was recorded in black people, followed by Indian, white and mixed-race people (Table 2).

Monthly frequencies for all groups

The mean number of suicides per month in 2006 was 36.0 (SD = 12.9) and that in 2007 was 41.1 (SD = 8.8). The monthly frequency peaked beyond 50 per month twice in 2006 (April and December) and once in October 2007 (Figure 1).

Monthly frequencies expressed as means for each race group within Durban per year also indicated a larger number for black people compared with the other race groups in both 2006 and 2007 (Table 3). The suicide rate per 100 000 had increased from 2006 to 2007 for all race groups except for white people (Table 3).

In terms of race and gender (Table 4 and Figure 2), the majority of suicides in both years were in black men and women, with a rise in the number of black men and a shift reduction in the number of black women between 2006 and 2007. There was a small increase in both mixed-race and Indian men and women, a decrease in white men and a small increase in white women.

The aggregated data indicates that most of the suicides occurred in people between the ages of 15 and 44 years (Figure 3). The majority of suicides took place amongst the 25–34 year olds, followed by the 15–24 and the 35–44 year age groups. In the under-14 age group, there were 13 boys (two in 2006 and 11 in 2007) and 10 girls (seven in 2006 and three in 2007). Most of the male age groups experienced an increase from 2006 to 2007 except in the 25–34 and 55–64 year olds. There was a decrease in the number of women between 2006 and 2007 in most categories except in the 35–44 and 55 years and older groups.

TABLE 2: Suicide frequencies by sex and race per year.

Suicide frequency variables	2006		2007	
	n	%	*n*	%
Sex				
Male	356	76.2	387	78.3
Female	111	23.8	107	21.7
Race				
Black	267	57.2	289	58.4
Mixed race	10	2.1	15	3.0
Indian	124	26.6	136	27.5
White	66	14.1	55	11.1

Source: Data collated from mortuary records

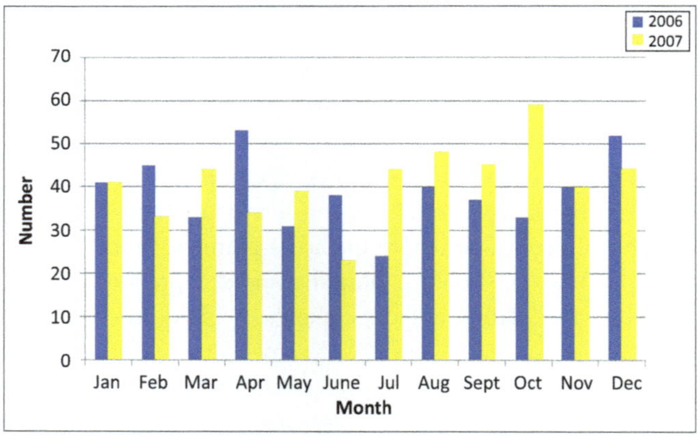

Source: Data collated from mortuary records

FIGURE 1: Suicide frequency by month and year.

TABLE 3: Suicide frequencies by race, monthly mean and rates per year of study.

Race group	2006		2007	
	Monthly Mean (SD)	Suicide Rate/100 000	Monthly Mean (SD)	Suicide Rate/100 000
Black	22.4 (6.0)	12	23.9 (6.4)	13
Mixed race	1.4 (0.8)	11	1.9 (1.1)	17
Indian	10.3 (4.2)	19	11.3 (3.8)	21
White	5.1 (3.0)	23	4.6 (2.3)	19

Source: Data collated from mortuary records
SD, standard deviation.

TABLE 4: Number of suicides by race and gender for 2006 and 2007.

Gender and year	Black	Mixed race	Indian	White	Gender Total	Gender %	Year total
Men 2006	202	7	91	53	353	75.9	465
Women 2006	63	3	32	14	112	24.1	
Men 2007	239	10	103	40	392	78.9	497
Women 2007	51	5	34	15	105	21.1%	
Total	**555**	**25**	**260**	**122**	**962**	-	-
% of Total	**58.0%**	**2.0%**	**27.0%**	**13.0%**	**100.0%**		

Source: Data collated from mortuary records

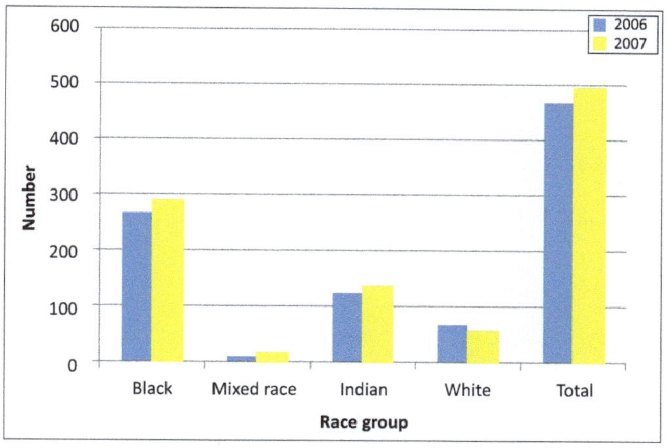

Source: Data collated from mortuary records

FIGURE 2: Number of suicides by race.

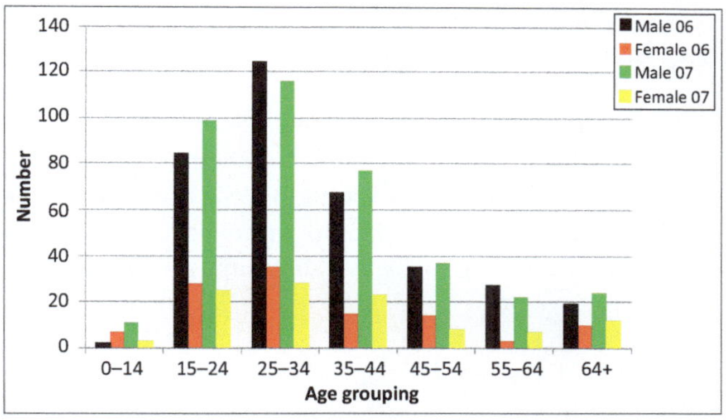

Source: Data collated from mortuary records

FIGURE 3: Suicide victims by gender and age.

The overall mean age (95% CI) at which people committed suicide was 34.14 years (95% CI 32.80–35.48) in 2006 and 34.63 (95% CI 33.29–35.97) in 2007. The lowest age had dropped from 9 years in 2006 to 5 years in 2007, as had the highest age from 98 to 95 (Table 5).

Of those for whom marital status was recorded, 60.6% in 2006 and 58.3% in 2007 were single (Table 6). Married persons accounted for 23.4% and 22.0% in 2006 and 2007 respectively.

In both 2006 and 2007, the majority of people who committed suicide were unemployed (43.4% in 2006 and 38.5% in 2007), followed by general workers (12.1% in 2006 and 14.1% in 2007), other varied occupations (11.2% in 2006 and 9.5% in 2007) and students (7.5% in 2006 and 5.6% in 2007).These figures are not shown in the Tables.

TABLE 5: Age descriptors of suicide victims by year.

Age	2006	2007
Mean age (95% CI) in years	34.1 (32.8–35.5)	34.6 (33.3–36.0)
Median age (SD) in years	30.0 (14.6)	31.0 (5.1)
Age range in years	9–98	5–95

Source: Data collated from mortuary records
SD, standard deviation; CI, confidence interval.

Breakdown of preferred methods of suicide

Overall, of the nine main methods used to commit suicide (Figure 4), hanging accounted for nearly two-thirds in both 2006 (61%) and 2007 (62%).This was followed by guns, jumping from heights and overdose. These four methods accounted for 88% of all suicides in 2006 and 94% of all suicides in 2007.

Hanging was the preferred method of suicide for all age groups except for those over 65 years in 2007, where jumping from high-rise buildings was the preferred method (Figure 5). In both the 15–24 and 25–34 year age groups, gun usage was the next most common method used, whilst in the 35–44 and 45–55 year age groups, overdose was the method of choice, followed by hanging and gun usage.

Discussion

This study was part of a larger study undertaken by the researcher during the period 2006–2011, some of the findings of which have been used in partial fulfilment of a doctoral degree.[1] The salient findings of this study in particular support and complement those found by Donson and others in 2007.[22] The total number of suicides confirmed in this study ($n = 495$) for Durban during 2007 was greater than that shown in the Donson study ($n = 398$).[22] The difference may be explained by the differing methodologies used in each study. There are no other recent relevant studies.

This study showed a gradient of increase in suicides over the two-year period studied, which is consistent with the reported gradual increase in suicide rates for the country as a whole from around 8% in 1999 to 11% currently.[6,23] Compared with suicide rates for the other major South African cities, the rates per 100 000 population in this study shows that Durban has a high suicide rate, which is also comparable with the average global rate.[22]

Although the results of the present study indicate that suicides occur throughout the year in Durban, there were discernible peaks at particular times, namely, early and

TABLE 6: Marital status of suicide victims by year of study.

Marital status	2006		2007	
	n	%	*n*	%
Single	282	60.6	290	58.3
Married	109	23.4	107	22.0
Separated	0	0	1	0.2
Divorced	15	3.2	18	3.4
Widowed	3	0.6	10	2.0
Not Recorded	55	11.8	71	14.1
Total	465	100%	497	100%

Source: Data collated from mortuary records

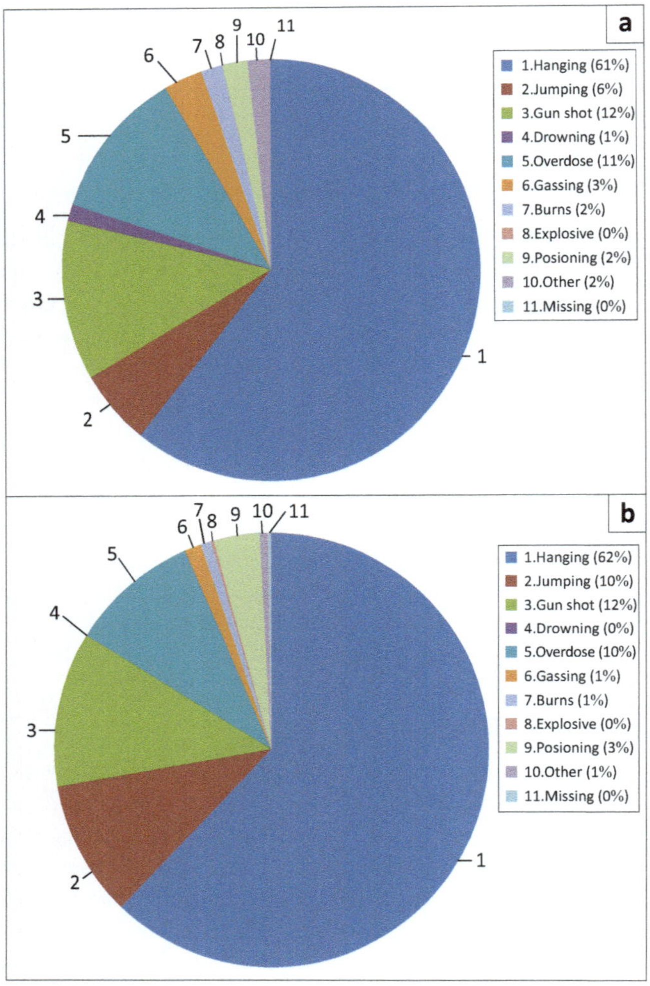

Source: Data collated from mortuary records

FIGURE 4: Most common suicide methods in (a)2006 and (b) 2007.

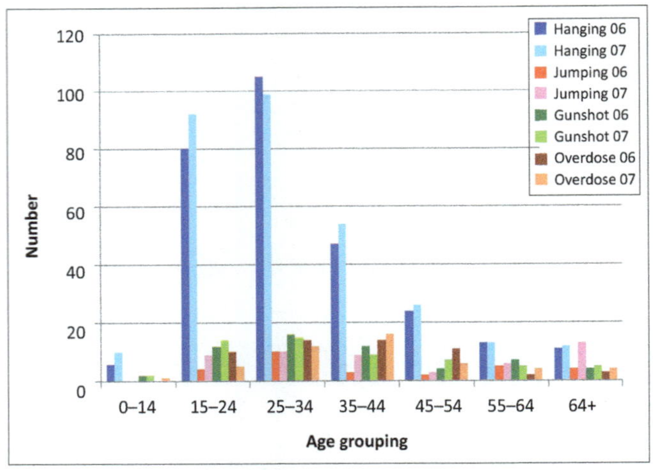

Source: Data collated from mortuary records

FIGURE 5: Age groupings and the four most common methods of suicide.

toward the end of the year, which is consistent with other findings for the country.[6,23] It has been postulated that this finding may be linked to high degrees of stress toward the year end, which have been precipitated by socio-economic difficulties and academic expectations, particularly amongst our youth.[6]

This study also demonstrated that the actual number of suicides per year of study varied considerably between racial groupings in Durban – it was twice as high for black people as for Indian people, the former constituting the largest racial or population group in the metropolitan area. Figures for mixed-race people and white people were much lower. These findings are in sharp contrast with earlier studies on suicide rates for the different race groups in South Africa, which showed that white South Africans consistently outnumbered black, Indian and mixed-race South Africans.[8,9,24] The suicide gradient amongst the different race groups per year showed an increase from 2006 to 2007 in all groups except for white South Africans.

The fact that the majority of suicides in both years were committed by men is consistent with those found in other studies.[9,15,25,26,27,28] At least two-thirds of the suicide victims in our research were unmarried, widowed or divorced. Similar findings have been reported in other studies with some reporting that separated men were at higher risk of committing suicide compared with separated women.[29,30]

In terms of age groupings, the majority of suicides in our study took place amongst 25–34 year olds, followed by 15–24 year olds and 35–44 year olds. Other local studies have reported comparable findings,[25,31] which is similar to the global trend of a shift to younger people committing suicide.[2] However, a study in Dar es Salaam, Tanzania, showed that the 45–59 year group had the highest suicide rate,[27] although varying figures are reported for Africa.[32] The high number of suicides committed by young students in the present study is a source of great concern and is consistent with previous South African research findings. Research findings have linked this trend to a variety of pre-disposing and risk factors. These include child abuse and neglect, interpersonal problems, peer pressure, substance abuse, family dysfunction and unrealistic academic expectations.[6,33,34,35]

The majority of suicide victims in our study were unemployed or casual workers. It is possible that socio-economic issues played a role in influencing a fatal suicidal outcome in these victims. This is supported by other studies which have shown an inverse relationship between income and psychological distress.[36] Also, a number of researchers have offered various related explanations regarding the deteriorating trend in suicides in South Africa. These include the inability to cope with new roles since the abolition of apartheid and the introduction of a democracy since 1994; acculturation and western lifestyle influences and moving away from protective traditional lifestyles; socio-economic pressures, with resulting interpersonal and family problems; inappropriate family and peer expectations; increasing urbanisation; increasing competitiveness; and rising unemployment in a changing South African society since democracy.[6,37,38]

The methods used in committing suicide depend on availability, knowledge of lethality and access to the method by the victim. In our study, hanging emerged as the dominant method in at least two-thirds of suicide victims, all racial groups, both genders and all ages, except in the over-65 year age group in 2007 where jumping was the chosen method. This was followed by other methods such as guns, jumping from heights and over-dosing of medicines. In general, hanging was the preferred method amongst unemployed victims (65.5%) compared with those who were employed at the time (56.6%). Interestingly, in the Eastern Cape Province of South Africa, hanging was reported to be the preferred method in uneducated (70%) and unemployed (64%) victims, whilst the more highly educated (17%) used firearms to commit suicide.[39] The prominence of suicide by hanging has also been documented in a number of other studies[13,40] and differs from those in a recent study conducted in Malawi where self-poisoning emerged as the being the most common method used by both men and women.[41]

Limitations

The data recorded in this study may not be truly representative for several reasons. Only data relating to confirmed suicides were extracted from mortuary registers and analysed in this study. It is possible that these registers may have contained administrative errors, omissions and inaccurate recordings, meaning that the number of suicides analysed may thus have been underestimated. The study also relied on the accuracy of the data entries recorded in mortuary registers in Durban. Some of the data may have been obtained from contacts other than next-of-kin and may not have been accurate. Missing data were noted in particular categories studied, such as marital status, occupation and method of suicide.

All suicides committed in Durban during the study period were analysed. This may have included persons not normally resident in Durban, therefore the figures presented in this study may not be truly representative of the residents domiciled in Durban.

The study design unfortunately precluded an exploration of precipitating factors and causes. Relatives and family members could not be interviewed. In instances where suicide notes were left by victims, details within these notes were filed in inquest files and not made part of the mortuary registers.

Conclusion

The actual rates of suicide per racial group showed a gradient increase from 2006 to 2007 for all groups except for white people. Health and education policy makers, counsellors and community leaders should respond to the disturbingly-high suicide figures recorded amongst certain categories of Durban residents such as black and Indian people, the unemployed and the youth, including scholars. This study endorses the call made by many researchers and policy makers for the enactment of a national policy framework in South Africa that would embrace a comprehensive multidisciplinary primary care approach to the current burden of suicidal behaviour in the country. Hanging emerged as the dominant method used by the majority of those committing suicide mainly because of its simplicity, proven effectiveness and easy access to structures within or adjacent to homes. There is therefore an urgent need for innovative employment strategies to help the unemployed, as well as greater awareness and education campaigns (amongst public health policy makers, low-cost housing developments and families) designed to restrict such easy access to any potential method by vulnerable individuals.

A larger and more extensive study over a longer period is recommended in order to confirm the reported trends.

Acknowledgements

The authors extend their gratitude to the KwaZulu-Natal Department of Health, the state mortuaries in Durban, South Africa, for their permission to view the mortuary records and to Ms T Esterhuizen and Mr Stephan van der Linde of the University of KwZulu-Natal for biostatistical support.

Competing interests

The authors declare that they have no financial or personal relationship(s) which may have inappropriately influenced them in writing this article.

Author's contributions

S.S.N. (Department of Family Medicine, University of KwaZulu-Natal) was responsible for all the work done in this study, including the study design, fieldwork and data analysis. L.S. (Department of Behavioural Medicine, University of KwaZulu-Natal), assisted with the editing of the final manuscript.

References

1. Naidoo SS. The impact of a brief intervention programme on suicidal behaviour in a South African community [unpublished Doctoral dissertation]. Durban: Department of Family Medicine, University of KwaZulu-Natal; 2012.

2. Bertolote JM, Fleischmann A. Suicidal behavior prevention: WHO perspectives on research. Am J Med Genet C Semin Med Genet. 2005;133C(1):8–12. http://dx.doi.org/10.1002/ajmg.c.30041, PMid:15645530

3. Phillips MR, Li X, Zhang Y. Suicide rates in China,1995–1999. Lancet 2002;359(9309):835–840. http://dx.doi.org/10.1016/S0140-6736(02)07954-0

4. Kong Y, Zhang J. Access to farming pesticides and risk for suicide in Chinese rural young people. Psychiatry Res. 2010;179(2):217–221. http://dx.doi.org/10.1016/j.psychres.2009.12.005, PMid:20483175, PMCid:PMC2925062

5. Burrows S, Schlebusch L. Priorities and prevention possibilities for reducing suicidal behaviour. In: A Van Niekerk, S Suffla, M Seedat, editors. Crime, violence and injury prevention in South Africa:data to action. Tygerberg: MRC-UNISA Crime,Violence and Injury Lead Programme, 2008; p. 173–201.

6. Schlebusch L. Suicidal behaviour in South Africa. Pietermaritzburg: University of KwaZulu-Natal Press; 2005. PMCid:PMC1287817

7. Matzopoulos R, Cassim M, Seedat M. A profile of fatal injuries in South Africa: Fourth Annual Report of the National Injury Mortality Surveillance System. Pretoria: Medical Research Council; 2003.

8. Burrows S, Vaez M, Butchart A, et al. The share of suicide in injury deaths in the South African context: sociodemographic distribution. Public Health. 2003;117(1):3–10. http://dx.doi.org/10.1016/S0033-3506(02)00019-7

9. Scribante L, Blumenthal R, Saayman G, et al. A retrospective review of 1018 suicide cases from the capital city of South Africa for the period 1997-2000. Am J Forensic Med Pathol. 2004;25(1):52–55. http://dx.doi.org/10.1097/01.paf.0000113862.03302.1d, PMid:15075690

10. Prinsloo M. A profile of fatal injuries in South Africa. Cape Town: South African Medical Research Council; 2002.

11. Asirdizer M, Yavuz MS, Aydin SD, et al. Suicides in Turkey between 1996 and 2005: general perspective. Am J Forensic Med Pathol. 2010;31(2):138–145. http://dx.doi.org/10.1097/PAF.0b013e3181cfc658, PMid:20110803

12. Dennis MS, Lindesay J. Suicide in the elderly: the United Kingdom perspective. Int Psychogeriatr. 1995;7(2):263–274. http://dx.doi.org/10.1017/S104161029500202X

13. Meel B. Epidemiology of suicide by hanging in Transkei, South Africa. Am J Forensic Med Pathol. 2006;27(1):75–78. http://dx.doi.org/10.1097/01.paf.0000202738.28446.4a, PMid:16501355

14. Meel BL. Suicide in HIV/AIDS in Transkei, South Africa. Anil Aggrawal's Internet Journal of Forensic Medicine and Toxicology. 2003;4(1):1–9.

15. World Health Organization. Report on a workshop on suicide prevention for countries in the African region. Geneva: Department of Mental Health, World Health Organization; 1999.

16. Flisher AJ, Parry CD. Suicide in South Africa. An analysis of nationally registered mortality data for 1984-1986. Acta Psychiatr Scand. 1994;90(5):348–353. http://dx.doi.org/10.1111/j.1600-0447.1994.tb01605.x, PMid:7872039

17. Sukhai A, Harris C, Moorad RG, et al. Suicide by self-immolation in Durban, South Africa: a five-year retrospective review. Am J Forensic Med Pathol. 2002;23(3):295–298. http://dx.doi.org/10.1097/00000433-200209000-00020, PMid:12198362

18. Roberts K, Wassenaar D, Canetto SS, et al. Homicide-suicide in Durban, South Africa. J Interpers Violence. 2010;25(5):877–899. http://dx.doi.org/10.1177/0886260509336964, PMid:19617417

19. Jena S, Mountany L, Muller A. A demographic study of homicide-suicide in the Pretoria region over a 5 year period. J Forensic Leg Med. 2009;16(5):261–265. http://dx.doi.org/10.1016/j.jflm.2008.12.009, PMid:19481707

20. Lester D. Personal violence (suicide and homicide) in South Africa. Acta Psychiatr Scand. 1989;79(3):235–237. http://dx.doi.org/10.1111/j.1600-0447.1989.tb10250.x, PMid:2711848

21. Statistics South Africa. South African population statistics In: Pretoria: Government Gazette; 2001.

22. Donson H, editor. A profile of fatal injuries in South Africa. Tygerburg: MRC/UNISA Crime, Violence and Injury Lead Programme; 2007. PMCid:PMC2659070

23. Schlebusch L, Govender RD. Age, Gender and Suicidal Ideation Following Voluntary HIV Counseling and Testing. Int J Environ Res Public Health. 2012;9(2):521–530.

24. Naidoo T, Kirk GM. Post-mortem analysis of all deaths. In: Faculty Research Day. Durban: University of Natal; 2004.

25. Matzopoulos R, Norman R, Bradshaw D. The burden of injury in South Africa: fatal injury trends and international comparisons. Tygerberg: Medical Research Council-University of South Africa, Crime, Violence and Injury Lead Programme; 2004.

26. Flisher AJ, Liang H, Laubscher R, et al. Suicide trends in South Africa, 1968--90. Scand J Public Health. 2004;32(6):411–418. http://dx.doi.org/10.1080/14034940410029469, PMid:15762025

27. Mgaya E, Kazaura MR, Outwater A, et al. Suicide in the Dar es Salaam region, Tanzania, 2005. J Forensic Leg Med. 2008;15(3):172–176. http://dx.doi.org/10.1016/j.jflm.2007.06.002, PMid:18313013

28. Bertolote JM. Suicide in the world: an epidemiological overview 1959–2000. London: Martin Dunitz; 2001. PMid:11431054

29. Kõlves K. Child suicide, family environment, and economic crisis. Crisis. 2010;31(3):115–117. http://dx.doi.org/10.1027/0227-5910/a000040, PMid:20573604

30. Masocco M, Pompili M, Vanacore N, et al. Completed suicide and marital status according to the Italian region of origin. Psychiatr Q. 2010;81(1):57–71. http://dx.doi.org/10.1007/s11126-009-9118-2, PMid:20041348

31. Bradshaw D, Masiteng K, Nannan N. Health status and determinants. Durban: Health Systems Trust; 2000.

32. Schlebusch L. An overview of suicidal behaviour in Africa. In: DM Ndetei, DM Szabo, editors. Contemporary psychiatry in Africa: a review of theory, practice and research. Nairobi, Kenya: Acrodile Publishing Limited, 2011; p. 375–396.

33. Pillay AL, Wassenaar DR. Recent stressors and family satisfaction in suicidal adolescents in South Africa. J Adolesc. 1997;20(2):155–162. http://dx.doi.org/10.1006/jado.1996.0073, PMid:9104651

34. Noor Mahomed SB, Selmer CA, Bosch BA. Psychological profiles of children presenting with suicidal behaviour, with a specific focus on psychopathology. In: L Schlebusch, BA Bosch, editors. Suicidal behaviour 4: Proceedings of the fourth Southern African conference on suicidology. Durban: University of Natal, 2000; p. 56–70.

35. Schlebusch L. Suicidal behaviour. In: A van Niekerk, S Suffla, M Seedat, editors. Crime, violence and injury in South Africa: enabling child safety. Pretoria, South Africa: Psychological Society of South Africa, 2012; p. 178–194.

36. McMillan KA, Enns MW, Asmundson GJ, et al. The association between income and distress, mental disorders, and suicidal ideation and attempts: findings from the Collaborative Psychiatric Epidemiology Surveys. J Clin Psychiatry. 2010;71(9):1168–1175. http://dx.doi.org/10.4088/JCP.08m04986gry, PMid:20441719

37. Wassenaar DR, Pillay AL, Descoins S, et al. Patterns of suicide in Pietermaritzburg 1982–1996: race, gender and seasonality. In: L Schlebusch, BA Bosch, editors. Proceedings of the fourth Southern African conference on suicidology: University of Natal, 2000; p. 97–111.

38. Vawda N. Suicidal behaviour among black South African children and adolescents. In: S Malhotra, editor. Mental disorders in children and adolescents: need and strategies for intervention. Delhi: CBS Publishers and Distributors, 2005; p. 94–100.

39. Meel BL. Determinants of suicide in the Transkei sub-region of South Africa. J Clin Forensic Med. 2003;10(2):71–76. http://dx.doi.org/10.1016/S1353-1131(03)00038-5

40. Burrows S, Laflamme L. Suicide mortality in South Africa: a city-level comparison across socio-demographic groups. Soc Psychiatry Psychiatr Epidemiol. 2006;41(2):108–114. http://dx.doi.org/10.1007/s00127-005-0004-4, PMid:16362168

41. Dzamalala CP, Milner DA, Liomba NG. Suicide in Blantyre, Malawi (2000–2003). J Clin Forensic Med. 2006;13(2):65–69. http://dx.doi.org/10.1016/j.jcfm.2005.08.006, PMid:16271492

10

Implementation of the principles of primary health care in a rural area of South Africa

Authors:
Surona Visagie[1]
Marguerite Schneider[2]

Affiliations:
[1]Centre for Rehabilitation Studies, University of Stellenbosch, South Africa

[2]Department of Psychology, Stellenbosch University, South Africa

Correspondence to:
Surona Visagie

Email:
surona@telkomsa.net

Postal address:
PO Box 40, Fraserburg, 6960

Background: The philosophy of primary healthcare forms the basis of South Africa's health policy and provides guidance for healthcare service delivery in South Africa. Healthcare service provision in South Africa has shown improvement in the past five years. However, it is uncertain as to whether the changes have reached rural areas and if primary healthcare is implemented successfully in these areas.

Objectives: The aim of this article is to explore the extent to which the principles of primary healthcare are implemented in a remote, rural setting in South Africa.

Method: A descriptive, qualitative design was implemented. Data were collected through interviews and case studies with 36 purposively-sampled participants, then analysed through Interpretative Phenomenological Analysis.

Results: Findings indicated challenges with regard to client-centred care, provision of health promotion and rehabilitation, the way care was organised, the role of the doctor, health-worker attitudes, referral services and the management of complex conditions.

Conclusion: The principles of primary healthcare were not implemented successfully. The community was not involved in healthcare management, nor were users involved in their personal health management. The initiation of a community-health forum is recommended. Service providers, users and the community should identify and address the determinants of ill health in the community. Other recommendations include the training of service managers in the logistical management of ensuring a constant supply of drugs, using a Kombi-type vehicle to provide user transport for routine visits to secondary- and tertiary healthcare services and increasing the doctors' hours.

La mise en œuvre des principes de soins de santé primaires dans une zone rurale d'Afrique du Sud

Contexte: La philosophie de soins de santé primaires (SSP) sont a la base de la politique de santé de l'Afrique du Sud. Meme si la prestation des services de santé a montré une amelioration, il y a des doutes que la SSP est mis en œuvre avec succès dans les zones rurales d'Afrique du Sud.

Objectifs: Cet article étudie a quelle mesure les principes de SSP sont mises en œuvre dans un cadre rurale d'Afrique du Sud.

Méthode: L'étude emploi une méthodologie qualitatif et descriptive. Les données ont été recueillies par des entrevues et études de cas avec 36 participants. La méthode d'analyse utilise la phénoménologie interprétative.

Résultats: Les résultats indiquent des défis dans la promotion de la santé, de la réadaptation individuel, organisation des soins, le rôle du médecin, les attitudes des travailleurs de la santé, des services de renvoi a d'autre niveau du service de santé et la gestion des conditions complexes.

Conclusion: Les principes de SSP n'ont pas été mis en œuvre avec succès. La communauté n'a pas été impliqué dans la gestion des services, ni les utilisateurs impliqués dans la gestion de leur santé personnelle. L'initiation d'un forum sur la santé dans la communauté est recommandé. Les fournisseurs de services, les utilisateurs et la communauté doivent identifier et agir sur les déterminants de la mauvaise santé. D'autres recommandations portent sur la formation des gestionnaires, amélioration des services de transport et une augmentation des heures to service par les medecins.

Introduction

The philosophy of primary healthcare (PHC) forms the basis of South Africa's health policy and provides guidance for healthcare service delivery in South Africa.[1] As such, the principles of primary healthcare should underpin healthcare delivery in South Africa.[2,3,4] These principles include equity; community participation; social and economic development; interventions focused on the determinants of poor health, health promotion, prevention, cure and rehabilitation; an integrated referral system to facilitate a continuum of care; teams of health professionals with specific and sophisticated biomedical- and social skills; adequate resources; and a client-centred approach.

A series of articles on health in South Africa published in The Lancet in 2009 reported challenges with regard to implementation of PHC in South Africa.[5,6] However, since then positive changes have been seen which resulted in an increase in life expectancy from 43 years in 2007 [7] to 60 years in 2012.[8] According to Mayosi et al. South Africa might for the first time be on track to meet millennium goals four to six.[8] This is ascribed to leadership changes in the Ministry of Health and policy changes in the management of HIV and tuberculosis, diseases of lifestyle, injury and violence as well as maternal- and child health. At the same time, these authors acknowledge specific challenges such as insufficient post-natal feeding support, an increase in non-communicable disease risk factors, high incidence of violence and accidents, race- and gender inequalities, challenges pertaining to social determinants of health such as low educational levels, poor housing and sanitation, limited public–private partnerships, as well as insufficient health surveillance and information systems.[8] In addition, Gaede and Versteeg[9] and Cooke, Couper and Versteeg[10] pointed out challenges to healthcare service provision in rural South Africa. They mentioned a shortage of healthcare service providers, transport challenges, distances, a loss of time and increased cost as being specific barriers.

The concept of rural is not a homogenous one[9,11,12] and healthcare service provision in rural areas are impacted on by the physical-, demographic-, economic-, social- and cultural contexts.[12] Physical harshness of the environment, climatic extremes and the landscape impact on healthcare access.[12,13,14] The size of the area can result in isolation and long distances from services.[9,11,14,15,16,17,18] The situation is exacerbated by demographic factors such as low population density, since this impacts negatively on the economic viability of services, with the result being that there are often fewer services available in rural communities,[9,11,18,19,20,21,22,23,24] meaning that users often have to travel long distances in order to access specialist care.[9,18]

In Africa (and South Africa), travelling distances are exacerbated by poor road infrastructure and meagre-, expensive-, inadequate- or nonexistent public transport.[20,21,25] This is confounded by unavailability or high cost of private transport.[20] Thus, in seeking healthcare, rural residents often incur an increased cost burden through travel and accommodation costs and time away from work.[18] In addition, people living in rural areas are often poorer than those in urban areas and have less resources to expend on healthcare.[12,19,20,21,22,23,24]

Socially, rural communities tend to be close-knit. This can make for high levels of support, but impacts negatively on privacy.[12,13,18] In addition, newcomers, including incoming healthcare providers, are seldom trusted immediately.[18] This situation can cause challenges in rural South Africa where community-service doctors and -therapists often rotate on a yearly basis. Finally, culture has a significant impact on how a person sees the world and determines one's perceptions and behaviour with regard to health- and healthcare seeking.[26]

As described above, healthcare service provision in South Africa is improving, but it is unclear as to what extent these improvements have reached remote, rural communities and whether it has made a difference in the health of people living in these communities. The aim of this article is to explore the extent to which the principles of PHC are implemented in a remote, rural setting in South Africa, as well as to identify gaps and possible solutions to the implementation of PHC in this setting.

Research method and design

Over the period of 2010–2013 a study on healthcare access for vulnerable groups in Africa, titled 'Enabling universal and equitable access to healthcare for vulnerable people in resource poor settings in Africa' (EquitAble),[27] was undertaken. The study consisted of three phases and data were collected in four sites in four African counties, as illustrated in Figure 1. The first phase of the study comprised analysis on international-, regional- and national policy documents.[28,29] The second- and third phases comprised an exploration of the access to healthcare by vulnerable groups through a series of qualitative interviews and a quantitative household survey within each site.

Findings presented in this article came from data collected during the qualitative exploration (Figure 1) in a rural Northern Cape Province town. The town was selected as a study site since it represented a rural setting with poor infrastructure and inequities amongst various social groups in the community.[30]

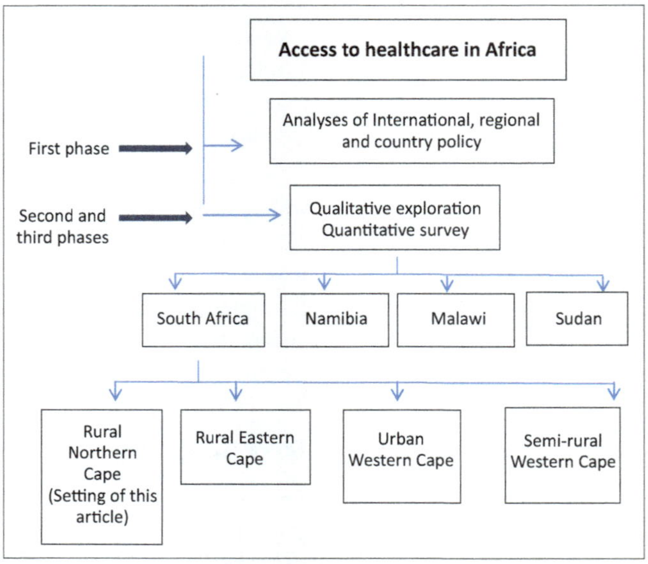

FIGURE 1: Schematic presentation of phases of the EquitAble study.[27]

The study setting

The Northern Cape Province is the largest province in South Africa and covers 30.5% of the country, but has, with just over 1.1 million people, the smallest population of the nine provinces and 2.2% of the total South African population.[31] The rural Northern Cape Province is sustained by farming, tourism and mining and contributes 2% of the national gross domestic product,[32] with 42% of the population living in poverty and 40% being unemployed.[33]

The study town is situated in an arid, rural, sheep-farming environment. The town and surrounding district covers roughly 10 000 km^2 with a population density of one person per 3 km^2. According to the EquitAble survey findings, tuberculosis, hypertension and joint pathology such as osteoarthritis were the most pressing health concerns in the community. Healthcare services to the community were provided by a nurse-driven Community Health-Care Centre (CHCC), supported by weekly outreach services from doctors and therapists. In addition, a private general practitioner visited the town every fortnight. Access to public secondary healthcare services are 200 km away, tertiary healthcare services 800 km away, private specialist healthcare services 400 km away and private pharmacies 200 km away. Access involves some driving on poorly-maintained gravel roads.

Study population, sampling and participants

All members of the study community and all persons that provide healthcare services to the community formed the study population. The primary author, a member of the community, used her knowledge of the community to identify possible participants. In addition, political and religious leaders in the community were asked to provide the names of possible participants. The primary author and the co-author reflected on these persons and selected the study participants through purposive sampling. Care was taken during sampling to include as wide a range of participants as possible and to include individuals that could shed the most light on the variables that impact on healthcare access.[34]

The group included users and non-users of government healthcare services, key informants, and healthcare service providers. Service users were sampled to include various groups such as persons with activity limitations, the elderly, children, people with low levels of education, people who are unemployed, people living far from services, woman-headed households and poor people. All of these groups are, according to the literature, vulnerable with regard to healthcare access. [19,22,25,35,36,37,38,39,40,41] Key informants were people who, by nature of their employment or other activities, had specific knowledge about healthcare services such as the hospital committee, clergy, municipal officers and old-age home staff. Healthcare service providers included those with direct client involvement, such as professional nurses, doctors, therapists and direct observation of therapy workers, as well as those without, such as general assistants. Further information on participants is provided in Table 1. Some participants fell into more than one category, for example, being coloured and a farm worker.

TABLE 1: Information on study participants.

Users/Non-users
• 4–65 years old • No to tertiary education • Four users lived more than 40 km from service • 10 users had activity limitations • Three Farmworkers • Six Unemployed • One Non-user
Providers' occupations
• Professional nurse • Doctors • Therapists • Emergency medical technician • General assistant • Direct observation of therapy worker
Role of key informants
• Lay preacher • Old-age-home representative • Community development worker • Member of the hospital committee • Farmer • Association for the physically disabled representative • Social worker

Data-collection procedure

Data were collected between April 2010 and July 2012 through semi-structured interviews, case studies, observations and document perusal. The primary author performed all data collection and was assisted by the co-author during the first week of interviews in April 2010 when 14 interviews were performed. In total, 22 semi-structured interviews were performed with 28 participants between April and June 2010. An additional eight case studies were performed with healthcare users between April 2010 and May 2012. Data were supplemented by field notes, observations at the CHCC and perusal of documents such as the municipality's Integrated Development Plan (IDP) and rough data from a community survey performed in 2009 by the municipality. All interviews were performed in Afrikaans, the language preferred by all participants. Interviews were recorded digitally with the written consent of the participants.

Data analysis

The primary author transcribed and analysed all data. Emerging themes were identified through interpretative phenomenological analysis (IPA).[42] The transcribed interviews were printed on the middle third of a page and the transcripts were read repeatedly. During the reading, key words or phrases, notes on linguistic and non-verbal aspects of data and conceptual comments were made in the left-hand column. Following this, emergent themes were penned in the right-hand column. The aim of this process was to distil the comments into themes that decreased the volume of information, whilst at the same time retaining complexity. Once the themes were identified, connections across themes were sought through ordering and re-ordering themes on a pin-up board to develop groups that fitted together. These groups were clustered into five superordinate themes through abstraction, subsumption, polarisation, contextualisation, numeration and/or function.[42] The superordinate themes were:

- Primary healthcare
- Healthcare management
- Disability approaches

- Rehabilitation
- Health, illness, personhood and the context

Under the superordinate theme of Primary Healthcare, seven themes were clustered. These seven themes are presented and discussed in this article. The other superordinate themes will be explored in separate papers.

Results

The seven themes clustered under the superordinate theme of Primary Healthcare are presented in Table 2. In addition, Table 2 shows the subthemes under each theme and how each theme can be associated with the principles of PHC.

The themes are illustrated through two case studies and additional narrative examples. The case studies were chosen because, in combination, the experiences of these healthcare users represent much of the essence of what was narrated by various participants. In the interests of privacy, aliases have been used to protect the identity of the participants.

Case study one – Jane and Rosy

The first case study tells the story of Jane and her granddaughter Rosie. Jane, a widow in her fifties, fostered three grandchildren amongst whom was Rosie, a four-year old on initial interview. Rosie was born without forearms and hands. She could not walk or talk, was incontinent and cognitively impaired. She was diagnosed with Cornelia de Lange syndrome, a genetic condition that does not preclude progress, but requires stimulation and input to facilitate it. The condition made her vulnerable to chest infections and they frequently accessed primary healthcare services, as explained by Jane:

> 'It seems to me her chest troubles her. She gets ill quickly. I cannot wait long when she is ill. I have to go to the clinic immediately.'

Jane said the following about their experiences at the CHCC:

Organisation of care

> 'It was always like this, when she got ill they assisted me immediately, but now it is a sad business. There is only one sister on duty and you have to wait for that sister. You go in the morning and sit there the entire day. Then they tell you to go away and come back in the afternoon. The way the clinic is now, on Monday they hand out pills, Wednesday is doctor's day. Then you cannot go to the clinic at all, because then they will not help you. And like today [*Friday*] then it is people from the farms, then you sit till late before they help you.'

Client-centred care

> 'I do not understand why sister took away the milk.'
>
> '...they did not tell me what was wrong with her.'
>
> 'I can understand that she lost weight, because she had a runny tummy and she vomited. She did not eat like she used to, but they [*nurses*] do not take notice of that.'
>
> '...they just want to help you quickly and quickly give some medication and ja well. I have to accept what they give.'
>
> 'I asked why they put her on a drip, but the sister spoke Xhosa and English and I could not understand what she said.'

Prevention

> 'They treated her with me to make sure that she did not catch it [*Jane had TB*].'

Attitudes

> 'I asked for pills, but they did not answer me. Then sister said don't you understand, do I have to speak German to you? They did not assist me that day.'

Referral services

Rosie was born in the tertiary hospital and went back there for further diagnostic tests in 2011. Her grandmother said the following:

TABLE 2: Themes, subthemes and their association with the principles of Primary Healthcare.

Themes	Subthemes	Primary Healthcare principles
Client-centred care	• Communication barriers • Little explanation given to users • Not seeking user's opinions • Not involving user in decisions • Users have little/no choice • Users left vulnerable	• Equity • 'People have the right and duty to participate individually and collectively in the planning and implementation of their healthcare'
Promotion, prevention, cure and rehabilitation	• Preventive and curative focus • Shortage of medication	• 'Addresses the main health problems in the community, providing promotive, preventive, curative and rehabilitative services' • '...provision of essential drugs'
Organisation of care	• Organisation of service delivery • Insufficient number of staff • Waiting times • Treatment protocols	• Adequate resources • Interventions focused on determinants of poor health
Doctor's role	• Availability of doctor services • Waiting times • Travel times • Role of nurses limited	• Teams of health professionals with specific and sophisticated biomedical and social skills
Attitudes	• Vary between individuals	• Equity
Referral services management of complex conditions	• Quality and standard of clinical services • Transport • Communication between primary and referral systems • Language barriers • Distance • Time loss • Teamwork • Users vulnerable • High staff turnover and decreased continuity • Poor compliance	• 'Integrated, functional and mutually supportive referral systems to facilitate a continuum of care • Adequate resources • Teams of health professionals with specific and sophisticated biomedical- and social skills • 'People have the right and duty to participate individually and collectively in the planning and implementation of their healthcare'

Source: Principles sourced from Declaration of Alma Ata, 1978 [2]

'We left here on Sunday morning just past eight. We got to Kimberley 6 o'clock Sunday night. The doctor saw us on the Wednesday. I was tired, flustered and sad. I do not know the place [*Kimberley*].'

Rehabilitation

Rosie did not receive rehabilitation, assistive devices or exercises and was not treated by the outreach physio-, occupational- and speech therapists who visited the town weekly:

'The doctor [*at tertiary level*] said that the people who give the exercises must come to her. Then she will get better…He talked about it but nothing further.'

Case two – Susan

Susan was a 62-year old lady on initial interview. She fell in March 2008, went to the CHCC with severe pain in her left hip and was immediately referred to the secondary hospital.

Referral services

'That same Sunday they took me to [*name of secondary hospital removed*] in the ambulance. There they took an x-ray of the leg. They said that nothing had broken and I can go home… I was treated very carelessly… They gave me a Brufen pill and told me there is nothing wrong, but I had so much pain. So much so that I was crying of pain that night… The next morning they told me to get up. They said I must get up and climb off; that I am a hypochondriac and other horrible things. Used bad language. I told them, I cannot get up. So they brought a wheelchair, and told me to get in. I could not get in, because I was in too much pain. Every movement was painful. So they helped me, but were very rough.'

'It wounded me terribly. I knew I had pain and was not a hypochondriac. It made me feel like a nothing. They brushed me aside.'

Management of complex conditions

At home, the pain persisted and her husband went back to the CHCC where they gave him pain medication for her. This did not provide respite and they decided to consult a private general practitioner. She said:

'When the doctor came, he picked up my legs and put them down again and said that there was a fracture. He immediately sent for the x-rays from [*name of secondary hospital removed*] and when he looked at them, he saw the fracture. He felt that I should actually go for an operation. He can't do it for me – I mean, he is a private doctor. He is expensive, and we cannot afford it. I had to do it through the state.'

But service providers at primary level refused to let her to go back for a second opinion:

'Every time they told him [*husband*] that I must stay in bed for 6 weeks. Then they give him pain pills for me. So I took the pain pills and it became what, 6 months. There was no improvement.'

[*Husband took over the narrative*] 'So I took her with my own private transport to [*name of secondary hospital removed*]. When we got there the specialist…told her that it was too late, they can't do anything for her. We decided that while they cannot do anything for her in the Northern Cape, we will go to the Western Cape. There they told me that it was cancer, and because of that she will not recover. They told me they cannot do anything for her. At that point they wrote her off and told me I must find a clinic or place where she can die. But, I said that I would not leave her there. I rented a pick-up and put her on a wooden board in the back. I took planks and hammered it together and put her on top of it, because she was not allowed to move and we drove home like that. I had to drag her into the house. I dragged her on a mattress, like an animal.'

Primary healthcare

Susan then said:

'…but she [*the outreach doctor*] said she is sorry, she will not touch me. She stood as far as that thing from the bed [*points to over-bed table, standing about a half meter from the bed*], because she did not want to touch me.'

'It's the second week now that I haven't got my Aldomed…we have been waiting.'

This was in 2009 and at the time of this being written in 2013 she was still alive. She suffers uncertainty with regard to the future as indicated in an interview in June 2012:

'For me there is always that question hanging. [*pause*] Why am I lying here? Do I really have cancer like the doctors said?'

Client-centred care

Both case studies illustrated challenges with regard to communication, explanations to users, seeking user's opinions, involving them in decision-making processes and a lack of choice. These challenges often left users vulnerable.

As illustrated in case study one, language barriers were experienced at primary level. However, this was not limited to primary level:

'The people [*users*] will tell you they were in Kimberley [*name of tertiary hospital removed*], but they have no idea what is wrong with them because the doctor spoke English and they do not understand English…it is also a problem in [*name of secondary hospital removed*] since two of the permanent doctors are from other countries and they have limited Afrikaans. They can cope, but only up to a certain point. This causes misunderstandings' (Male, provider, age mid-twenties).

Case study one further illustrates that the users' opinions were not sought and that they did not receive explanations around management strategies. Other results indicated that users were not told or did not understand what was wrong with them: '….they do not know what the diagnosis is' (Female, user, 43 years old).

Users had no choice with regard to which professional they could consult or to which hospital they were referred. They could not consult a doctor without the referral of a sister or a specialist without the referral of a doctor. In addition, users were not allowed to ask for a second opinion, as was illustrated in case study two.

Promotion, prevention, cure and rehabilitation

The focus of healthcare services in the study setting seemed to be on prevention and cure, with good management of common conditions. Little evidence was found regarding health-promotion activities and rehabilitation.

Even prevention and cure were hampered by a shortage of medication:

> 'The provision of drugs is uncertain, especially with diabetes and hypertension' (Male, provider, age unknown).
>
> 'Sometimes we only have one or two types of antibiotics and not necessarily the one you need to treat the condition that the person suffers from. Today we had no fever syrup for children at the clinic. If the child has a fever there is nothing we can give him' (Male, provider, age unknown).

The causes of the problem were unclear, but seemed to be connected to ordering and delivery systems as well as payment and insufficient stock in the depots:

> 'The depot say they have medication, but were not paid. Then the blame is shifted to the facilities for not submitting orders on time. But our order went through on time. Somewhere is a delay' (Female, provider, age unknown).

The lack of medication can impact on continuity of care, can increase the risk of side effects and can cause complications and permanent impairments:

> '....a five-year old child who has to wait a month will sustain damage just because there is no money to buy ten rand's worth of eye ointment' (Male, provider, age unknown).

With regard to the skills of the service providers it seems that the quality of care given and the clinical skills varied between different providers as well as from condition to condition. However, in general, the standard of primary care at clinic level was good. In addition, results like those in case study two pointed toward sisters referring appropriately to doctors and referral services.

Organisation of care

Service provision at the CHCC was organised in such a way that certain users received preferential treatment on specific days as illustrated in case study one. CHCC staff said that nobody will be turned away on those days, but that they will have to wait longer. Users, however, experienced the situation differently:

> '....it was a day that the doctor was there...then all shutters go up. Nobody can see no-one for nothing [*sic*]. You cannot even mention the problem – how do they know whether it is a crisis or not? I had to turn around...they did not see him [*her son*] at all that day' (Female, user, 43 years old).

In addition, case study one illustrates long waiting times and a shortage of staff.

Another aspect that related to organisation of care was treatment protocols:

> 'According to protocol you cannot start treating PTB [*pulmonary tuberculosis*] before it has been confirmed through sputum. But the problem is often, especially with HIV positive patients the sputum yield, the positive results are low [*sic*]. The person might have full blown PTB, but the sputum might be empty [*sic*] under the microscope. Then you have to grow a culture for six weeks. I feel there have [*sic*] to be room for doctors to use their clinical judgement' (Male, provider, age unknown).

Doctor's role

Outreach doctors visited the community for eight hours per week. All participants agreed that this was not enough:

> '....the appointment of many of the people whose condition is not an emergency was postponed for a week or two. It is not ideal, but some people have to wait for a period of time' (Male, provider, age unknown).

Users have died whilst waiting:

> 'I took my daughter, who was very sick to the clinic on Thursday. The sister said I must come back on the Monday to see the doctor. The Sunday morning I found her dead in her bed. She died' (Male, user, 65 years old).

In the case of an emergency, the user was transported to the secondary hospital. However, this took time and impairments could worsen:

> 'My one son was in an accident. An airplane had to come that night to pick him up. They saved his life. They say his one leg had gotten too cold and now he is a cripple for the rest of his life. I wonder what could have happened if a doctor were there at the scene. By that I don't mean that doctors save lives – the Lord is in control. One is just reassured by the fact that there is a doctor' (Female, user, 73 years old).

Other issues mentioned included that rape victims and women experiencing labour complications must travel to the secondary hospital. In addition, professional nurses cannot issue a death certificate. Healthcare providers were ambivalent on the subject:

> 'There is not enough work for a doctor. He will be sitting around' (Female, provider, age unknown).
>
> 'We will appreciate a permanent doctor. Sometimes we have to treat cases. Och!! It makes your hair stand on end. And you are on your own...and you have to take such serious decisions' (Female, provider, age unknown).

Attitudes

Both case studies illustrated attitudinal challenges amongst healthcare service providers. However, the findings indicated that the attitudes of service providers depended on the individual person, with some being respectful, courteous, helpful and friendly and others less so.

Referral services

Dissatisfaction with referral services was voiced. Case study two provides some insight into possible causes of the dissatisfaction. Challenges included the standard of clinical services, transport, loss of time, loss of feedback and logistical issues.

One healthcare provider felt that the skills of doctors at the referral centres were substandard:

> '...no support on secondary level and quality of medicine practice by outreach specialists poor' (Male, provider, age unknown).

Some users preferred not to be referred to tertiary services:

> 'A lot of patients do not want to go to Kimberley or Upington anymore. They ask me with tears in their eyes to rather keep them here. They will rather die here before I refer them again' (Male, provider, age unknown).

Reasons for this unwillingness included aspects such as poor quality of care ('the guys come back with pressure sores' [Male, provider, age unknown]), language ('language is a big issue' [Male, provider, age unknown]), lack of support systems, the poor living conditions in the overnight facilities ('You have to overnight in an out of the way place. You have to take your own duvet or blanket. Sometimes the mattresses are covered in blood. It is not pleasant at all' [Male, user, 58 years old]) and transport.

Transport to the secondary hospital was provided through stretcher ambulances. Users had misgivings about this form of transport and complaints included the poor condition of the roads, fast and reckless driving, disrespect for users and that it was unsafe and uncomfortable:

> '...to sit on a stretcher in an ambulance is life threatening. These are gravel roads, and if the driver suddenly steps on the brake, there is nothing to hold on to. So you are going to get hurt in that ambulance...' (Male, user, 58 years old).

The same ambulances used to transport users to the secondary hospitals for appointments are used for emergency transport and are thus not always available in town: 'I had the baby on the farm...when the birth pains started I told him [*husband*] to phone' (Female, user, 37 years old). However, the ambulance had left on a routine trip to the secondary hospital and could not come to fetch her. This user delivered the baby on the farm unattended by anyone but her husband.

When patients visited the tertiary hospital, notes were often mislaid:

> 'Sometimes they come back with a letter, but at other times, I do not know what happens, whether they lose it in the ambulance. When you phone the specialist they said they always give a letter. Either the patients lose it, or the ambulance lose it [*sic*] and the patient cannot tell you what was said' (Male, provider, age unknown).

Management of complex conditions

User outcomes pointed to a problem with regard to the management of complex conditions, as illustrated by case study two. This impression was also confirmed by health service providers. According to the providers, the need for teamwork and specialist support in complex cases made it difficult since consulting a specialist involved travelling long distances. Distances and the low population density, with the resultant limited availability of services, caused loss of time:

> '...the Northern Cape has its challenges, because it is far from most things... It often takes a week or two to finish the work up of a patient and come to a decision. X-rays, blood results are not completed on the same day, so the patient has to come back' (Male, provider, age unknown).

> 'In an emergency our biggest challenge is the distances. If somebody has been shot and has to go to Kimberley the road is just too long and there is a good chance that he might die on the way' (Male, provider, age unknown).

Other aspects mentioned included a lack of compliance on the part of the patients – 'They do not attend the appointments' (Female, provider, age unknown) – and high staff turnover:

> 'I think a big problem with continuity is that every year there is someone different, for example with occupational therapy the one person leave in December and the next one only come in January [*sic*]. Thus there is not handover' (Female, provider, age unknown).

Ethical considerations

The study received ethical clearance from the Committee for Human Research of the University of Stellenbosch (clearance reference number N09/10/270) and permission to access the CHCC in the study setting was obtained from the Northern Cape Department of Health. Participation in the study was voluntary and all participants signed an informed consent form. All data will be kept confidential.

Trustworthiness

Rigour

Rigour was achieved through prolonged engagement, persistent observation, triangulation, reflection and maintenance of a chain of evidence.[43] Prolonged engagement should assist researchers to develop a comprehensive understanding of the study context and phenomena under study. The primary author collected data for various lengths of time during a three-year period. In addition, she is a member of the study community. During data collection the primary author focused on being constantly aware of what was meant by the participants and made notes on her observations throughout in an attempt to capture the mood and feelings of participants. Statements were probed by asking for explanations in a quest for better understanding. Depth of understanding was enhanced by going back to the participants to further explore issues that were found to be unclear during data analysis.[34] Triangulation was used in order to ensure a rich and comprehensive account of study phenomena.[43,44] Triangulation of sources was achieved by interviewing the same person at different points in time and by interviewing people with different interests in the phenomena under study such as healthcare users, key informants and healthcare service providers. In addition, data were collected in various ways such as interviews, case studies and through observation. The primary author kept a journal on her thoughts and reflections throughout the study process. Through this she tried to remain aware of her own values and background whilst seeking participants' interpretation of various situations. Finally, all data, field notes, reflections, documents and notes on discussions with the co-author and EquitAble team were kept in order to allow for independent analysis or review should anyone wish to conduct one in order to verify findings and conclusions.

Discussion

The declaration of Alma Ata states that PHC must be '... accessible to individuals and families in the community through their full participation'.[2] No evidence of user participation in healthcare service management was found in the current study. Key to ensuring equity and quality of primary healthcare services is building relationships with communities and involving community members in healthcare services. A starting point might be service monitoring through consumer groups.[45]

Furthermore it seems that care in this setting was not client-centered and that individual users were not enabled to allow them to manage their conditions. Literature indicates that empathetic healthcare providers enable users by listening to their opinions and explaining the cause, prevention and management of the disease.[46] However, language barriers, rigid protocols, insufficient explanations, some attitudinal challenges and a failure to seek the opinions of users and include users in the planning of management strategies point towards a lack of client-centered services in the current study and might, at least in part, have caused the non-compliance pointed out by a provider. Goudge et al. connected a lack of understanding of the condition, whether due to poor or no explanations or language barriers, to incorrect or no adherence to treatment regimes.[40] In addition, providers must be allowed flexibility in clinical decision making instead of having to follow rigid protocols which, according to Schaay & Sanders, might reduce the scope of primary healthcare to a set of technical curative interventions with little attention being given to the determinants of ill health.[4]

The results showed that prevention and cure were covered in the study setting, but the efforts were hampered by a lack of medication. This finding is in keeping with findings from other South African studies.[40,41,47,48] However, participants in other settings, even rural settings, could access pharmacies or secondary hospitals for supplies in instances where the clinic was out of stock.[40] The closest private pharmacy and secondary hospital to the current study setting is 200 km away, making this solution less feasible for the study population. From the data it seems as if the problem was caused by logistical issues such as orders, payment and deliveries. One way of addressing the problem could be through standard pre-packed kits. However, these do not take into account variations in morbidity patterns.[38] A more viable long-term solution, which at the same time invests in human-resource development, is to train managers at district level with regard to dealing with these logistical issues, coupled with monitoring and evaluation processes to ensure long-term adherence to minimum standards.

The professional nurses at the CHCC seemingly provided curative care within the spectrum of what they were used to, namely, the everyday ailments most often seen at primary level,[49] but had inadequate skills to deal with more complex conditions and might have been supported inadequately at secondary level, as indicated by Susan's case. A study from rural Australia reported similar challenges and found that it took a long time to arrive at a diagnosis. They ascribed this time lapse to limited availability of doctors in rural areas.[11] This study would like to echo this sentiment and say that even if the doctor at primary level could not made the diagnosis, the increased authority[49] that goes with being a doctor might have facilitated more timely second opinions.

It seems that time loss, delayed treatment and other challenges with regard to curative care mentioned in the results could be addressed, to some extent, through appointing a doctor in this setting. In addition, according to PHC policy, service providers – including doctors – are to focus on communities and health promotion through addressing the social determinants of disease as well as focusing on curative healthcare. Thus a permanent doctor in this community would, as traditional leader of the healthcare team in South Africa, be ideally placed to initiate health promotion in the study setting. The team can expand promotive and preventative services in accordance with primary healthcare principles and, as urged by previous authors, through identifying community-specific determinants of the burden of disease and assisting the community to develop and implement health-promotion programmes to address this within the context of the family, community and culture.[50]

Furthermore, primary healthcare is dependent on an integrated referral system to facilitate a continuum of care through all levels and places of healthcare in the system.[3,4] The results of this study imply a lack of an adequate referral system and show that PHC, even in instances where users were satisfied with the services delivered at primary level, can fail if not supported by a well-functioning referral structure. Users expressed satisfaction with the management of common conditions at PHC level, whilst dissatisfaction with the management of conditions that needed more intervention than what could be provided at the CHCC was also expressed. Dissatisfaction was severe enough to make users choose not to access government-provided referral services, even in the face of adverse health outcomes.

Another aspect that requires attention is the way the ambulance is used. A baby was born unattended since the ambulance was used to drive users for routine visits to referral services. These routine trips occur three or four days a week and any number of emergencies requiring the urgent use of an ambulance can happen in town during that time. In addition, users sat on stretchers with no safety belts and nowhere to hold on whilst being driven at speed over gravel roads in poor condition. One of the study participants suggested the use of a small bus for routine trips to secondary- and tertiary-care institutions, which would leave the ambulance and trained emergency medical technicians free to attend to emergencies.

Limitations of the study

This was a qualitative study performed in one rural town. Recommendations can thus only be applied to other rural settings after careful comparison of demographic and contextual details.

It is also a limitation that the views of managers were not sought during data collection. Although some of the findings were discussed with two managers, one from district and one from provincial level, no interviews were conducted with managers *per se*.

Data were analysed by one researcher only. Although all findings and interpretations were discussed with other members of the EquitAble team, the credibility of findings could have been enhanced if data had been analysed by more than one person.

Conclusion

According to the findings, the principles of PHC were not implemented with complete success in this rural setting. The community was not involved in service management and individual clients were not involved adequately in their healthcare. Services were curative and preventative in nature, with little evidence of health promotion, and although the need for rehabilitation was acknowledged, it was not provided. In order to develop health-promotion strategies the burden of disease and the determinants of ill health in the study community must be explored through further study. In that way, service providers, users and the community would be able to act on the information and focus on addressing the determinants of ill health in this community through health-promotion activities. The delivery of rehabilitation services to the community will be explored in a separate article.

Recommendations

The initiation of a community-health forum through which community members can voice their pleasure, frustration and hopes for healthcare and which can assess services against predetermined minimum standards and criteria for quality is recommended.[45] It is also recommended that a doctor be appointed in the community to assist with curative work and to drive a process focused on determining and addressing the determinants of ill health in the community.

Other recommendations include the training of district- and local service managers in the logistical management of ensuring a constant supply of drugs, using a Kombi-type vehicle to provide user transport for routine visits to secondary- and tertiary healthcare services and providing translators in instances where service providers cannot speak Afrikaans.

Acknowledgements

This research was funded by the European Commission Framework Programme 7, Project Title: 'Enabling universal and equitable access to healthcare for vulnerable people in resource-poor settings in Africa', grant agreement number 223501. Thanks are also extended to Martha Geiger for reviewing a draft of this article and providing valuable input.

Competing interests

The authors declare that they have no financial or personal relationship(s) which may have inappropriately influenced them in writing this article.

Authors' contributions

S.V. (University of Stellenbosch) was involved in project design, did the data collection and analysis and drafted the article. M.S. (University of Stellenbosch) was involved in project design, data collection and made conceptual contributions to the article.

References

1. Naledi T, Barron P, Schneider H. Primary health care in SA since 1994 and implications of the new vision for PHC Re-engineering. In: Padarath A, English R, editors. South African Health Review 2011. Durban: Health Systems Trust, 2011. p. 17–28.
2. Declaration of Alma Ata. International conference on primary health care. Alma Ata, USSR, 6–12 September, 1978.
3. World Health Organization. The World Health Report 2008 – primary health care (now more than ever). Geneva: World Health Organization; 2008.
4. Schaay N, Sanders D. International perspective on primary health care over the past 30 years. In: Barron P, Roma-Reardon J, editors. South African Health Review 2011. Durban: Health Systems Trust, 2008. p. 3–16.
5. Kleinert S, Horton R. South Africa's health: departing for a better future? Lancet. 2009;374(9692):759–760. http://dx.doi.org/10.1016/S0140-6736(09)61306-4
6. Coovadia H, Jewkes R, Barron P, et al. The health and health system of South Africa: historical roots of current public health challenges. Lancet. 2009;374(9692):817–834. http://dx.doi.org/10.1016/S0140-6736(09)60951-X
7. Katzenellenbogen J, Hoffman M. Levels of prevention. In Joubert G, Ehrlich R, editors. Epidemiology: A research manual for South Africa. 2nd ed. Cape Town: Oxford University Press; 2007. p. 16–17.
8. Mayosi BM, Lawn JE, Van Niekerk A, et al. Health in South Africa: changes and challenges since 2009. Lancet. 2012;380(9858):2029–2043. http://dx.doi.org/10.1016/S0140-6736(12)61814-5
9. Gaede B, Versteeg M. The state of the right to health in rural South Africa. In: Padarath A, English R, editors. South African Health Review 2011. Durban: Health Systems Trust, 2011. p. 99–106.
10. Cooke R, Couper I, Versteeg M. Human resources for rural health. In: Padarath A, English R, editors. South African Health Review 2011. Durban: Health Systems Trust, 2011. p. 107–118. PMid:21872609 PMCid:PMC3191284
11. FitzGerald M, Pearson A, McCutcheon H. Impact of rural living on the experience of chronic illness. Aust J Rural Health. 2001;9(5):235–240. http://dx.doi.org/10.1046/j.1440-1584.2001.00398.x, PMid:11736847
12. Philo C, Parr H, Burns N. Rural madness: a geographical reading and critique of the rural mental health literature. J Rural Studies. 2003;19(3):259–281. http://dx.doi.org/10.1016/S0743-0167(03)00005-6
13. Goins RT, Williams KA, Carter MW, et al. Perceived barriers to health care access among rural older adults: a qualitative study. J Rural Health. 2005;21(3):206–213. http://dx.doi.org/10.1111/j.1748-0361.2005.tb00084.x, PMid:16092293
14. Brems C, Johnson ME, Warner TD, et al. Barriers to healthcare as reported by rural and urban interprofessional providers. J Interprof Care. 2006;20(2):105–118. http://dx.doi.org/10.1080/13561820600622208, PMid:16608714
15. Arcury TA, Gesler WM, Preisser JS, et al. The effects of geography and spatial behavior on health care utilization among the residents of a rural region. Health Serv Res. 2005;40(1):135–156. http://dx.doi.org/10.1111/j.1475-6773.2005.00346.x, PMid:15663706, PMCid:PMC1361130
16. Buchanan RJ, Stuifbergen A, Chakravorty BJ, et al. Urban/rural differences in access and barriers to health care for people with multiple sclerosis. J Health Hum Serv Adm. 2006;29(3):360–375. PMid:17571473
17. Cummins P. Access to health care in the Western Cape. Lancet. 2002;360(Suppl):S49–S50. http://dx.doi.org/10.1016/S0140-6736(02)11820-4
18. Elliot-Schmidt R, Strong J. The concept of well-being in a rural setting: understanding health and illness. Aust J Rural Health. 1997;5(2):59–63. http://dx.doi.org/10.1111/j.1440-1584.1997.tb00239.x
19. Hjortsberg CA, Mwikisa CN. Cost of access to health services in Zambia. Health Policy Plan. 2002;17(1):71–77. http://dx.doi.org/10.1093/heapol/17.1.71
20. Obrist B, Iteba N, Lengeler C, et al. Access to health care in contexts of livelihood insecurity: a framework for analysis and action. PLOS Med. 2007;4(10):1584–1588. http://dx.doi.org/10.1371/journal.pmed.0040308, PMid:17958467, PMCid:PMC2039761
21. Kiwanuka SN, Ekirapa EK, Peterson S, et al. Access to and utilisation of health services for the poor in Uganda: a systematic review of available evidence. Trans R Soc Trop Med Hyg. 2008;102(11):1067–1074. http://dx.doi.org/10.1016/j.trstmh.2008.04.023, PMid:18565559
22. Peters DH, Garg A, Bloom G, et al. Poverty and access to health care in developing countries. Ann N Y Acad Sci. 2008;1136:161–171. http://dx.doi.org/10.1196/annals.1425.011, PMid:17954679
23. Ansah EK, Narh-Bana S, Asiamah S, et al. Effect of removing direct payment for health care on utilisation and health outcomes in Ghanaian children: a randomised controlled trial. PLOS Med. 2009;6(1):e1000007. http://dx.doi.org/10.1371/journal.pmed.1000007, PMid:19127975, PMCid:PMC2613422
24. Bakeera SK, Wamala SP, Galea S, et al. Community perceptions and factors influencing utilization of health services in Uganda. Int J Equity Health. 2009;8:25. http://dx.doi.org/10.1186/1475-9276-8-25, PMid:19602244, PMCid:PMC2717964
25. Lee S, Martinez G, Ma GX, et al. Barriers to health care access in 13 Asian American communities. Am J Health Behav. 2010;34(1):21–30. http://dx.doi.org/10.5993/AJHB.34.1.3, PMid:19663748

26. Helman CG. Culture, health and illness. 5th ed. London: Hodder Arnold; 2007.

27. Mannan H. Enabling universal and equitable access to healthcare for vulnerable people in resource poor settings in Africa: EquitAble. Dublin: Centre for Global Health, Trinity College Dublin; 2008.

28. Mannan H, Amin M, MacLachlan M, The EquitAble Consortium. The EquiFrame Manual: A tool for evaluating and promoting the inclusion of vulnerable groups and core concepts of human rights in health policy documents. Dublin: The Global Health Press; 2011.

29. Schneider M, Eide AH, Amin M, et al. Inclusion of vulnerable groups in health policies: Regional policies on health priorities in Africa. African Journal of Disability. 2013;2(1). http://dx.doi.org/10.4102/ajod.v2i1.40

30. Karoo Hoogland municipal integrated development plan, 2009–2011; 2009.

31. Statistics South Africa. Census 2011 Statistical release – P0301.4. Pretoria: Statistics South Africa [document on internet]. [c2012] [cited 2012 Nov.]. Available from: www.statssa.gov.za

32. Anonymous. World atlas for South Africans. 2nd ed. Cape Town: Sunbird Publishers, South Africa; 2008.

33. Leon J. Gaffney's Local Government in South Africa2007–2008: official yearbook. Johannesburg: The Gaffney Group.

34. Domholdt E. Rehabilitation research: principles and applications. 3rd ed. San Francisco: Elsevier Saunders; 2005. PMid:15944880

35. Khan MM, Hotchkiss DR, Berruti AA, et al. Geographic aspects of poverty and health in Tanzania: does living in a poor area matter? Health Policy Plan. 2005;21(2):110–122. http://dx.doi.org/10.1093/heapol/czj008, PMid:16361350

36. McGibbon E, Etowa J, McPherson C. Health-care access as a social determinant of health. Can Nurse. 2008;104(7):22–27. PMid:18856224

37. Leight SB. The application of a vulnerable populations conceptual model to rural health. Public Health Nurs. 2003;20(6):440–448. http://dx.doi.org/10.1046/j.1525-1446.2003.20604.x, PMid:14629675

38. Mamdani M, Bangser M. Poor people's experiences of health services in Tanzania: a literature review. Reprod Health Matters. 2004;12(24):138–153. http://dx.doi.org/10.1016/S0968-8080(04)24135-0

39. Mechanic D, Tanner J. Vulnerable people, groups, and populations: societal view. Health Aff (Millwood). 2007;26(5):1220–1230. http://dx.doi.org/10.1377/hlthaff.26.5.1220, PMid:17848429

40. Goudge J, Gilson L, Russell S, et al. The household costs of health care in rural South Africa with free public primary care and hospital exemptions for the poor. Trop Med Int Health. 2009;14(4):458–467. http://dx.doi.org/10.1111/j.1365-3156.2009.02256.x, PMid:19254274

41. Uys LR. Universal access to health care: if not now, when? Reflect Nurs Leadersh. 2001;27(2):20–23.

42. Smith JA, Flowers P, Larkin M. Interpretative phenomenological analysis: theory, method and research. London: Sage; 2009.

43. Cohen D, Crabtree B. Qualitative research guidelines project. July 2006. [page on internet]. [c2006] [cited 2013 Aug 18]. Available from: http://www.qualres.org/HomeExam-3705.html

44. Denzin NK, Lincoln YS. Introduction. In: Denzin NK, Lincoln YS, editors. The SAGE handbook for qualitative research. 3rd ed. Thousand Oaks, California: Sage Publications; 2005. p. 1–31.

45. Logie DE, Rowson M, Mugisha NM, et al. Affordable primary health care in low-income countries: Can it be achieved? Afr J Prm Health Care Fam Med. 2010;2(1).

46. Birhanu Z, Woldie MK, Assefa T, et al. Determinants of patient enablement at primary health care centres in central Ethiopia: a cross-sectional study. Afr J Prm Health Care Fam Med. 2011;3(1).

47. Mashia EO, Van Wyk NC. Accessibility of district health nursing services in the greater Bronkhorstspruit. Health SA Gesondheid. 2004;9(1).

48. Walker L, Gilson L. 'We are bitter but we are satisfied': nurses as street-level bureaucrats in South Africa. Soc Sci Med. 2004;59(6):1251–1261. http://dx.doi.org/10.1016/j.socscimed.2003.12.020, PMid:15210096

49. Reid S, Mash B, Thigiti J, et al. Names and roles for the generalist doctor in Africa. Afr J Prm Health Care Fam Med. 2010;2(1).

50. Hugo JFM, Couper ID, Thigiti J, et al. Equity in health care: Does family medicine have a role? Afr J Prm Health Care Fam Med. 2010;2(1).

11

Overweight and obesity profiles in Niger Delta Region, Nigeria

Authors:
Alphonsus U. Idung[1]
Festus Abasiubong[2]
Sunday B. Udoh[1]
Uwemedimbuk S. Ekanem[3]

Affiliations:
[1]Faculty of Clinical Sciences, Department of Family Medicine, College of Health Sciences, University of Uyo, Nigeria

[2]Faculty of Clinical Sciences, Department of Psychiatry, College of Health Sciences, University of Uyo, Nigeria

[3]Department of Community Health, Faculty of Clinical Sciences, College of Health Sciences, University of Uyo, Nigeria

Correspondence to:
Alphonsus Idung

Email:
dridung@yahoo.com

Postal address:
Department of Family Medicine, University of Uyo, c/o P.O. Box 4208, University of Uyo Post Office, Uyo, Akwa Ibom State, Nigeria, 520003

Introduction: Overweight and obesity are global public health problems because of their effect on individuals, families and communities. The objective of this study was to describe the profile of overweight and obesity amongst adult outpatients in Uyo in the Niger Delta region of Nigeria.

Method: This was a cross-sectional descriptive study done between October 2011 and March 2012. Using a systematic sampling technique, 584 subjects aged 18–65 years were recruited; data were collected with a structured questionnaire. Subjects were measured for height, weight, waist and hip circumferences. Body mass index (BMI) and waist–hip ratio (WHR) were calculated. Subjects with a BMI of 25.0 kg/m² – 29.9 kg/m² were regarded as being overweight whilst a BMI of > 30.0 kg/m² was regarded as obese. Subjects with a WHR of > 0.90 for men or > 0.85 for women were regarded as having abnormal WHR.

Results: Of the 584 subjects, 196 (36.6%) were men and 388 (66.4%) women. The mean age for men and women was 43.3 ± 17.8 years and 50.2 ± 13.6 years, respectively. The prevalence of overweight amongst men was 39.8% versus 31.7% for women; obesity in men was 28.0% versus 52.0% in women. Overweight and obesity were more prevalent in subjects aged 25–54 years and amongst married subjects. There was a significant relationship between obesity and television viewing ($p = 0.003$). Hypertension ($p = 0.008$) and osteoarthropathies ($p = 0.043$) were more prevalent amongst the obese than the non-obese subjects.

Conclusion: Overweight and obesity are now common in our environment. There is therefore a need for more public education about the health consequences of big body size.

Profils de surpoids et d'obésité dans la région du delta du Niger au Nigeria

Introduction: Le surpoids et l'obésité sont des problèmes mondiaux de santé publique du fait de leur effet sur les individus, les familles et les communautés. L'objectif de cette étude était de décrire le profil de surpoids et d'obésité parmi les patients ambulatoires adultes à Uyo, dans la région du delta du Niger, au Nigeria.

Méthode: Il s'agissait d'une étude descriptive transversale effectuée entre octobre 2011 et mars 2012. 584 sujets de 18-65 ans ont été recrutés selon une technique d'échantillonnage systématique; les données ont été obtenues à l'aide d'un questionnaire structuré. La taille, le poids, les tours de taille et de hanches ont été mesurés. L'Indice de masse corporelle (IMC) et le Rapport taille-hanches (RTH) ont été calculés. Les sujets présentant un IMC compris entre 25.0 et 29.9 kg/m² étaient considérés comme étant en surpoids, alors qu'un IMC > 30.0 kg/m² était considéré comme de l'obésité. Les sujets présentant un RTH > 0.90 pour les hommes ou > 0.85 pour les femmes étaient considérés comme présentant un RTH anormal.

Résultats: Parmi les 584 sujets, 196 (36.6%) étaient des hommes et 388 (66.4%) des femmes. L'âge moyen pour les hommes et les femmes était respectivement de 43.3 ± 17.8 ans et 50.2 ± 13.6 an. La prévalence de surpoids parmi les hommes était de 39.8% contre 31.7% pour les femmes; l'obésité chez les hommes était de 28.0% contre 52.0% chez les femmes. Le surpoids et l'obésité étaient plus répandus chez les sujets âgés entre 25 et 54 ans et parmi les sujets mariés. On a pu observer une relation significative entre l'obésité et le fait de regarder la télévision ($p = 0.003$). L'hypertension ($p = 0.008$) et les ostéo-arthropathies ($p = 0.043$) étaient plus répandues parmi les sujets obèses que chez les non-obèses.

Conclusion: Le surpoids et l'obésité sont maintenant courants dans notre environnement. Il est donc nécessaire d'éduquer davantage le public à propos des conséquences sur la santé d'une grande taille corporelle.

Introduction

Overweight and obesity are a global public health problem because of their effect on individuals, families and communities. It is estimated that about one billion people are overweight and more than 300 million obese worldwide.[1]

Overweight and obesity are reported to account for 44% of the global burden of diabetes mellitus, 23% of ischaemic heart disease and 7% – 41% of some malignancies.[1] It is estimated that of the projected 64 million deaths worldwide in 2015, 41 million (64%) will result from non-communicable diseases (NCDs), of which obesity is a major contributor.[2]

The World Health Organization (WHO) defines 'overweight' as a body mass index of 25.0 kg/m^2 – 29.9 kg/m^2 and 'obesity' as a body mass index of > 30.0 kg/m^2.[2] The body mass index (BMI) is usually calculated by dividing the weight in kilograms by the square of the height in metres (BMI = Wt [kg] / Ht^2 [m]).[3] Its flaw lies in the fact that it may misclassify a very muscular person as obese and it may also overestimate fatness in hypertrophied athletes or underestimate fatness in the elderly.[4] Body mass index also cannot estimate intra-abdominal fat which is an independent predictor of health risk.[5]

The waist-hip ratio (WHR) as a measure of obesity has been judged to be very valuable as it provides an index of the proportion of intra-abdominal fat.[4,5] The normal waist circumference for women is 88 cm or less, whilst the normal waist circumference for men is 102 cm or less. Average waist-hip ratio values for men and women are about 0.93 (range 0.75–1.10) and 0.83 (range 0.70–1.0),[4,5] respectively. Some have, however, combined BMI with the measure of waist circumference in order to predict disease risk in patients.[6]

The aetiology of obesity is poorly understood, but genetic, environmental, socioeconomic and viral factors have been implicated.[7,8] Other factors include lack of sufficient physical exercise arising from unplanned urbanisation, the lure of technology and safety fears. It has also been documented that adults who watch four or more hours of television each day are four times more likely to be overweight or obese than those who spend less time in this pursuit.[8] Overweight and obesity are on the increase in Africa and might assume an epidemic dimension in the near future.[9] The reported prevalence of overweight and obesity amongst urban dwellers in Africa is 35% and it is estimated that by 2025, 75% of the obese people worldwide will reside in the developing world.[1,9]

The reported prevalence of overweight and obesity amongst urban dwellers in Jos, North Central Nigeria is 21.4%, made up of 19.4% males and 23.5% females, of whom 17.2% were overweight whilst 4.2% were obese.[10] Another study from Lagos, South-West Nigeria, reported the prevalence of obesity amongst urban dwellers to be 6.9%.[11]

Published reports on the prevalence of overweight and obesity in Uyo, a community in the Niger Delta Region, South-South Nigeria are, however, scarce in the scientific literature. This study is therefore aimed at describing the occurrence of overweight and obesity amongst family medicine outpatient clinic attendees in Uyo.

It is hoped that the findings will add to the pool of available knowledge, for the purpose of increasing awareness on lifestyle issues in the region which could help prevent the epidemic of overweight and obesity with its attendant health consequences.

Research methods and design

Location of the study

This study was carried out at the family medicine outpatient clinic of the University of Uyo Teaching Hospital (UUTH). UUTH is located on the outskirts of Uyo, the capital of Akwa Ibom State in Nigeria. Nigeria is divided into six geopolitical zones as follows: North-East, North-West, North-Central, South-East, South-West and South-South. Uyo is located in the South-South geopolitical zone, which is often referred to as the Niger Delta Region of Nigeria. It is one of the major oil-producing areas in the region. UUTH is the only tertiary and referral health institution in the State and its environs, serving a population of approximately 3.9 million people.

Subjects

The study was carried out amongst outpatients attending the family medicine clinic for various medical problems. They were recruited using a systematic random-sampling method with a sampling interval of six. Each recruited subject was given information regarding the research objectives after written informed consent was obtained. Numbers ranging from one to six were assigned to the first six subjects who met the inclusion criteria. The first respondent was chosen by simply balloting one of the numbers from a basket containing the assigned numbers. Subsequently, every sixth subject was recruited into the study. Where, however, a subject was judged to be too ill at the point of recruitment into the study, that subject was dropped and the next subject who met the inclusion criteria was recruited. Other exclusions included pregnant women as well as subjects who were below the age of 18 or above 65 years of age.

Methods

This study, with a sample of 584 consenting male and female subjects, took place between October 2011 and March 2012. Weight was measured in kilograms to the nearest 0.5 kg using a Hanna-calibrated bathroom scale, model BR9011. Each subject was weighed wearing light clothing without shoes or stockings. The height of the subjects was measured using an improvised wooden stadiometer mounted on a vertical wall with the respondent standing erect against the wall on a horizontal floor without shoes. The head was placed so as to ensure that the external auditory meatus and the angle of the eye were on a horizontal line. The height was measured in metres to the nearest 0.1 cm. BMI was calculated as the weight (kg) / (height [m])^2 (i.e. kg/m^2).

A non-stretch tape was used to measure the body circumference. The smallest circumference between the xiphisternum and the umbilicus on expiration was taken as being the waist circumference. Measurements were taken to the nearest 0.1 cm after normal expiration with the subject in an upright position. Hip circumference was measured to the nearest 0.1 cm at the maximum posterior protuberance of the buttocks whilst the subject was standing upright with feet together.

Moreover, each of the subjects was assessed using an interviewer-administered structured questionnaire containing such information as age, marital status, highest level of education attained, income (in Nigerian Naira denomination) using the approved wage structure in the Nigerian public service.[12] Other information contained in the questionnaire included the occupational status of the respondents, which was classified as non-skilled (including labourers, pensioners and students), skilled (including tailors and teachers without a University degree) and professional (including lawyers, teachers with University degree and soldiers). The questionnaire also elicited information with regard to the average number of hours spent each day watching television and the number of days spent each week engaging in any form of structured physical exercise such as cycling, rope-skipping, trekking and/or hiking and other forms of aerobic physical exercise.

Data analysis

The statistical analysis was done using SPSS Statistics version 17.0 (IBM Corporation), distribution and cross-tabulation data were generated, the *t*-test was used to compare means and Chi-square was used to compare proportions. A *p*-value of 0.05 was used to determine the level of statistical significance.

Ethical considerations

Ethical approval for the study was obtained from the UUTH ethical committee (UUTH/AD/S/96/VOL.1X/969). A pretest of the research questionnaire was performed in order to determine its applicability, experience and logistical problems.

Results

Of the 584 subjects recruited into the study, 36.6% (n = 196) were men, whilst 66.4% (n = 388) were females.

Table 1 shows the sociodemographic and clinical characteristics of the subjects. There was a statistically-significant difference between the mean age of women (50.2 [SD = 3.6]) and men (43.3 [SD = 17.8]) (p = 0.000). Subjects between the ages of 25 and 54 were more obese (p = 0.000). Overweight and obesity was more prevalent amongst the married respondents in this study (p = 0.002). Women had a mean BMI of 30.7 kg/m^2 (SD = 5.7) versus 27.6 kg/m^2 (SD = 4.5) for men (p = 0.000). Women had a mean waist circumference of 95.3 cm (SD = 12.4) versus 91.2 cm (SD = 11.2) for men (p = 0.000). The mean hip circumference for women was 109.4 cm (SD = 14.2), whilst the mean hip circumference for men was 103.3 cm (SD = 10.4) (p = 0.000). Approximately 65.0% of the women had an abnormal WHR compared with 37.8% of the men.

Table 2 shows the lifestyle characteristics of the respondents. The number of hours spent watching television each day was a significant contributor to obesity in this study (p = 0.003). Conversely, the number of days spent doing structured physical exercise did not contribute significantly to obesity in this study (p = 0.72).

Table 3 shows the prevalence of medical conditions amongst the respondents in this study. There was a statistically-significant difference (p = 0.008) between the presence of hypertension and the presence of osteoarthropathies (p = 0.043) when comparing the obese versus the non-obese subjects in this study.

TABLE 1: Characteristics of the study population.

Variables	Subjects	
	Female (F) (n = 388 [%])	Male (M) (n = 196 [%])
Socio demographic age in years		
18–24	9 (2.3)	12 (6.1)
25–34	120 (30.9)	38 (19.4)
35–44	118 (30.4)	58 (29.6)
45–54	94 (24.2)	56 (28.6)
55–64	42 (10.8)	20 (10.2)
65	5 (1.3)	12 (6.1)
Marital status		
Single	64 (16.5)	45 (23.0)
Married	281 (72.4)	145 (74.0)
Divorced and/or separated	8 (2.1)	2 (1.0)
Widow	35 (9.0)	4 (2.0)
Educational level		
No formal education	8 (2.1)	1 (0.5)
Primary school	54 (13.9)	25 (12.8)
Secondary school	92 (23.7)	51 (26.0)
Post-Secondary school	234 (60.3)	119 (60.7)
Income		
Low	217 (56.0)	96 (49.0)
Middle	108 (27.8)	65 (33.2)
High	63 (16.2)	35 (17.8)
Occupation		
Non-skilled	75 (19.3)	28 (14.3)
Skilled	115 (29.7)	69 (35.2)
Professional	198 (51.0)	99 (50.5)
Place of residence		
Urban	244 (62.9)	123 (62.8)
Rural	144 (37.1)	73 (37.2)
Body Mass Index (kg/m^2)		
< 18.5	-	-
18.5–24.9	63 (16.2)	63 (32.1)
25.0–29.9	123 (31.7)	78 (39.8)
30.0–34.9	108 (27.8)	44 (22.4)
35.0–39.9	69 (17.8)	9 (4.6)
≥ 40.0	25 (6.4)	2 (1.0)
Waist circumference		
≤ 88 cm (F)	84 (21.6)	-
≤ 102 cm (M)	-	171 (87.2)
≥ 88 cm (F)	304 (78.4)	-
≥ 102 cm (M)	-	25 (12.8)
Quartiles of waist–hip- ratio		
≤ 0.84	136 (35.0)	57 (29.1)
0.85–0.89	142 (36.6)	65 (33.1)
> 0.93	110 (28.4)	74 (37.8)

TABLE 2: Lifestyle characteristics of the subjects.

Lifestyle characteristics	Subjects		
	Non-obese (n = 327 [%])	Obese (n = 257 [%])	p-value
How many hours do you spend to watch television each day?			
< 4 hours	273 (83.5)	189 (73.5)	0.003*
≥ 4 hours	54 (16.5)	68 (26.5)	-
How many days do you engage in structured physical exercise per week?			
None	201 (61.5)	150 (58.4)	-
1–4 days (each episode lasting up to 30 minutes)	94 (28.7)	78 (30.4)	0.72
> 5 days (each episode lasting up to 30 minutes)	32 (9.8)	29 (11.2)	-

*, Statistically significant.

TABLE 3: Prevalence of medical conditions of subjects.

Medical history	Subjects		
	Non-obese (n [%])	Obese (n [%])	p-value
Hypertension	104 (31.8)	110 (42.8)	0.008*
Diabetes mellitus	48 (14.7)	48 (18.7)	0.24
Osteoarthropathies	25 (7.6)	33 (12.8)	0.043*
Others (malaria, dyspepsia, enteric fever etc.)	24 (7.3)	23 (8.9)	0.58

*, Statistically significant.

Discussion

Malnutrition, particularly undernutrition and starvation, have long been a major problem in Africa, particularly amongst the inhabitants of rural areas. Interestingly, however, in our study we found a high prevalence of obesity amongst our subjects (52.0% for the women versus 28.0% for the men). This figure is, however, still lower than the prevalence rates of 71.6% in female and 50.5% in male hypertensive patients in Nigeria.[13]

In another population-based study, obesity was reported amongst 21% of the male and 28% of the female respondents.[14] The differences in the prevalence of obesity amongst different workers in Nigeria might be due to the differences in the study design as well as the study subjects, but it is nonetheless important to take note of the fact that obesity is no longer only a problem of the affluent or of those in developed countries.

The reasons for the increasing prevalence of obesity amongst the respondents in this study may be due to the fact that Uyo and its environs, which were predominantly an agrarian subsistent farming community less than a decade ago, are now changing into a modern metropolis because of Uyo's currents status as a State capital, coupled with rapid but unplanned urbanisation as well as a possible change from local dietary patterns.

The high prevalence of overweight women (31.7%) and men (39.8%) in this study suggests that the obesity rate will continue to rise unless drastic action is taken. The prevalence of obesity was higher in women than men, a finding that is consistent with other studies in Nigeria and various parts of Africa.[10,13,14,15]

In Ghana, obesity is reported to be six times more common in women than in men and in Morocco, four times more common.[16] Amongst Africans, including Nigerians, being overweight or obese is thought to reflect affluence and happiness, a factor that may seriously militate against any effort toward managing the problem. Married women were more obese than others in this study, a finding that is also consistent with reports from other studies.[17,18] The reason for this is that being overweight or obese is thought to reflect a husband's ability to take care of his wife and family – a serious misconception that needs to be addressed properly amongst those who are vulnerable.

Although it has been shown to be a possible contributor to overweight and obesity in this study, the role of television viewing, a largely sedentary activity, as a factor in the aetiology of overweight and obesity should be interpreted with caution.[8] The reason for this is that other factors, such as the environment and genetics, must not be overlooked. Further studies in this regard are hereby advocated.

Finding from this study also show a high prevalence of chronic medical conditions amongst the respondents, which is consistent with reports from other studies.[13,14,19,20]

The health consequences of obesity are real and serious. In addition, the economic burden in both the private and public sector is enormous, because the cost of treatment of obesity-related diseases are borne not only by the obese and their families, but also by all tax payers or contributors to the Nigerian National Health Insurance Scheme.

Limitations

One limitation of this study is that the data used is cross-sectional – it would have been more appropriate to follow up with individuals over time so as to ascertain the changes in their BMI over time as well as the presence of other risk factors. Moreover, the population used in this study does not represent the entire adult population in the Niger Delta Region of Nigeria, as it is derived only from patients attending an outpatient clinic.

Conclusion

The findings of this study have shown that overweight and obesity are prevalent amongst the outpatients seen in our hospital.

Considering the chronic nature of most disease associated with obesity as well as the enormous cost of treatment, the prospect of taking on a larger disease burden is alarming for the already poorly-funded and ill-equipped healthcare delivery system in the Niger-Delta Region of Nigeria, which is still grappling with the scourge of HIV. The scientific community is therefore encouraged to join in efforts to create more responsible solutions for the obesity epidemics at the societal level.

In view of the alarming presence of overweight and obesity amongst our respondents in particular and Nigerians in general, we recommend that citizens be encouraged to adopt a healthier lifestyle through good public sensitisation and education. Physicians and caregivers need some more training on motivational interview techniques in order to become more effective in motivating their overweight and obese patients to adopt healthier lifestyle. There is also a need to establish acceptable BMI cut-offs for overweight and obesity for Nigerians.

Family physicians should interact more with local health educators in order to promote collaboration amongst care providers and communities and to identify the most sustainable and community-friendly strategies to promote healthy weight.

There is also a need for interdisciplinary and collaborative research from family medicine, community health and urban planning so as to facilitate practice and policy changes that could foster broad population-level behavioural changes.

Acknowledgements

Competing interests

The authors declare that they have no financial or personal relationship(s) which may have inappropriately influenced them in writing this article.

Authors' contributions

A.U.I. (Department of Family Medicine, University of Uyo), F.A. (Department of Psychiatry, University of Uyo) and S.B.U. (Department of Family Medicine, University of Uyo) wrote the manuscript and U.S.E. (Department of Community Health, University of Uyo) performed the statistical analysis.

References

1. World Health Organization. WHO Technical Report Series 894; Obesity: Preventing and managing the global epidemic. [document on Internet]. c2000 [cited 2012 Nov. 05]. Available from: http://whqlibdoc.who.int/trs/WHO_TRS_894.pdf
2. World Health Organization. Preventing chronic diseases: a vital investment. Geneva: World Health Organization; 2005.
3. Garrew JS, Webster J. Quetelet's Index (Wt/Ht^2) as a measure of fatness. Int J Obes. 1985;9(2):147–153.
4. Njoku CH. Obesity measurement and management: a review. Nigerian Medical Practitioner. 2006;49(6):144–147. http://dx.doi.org/10.4314/nmp.v49i6.28821
5. Screening for obesity. Guide to clinical preventive service: Report of the Task Force, 2nd edition. Maryland: US Preventive Services Task Force; 1996. p. 219–229.
6. Finer N. Obesity. Clin Med. 2003;3(1):23–27. http://dx.doi.org/10.7861/clinmedicine.3-1-23, PMid:12617409
7. Oyekan AO. Genetics of food intake, body weight and obesity – role of leptin. Nigerian Medical Practitioner. 2005;47(6):108–112.
8. Jeffery RW, French SA. Epidemic obesity in the United States: are fast foods and television viewing contributing? Am J Public Health. 1998;88(2):277–280. http://dx.doi.org/10.2105/AJPH.88.2.277
9. Ziraba AK, Fotso JC, Ochako R. Overweight and obesity in urban Africa: a problem of the rich or the poor? BMC Public Health. 2009;9:465. http://dx.doi.org/10.1186/1471-2458-9-465, PMid:20003478, PMCid:PMC2803188
10. Puepet FH, Zoakah AI, Chuwak EK. Prevalence of overweight and obesity among urban Nigerian adults in Jos. Highland Medical Research Journal. 2002;1(1):13–16.
11. Johnson TO. Prevalence of overweight and obesity among adult subjects of an urban African population sample. Br J Prev Soc Med. 1970;24(2):105–109. PMid:5431067, PMCid:PMC1059263
12. National Minimum Wage Act, Cap N61, Laws of the Federation of Nigeria 2004, as amended, further amended by National Minimum Wage (Amendment) Act, 2011.
13. Amodu PH, Mbah IO, Lawson L. Prevalence of obesity and dyslipidaemia in hypertensives in Abuja, Nigeria. Scand J Clin Lab Invest Suppl. 2005;240:14–17. http://dx.doi.org/10.1080/00365510500236069, PMid:16112955
14. Kadiri S, Salako BL. Cardiovascular risk factors in middle aged Nigerians. East Afr Med J. 1997;74(5):303–306. PMid:9337008
15. Etukumana EA, Puepet FH, Obadofin M. Prevalence of overweight and obesity among rural adults in North Central Nigeria. Nigerian Journal of Family Practice. 2013;3(2):41–46.
16. Biritwum R, Gyapong J, Mensah G. The epidemiology of obesity in Ghana. Ghana Med J. 2005;39(3):82–85. PMid:17299549, PMCid:PMC1790818
17. Siervo M, Grey P, Nyan OA, et al. A pilot study on body image, attractiveness and body size in Gambians living in an urban community. Eat Weight Disord. 2006;11(2):100–109. PMid:16809982
18. Mvo Z, Dick J, Steyn K. Perceptions of overweight African women about acceptable body size of women and children. Curationis. 1999;22(2):27–31. http://dx.doi.org/10.4102/curationis.v22i2.719, PMid:11040616
19. Pi-Sunyer FX. Comorbidities of overweight and obesity: current evidence and research issues. MedSci Sports Exerc. 1999;31(11 Suppl):S602–608. http://dx.doi.org/10.1097/00005768-199911001-00019, PMid:10593535
20. Peeters A, Bonneux L, Nusselder WJ, et al. Adult obesity and the burden of disability throughout life. Obes Res. 2004;12(7):1145–1151. http://dx.doi.org/10.1038/oby.2004.143, PMid:15292479

12

The characteristics of HIV and AIDS patients with deep vein thrombosis at Dr. George Mukhari Academic Hospital

Authors:
Indiran Govender[1]
Honey L. Mabuza[1]
Gboyega A. Ogunbanjo[1]

Affiliations:
[1]Department of Family Medicine & PHC, Sefako Makgatho Health Sciences (formerly known as the University of Limpopo, Medunsa Campus), South Africa

Correspondence to:
Indiran Govender

Email:
indiran.govender@gmail.com

Postal address:
PO Box 222, Medunsa 0204, South Africa

Background: Deep vein thrombosis (DVT) is 10 times more prevalent in HIV and AIDS patients than in the general population and is more common in patients with severe immune suppression (CD4 < 200 cells/mL). Opportunistic infections render HIV and AIDS patients susceptible to a hypercoaguable state, including lower protein S levels.

Aim and setting: To present the profile of HIV and AIDS patients who developed DVT in the primary care wards of Dr. George Mukhari Academic Hospital (DGMAH), Garankuwa.

Methods: Cross-sectional study of clinical records of admitted HIV and AIDS patients without DVT to the primary care wards, DGMAH, from 01 February 2010 to 31 January 2011.

Results: Two hundred and twenty-nine patients were admitted and 17 (7.4%) developed DVT. Of those that developed DVT, eight (47%) had infection with tuberculosis (TB), four (24%) had pneumonia and four (24%) had gastroenteritis. The risk of developing DVT was 8/94 (8.5%) in those with TB, 4/53 (7.5%) in those with gastroenteritis and 4/75 (5.3%) in those with pneumonia. The mean duration of stay was 14.1 days in those with DVT versus 4.0 days in those without.

Conclusion: HIV (and AIDS) is a hypercoaguable state and the risk of DVT is relatively high in patients with opportunistic infections. HIV and AIDS patients who are admitted to hospital with opportunistic infections may benefit from anti-thrombotic prophylaxis and further studies are needed to evaluate this.

Caractéristiques des patients atteints du VIH et du SIDA souffrant de thrombose veineuse profonde à l'hôpital universitaire Dr. George Mukhari.

Contexte: Les thromboses veineuses profondes (DVT) sont 10 fois plus répandues chez les patients atteints du VIH et du SIDA que dans la population en général, et sont plus courantes chez les patients souffrant de suppression immunitaire grave (CD4 < 200 cellules/mL). Les infections opportunistes rendent les patients atteints du VIH et du SIDA plus susceptible à l'hyper-coagulation, y compris à des niveaux de protéine S plus faibles.

Objectif et cadre: Présenter le profil des patients atteints du VIH et du SIDA qui ont développé une DVT dans les services de soins primaires de l'hôpital universitaire Dr. George Mukhari (DGMAH), à Garankuwa.

Méthodes: Etude transversale des dossiers cliniques des patients atteints du VIH et du SIDA sans DVT admis dans les services de soins primaires du DGMAH, du 1er février 2010 au 31 janvier 2011.

Résultats: Sur les deux cent vingt et un patients admis, 17 (7.4%) ont eu une DVT. Parmi ceux qui ont eu une DVT, huit (47%) avaient la tuberculose (TB), quatre (24%) avaient une pneumonie et quatre (24%) avaient une gastroentérite. Le risque de développer une DVT était de 8/94 (8.5%) chez ceux qui avaient la tuberculose, 4/53 (7.5%) chez ceux avec une gastroentérite et 4/75 (5.3%) chez ceux qui avaient une pneumonie. La durée moyenne de l'hospitalisation était de 14.1 jours chez ceux souffrant d'une DVT contre 4.0 jours chez ceux sans DVT.

Conclusion: Le VIH (et le SIDA) est une condition d'hyper-coagulation et le risque de DVT est assez élevé chez les patients avec des infections opportunistes. Les patients atteints du VIH et du SIDA qui sont hospitalisés avec des infections opportunistes peuvent profiter d'une prophylaxie anti-thrombotique, et des études supplémentaires sont nécessaire pour l'évaluer.

Introduction

Deep vein thrombosis (DVT) is 10 times more common in HIV and AIDS patients, particularly in those with severe immune suppression (CD4 < 200 cells/mL).[1,2,3] Opportunistic infections increase the risk of HIV and AIDS patients having a thromboembolic event by lowering protein S levels and through immobility.[4,5] Such chronic inflammation in patients with HIV can elevate C4b-binding protein, which binds protein S and decreases free levels.[6] Patients seen with DVT are also more likely to be HIV-positive.[7]

The increased risk of DVT might require prophylactic management in hospitalised HIV-positive patients, but there are currently no studies to guide clinical practice. We present a profile of HIV and AIDS patients with concomitant DVT in the primary care wards of Dr. George Mukhari Academic Hospital (DGMAH), GaRankuwa.

Research methods and design

This was a cross-sectional study of clinical records of HIV and AIDS patients admitted to the primary care wards at DGMAH without concomitant DVT from 01 February 2010 to 31 January 2011. Only patients with laboratory-confirmed HIV (ELISA blood test) and who developed DVT (confirmed by D-dimer levels and ultrasound) were included in the study. Data were entered into an Excel® spreadsheet, analysed using SAS (Statistical Analysis System) software, then frequencies and proportions were computed. The Medunsa Research Ethics Committee provided ethical clearance (MREC/M/69/2010: IR).

Results

Seventeen out of 229 patients with HIV and AIDS developed DVT during the study period, which implies that 7.4% of patients developed a DVT. Six patients (35%) were on highly-active antiretroviral therapy (HAART), nine (53%) had a DVT in the right leg, 16 (94%) showed improvement on treatment and 17 (100%) were discharged on warfarin. The majority were women (n = 11; 65%) and the mean age was 40 years. Table 1 shows the reasons for admission in those who developed DVT; tuberculosis (TB) (47%), pneumonia (24%) and gastroenteritis (24%) were the most common opportunistic infections.

Table 2 shows the reasons for admission for all 229 patients and the percentage that developed DVT in each category.

TABLE 1: Morbidity in patients with HIV and AIDS and deep vein thrombosis (N = 17).

Reason for admission	Frequency n (%)
Tuberculosis	8 (47)
Pneumonia (not Tuberculosis)	4 (24)
Gastroenteritis	4 (24)
Attempted suicide	2 (12)
Anaemia	2 (12)
Cerebrovascular accident	1 (6)
Postpartum	1 (6)

TABLE 2: Risk of deep vein thrombosis with different reasons for admission of patients with HIV and AIDS (N = 229).

Reason for admission	Total number of patients n	Patients developing DVT in each category n (%)
Tuberculosis	94	8 (8.5)
Gastroenteritis	53	4 (7.5)
Stroke (Cerebrovascular accident)	1	1 (100.0)
Pneumonia (not Tuberculosis)	75	4 (5.3)
Attempted suicide	3	2 (66.7)
Diabetes Mellitus	2	0 (0.0)
Hypertension	1	0 (0.0)
Hepatitis	4	0 (0.0)
Anaemia	5	2 (40.0)
Postpartum	1	1 (100.0)

Amongst the three most common opportunistic infections and reasons for admission, the risk of developing DVT ranged from 5.3% to 8.5%, with a mean risk of 7.2%.

Patients with HIV and AIDS complicated by DVT had a mean hospital stay of 14.1 days, compared to a mean of 4.0 days for those without DVT.

Discussion

The overall risk of developing DVT in patients admitted with HIV and AIDS was 7.4% and, amongst the three most common opportunistic infections, the risk was highest in those with TB. The risk in this study group was much lower than that reported in a specialist haematology service (84%), but higher than rates reported in their controls (4%).[6] A high risk was also found in those with stroke, severe anaemia and attempted suicide, although the absolute numbers of such patients were very small. Of all those who developed DVT, the most commonly-associated condition was TB (in almost half the cases), a finding that was also reported in Brazil.[2]

Whereas 25% of the patients had more than one DVT and 6% developed pulmonary embolism in a study conducted at Mount Sinai Hospital,[1] none of our patients developed clinical pulmonary embolism. Nevertheless, the patients with DVT had a much longer hospital stay and required ongoing treatment with warfarin. Because of this study, the clinical team introduced a policy on prophylaxis with low molecular weight heparin for DVT amongst high-risk patients.

Further studies are needed to develop evidence-based clinical guidelines on the use of DVT prophylaxis in patients admitted with HIV and opportunistic infections.

Conclusion

HIV (and AIDS) is a hypercoaguable state and the risk of developing DVTs in patients with opportunistic infections is high amongst patients, particularly those with TB, admitted in our wards. These patients may benefit from anti-thrombotic prophylaxis, however further research is required in order to develop evidence-based clinical guidelines.

Acknowledgements

The authors would like to thank Dr Barua and Dr Andre Marais who assisted in the data collection.

Competing interests

The authors declare that they have no financial or personal relationship(s) that may have inappropriately influenced them in writing this article.

Authors' contributions

I.G. (Sefako Makgatho Health Sciences) was involved in the contemplation of the research idea, protocol write-up, data collection and research write-up. H.L.M. and G.A.O. (both Sefako Makgatho Health Sciences) were involved in the protocol write-up, data analysis and research write-up.

References

1. Saber AA, Aboolian A, LaRaja RD, et al. HIV/AIDS and the risk of deep vein thrombosis: A study of 45 patients with lower extremity involvement. Am Surg. 2001;67(7):645–647.
2. Cortez-Escalante JJ, Castro C, Romero GA, et al. Pulmonary thromboembolism in AIDS patient with chronic venous insufficiency, pulmonary tuberculosis and breast cancer: A case report and pathophysiology review. Rev Inst Med Trop Sao Paulo. 2006;48(2):105–108. http://dx.doi.org/10.1590/S0036-46652006000200010
3. Shen YM, Frenkel EP. Thrombosis and a hypercoagulable state in HIV-infected patients. Clin Appl Thromb Hemost. Jul;10(3):277–280.
4. Saif MW, Bona R, Greenberg B. AIDS and thrombosis: Retrospective study of 131 HIV-infected patients. AIDS Patient Care STDs. 2001;15(6):311–320. http://dx.doi.org/10.1089/108729101750279687
5. Goldstein KM, Gluckman S, Mounzer K. Challenge of coadministering antitretroviral therapy and oral anticoagulants in HIV-positive patients. AIDS Read. 2008;18(9):480–482, 486–489.
6. Hall IE, Andersen MS, Krumholz HM, Gross CP. Predictors of venous thromboembolism in patients with advanced common solid cancers. J Cancer. 2009;Article ID 182521, 9 pages.
7. Dolin R, Masur H, Saag MS. AIDS therapy e-dition. 3rd ed. Philadelphia, PA: Churchill Livingstone Elsevier; 2008.

13

Midwifery workforce profile in Limpopo Province referral hospitals

Authors:
Sam T. Ntuli[1]
Gboyega A. Ogunbanjo[2]

Affiliations:
[1]Department of Public Health Medicine, University of Limpopo, Polokwane Campus, South Africa

[2]Department of Family and Primary Health Care, University of Limpopo, Medunsa Campus, South Africa

Correspondence to:
Thembelihle Ntuli

Email:
tsntuli@hotmail.com

Postal address:
Postal Bag X9537, Polokwane 0699, South Africa

Background: In sub-Saharan Africa including South Africa, maternal mortality rates remain unacceptably high due to a shortage of registered nurses with advanced midwifery diplomas.

Objective: To determine the profile of registered nurses (RNs) involved in maternity care in public referral hospitals of the Limpopo Province, South Africa.

Method: A cross-sectional descriptive study was conducted in all maternity units of Limpopo's public referral hospitals. The study population comprised of 210 registered nurses, who became the study sample. Data on their educational profile and work experience in midwifery was analysed using STATA version 9.0.

Results: The mean age of the 210 registered nurses was 44.5 ± 9.1 years (range 21 to 62). The majority (152/210; 70%) were 40 years and older, 56% (117/210) had been working for more than 10 years, and 63/210 (30%) were due to retire within 10 years. Only 22% (46/210) had advanced midwifery diplomas, i.e. after their basic undergraduate training. Only six (2.9%) of the RNs providing maternity care in these referral hospitals were studying for advanced midwifery diplomas at the time of the study.

Conclusion: This study demonstrated a shortage of registered nurses with advanced midwifery training/diplomas in referral hospitals of the Limpopo Province. This has a potentially negative effect in reducing the high maternal mortality rate in the province.

Le profil de la pratique de sage-femme dans les hôpitaux de recours.

Présentation: En Afrique subsaharienne, Afrique du Sud comprise, les taux de mortalité maternelle reste à des niveaux élevés inacceptables en raison d'un manque d'infirmières qualifiées disposant également d'un diplôme de sage-femme.

Objectif: Déterminer le profil des infirmières qualifiées (IQ) impliquées dans les soins de santé maternelle dans les hôpitaux de recours publics de la province du Limpopo, en Afrique du Sud.

Méthode: Une étude descriptive transversale a été réalisée dans tous les services de maternité des hôpitaux de recours publics de la province du Limpopo. La population de l'étude était composée de 210 infirmières qualifiées (IQ), qui ont constitué l'échantillon de l'étude. Les données relatives à leur profil éducatif et à leur expérience professionnelle dans la profession de sage-femme ont été analysées à l'aide du logiciel STATA version 9.0.

Résultat: Les 210 infirmières qualifiées étaient en moyenne âgées de 44,5 ± 9,1 ans (fourchette allant de 21 à 62 ans). La majorité d'entre elles (152/210; 70%) était âgée de 40 ans et plus, 56% (117/210) d'entre elles exerçaient depuis plus de 10 ans, et 63/210 (30%) devaient prendre leur retraite dans les 10 années suivantes. Seules 22% (46/210) d'entre elles étaient titulaires de diplômes de sage-femme d'un niveau supérieur à leur formation de premier cycle de base. Seulement six (2.9%) IQ fournissant des soins de santé maternelle dans ces hôpitaux de recours suivaient des études pour obtenir leur diplôme de sage-femme au moment de l'étude.

Conclusion: Cette étude a mis en avant un manque d'infirmières qualifiées disposant également d'une formation/d'un diplôme de sage-femme dans les hôpitaux de recours de la province du Limpopo. Ceci a un impact potentiellement négatif sur la réduction du fort taux de mortalité maternelle dans la province.

Introduction

The World Health Organization (WHO) reported a global reduction of maternal mortality ratio (MMR) from 400 to 210 per 100 000 live births between 1990 and 2010.[1] Relatively acceptable MMR is between 12 and 15 deaths per 100,000 live births based on available USA data obtained between 2003 and 2007.[1] Progress is being made in both developed and developing countries, however, MMR remains unacceptably high in sub-Saharan Africa, despite average reductions from 850 to 500 per 100 000 live births.[2] The global decrease in MMR has been attributed to an increase in the proportion of deliveries attended to by skilled health personnel.[2] In South Africa (SA), the National Committee for the Confidential Enquiries into Maternal Deaths (NCCEMD) reported a 22% increase in MMR between 2005/2007 and 2008/2010, with the leading causes of death remaining unchanged, namely non-pregnancy related infections (HIV/AIDS), obstetric haemorrhage and hypertension.[3] This implies that SA may probably miss its Millennium Development Goal (MDG) 5 target of reducing its MMR by 75% by 2015. The Limpopo province recorded a district MMR of 275.9 per 100 000 live births (Capricorn district) and 616 maternal deaths (12% of the country's total maternal deaths) between 2008 and 2010.[3] In South Africa, a total number of 4867 maternal deaths was reported between 2008 and 2010.[3]

In South Africa, nursing education and practice have undergone changes in response to the demands of current clinical practice. Amongst the strategies used by SA to reduce MMR in meeting its MDG5 target, has been to improve the knowledge and skills of healthcare workers involved in maternal care.[3] The Department of Health (DoH) initiated a programme of diploma and master's degree to train registered nurses known as 'clinical nurse specialists' (advanced midwives) who will be able to function with the increased responsibility of working independently in maternity units. However, little information is available on the proportion of RNs with advanced midwifery training involved in maternal care. In order to assist local healthcare teams to plan the training requirements for an advanced midwifery workforce, there is a need to identify the proportion of registered nurses with advanced midwifery training who provide maternity services in their settings.

A cross-sectional, descriptive study was undertaken to establish the profile of registered nurses (RNs) involved in maternity care in referral hospitals of the Limpopo Province, South Africa. These referral facilities were chosen because health care providers at lower levels of the health system, who may lack midwifery skills, seek the assistance of health care providers at higher levels of care. These health care providers are supposed to be better equipped or specially trained to provide guidance in the management, or to take over the responsibility of care for a particular episode of a patient's clinical condition.

Method

The study was carried out in all maternity units of the referral hospitals in Limpopo Province, South Africa. A questionnaire which was initially piloted to ensure validity and reliability was distributed to all referral hospitals comprising of (4) four regional hospitals and (1) one tertiary hospital complex (comprising of two hospitals situated 30 km apart). Data was collected from either the maternity nursing manager, sister in charge of the maternity unit or the nursing manager of the various referral hospitals who signed consent forms before providing the required information on their nursing staff. Data reflected the demographic and educational profile of registered nurses practicing midwifery in March 2013. The statistical software, STATA version 9.0 was used for data analysis.

Ethical considerations

Ethics approval was obtained from the Polokwane/Mankweng hospital complex Research Ethics Committee (PMREC) of the University of Limpopo (Polokwane Campus) in South Africa (Ethics clearance certificate number: PMREC 50/2013). Permission to obtain the demographic and educational data of the nurses was obtained from the Limpopo Province Research Committee. Anonymity and confidentiality of data was assured by group data analysis without any personal identifiers.

Results

There were 210 registered nurses working in the various maternity units of the referral hospitals in the Limpopo Province during March 2013. Figure 1 shows the age distribution of the RNs who provided maternal care in these referral hospitals during the study period. The mean age of these nurses was 44.5 ± 9.1 years (range 21 to 62 years). The majority (152/210; 70%) were 40 years and older.

Analysis of work experience is presented in Figure 2, and shows that 56% (117/210) had been working for more than 10 years as registered nurses involved in maternity care. Almost 14% (30/210) had less than 5 years' work experience. Of these (n = 30), 60% (18/30) were younger than 30 years of age.

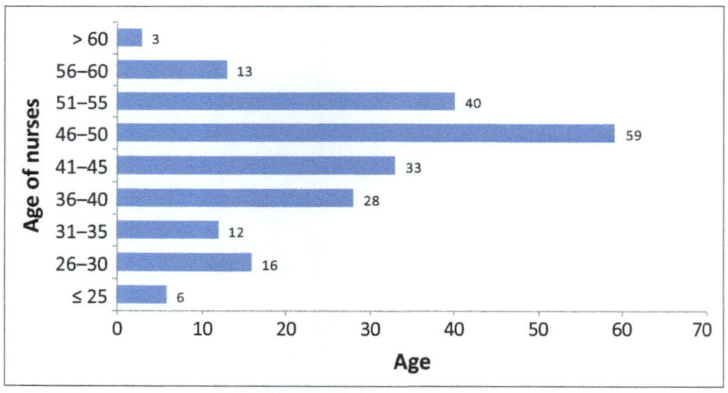

FIGURE 1: Age differences for registered nurses.

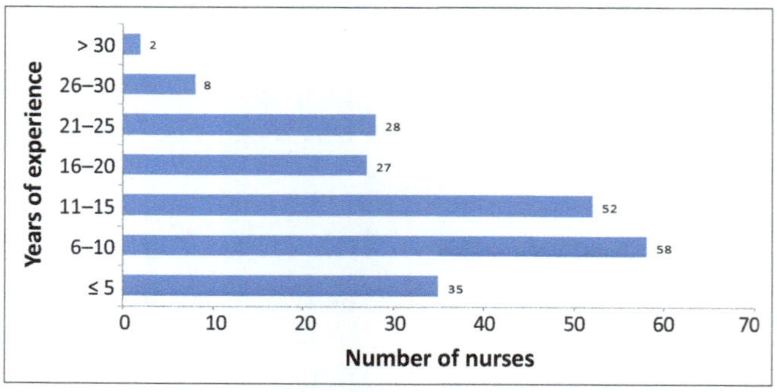

FIGURE 2: Years of experience of registered nurses (RNs) working in maternity facility.

TABLE 1: Distribution of registered nurses with advanced midwifery training per facility.

Registered Nurses (RNs)	Tertiary Complex		Regional Hospitals			
	Hospital A	Hospital B	Hospital C	Hospital D	Hospital E	Hospital F
Number of RNs in maternity units	28	37	18	33	29	65
Number of RNs with advanced midwifery diplomas N (%)	6 (21%)	5 (14%)	8 (44%)	10 (30%)	6 (21%)	11 (17%)

Note: Fewer than 3% (6/210) of the RNs were studying for a postgraduate diploma in midwifery.

Table 1 shows a brief profile of the postgraduate education levels achieved by the RNs involved in maternity care per health facility. Only 21.9% (46/210) of them had advanced midwifery diplomas obtained from various colleges of nursing or universities. Less than 3% (6/210) of the RNs based at the referral hospitals were studying for an advanced diploma in midwifery at the time of the study.

Discussion

From our study, a small proportion, that is, approximately 22% (46/210) of the RNs had completed advanced midwifery training. This finding is in contrast to those studies conducted in a number of developed countries, which showed that more than 50% of midwives had completed postgraduate training in midwifery.[4,5] In addition, previous studies have shown that having a skilled attendant present at every maternal delivery reduces maternal deaths.[6,7] A recent global review suggests levels of maternal mortality in developing regions have fallen since 1990, but it has become increasingly clear that significant improvements in health care for women are required if the goal is to be achieved.[8] This is the case for sub-Saharan Africa and South Asia, in which at least 87% of the estimated annual 342 900 maternal deaths worldwide occur according to recent estimates, with over 50% of all maternal deaths occurring in only six countries, namely India, Nigeria, Pakistan, Afghanistan, Ethiopia and the Democratic Republic of Congo. [8]

From the questionnaire, the following were given as possible reasons for the high number of midwives without advanced midwifery training: shortage of staff due to high staff turnover and unavailability of training spaces at the nursing colleges. However, a study on job satisfaction amongst registered nurses (n = 34) in a community hospital in Limpopo Province, South Africa found that more than half (54%; 18/34) were dissatisfied with personal growth and development of staff.[9] Another study reported that 69% (65/94) of registered nurses were absent from work because they had to do jobs that required more skills than they had.[10]

In addition to these challenges, the nursing population is also ageing. Our findings indicate that more than two-thirds of the registered nurses were 40 years and older, which means that half of the current group will retire within 10 to 15 years' time. These findings concur with reports by Sipe and co-workers,[4] as well as Bogossian and collaborators[5], which reported that clustering occurred in the age range of 51–54 years and, that 73% (534/729) of practicing midwives were over 40 years of age respectively. It was interesting to note that 60% (126/210) of the registered nurses had been working in maternity wards for more than ten years, of whom only 22% had advanced midwifery diplomas. This indicates that registered nursing education and training in 'maternal care' in the Limpopo province occurs primarily through 'on the job' experience. Bogossian *et al.*[4] indicated that the majority of midwives (61%; 305/729) in their study were working part-time, an average of 35 hours per week. In contrast, our study showed that all midwives worked full-time for an average of 40 hours per week. The implication of the latter is that the nurses working in these maternity units are relatively overworked and only slightly over a fifth had the advanced midwifery training to deal with the possible complications associated with maternal morbidity and mortality. Crowe *et al.*[11] conservatively estimate that there will be between 130 and 180 million non-skilled birth attendant (SBA) births in South Asia and sub-Saharan Africa from 2011 to 2015 with 90% of these in rural areas. This means that there is an urgent need to step up advanced midwifery training of nurses if the province (with its high maternal mortality ratio) and South Africa are to achieve the MDG5 target by 2015.

Limitations of the study

The findings of this study cannot be generalised as it did not extend to registered nurses providing maternal care in Primary Health Care (PHC) clinics/health centres and district hospitals. Nevertheless, the study demonstrates the level of training of RNs managing maternal cases in the maternity units of the referral hospitals where complicated or high risk maternal cases are sent from the primary care facilities.

Conclusion

This study demonstrated a shortage of registered nurses with advanced midwifery training/diplomas in referral hospitals of the Limpopo Province. This has a potential negative effect in reducing the high maternal mortality rate in the province. The challenges raised in this study in terms of the profile of RNs managing these maternity units require urgent interventions to fast track advanced midwifery training programmes to upskill the RNs currently employed in the province. Additional research is needed to examine the profile of registered nurses providing maternal care in the Primary Health Care (PHC) and district hospitals, as this will give a comprehensive picture of the training needs in advanced midwifery for Limpopo province.

Acknowledgements

The authors acknowledge the support of the maternity nursing managers, sisters in charge of the maternity wards, and nursing managers of the various referral hospitals in Limpopo province who assisted with the data collection.

Competing interests

The authors declare that they have no financial or personal relationship(s) which may have inappropriately influenced them in writing this article.

Authors' contributions

S.T.N. (University of Limpopo) conceptualised the research idea; S.T.N. and G.A.O. (University of Limpopo) drafted the manuscript; G.A.O. reviewed and approved the final manuscript.

References

1. Xu J, Kochanek KD, Murphy SL, Tejada-Vera B. Final data for 2007, in National vital statistics reports. Hyattsville (MD): National Center for Health Statistics; 2010.
2. World Health Organization. Maternal mortality 1990–2010: WHO, UNICEF, UNFPA and the World Bank. Trends in maternal mortality: 1990 to 2010. Geneva: World Health Organization; 2012. [cited 2013 Sept 06] Available from: http://www.who.int
3. National Department of Health. South Africa saving mothers 2008–2010: Fifth report on confidential enquiries into maternal deaths in South Africa. Pretoria: National Department of Health; 2012. [cited 2013 June 05] Available from: http://www.doh.gov.za
4. Sipe TAN, Fullerton JT, Schuiling KD. Demographic profile of certified nurse-midwives, certified registered nurse anesthetists, and nurse practitioners: Reflections on implications for uniform education and regulation. J Prof Nurs. 2009;25(3):178–185. http://dx.doi.org/10.1016/j.profnurs.2009.01.002
5. Bogossian, FE, Long MH, Benefer C, et el. A workforce profile comparison of practising and non-practising midwives in Australia: Baseline data from the midwives and nurses e-cohort study. Midwifery. 2011;27(3):342–349. http://dx.doi.org/10.1016/j.midw.2011.03.001
6. Graham WJ, Bell JS, Bullough CHW. Can skilled attendance at delivery reduce maternal mortality in developing countries? Studies in Health Service Organization and Policy. 2001;17:97–130.
7. Liang J, Li X, Dai L, et el. The changes in maternal mortality in 1000 counties in mid-Western China by a government-initiated intervention. PLoS One. 2012;7(5). http://dx.doi.org/10.1371/journal.pone.0037458
8. Hogan MC, Foreman KJ, Naghavi M, et el. Maternal mortality for 181 countries, 1980–2008: A systematic analysis of progress towards Millennium Development Goal 5. Lancet. 2010;375:1609–1623. http://dx.doi.org/10.1016/S0140-6736(10)60518-1
9. Kekana HP, Du Rand EA, van Wyk NC. Job satisfaction of registered nurses in a community hospital in the Limpopo Province in South Africa. Curationis. 2007;30(2):24–35. http://dx.doi.org/10.4102/curationis.v30i2.1068
10. Nyathi M, Jooste K. Working conditions that contribute to absenteeism among nurses in a provincial hospital in the Limpopo Province. Curationis. 2008;31(1):28–37. http://dx.doi.org/10.4102/curationis.v31i1.903
11. Crowe S, Utley M, Costello A, Pagel C. How many births in sub-Saharan Africa and South Asia will not be attended by a skilled birth attendant between 2011 and 2015? BMC Pregnancy Childbirth. 2012 Jan 17;12:4. http://dx.doi.org/10.1186/1471-2393-12-4

14

Blood pressure control amongst patients living with hypertension presenting to an urban district hospital outpatient clinic in Kwazulu-Natal

Authors:
Folafolu A. Adebolu[1]
Mergan Naidoo[1]

Affiliations:
[1]Department of Family Medicine, University of Kwazulu-Natal, South Africa

Correspondence to:
Folafolu Adebolu

Email:
folagreat2000@yahoo.com

Postal address:
PO Box 50477, Musgrave 4062, Durban

Background: The prevalence of hypertension in South Africa has been estimated to be 20% of the adult population with over six million people being affected. Poor adherence to treatment plans lead to inadequate blood pressure control and high morbidity. Many studies have looked at factors contributing to poor blood pressure control in South Africa but few studies actually focus on district hospitals in Kwazulu-Natal in particular, despite the fact that the province has the most heterogeneous population in South Africa.

Method: The study was a descriptive cross-sectional study conducted at the chronic outpatient clinic of an urban district hospital involving 370 participants aged 18–90 years.

Result: The study showed poorly controlled blood pressure in 58% of the participants. Only 35% knew their blood pressure results on the day of interview and 19.2% were aware of their target blood pressure. Good adherence was self-reported by 95% of the participants, whist 51.4% reported significant side-effects to medication.

Conclusion: The majority of patients had poor knowledge about blood pressure and little awareness of their blood pressure reading. These may be precursors to poor blood pressure control and this needs further investigation. A high level of self-reported adherence to medication did not translate into effective blood pressure control. A significant number reported medication side-effects which may have contributed to the poor blood pressure control. The high adherence rate may therefore have been over reported. An objective way to measure adherence will be necessary for future research.

Contrôle de la tension artérielle des patients souffrant d'hypertension qui se rendent aux consultations externes d'un hôpital urbain de district au Kwazulu-Natal.

Contexte: La prévalence de l'hypertension en Afrique du Sud est estimée à 20% de la population adulte, soit plus de six millions de personnes. La non-observation du plan de traitement mène au contrôle insuffisant de la tension artérielle et à un taux élevé de décès. De nombreuses études ont examiné les facteurs contribuant au contrôle insuffisant de la tension artérielle en Afrique du Sud, mais peu d'études se sont réellement penchées sur les hôpitaux de district du Kwazulu-Natal en particulier, en dépit du fait que la province a la population la plus hétérogène d'Afrique du Sud.

Méthode: L'étude descriptive et transversale a été menée à la clinique de consultations externes pour malades chroniques d'un hôpital urbain de district, parmi 370 participants âgés de 18 à 90 ans.

Résultat: L'étude a révélé une tension artérielle mal contrôlée chez 58% des participants. Seuls 35% d'entre eux savaient quelle était leur tension artérielle le jour de l'entrevue et 19.2% savaient la tension artérielle visée. 95% des patients ont déclarés qu'ils suivaient le traitement, tandis que 51.4% ont déclarés que le médicament avait des effets secondaires significatifs.

Conclusion: La majorité des patients avait peu de connaissances sur la tension artérielle et ils n'étaient pas au courant de leur taux de tension. Cela peut être l'indication d'un mauvais contrôle de la tension artérielle et doit faire l'objet de recherches supplémentaires. Le taux élevé d'adhésion auto-déclarée au traitement ne se traduit pas par un contrôle efficace de la tension artérielle. Un nombre significatif de patients a déclaré avoir des effets secondaires au traitement, ce qui peut avoir contribué au mauvais contrôle de la tension. Ainsi, le taux élevé d'adhérence peut avoir été sur-déclaré. Pour les recherches futures il faudra trouver une manière plus objective de mesurer l'adhésion aux médicaments.

Introduction

Hypertension is a major worldwide health challenge and a key risk factor responsible for adverse cardiovascular events. Although, largely preventable and modifiable, uncontrolled hypertension has been reported to negatively affect the global population's health, causing cerebrovascular accidents and cardiac diseases.[1]

Hypertension 'accounts for greater than 5.8% of the total deaths, 11.9% of the years of life lost, and 1.4% of the disability-adjusted life years worldwide'.[2] It has a major influence in the development of cardiac and vascular diseases. Despite being a highly treatable condition, studies have shown that hypertension remains poorly controlled.[3] In addition, the diagnosis, management, and control of hypertension pose a great challenge for physicians and researchers.[4]

Hypertension affects approximately one billion individuals worldwide and fifty million individuals in the United States of America.[5] A number of clinical trials have shown that optimal blood pressure (BP) control can be achieved in most hypertensive patients using multiple antihypertensive medications.[6] A retrospective study conducted in community-based settings in the USA indicated that 70% of the population had blood pressure levels that were optimally controlled. This was similar to the National Health and Nutrition Examination Survey (NHANNES) study done between 2007 and 2008, which indicated that 69% of patients in this cohort had controlled blood pressure. This study showed that optimally controlled patients living with hypertension were significantly more likely to be younger and have less co-morbidity.[7] A study which looked at uncontrolled hypertension in the United States concluded that the majority of cases were due to systolic hypertension. This report reaffirms the need to assess the extent to which patients are aware of their systolic blood pressure as systolic blood pressure awareness and education is an important component of the interventional programme that is used in the control of hypertension.[7,8]

Hypertension control has been positively linked to adequate knowledge about blood pressure goals. A recent study done on 7649 participants across Europe showed that poor blood pressure control bears a strong correlation to lack of knowledge of target blood pressure. The study found that 50.4% of participants had controlled blood pressure and 49.4% had knowledge of their target blood pressure.[9] Numerous studies have concluded that poor medication adherence, lack of patient awareness about their target blood pressure levels, physician inertia as well as the presence of drug side-effects should be considered as possible causes of inadequately controlled blood pressure.[3]

Adequate assessment and treatment of hypertension has always been a major challenge for public health care workers.[5] An article in Time magazine in 2004 stated that 'with sub-Saharan Africa's population of 650 million and increasing longevity and westernization, hypertension has now changed from a relatively rare condition to a major problem. This observation necessitated the African Union to regard hypertension as one of the continent's greatest challenges after AIDS'.[10] The prevalence of hypertension in rural studies undertaken in sub-Saharan Africa in the 1970s, 1980s and 1990s using the previous definition of blood pressure of 160/95 mmHg found hypertension to be as low as 4.1% in Ghana, 7.0% in Lesotho, 5.9% in Nigeria, and 7.37% in rural Zululand in South Africa.[11]

Estimates based on the 1998 demographic survey put the prevalence of hypertension at 11% and 14% of South African males and females respectively. This implies that there were six million hypertensive persons in South Africa.[12] This number is likely to be even higher in 2012 because of population growth and growing urbanisation.[13] In the year 2000, 47 000 deaths in South Africa were attributed to high blood pressure, and elevated blood pressure was the second leading contributory cause of death.[14]

A study amongst Durban adults reporting hypertension trends using the WHO criteria of 160/90 mmHg found hypertension to be more common in urban black South Africans of Zulu origin (25%), moderate in white South Africans (17%), and Indian populations (14%), and the lowest in rural black South Africans.[15] The 2011 South African Hypertension Guidelines recommend that the target blood pressure for patients on hypertensive therapy should be below 140/90.[16] In patients with major cardiovascular risks such as those with diabetes mellitus, associated clinical conditions or established target organ damage, the optimal blood pressure should be 130/80 mmHg.[16]

In well conducted clinical trials, antihypertensive drugs either as mono-therapy or combination therapy have been shown to effectively control blood pressure and reduce cardiovascular morbidity and mortality.[17] However, outside of clinical trials, control of hypertension remains disappointing with an estimated 30% of patients on treatment being effectively controlled.[16,18]

Despite the availability of multiple effective antihypertensive drugs, control of hypertension remains poor.[5,19] In both high and low income countries, less than 27% and 10% respectively of hypertensive patients have achieved their target blood pressure.[5,19]

Many reasons have been ascribed for the poor control of hypertension worldwide. Patient knowledge of hypertension also plays an important role in the ability to achieve successful control.[17] In addition, poor treatment adherence, inappropriate prescriptions, therapeutic inertia and unhealthy lifestyle contribute to poor control.[3,20,21] The 2011 South African Hypertension Guidelines emphasised poor adherence to medication as one of the main causes of uncontrolled blood pressure and was thought to be due to treatment factors, patient factors and illness related factors.[16] Other factors identified as contributors to uncontrolled hypertension include sex, age, and race.[8] In South Africa, white and Asian individuals have been noted to have better blood pressure control compared to their black counterparts.[12] Black individuals also develop hypertension earlier in life, have more severe hypertension related complications and respond differently to antihypertensive medication.[22]

In the first South African Demographic and Health Survey (1998), awareness, treatment status, and control varied substantially between men and women, as well as between different ethnic groups.[12] Women were substantially more likely to be aware of their hypertension than men, 51% and 26% respectively. The population survey also found that 36% of women and 21% of men had hypertension but were not on treatment. Amongst those on treatment, only 18% were controlled. With respect to ethnic differences, black South Africans had the lowest rates of awareness, treatment rates and control of hypertension.[12]

There is little published data on hypertension control amongst patients attending district hospitals in the KwaZulu-Natal Province, South Africa. The aim of this research was to describe the pattern of blood pressure control amongst patients attending a busy outpatient clinic in an urban district hospital. The specific objectives were to describe the demographic and clinical characteristics, knowledge of hypertension targets, degree of adherence to medication and knowledge of side-effects to antihypertensive medications. Approval for the study was granted by the Bioethics Research Committee of the University of KwaZulu-Natal (UKZN), the postgraduate education committee, hospital management and the KwaZulu-Natal Department of Health. Written consent was obtained from all study participants.

Methods

This was a descriptive, cross-sectional study done at the chronic outpatient clinic at a busy urban public health district hospital. An average of 1375 hypertensive patients was seen monthly at the outpatient clinic in 2011. A sample size of 370 was selected as being appropriate for an observational descriptive study as confirmed with a biostatistician. Hypertensive patients visiting the outpatient clinic were systematically sampled by selecting every third patient that met the inclusion criteria over a three month period commencing October 2012. Sampling was stopped when the sample size was attained. The inclusion criteria were all patients living with hypertension older than 18 years attending the chronic clinic, and on treatment for hypertension for at least one year. Excluded from the study were pregnant women and cognitively impaired patients. Patients' clinical records were reviewed and an exit structured interview was conducted with each participant by the principal investigator after the participant had consulted the hospital medical officer. The study tool captured demographic data, anthropometric data and, clinical information from the clinical record. Patients were asked specific questions about their hypertension, co-morbid conditions, and habits. Blood pressure readings from the last two clinic visits plus current blood pressure readings were captured. Poor control was defined as blood pressures greater than 140 mmHg systolic or 90 mmHg diastolic. Patients who had two of the three readings elevated were considered to be poorly controlled. Data was captured and analysed using SPSS Statistics for Window Version 21.0. (Armonk, NY: IBM Corp 2012). Results were summarised by frequencies and percentages (categorical variables) and mean, median, standard deviation and percentiles (numerical variables) as appropriate. Wilcoxon signed rank test was used in analysing the variations and trends between the categorical data.

Results

Forty-nine percent of the participants were black South Africans, 25.4% were Indians, 17.8% were Mixed race and 7.6% were white South Africans with their age groups being presented in Table 1. Approximately 62.3% of the participants had secondary and tertiary education, 59.1% were pensioners or patients collecting a social grant. Sixty percent of the participants were either overweight or obese.

The study showed uncontrolled blood pressure (BP) in 58% of the participants during the preceding three months. Other determinants of blood pressure control are shown below in Table 2. Eighty percent had other co-morbid diseases such as diabetes mellitus, asthma or arthritis and 60% were either obese or overweight. Approximately 81% did not know what their target blood pressure should be, and 65% could not recall what their blood pressure for the current visit was.

TABLE 1: Demographic details (*n* = 370).

Variables	Number	% of uncontrolled BP in each group
Age		
18–37	19	57.8
38–57	132	51.5
58–77	187	63.6
78–97	32	56.2
Sex		
Male	111	56.7
Female	259	59.0
Marital status		
Single	111	62.1
Married	160	60.0
Divorced	30	60.0
Widowed	69	59.4
Race		
Black South African	182	65.9
White South African	28	35.7
Mixed Race	66	62.1
Indian	94	47.8
Education level		
No education	44	63.6
Primary	95	58.9
Secondary	203	56.6
Tertiary	28	57.1
BMI (Kg/m^2)		
< 18	34	2.94
18–24	113	61.0
25–29	89	61.7
> 30	134	67.9

BP, blood pressure; BMI, body-mass index.

TABLE 2: Determinants of blood pressure control.

Variables	Number	%
Blood pressure		
Controlled	155	41.9
Not controlled	215	58.1
No of antihypertensive medication		
One	13	3.5
Two	70	18.9
Three	108	29.2
> Three	179	48.4
Naming of antihypertensive medications		
Adequate knowledge	77	20.8
Partial knowledge	88	23.7
No knowledge	205	55.5
Adherence		
> 95%	327	88.4
< 95%	43	11.6
Side effects to medication		
Yes	190	51.4
No	180	48.6
Knowledge of target blood pressure		
Adequate knowledge	71	19.2
No knowledge	299	80.8
Presence of co-morbidity		
Yes	297	80.3
No	73	19.7
Investigations		
No investigation in clinical record	171	46.2
Partially investigated	120	32.4
Investigated according to guidelines	79	21.4
Patients view about their weight		
Normal	237	64.1
Obese	120	32.4
Underweight	13	3.5
Knowledge about DASH diet		
Adequate knowledge	178	48.1
No knowledge	192	51.9
Presence of stress		
Stress present	245	66.2
Stress absent	125	33.8
Knowledge of BP reading at this consultation		
Adequate knowledge	127	34.3
No knowledge	243	65.7

BP, blood pressure.

TABLE 3a: Crosstabs of blood pressure control versus determinant factors.

BP versus adherence	Adherence > 95%	Adherence < 95%	*p*-value
BP controlled (%)	36.5	5.4	0.514
BP not controlled (%)	51.9	6.2	

BP, blood pressure.

TABLE 3b: Crosstabs of blood pressure control versus determinant factors.

BP versus associated co-morbidity	Co-morbidity present	Co-morbidity absent	*p*-value
BP controlled (%)	31.6	9.4	0.068
BP not controlled (%)	48.6	10.3	

BP, blood pressure.

TABLE 3c: Crosstabs of blood pressure control versus determinant factors.

BP versus presence of side effect	Side effect of drug reported	Side effect of drug not reported	*p*-value
BP controlled (%)	17.6	24.9	0.004
BP not controlled (%)	33.8	23.8	

BP, blood pressure.

TABLE 3d: Crosstabs of blood pressure control versus determinant factors.

BP control versus knowledge of target BP	Good knowledge of target BP	No knowledge of target BP	*p*-value
BP controlled (%)	17.5	82.5	0.585
BP not controlled (%)	29.9	79.1	

BP, blood pressure.

TABLE 3e: Crosstabs of blood pressure control versus determinant factors.

BP versus determinant	Medications prescribed				*p*-value
	Number of medicine	Number of medicine	Number of medicine	Number of medicine	
BP versus number of medicine	1	2	3	> 3	0.527
BP controlled (%)	1.6	9.1	12.4	18.6	
BP not controlled (%)	1.9	9.7	16.8	29.7	

BP, blood pressure.

TABLE 3f: Crosstabs of blood pressure control versus determinant factors.

BP versus determinant	Black people	White people	Mixed race	Asian	*p*-value
BP controlled (%)	40.3	11.0	16.9	31.8	0.004
BP not controlled (%)	55.6	4.6	19.0	20.8	

BP, blood pressure.

Most participants claimed that they were not told what their blood pressure was by the health care providers managing their hypertension. Eighty-eight percent of participants claimed a 95% adherence to treatment. This information was not verified. Fifty-one percent of the participants reported significant side-effects ranging from cough, dizziness, skin rashes and urinary frequency, but almost 60% of these did not know if the drug treatment was causing these side-effects. More than 70% of the study participants indicated that they practiced at least one form of exercise to decrease their weight. Only 48% of the hypertensive patients could describe what a DASH diet was and these participants claimed to adhere to it. Sixty-six percent of the participants claimed to be psychologically stressed.

The associations between the various factors contributing towards blood pressure control are shown in Table 3 A and B below. There was no statistically significant difference between blood pressure control, and adherence ($p = 0.514$). There was no statistically significantly association between blood pressure control and increase in number of antihypertensive medications used ($p = 0.527$).There was a statistically significant association between side- effects to medication and blood pressure control ($p = 0.004$). There was a statistically significant association between BP control and ethnic group ($p = 0.004$).

Discussion

The study showed a blood pressure control rate of 41.9% amongst the patients attending a district hospital in Kwazulu-Natal. The control rate was slightly higher than the average rate of 40% that was previously reported in South Africa but consistent with a global control rate of 19% – 54%.[23] However, this degree of control is too low considering the complications of hypertension. Poor blood pressure control translates into increased cardiovascular morbidity and mortality such as ischemic heart diseases which affects the burden placed on health care services in South Africa.

The demographics of the study group presented in Table 1 showed that the predominant racial group in this study was black South African people and the predominant gender was female. The cross tabulation for BP control versus race showed a significant relationship (p = 0.004.) These further affirm findings of earlier studies which showed highest reported cases to be amongst urban black South Africans and females when viewed along ethnic and gender lines.[12,15]

It has been argued that greater medication adherence and better blood pressure control improves with patients' knowledge of hypertension.[24] This study showed that only 19.2% of the participants had knowledge of their target blood pressure and the cross tabulation for the blood pressure control vs. knowledge of target blood pressure did not show a statistically significant relationship (p = 0.585).

The self-reported adherence rate of 88.4% does not correlate with the degree of control noted (42%). A high adherence should translate into a well-controlled blood pressure. The cross tabulation between BP control and side-effects indicated that there is a statistically significant association between side- effects reported and BP control. This would suggest that patients who experienced side- effects to drugs may have over reported their adherence rates. This over reporting of adherence is consistent with findings from other studies.[25,26]

This study showed that 51% of the participants reported side-effects to antihypertensive medications but 60% of these participants could not identify which drugs caused the side-effects. It has been reported that 35% of hypertensive patients will stop taking their drugs in the first six months if they experience a side-effect. Another reported reason for stopping medication was patient dissatisfaction with treatment.[27] The significantly higher proportion of side-effects noted in this study was associated with multiple antihypertensive medications and this was statistically significant (p = 0.042).

This study showed that 70% of the participants were using more than three medications, which is of concern as they constituted the largest percentage of uncontrolled hypertensive patients. These participants would be classified as having resistant hypertension and in South Africa should have been managed at a regional level hospital. The study also showed that 80.3% of the participants had other co-morbid diseases necessitating poly-pharmacy, which increased the possibility of adverse drug-drug interactions.

Implications of the research

The findings of this study support previous studies which demonstrated that only about 40% of hypertensive patients attain blood pressure control in South Africa. A plan to improve the control of blood pressure from the current 42% to greater than 80% is urgently required. The poor knowledge of blood pressure control and hypertensive targets amongst this cohort of participants should be addressed by clinicians through improved patient education. The high number of reported side-effects to anti-hypertensive medication should alert physicians that prescription practices in hypertensive patients may need reviewing. In addition, quality assurance teams at district level should be encouraged to do regular clinical audits of the management of hypertensive patients and monitor outcomes. Regular monitoring and evaluation of hypertension should be part of routine clinical practice and poorly controlled patients with resistant hypertension must be referred to higher levels of care. This study supports the development and implementation of educational programmes that improve the knowledge of hypertension in patients.

Recommendations

Educational intervention aimed at counselling patients about the cardiovascular implications should be instituted. Pharmacists, nurses and doctors managing hypertensive patients should aim to address the gaps in the management of hypertension identified by this study. There is need for future research on patients' adherence rates using a more objective approach than self-reporting.

Limitations

It is worth mentioning that a degree of bias may exist in this study. Adherence rates may have been over reported as the investigator is a doctor known to patients at the clinic. The predominant age group are elderly with multiple co-morbidities, which might have made hypertension control more difficult. The generalisation of these results should be limited to urban district hospitals and communities with heterogeneous ethnic populations.

Acknowledgements

Dr Mergan Naidoo supervised the research. Dr Andrew Ross provided useful critiques and was very supportive. Mr B Tlou provided the statistician services required at different stages of the research whilst Mr H.O Ojugbele also gave tremendous support.

Competing interests

The authors declare that they have no financial or personal relationship(s) which may have inappropriately influenced them in writing this article.

Authors' contributions

F.A.A. (University of Kwazulu-Natal) was the principal researcher, whilst the research was supervised by M.N. (University of Kwazulu Natal).

References

1. Williams B. The year in hypertension. J Am Coll Cardiol. 2009;55(1):65–73. http://dx.doi.org/10.1016/j.jacc.2009.08.037
2. Machado M, Bajcar J, Guzzo GC, Einarson TR. Sensitivity of patient outcomes to pharmacist interventions. Part II: Systematic review and meta-analysis in hypertension management. The Annals of Pharmacotherapy. 2007;41(11):1770–1781. http://dx.doi.org/10.1345/aph.1K311
3. Morgado M, Rolo S, Macedo AF, Pereira L, Castelo-Branco M. Predictors of uncontrolled hypertension and antihypertensive medication nonadherence. Journal of Cardiovascular Disease Research. 2010;1(4):196–202. http://dx.doi.org/10.4103/0975-3583.74263

4. Kannel WB. Blood pressure as a cardiovascular risk factor: Prevention and treatment JAMA: The Journal of the American Medical Association. 1996;275(20):1571–1576. http://dx.doi.org/10.1001/jama.1996.03530440051036
5. Chobanian AV, Bakris GL, Black HR, Cushman WC, Green LA, Izzo JL, et al. Seventh Report of the Joint National Committee on Prevention, Detection, Evaluation, and Treatment of High Blood Pressure. Hypertension. 2003;42(6):1206–1252. http://dx.doi.org/10.1161/01.HYP.0000107251.49515.c2
6. Black HR, Elliott WJ, Neaton JD, Grandits G, Grambsch P, Grimm RH, et al. Baseline characteristics and early blood pressure control in the CONVINCE trial. Hypertension. 2001;37(1):12–18. http://dx.doi.org/10.1161/01.HYP.37.1.12
7. Knight E, Bohn R, Wang P, Glynn R, Mogun H, Avorn J. Predictors of uncontrolled hypertension in ambulatory patient. Hypertension. 2001;38(4):809–814. http://dx.doi.org/10.1161/hy0901.091681
8. Hyman DJ, Pavlik VN. Characteristics of patients with uncontrolled hypertension in the United States. New England Journal of Medicine. 2001;345(7):479–486. http://dx.doi.org/10.1056/NEJMoa010273
9. Pruggera C, Keila U, Wellmanna Jr, Bacquerb DD, Backerb GD, Ambrosioc GB, et al. Blood pressure control and knowledge of target blood pressure in coronary patients across Europe: Results from the EUROASPIRE III survey. Journal of Hypertension 2011;29(8):1641–1648. http://dx.doi.org/10.1097/HJH.0b013e328348efa7
10. Kluger J. Blowing a gasket. Time. 2004;December. 164(23):34–40.
11. Seedat Y. Hypertension in developing nations in sub-Saharan Africa. Journal of Human Hypertension. 2000;14(10–11):739–747. http://dx.doi.org/10.1038/sj.jhh.1001059
12. Steyn K, Gaziano TA, Bradshaw D, Laubscher R, Fourie J. Hypertension in South African adults: Results from the Demographic and Health Survey, 1998. Journal of Hypertension. 2001;19(10):1717–1725. http://dx.doi.org/10.1097/00004872-200110000-00004
13. Twagirumukiza M, Van Bortel LM. Management of hypertension at the community level in sub-Saharan Africa (SSA): towards a rational use of available resources. J Hum Hypertens. 2011;25(1):47–56. http://dx.doi.org/10.1038/jhh.2010.32
14. Norman R, Gaziano T, Laubscher R, Steyn K, Bradshaw D, Collaboration SACRA. Estimating the burden of disease attributable to high blood pressure in South Africa in 2000. South African Medical Journal. 2007;97(8):692–698.
15. Seedat YK. Race, environment and blood pressure: The South African experience. Journal of Hypertension. 1983;1(1):7–12. http://dx.doi.org/10.1097/00004872-198306000-00003
16. Seedat YK, Rayner BL. South African hypertension guideline 2011. South African Medical Journal. 2012;102(1):60–83.
17. Ragot S, Sosner P, Bouche G, Guillemain J, Herpin D. Appraisal of the knowledge of hypertensive patients and assessment of the role of the pharmacists in the management of hypertension: Results of a regional survey. J Hum Hypertens. 2005;19(7):577–584. http://dx.doi.org/10.1038/sj.jhh.1001859
18. Ly N, McCaig L. National Hospital Ambulatory Medical Care Survey: 2000 outpatient department summary. Maryland, USA: 2000.
19. Pereira M, Lunet N, Azevedo A, Barros H. Differences in prevalence, awareness, treatment and control of hypertension between developing and developed countries. Journal of Hypertension. 2009;27(5):963–975 http://dx.doi.org/10.1097/HJH.0b013e3283282f65
20. Ong KL, Cheung BMY, Man YB, Lau CP, Lam KSL. Prevalence, awareness, treatment, and control of hypertension among United States adults 1999–2004. Hypertension. 2007;49(1):69–75. http://dx.doi.org/10.1161/01.HYP.0000252676.46043.18
21. Rodríguez Pérez MC, Cabrera de León A, Morales Torres RM, Domínguez Coello S, Alemán Sánchez JJ, Brito Díaz B, et al. Factors associated with knowledge and control of arterial hypertension in the Canary Islands. Revista Española de Cardiología. 2012;65(3):234–240. http://dx.doi.org/10.1016/j.recesp.2011.09.021
22. Opie LH, Seedat YK. Hypertension in sub-Saharan African populations. Circulation. 2005;112(23):3562–3568. http://dx.doi.org/10.1161/CIRCULATIONAHA.105.539569
23. Rayner B. Combination therapy in hypertension. SA Pharmaceutical Journal. 2007;74(6):30–34.
24. Kim E-Y, Han H-R, Jeong S, Kim KB, Park H, Kang E, et al. Does knowledge matter?: Intentional medication nonadherence among middle-aged Korean Americans with high blood pressure. Journal of Cardiovascular Nursing. 2007;22(5):397–404 http://dx.doi.org/10.1097/01.JCN.0000287038.23186.bd
25. Voils CI, Hoyle RH, Thorpe CT, Maciejewski ML, Yancy Jr WS. Improving the measurement of self-reported medication nonadherence. Journal of Clinical Epidemiology. 2011;64(3):250–254. http://dx.doi.org/10.10Svarstad BL, Chewning BA, Sleath BL, Claesson C. The brief medication questionnaire: A tool for screening patient adherence and barriers to adherence. Patient Education and Counseling. 1999;37(2):113–124. http://dx.doi.org/10.1016/S0738-3991(98)00107-4
26. Trinder YA. Common and less common adverse effects of antihypertensives: A general practitioner's perspective. South African Family Practice. 2012 54(2):31–32.

15

Injustice to transsexual women in a hetero-normative healthcare system

Authors:
Douglas Newman-Valentine[1]
Sinegugu Duma[1]

Affiliations:
[1]Division of Nursing and Midwifery, University of Cape Town, South Africa

Correspondence to:
Douglas Newman-Valentine

Email:
douglas.newman-valentine@uct.ac.za

Postal address:
University of Cape Town F45 Old Main Building, Groote Schuur Hospital, Observatory 7925, South Africa

Background: Transsexual women who are on the journey of sexual re-alignment will experience various health problems. These problems are related directly to the treatment regime that they are following in order to attain and maintain their physical embodiment as a woman. They are forced to negotiate a hetero-normative healthcare system in order to receive assistance and care for their health problems related to their sexual re-alignment process.

Aim: The questions posed were: What are the unique health problems that transsexual women experience whilst on the journey of sexual re-alignment? What is the current context of the South African healthcare system in which transsexual women should negotiate healthcare? These questions were asked in order to explore the health problems with which transsexual women are faced and to describe the hetero-normative healthcare system in South Africa.

Method: An electronic literature search was executed via the EBSCO host with specific inclusion and exclusion criteria. The search words that were used were: Transsexual/s and Health/Healthcare. All studies had to be peer reviewed and published in the English language, from January 1972 up until February 2013. Literature on transsexual children was excluded.

Results: Transsexual women have the potential to suffer significant side-effects from their sexual re-alignment treatment, including cardio-vascular problems, endocrine problems and mental ill-health. They are also vulnerable to HIV infection. They have poor access to quality holistic healthcare and this may lead an increase in the mortality and morbidity figures of women.

Conclusion: A hetero-normative healthcare system has a negative impact on the health of transsexual women and will cause them to be marginalised. This could contribute to both homo- and trans-phobia that will in turn strengthen the belief that transsexual women are un-African.

Injustice envers les femmes transsexuelles dans un système de santé aux normes hétérosexuelles.

Contexte: Les femmes transsexuelles qui sont sur le chemin du réalignement sexuel souffriront de différents problèmes de santé. Ces problèmes proviennent directement du traitement qu'elles suivent pour atteindre et maintenir leur corps de femme. Elles doivent surmonter un système de santé aux normes hétérosexuelles pour recevoir de l'aide et des soins pour leurs problèmes de santé liés au processus de réalignement sexuel.

Objectif: Les questions posées étaient: Quels sont les problèmes de santé particuliers que les femmes transsexuelles rencontrent sur le chemin du réalignement sexuel? Quel est le contexte actuel du système de santé sud-africain avec lequel les femmes transsexuelles doivent négocier leurs soins? On a posé ces questions pour examiner les problèmes de santé auxquels les femmes transsexuelles sont confrontées et décrire le système de santé hétéro-normatif en Afrique du Sud.

Méthode: On a effectué une recherche de littérature électronique par l'hôte EBSCO avec des critères spécifiques d'inclusion et d'exclusion. Les mots de recherche utilisés sont: Transsexuel/s et Santé/Services de santé. Toutes les études ont été vérifiées par les pairs et publiées en anglais, de janvier 1972 à février 2013. On a exclu la littérature sur les enfants transsexuels.

Résultats: Les femmes transsexuelles peuvent ressentir des effets secondaires significatifs de leur traitement de réalignement sexuel, tels que des problèmes cardio-vasculaires, endocrines et de santé mentale. Elles sont aussi vulnérables à l'infection par le VIH. Elles n'ont pas accès à des soins de santé de qualité ce qui peut augmenter les chiffres de mortalité et de morbidité des femmes.

Conclusion: Un système de santé hétéro-normatif a un impact négatif sur la santé des femmes transsexuelles et les amènera à être marginalisées. Cela pourra contribuer à l'homo- et trans-phobie qui à leur tour renforceront la croyance que les femmes transsexuelles sont contraires à la mentalité africaine.

Introduction

Transsexual women experience significant health problems which are related directly to their gender re-alignment journey. They have to negotiate care in a hetero-normative healthcare system, which is exclusive.

The reviewed literature in this article explores the health problems which transsexual women experience and makes a description of the hetero-normative health care system in South Africa, after which appropriate recommendations for practice and research are made.

Transsexual woman: A definition

The term Transsexual describes someone who identifies psychologically and emotionally as having a gender identity in opposition to that which was assigned at birth. Someone who identifies as transsexual or transgender may want to make changes to their body using hormones or gender confirming surgeries to transition their physical features to match their internal sense of gender.[1]

A transsexual individual can further be described as a person who wishes to be of the opposite sex and is in the process of gender re-alignment.[2]

A transsexual woman is a person who was sexually defined and registered as male at birth, but identifies psychologically as female. She will seek medical help to align her physical embodiment with her gender and will be placed on a regime of lifelong hormonal therapy and various gender-confirming surgeries.

Hetero-normativity explained

Hetero-normativity can be described as the belief that heterosexuality is the ideal and that all other sexualities are inferior. Legal and social structures are thus designed to accommodate heterosexuality, thus denying rights and status to different sexualities.[3]

The phenomenon of hetero-normativity is evident in all sectors of daily life. In most of the African countries, marriage is only recognised between a man and a woman. This immediately gives a superior status to the heterosexual union. At government institutions, banks, schools and universities, one of the first categories in which people are placed is either male or female. Even in culture, hetero-normativity is so deeply ingrained that it is often missed. When a child is born, the first information that a midwife or doctor will give a mother is the sex of the child. Family will usually enquire about the sex of a child before they question the health and well-being of the mother and the baby. This will be followed by 'gender appropriate' gifts and toys, as people naturally see gender and sex as being interchangeable.

Methods

The literature review was done in a systematic manner. The search for the literature was done electronically via the EBSCO host with specific inclusion and exclusion criteria. The search words that were used were: Transsexual/s and Health/Healthcare. All studies had to be peer reviewed and published in the English language, anywhere from January 1972 up until February 2013.

All studies that were published in the Cinhal, Health Source, Humanities International Complete, Medline, Psyc Articles and Soc Index databases and which were found to be relevant to transsexuals and healthcare were included in the study. All studies that were specific to transsexual children under the age of 18 were automatically excluded.

The initial search yielded 172 studies. A total of 105 of the studies were excluded because of both the inclusion and exclusion criteria and repetition of studies on the databases. This exclusion process yielded 67 studies that were selected for the critical appraisal process.

A CASP (Critical Appraisal Skills Programme) critical appraisal tool was utilised to measure the quality of the 67 studies that were selected.[4] After this process, another 37 studies were excluded because of insufficient rigour or reliability, leaving 23 studies which were finally selected for review.

Appropriate grey literature, such as acts and policies, was also included in this article.

Review findings

The South African healthcare system in context

Chapter two of the *Constitution of the Republic of South Africa* proclaims that healthcare is a human right for all citizens. It states that each citizen has a right to healthcare services, including reproductive healthcare.[5] Furthermore, the *National Health Act* 2004 aims to provide the best possible health services to citizens. It is written that it protects and promotes the rights of vulnerable groups, including women, children, older persons and the disabled.[6]

Both the *Constitution* and the *National Health Act* are specific regarding who exactly would be defined as a vulnerable group, however, transsexual women are get specified. The National Department of Health has initiated and implemented various strategies in order to improve the health status of the South African population, but all of these initiatives are silent with regard to transsexual women.

The latest reform in the South African healthcare system is the National Health Insurance (NHI). The main objectives for the implementation of the NHI in South Africa are to bring reform, improve service and to promote equity and efficiency in the healthcare system.[7] Throughout this document, the issue of equity is discussed in detail, yet transsexual women seem to be excluded in this latest plan of the South African government.

In the South African healthcare system, a person is treated as either male or female and there are various health programmes that place the focus of care on either men or women, such as the women's health and men's health programmes. This rigid form of gender identification within the health system will place people into two distinct boxes of care, with no space for people who are identified as different. With the definition of hetero-normativity in mind, where heterosexuality is seen as the norm, the South African healthcare system in effect treats people strictly as heterosexual men and/or women.

Hetero-normativity is a form of discrimination that is present in the healthcare system of South Africa, but it is not accepted as such. This leads to an exclusive healthcare system which denies a subset of the population, such as transsexual women, access to quality appropriate healthcare.

The silence with regard to the protection of sexual minority groups in the healthcare system might result in an increase in the morbidity and mortality figures of the country and is in direct conflict with the aims and objectives of the health legislation of South Africa.

Health problems of transsexual women

Literature shows that the life-long administration of feminising hormones used by transsexual women has the potential to lead to an increase in both systolic and diastolic blood pressure. Furthermore, it can increase insulin resistance in transsexual women.[8] Pulmonary embolism, deep venous thrombosis and osteoporosis may also occur.[9] Transsexual women require chronic management to treat conditions such as diabetes and hypertension. What makes these chronic conditions unique to transsexual women, is that they are subjected to a regimen of lifelong hormonal treatment in order to facilitate and maintain their transitioning and sexual re-alignment.

The chronic infection, HIV, may also affect transsexual women. Two large studies, conducted in the United States of America (USA), identified that 40% of the participants reported inconsistent condom use. Less than half of the respondents made use of protection during their last sexual encounter, whilst 64% of the respondents reported having engaged in high-risk sexual activity during the past three months.[10,11]

Transsexual women are anatomically more vulnerable to HIV because of the vulnerability of the tissue in the neo-vagina and the rectal mucosa.[11] The immediate question asked would be why this subset of the community would take such health risks knowing that they might become infected with either HIV or other sexually-transmitted infections (STIs). It is not clear if their attending health providers inform these women about the dangers of contracting HIV and other STIs.

In 2002, Kenagy found, in a needs assessment survey, that male-to-female (MTF) transsexual women believe that they will not become infected with HIV and thus indulge in risky behaviour.[12] HIV prevention programmes in South Africa target groups other than transsexual women. It is possible that the absence of health education for this group perpetuates the belief on the part of transsexual women that they are not at risk for HIV infection.

Two USA-based qualitative studies concluded that transsexual women have a need to be accepted. They participate in high-risk sexual encounters in order to avoid rejection.[13]

Two surveys conducted in Rome and California, reported that 20% and 52%, respectively, of the transsexual women surveyed were HIV positive. It was noted that this was possibly an underestimation, since the respondents self-reported their HIV status.[14,15]

South Africa has a female HIV prevalence rate of approximately 17.4%,[16] which is high in comparison with international statistics. This elevated prevalence of HIV amongst women is a concern and could suggest an even higher infection rate amongst transsexual women because of their vulnerability.

Apart from their physical healthcare needs, transsexual women are at great risk of mental ill-health as a result of the dramatic changes they experience during their transitioning process. A USA-based survey, which looked at 446 transsexual individuals, found that transsexual women have diminished mental health as opposed to their heterosexual counterparts.[17] In 2010, Hoshiai and others, identified that 72% of transsexual women had suicidal ideation, which can be correlated directly with the poor state of their mental wellness. Furthermore, androgen deprivation, which forms an integral part of the treatment toward gender re-alignment, can lead to depression.[18]

The prevalence of homophobia against Lesbian, Gay, Bi-Sexual, Transgendered and Intersex (LGBTI) youth is high[19] and it is recognised that a higher suicide risk is present in this group.[20] It can be concluded that transsexual women may potentially be at higher risk for suicide because they are even more marginalised than other people of the Lesbian, Gay, Bi-Sexual (LGB) community and often suffer internalised stigma.[21]

From the above, it is clear that supporting the mental well-being of this subset of the community is challenging. It is exacerbated by homo- and trans-phobia, stigma and depression, possibly caused by androgen deprivation.

The available literature demonstrates that transsexual women are at risk of the development of hypertension, diabetes, embolism, osteoporosis, HIV and mental illness amongst others. These conditions are directly related to their journey of sexual transition and will require them to seek appropriate healthcare at all available levels of care.

Access to appropriate healthcare services

Literature from North and South America shows that access to available services for the LGBTI community remains largely limited, or that there is a complete absence of healthcare services available to the transsexual community.[22,23] In the USA, both African-American and uninsured, impoverished, foreign-born transsexual women, are reported to have the least access to healthcare services.[22,24]

Adequate access to healthcare and provision of hormone therapy significantly increase the quality of life of transsexual women. Of critical importance is the availability of trans-specific health education, which could have a positive influence on their health risk behaviour patterns.[16,25] The knowledge of healthcare providers regarding transsexual health issues is vital for their access to and utilisation of appropriate healthcare services.

In the USA, a study of 101 MTF transsexual women found that a barrier to effective healthcare is the limited access to a healthcare provider that has adequate knowledge about the specifics of transsexual health.[26]

Another smaller study showed that specific health programmes do not acknowledge the LGBTI community,[19,20] but in a patient satisfaction survey of 180 transsexual women, it was confirmed that transsexual women consider their healthcare needs to be important.[27]

Health professionals' attitude, such as respect and sensitive care, is another critical factor toward increasing access and utilisation of healthcare services by the transsexual women. This was highlighted in a study where it was found that transsexual women from Australia, America and Europe choose to have trans-related procedures performed in Thailand. The Thai healthcare system is more accepting of the needs of transsexual women.[28]

Evidence suggests that having adequate access to trans-related healthcare is directly proportional to positive health outcomes for transsexual women. An improvement in the quality of healthcare provided to transsexual women will have a positive impact on the morbidity and mortality statistics of this group.

Transsexual women in Africa

Research in Africa is silent with regard to access to healthcare for transsexual women. It is assumed that the reason for this silence is because of the fact that any sexuality other than heterosexuality is deemed illegal in the significant majority of African countries and Africa has a very strong hetero-normative culture. It is then further assumed that African transsexual women will have poor access to quality healthcare and will contribute to the already high mortality and morbidity figures.

The population of transsexual women in South Africa is unknown. Hetero-normative census data does not make provision for documenting a transsexual woman as such. Through working with transsexual women, it has been observed that the community of transsexual women is fluid in nature. They will often move to protect their safety as they are under constant threat of transphobic violence, including rape. The violence and rape are a result of the society's hetero-normative belief and people will condone the violence and rape of these women because they are seen as lesser beings that can be treated in any manner.

With little known about the population of transsexual women, transsexual women indeed contribute to the mortality and morbidity figures of women. International literature clearly states that these women will experience health problems that may lead to death and chronic illness if not managed appropriately.

The difficulty arises in the reporting of mortality and morbidity figures of transsexual women, as there is no provision made in the hetero-normative reporting system for the reporting of this data. Even after death, transsexual women remain silent in the healthcare system. Without adequate reporting systems, audits are impossible and no evidence will be available to influence positive change in healthcare services for these women.

Conclusion

Literature suggests that transsexual women could potentially suffer significant chronic side-effects as a result of their treatment, such as diabetes, hypertension, osteoporosis and cancer, amongst others. These side-effects could be managed successfully should health practitioners have enough knowledge regarding trans-related healthcare. It is recommended that health practitioners be trained to manage these clients who would present at primary healthcare clinics with their trans-related health problems. This will ensure holistic care for these women.

Transsexual women are silent in health reporting systems. It is recommended that transsexual women should be noted as such on admission to any healthcare institution and should form part of data collected in healthcare systems.

Trans-phobia is a common phenomenon. This might lead to violence in the form of physical and sexual abuse of transsexual women. These violations should be noted as 'Transphobic violence' in order to have focused treatment and to influence prevention campaigns.

Amongst various factors, the vulnerability of the neo-vagina of transsexual women and the susceptibility of the rectal mucosa will make them vulnerable to the contraction of HIV. It is recommended that health education programmes that place a focus on the prevention of HIV should include transsexual women. This could increase awareness amongst transsexual women themselves and could also inform the broader population regarding the existence of transsexual women. It is also recommended that transsexual women be included in all other health education programmes in order to reduce stigma.

Research needs to be done to describe transsexual women in Africa. Their health problems should be investigated and reported. The phenomenon of homophobic violence, which includes rape, should also be investigated and reported as such.

These strategies will give a voice to an otherwise marginalised people, it will create awareness of the problems that a silenced community experience and it may start to break the stigma that any sexuality other than heterosexuality is un-African.

Acknowledgements

Competing interests

The authors declare that they have no financial or personal relationship(s) that may have inappropriately influenced them in writing this article.

Authors' contributions

D.N-V. (University of Cape Town) did this review as part of his PhD study at the University of Cape Town. S.D. (University of Cape Town) is the supervisor of this study and made significant intellectual contributions to this article.

References

1. Spicer SS. Healthcare needs of the transgender homeless population. J Gay Lesbian Ment Health. 2010;14(4):320–339. http://dx.doi.org/10.1080/19359705.2010.505844
2. Sobralske M. Primary care needs of patients who have undergone gender reassignment. J Am Acad Nurse Pract. 2005;17(4):133–138. http://dx.doi.org/10.1111/j.1041-2972.2005.0021.x
3. Pennington J, Knight T. Through the lens of hetero-normative assumptions: Re-thinking attitudes towards gay parenting. Cult Health Sex. 2011;13(1):59–72. http://dx.doi.org/10.1080/13691058.2010.519049
4. CASP International Network. Appraisal tools [page on the Internet]. c2014 [cited 2014 Apr 19]. Available from: http://www.caspinternational.org/?o=1012
5. Constitution of the Republic of South Africa [No. 108 of 1996], South Africa. Pretoria: Government Printers; 1997.
6. National Health Act [No.61 of 2003], South Africa. Pretoria: Government Printers; 2004.
7. Department of Health. National Health Insurance in South Africa [document on the Internet]. c2011 [cited 2014 Sep 14]. Available from: http://www.hst.org.za/sites/default/files/2bcce61d2d1b8d972af41ab0e2c8a4ab.pdf
8. Elbers JMH, Giltay EJ, Teerlink T, et al. Effects of sex steroids on components of the insulin resistance syndrome in transsexual subjects. Clin Endocrinol (Oxf). 2003;58(5):562–571. http://dx.doi.org/10.1046/j.1365-2265.2003.01753.x
9. Persson DI. Unique challenges of transgender aging: Implications from the literature. J Gerontol Soc Work. 2009;52(6):633–646. http://dx.doi.org/10.1080/01634370802609056
10. Kenagy GP, Hsieh CM. The risk less known: Female-to-male transgender persons' vulnerability to HIV infection. AIDS Care. 2005;17(2):195–207. http://dx.doi.org/10.1080/19540120512331325680
11. Sevelius JM, Reznick OG, Hart SL, et al. Informing interventions: The importance of contextual factors in the prediction of sexual risk behaviors among transgender women. AIDS Educ Prev. 2009;21(2):113–127. http://dx.doi.org/10.1521/aeap.2009.21.2.113
12. Kenagy G. HIV among transgendered people. AIDS Care. 2002;14(1):127–134. http://dx.doi.org/10.1080/09540120220098008
13. Melendez RM, Pinto R. 'It's really a hard life': Love, gender and HIV risk among male-to-female transgender persons. Cult Health Sex. 2007;9(3):233–245. http://dx.doi.org/10.1080/13691050601065909
14. Edwards JW, Fisher DG, Reynolds GL. Male-to-female transgender and transsexual clients of HIV service programs in Los Angeles County, California. Am J Public Health. 2007;97(6):1030–1033. http://dx.doi.org/10.2105/AJPH.2006.097717
15. Verster A, Davoli M, Camposeragna A, et al. Prevalence of HIV infection and risk behaviour among street prostitutes in Rome, 1997–1998. AIDS Care. 2001;13(3):367–372. http://dx.doi.org/10.1080/09540120120044017
16. Statistics South Africa. P0302 – Mid-year population estimates, 2013 [document on the Internet]. c2013 [cited 2014 Sep 14]. Available from: http://beta2.statssa.gov.za/?page_id=1854&PPN=P0302&SCH=5500
17. Newfield E, Hart S, Dibble S, et al. Female-to-male transgender quality of life. Qual Life Res. 2006;15(9):1447–1457. http://dx.doi.org/10.1007/s11136-006-0002-3
18. Hoshiai M, Matsumoto Y, Sato T, et al. Psychiatric comorbidity among patients with gender identity disorder. Psychiatry Clin Neurosci. 2010;64(5):514–519. http://dx.doi.org/10.1111/j.1440-1819.2010.02118.x
19. McDermott E, Roen K, Scourfield J. Avoiding shame: Young LGBT people, homophobia and self-destructive behaviours. Cult Health Sex. 2008;10(8):815–829. http://dx.doi.org/10.1080/13691050802380974
20. Scourfield J, Roen K, McDermott L. Lesbian, gay, bisexual and transgender young people's experiences of distress: Resilience, ambivalence and self-destructive behaviour. Health Soc Care Community. 2008;16(3):329–336. http://dx.doi.org/10.1111/j.1365-2524.2008.00769.x
21. James C, Haye DL. Challenges and treatment of a transsexual in Jamaica. Social & Economic Studies. 2011;60(1):137–153.
22. Harawa NT, Bingham TA. Exploring HIV prevention utilization among female sex workers and male-to-female transgenders. AIDS Educ Prev. 2009;21(4):356–371. http://dx.doi.org/10.1521/aeap.2009.21.4.356
23. Infante C, Sosa-Rubi S, Cuadra SM. Sex work in Mexico: Vulnerability of male, travesti, transgender and transsexual sex workers. CultHealth Sex. 2009;11(2):125–137. http://dx.doi.org/10.1080/13691050802431314
24. Sanchez NF, Sanchez JP, Danoff A. Health care utilization, barriers to care, and hormone usage among male-to-female transgender persons in New York City. Am J Public Health. 2009;99(4):713–719. http://dx.doi.org/10.2105/AJPH.2007.132035
25. Bockting WO, Robinson BE, Forberg J, et al. Evaluation of a sexual health approach to reducing HIV/STD risk in the transgender community. AIDS Care. 2005;17(3):289–303. http://dx.doi.org/10.1080/09540120412331299825
26. Sánchez FJ, Vilain E. Collective self-esteem as a coping resource for male-to-female transsexuals. J Couns Psychol. 2009;56(1):202–209. http://dx.doi.org/10.1037/a0014573
27. Bockting W, Robinson B, Benner A, et al. Patient satisfaction with transgender health services. J Sex Marital Ther. 2004;30(4):277–294. http://dx.doi.org/10.1080/00926230490422467
28. Aizura AZ. Feminine transformations: Gender reassignment surgical tourism in Thailand. Med Anthropol. 2010;29(4):424–443. http://dx.doi.org/10.1080/01459740.2010.501314

16

Patient knowledge of HIV and its treatment in South Africa

Authors:
Lauren M. Terblanche[1]
Ethelwynn L. Stellenberg[1]

Affiliations:
[1]Division of Nursing, Department of Interdisciplinary Health Sciences, Faculty of Medicine and Health Sciences, Stellenbosch University, South Africa

Correspondence to:
Lauren Terblanche

Email:
laurenterblanche@sun.ac.za

Postal address:
P.O. Box 19063, Tygerberg, 7500

Background: Patients on antiretroviral therapy (ART) need to achieve a 90% adherence rate to ART in order to prevent disease progression and drug resistance. The patients' knowledge of ART and HIV is thus crucial to ensuring good adherence, decreased risk for drug resistance and cost-effective treatment for these patients.

Aim: To determine the knowledge of infected patients with regard to HIV and the ART they were receiving.

Setting: The study was conducted at a comprehensive community health centre in a developing low socio-economic community near Cape Town, South Africa.

Methods: A quantitative descriptive correlative research design was applied. A sample consisting of 200 (8.5%) respondents was selected from a population of 2349. A multiple-choice questionnaire, comprising 29 questions, including 14 critical knowledge testing questions, was used in individual interviews conducted by either the researcher or fieldworker who assessed the respondents' knowledge regarding various key aspects of HIV and ART.

Results: Misconceptions regarding HIV and ART were revealed and scores for the 14 critical knowledge testing questions in the questionnaire revealed that 0% of the respondents had good knowledge, 20% had average knowledge and 80% had poor knowledge.

Conclusion: The respondents on ART in this particular community health centre had poor knowledge of HIV and ART. This may contribute to poor adherence rates, increased drug resistance, disease progression and increased costs for the government with regard to treating such patients. Increased attention needs to be given to patient education.

Le savoir est essentiel: La Connaissance du VIH et de son traitement par les patients sous traitement antirétroviral.

Contexte: Les patients sous traitement antirétroviral (ART) ont besoin d'atteindre un taux d'observance de 90% à la thérapie antirétrovirale pour prévenir la progression de la maladie et la résistance aux médicaments. Par conséquent, la connaissance de l'ART et du VIH par les patients est essentielle pour assurer une bonne adhérence, réduire le risque de résistance aux médicaments et assurer un bon rapport coût-efficacité du traitement de ces patients.

Objectif: Déterminer les connaissances des patients infectés sur le VIH et l'ART administré.

Cadre: Cette étude a été menée dans un centre de santé communautaire polyvalent dans une communauté au statut socioéconomique faible près du Cap, en Afrique du Sud.

Méthodes: Un modèle d'étude quantitative descriptive et corrélative a été utilisé. Un échantillon constitué de 200 (8.5%) répondants a été sélectionné parmi une population de 2349 individus. Un questionnaire à choix multiples composé de 29 questions, dont 14 questions testant les connaissances essentielles, a été administré au cours d'entretiens individuels menés par le chercheur ou l'agent de terrain chargé d'évaluer les connaissances des répondants sur divers aspects clés du VIH et de l'ART.

Résultats: Des idées fausses concernant le VIH et l'ART ont été révélées et les scores pour les 14 questions du questionnaire testant les connaissances essentielles ont révélé que 0% des personnes interrogées disposaient de bonnes connaissances, 20% de connaissances moyennes et 80% de mauvaises connaissances.

Conclusion: Les personnes sous antirétroviraux interrogées dans ce centre de santé communautaire particulier disposaient de mauvaises connaissances sur le VIH et l'ART. Cela peut contribuer à de faibles taux d'observance, à une augmentation de la résistance aux médicaments, à la progression de la maladie et à l'augmentation des coûts liés au traitement de ces patients pour le gouvernement. Une attention accrue doit être accordée à l'éducation des patients.

Introduction

Despite the call for better coordination and monitoring in South Africa, the number of people living with HIV has shown a constant increase every year since the first diagnosis in the 1980s,[1] with more and more people being affected by this debilitating disease. Studies have shown that the number of patients receiving antiretroviral therapy (ART) in South Africa has increased from less than 50 000 in 2004 to 1.79 million in 2011.[2]

Various interventions have been introduced with regard to reducing the vulnerability to HIV infection and the impact of acquired immune deficiency syndrome (AIDS) in order to increase awareness and knowledge of the disease, including:

- prevention of the sexual transmission of HIV through distribution of free condoms
- an increase in coverage for voluntary counselling and testing promotion of regular HIV testing
- the placement of non-profit organisation (NPO)-funded counsellors within community health centres (CHCs) to provide education and information in adherence classes as well as continuous HIV counselling and support to patients.[1]

However, research shows that South Africa's main contributing factors in the spread of this disease are rooted in poverty, underdevelopment, the low status of women and gender-based violence in the communities.[1]

The standard treatment of choice for people living with HIV is ART which functions by suppressing the replication of HIV.[3] It has been confirmed (Mouton J. 2013, personal communication, January 16) that it currently costs the South African government approximately R124.00 per month to treat a patient with first-line ART and, once they move to second-line ART, approximately R547.00 per month. As there are currently only two lines of drug treatment in South Africa, it is important that patients adhere to their treatment, bearing in mind that patients who fail second-line therapy have few treatment options left to them.[3] Adherence to ART is thus important with regard to containing the disease because incomplete adherence may lead to poor treatment outcomes and an increased risk for HIV-related mortality.[4] Adherence of more than 90% needs to be achieved in order for ART to be effective.[5] If ART is not adhered to correctly, HIV is not controlled optimally within the body – the viral load in the blood increases, thus aiding disease progression which poses a higher risk for opportunistic infections such as tuberculosis (TB).[6] Poor adherence could also lead to ART resistance.[6]

Adherence rates are not always optimal, as was identified in a study conducted in South Africa[7] which found that only 62.5% of patients had an adherence rate of more than 90% and, therefore, 37.5% of the respondents were at risk of developing resistance because of unacceptable adherence levels.[8]

It is believed that knowledge of the disease has an influence on adherence levels. Various studies have been focused on improving adherence through changing behaviour patterns and other interventions,[7] such as patient education; however, there are few studies available that report on patients' knowledge about various factors relating to HIV.[4] Some studies conducted in specialised HIV clinics have shown that patients demonstrated good knowledge of HIV and the transmission thereof,[9] but it has also been identified that adherence rates to ART are influenced strongly by misconceptions regarding HIV.[10]

Some misconceptions identified in studies conducted in Botswana were that out of 400 respondents, both male and female, 40.3% did not believe that they could be re-infected with HIV through sexual intercourse or any other means.[10] Another misconception was that some people (n = 122; 30.5%) believed that HIV could be cured.[10] In the same study it was indicated that 9.3% of the respondents believed that HIV did not even really exist.[10]

Another misconception revealed in a study conducted in KwaZulu-Natal, South Africa, was that showering after sex can be used as a preventative measure.[11]

It is believed that, with improved insight and knowledge about the disease and the management thereof, an improvement in adherence may result as patients with inadequate knowledge of HIV and its transmission would be more likely to report not taking ART.[12]

Orisakwe, Ross and Ocholla[11] state that adherence classes provided by healthcare workers are vital for adherence to ART as they provide patients with information about the disease, correct doses of medication and possible side effects. It is believed that knowledge of ART and HIV will empower the HIV-positive individual. This is substantiated by the Health Belief Model which suggests that knowledge, attitudes and perceptions of risk affect the behaviour of individuals.[13] HIV health education policies have been put in place by the South African government in order for healthcare workers and HIV counsellors to continue with HIV health education throughout the treatment of their patients.[1] It is believed that the individual will consequently be motivated to be part of the collaborative process because initiation of ART is a clinical decision which should always be made jointly between the informed patient and the healthcare provider.[14]

Adequate patient education is specifically required when treating a patient infected with HIV as it comprises many facets that need constant attention. Patients need to be informed in full about their disease in order to be able to make informed decisions and to adhere effectively to treatment which would allow them to contain the disease. Patients may adhere to education given to them regarding prevention of HIV transmission through safe sex practices, taking medication as prescribed and accepting responsibility for their own health. This may, ultimately, contribute to an improvement in the quality of life of patients with HIV, as well as contributing positively to the strategic plan that the South African government has made in order to tackle the HIV problem in the country. For this reason, determining the knowledge that patients have regarding HIV may assist in determining whether or not the current patient education model being implemented in CHCs is successful and, if not, which measures can be put in place in order to improve the current model or implementation thereof.

The principle investigator (PI) identified during her clinical practice that the high burden of HIV in South Africa, combined with overcrowded CHCs, aggravated the daily management of patients. The high influx of patients into clinics every day increases time constraints and minimises consultation time, thereby diminishing the opportunity for effective patient education regarding HIV.[15]

With this in mind, this study set out to determine what knowledge infected patients receiving ART had with regard to HIV and the treatment they were receiving at the particular CHC, as well as to determine which demographic factors, if any, influenced this knowledge.

Research methods and design

Study design

This study followed a quantitative descriptive correlative research design.

Setting

The study was conducted at a comprehensive CHC with a newly-built ART clinic in a developing low socio-economic community near Cape Town, South Africa with a population of 66 667.[16] The ART clinic was equipped with doctors, nurses, HIV counsellors and other allied staff. The CHC managed an average number of 1200 patients daily presenting with a variety of medical conditions. This setting was chosen as it ensured a homogenous group of patients from the same socio-economic level.

Study population and sampling strategy

The specific criteria for the target population for this study included all ART recipients who were above the age of 18, who had been on ART for at least three months and who were attending the particular CHC. The total number of patients who met the specific criteria for this study at the time was 2349.

As guided by a statistician, a convenience sample of 200 (8.5%) respondents was selected. It was decided that the first 200 respondents who voluntarily gave written consent to participate in the study and who complied with the specific criteria would be included in the sample.

Convenience sampling was best suited for this study because of the profile of the patients attending this CHC. Patients received booked appointments; however, various factors influenced the regular attendance of patients to the clinics (such as the availability of transport, unemployment and finances) and it could therefore not be relied upon that patients would attend their follow-up appointments.

Data collection

A structured and pre-tested multiple-choice questionnaire which was designed by the PI was used for collecting the data. The questionnaire comprised two sections: Section A covered demographic data such as age and gender and also included the length of time living with HIV and the length of time on ART. Section B comprised 26 multiple-choice questions and three closed-ended questions which tested the knowledge of key aspects of HIV and ART such as modes of transmission, the duration of the window period as well as whether or not ART can cure HIV.

Twenty questions tested knowledge of HIV and ART, 14 of which were designated 'critical questions'. The critical questions were identified in consultation with various HIV specialists as being the basic questions that all ART recipients should know and be able to answer.

The questionnaire was designed by the PI after an extensive literature review had been conducted on various aspects of the subject. The content validity was validated by the study supervisor, an expert in the field of research methodology and nursing, as well as by three additional experts in the fields of nursing, HIV and research. The questionnaire was then also reviewed by a statistician to ensure the suitability of the questionnaire for data analysis. A pilot study was conducted on 20 respondents in order to test the validity and reliability of the study. The questionnaire and methodology proved to be reliable and valid throughout both the pilot study and the main study.

The data was collected at the CHC over a period of three weeks in August 2011 by means of individual interviews with each of the respondents.

The fieldworker, a known educated Xhosa member of the community and a volunteer at the CHC, was trained. This included sitting in during five interviews conducted by the PI, which was done with the consent of the respondents. The fieldworker then conducted two individual interviews in the presence of the researcher before she was allowed to conduct interviews on her own. The fieldworker was fluent in both Xhosa and English.

Respondents were selected according to their availability and the willingness of each respondent to present for ART follow-up on a particular day; namely, those who complied with the specific criteria set for the study. Participation was completely voluntary and no incentive was given for taking part in the study.

Each respondent was provided with an information leaflet as well as a written informed consent document. Written informed consent was then obtained from each of the respondents, in their preferred language (English, Afrikaans or Xhosa) and, thereafter, the PI or trained fieldworker conducted an individual interview with each respondent, finally completing 200 interviews. It was stressed that participation was entirely voluntary and that, should the respondents agree to take part, they were free to withdraw at any time without having to give an explanation. Only two respondents excluded themselves because of time constraints.

The questionnaire was presented and completed by the PI or trained fieldworker during individual, structured interviews by reading questions in a language (English or Afrikaans) which the respondent understood, as well as providing all possible answers from the questionnaire from which the respondent could select answers. Interviewer bias was prevented by allowing the PI or trained fieldworker only to read a question and read out the set of answers slowly as stated in the questionnaire. The respondent was then given an opportunity to select an answer (or answers) which was marked off on the questionnaire by the interviewer. To ensure confidentiality, all documentation was anonymous, with no identification. Once the interview was completed, the completed questionnaire was placed in a box, which was with the fieldworker or PI at all times during the interviews. The PI collected the completed questionnaires from the fieldworker on a daily basis.

The data gathered from the study were handled only by the PI and the fieldworker, then coded and stored in a secure location.

Given the nature of the questions in the questionnaire, potential psychological stress was anticipated and there was always a counsellor available should respondents have required some assistance. However, none of the respondents experienced any stress during the process.

Data analysis

Data were captured on an Excel spreadsheet by the PI and the document was then analysed with the help of a statistician, using the computerised data analysis programme, STATISTICA Version Nine (StatSoft, Tulsa, OK, 2009). For descriptive purposes frequency tables, histograms, means and standard deviations were used. Knowledge testing questions were correlated with the demographic variables. For comparison of variables, this included cross tabulation using the Chi-square test, correlation analyses or ANOVA. A 95% confidence interval with a significance level of ($p \leq 0.05$) was used to establish statistically-significant associations between variables as discussed.

The questionnaire consisted of a total of 29 questions of which 20 tested HIV and ART knowledge. In consultation with various professionals in the field of HIV, 14 questions in the questionnaire were identified as critical questions (Tables 2 and 3) and it was expected that respondents should be able to answer these basic but important questions correctly. The other questions, however, were seen as 'good to know'.

These 14 questions were identified to be the basis for deciding whether or not the respondents in the study had good, average or poor knowledge of HIV and ART. Respondents were considered to have good knowledge if they had all 14 critical questions correct, average if they had 11 to 13 correct and poor if they had 10 or fewer correct.

Ethical considerations

Respondents were not exposed to any physical risks and permission to conduct this study was obtained in writing from the Health Research Ethics Committee of Stellenbosch University on 8 April 2011 (ref. N11/02/056) and from the Provincial Regional Head for Primary Health Care Services on 8 August 2011 (ref. LSB/ELS/08/11). Verbal permission was obtained on 9 August 2011 from the head of the CHC where the data collection took place.

Results

The data indicated that 72.5% (n = 145) of the respondents were female and 75% (n = 150) were Xhosa speaking. The mean age was 37.5 years and, although the study was conducted in a low socio-economic area, 196 (98%) were literate with 78.5% (n = 157) having a highest education level between grades 8 and 12. Table 1 contains the demographic data from the study.

TABLE 1: Demographic characteristics and education of the study population (N = 200).

Variables	%	*n*
Gender		
Male	27.5	55
Female	72.5	145
Home language		
Xhosa	75	150
English	3.5	7
Afrikaans	18	36
Zulu	2	4
Other	2	4
Literacy level		
Can read and write	98	196
Highest education level		
No Schooling	1	2
Grade 1–7	20.5	41
Grade 8–9	22.5	45
Grade 10–12	56	112
Length of time living with HIV		
< 1 year	7.5	15
1–3 years	30	60
3–5 years	25.5	51
> 5 years	36.5	73
Don't know	0.5	1
Length of time on antiretroviral therapy		
< 1 year	23.5	47
1–3 years	39	78
3–5 years	20	40
> 5 years	17.5	35

Note: Minimum age 37.5; Mean age 37.5 years; Maximum age 62 years.

Knowledge regarding the action of HIV compromising the immune system was only answered correctly by 57% (*n* = 114) of the respondents and many of the respondents thought HIV merely destroys your organs; however, the spread of HIV was relatively well understood by most of the respondents (Table 2).

What is of concern, however, is that 1% (*n* = 2) of the respondents indicated that HIV cannot be spread through sexual intercourse and 6% (*n* = 12) stated that HIV cannot be spread through HIV-infected body fluids. Some had the mistaken belief that HIV could be spread through coughing and mosquitoes – this was observed during analysis (Table 2), which corresponded with previous studies conducted.

The knowledge of the window period was poor, with only 42.5% (*n* = 85) of the respondents knowing what it was.

Patients became very confused with the difference between a CD4 count and a viral load, giving the answer for what a viral load is under the question of CD4 count and *vice versa*. Only 71% (*n* = 142) of the respondents knew what a CD4 count was and only 60% (*n* = 120) knew what a viral load was. The majority (*n* = 159; 80%) of the respondents knew when their last CD4 count was done; however, few (*n* = 23; 11.5%) indicated correctly that their CD4 count should be measured every 12 months.

Most of the respondents were aware that HIV could be transmitted intrauterinally and 93.5% (*n* = 187) also knew that they could still have HIV-negative children with the help of ART.

The open questions allowed themes to be identified as to the reasons why respondents started on ART. It is interesting to note that, as previously mentioned, only 71% (*n* = 142) knew what a CD4 count was, but that 80% (*n* = 160) said that they were placed on ART because of a low CD4 count.

Respondents (*n* = 197; 98.5%) knew that ART could not cure HIV and that treatment was likely to be lifelong; however, only 93.5% (*n* = 189) of the respondents understood the actual function of ART. A misconception was identified in that 1% (*n* = 2) of the respondents indicated that ART has the function of making unprotected sex safe (Table 3).

Education on side effects seemed to be lacking as many of the respondents indicated that they had not had any education on the side effects of ART.

Only 10.5% (*n* = 21) could name two danger signs and, although not all respondents (*n* = 126; 63%) could name the danger signs, they knew that if something abnormal did occur, they should stop the medication and go to the clinic as soon as possible. However, 33% (*n* = 66) did not know what to do at all.

The majority (*n* = 153; 76.5%) of the respondents knew that if they forgot to take their medication that they should take it as soon as possible thereafter.

Many of respondents indicated that ART did not cure HIV and when asked the question, 'what will happen if you stop taking your medication?', 94.5% (*n* = 189) of the respondents indicated correctly that 'the ART will become less effective and the HI-Virus will increase in your blood' (Table 3).

TABLE 2: Assessment of knowledge of HIV.

Questions	%	*n*
Action of HIV (cc)		
Kills the immune system†	57	114
HIV is spread by (cc)		
Kissing	96.5	193
Hugging	99	198
Sexual intercourse†	99	198
Mosquitoes	90	180
Coughing	88.8	177
Blood transfusion†	100	200
Infected bodily fluids†	94	188
The window period is (cc)		
When HIV cannot be seen in the blood†	42.5	85
Duration of the window period (cc)		
3 months†	41	82
A CD4 count is (cc)		
Number of fighter cells in the blood†	71	142
How often a CD4 count should be monitored (cc)		
12 monthly†	11.5	23
Importance of monitoring the CD4 count		
To monitor if treatment is effective†	69.5	139
A viral load is		
Number of HIV cells in the blood	35	70
If you are HIV positive your children will definitely be positive (cc)		
No	93.5	187

n, Results expressed as number of respondents with the correct answer; %, Results expressed as percentage of respondents with the correct answer; †, All correct answers; cc, Critical questions.

TABLE 3: Assessment of knowledge of antiretroviral therapy.

Questions	%	*n*
Antiretroviral therapy can cure HIV (cc)		
No†	98.5	197
Action of antiretroviral therapy (cc)		
Kills the virus	2	4
Reduces the viral load in the blood†	94.5	189
Makes it safe to have unsafe sex	1	2
Don't know	2.5	5
Patient received education on antiretroviral side effects		
Yes	61	122
No	39	78
Antiretroviral therapy can cause dangerous side effects (cc)		
Yes†	36.5	73
Name two danger signs (cc)		
Could name two	10.5	21
Action to take if experience danger signs (cc)		
Stop and go to the clinic immediately†	63	126
Continue medication	3	6
Skip a day and continue	1	2
Don't know	33	66
What should be done if medication is forgotten (cc)		
Drink immediately when you remember†	76.5	153
Result from ceasing to take medication (cc)		
Antiretroviral therapy becomes less effective, HIV will increase	94.5	189

n, Results expressed as number of respondents with the correct answer; %, Results expressed as percentage of respondents with the correct answer; †, All correct answers; cc, Critical questions.

What was interesting is that most (n = 167; 83.5%) of the respondents indicated that they had gained their HIV and ART knowledge from the HIV 'sister' i.e. the professional registered nurse or the doctor (n = 11; 5.5%) in the clinic and not from other sources such as the HIV counsellors.

Respondents' scoring

Analysis of the data revealed that the average score of all 200 respondents for all 20 knowledge testing questions in the questionnaire, including the 'good to know' questions, was 63%. Analysis of the 14 critical questions revealed that none of the respondents had good knowledge, only 20% (n = 40) of the respondents had average knowledge and 80% (n = 160) of the respondents had poor knowledge (Figure 1).

Discussion

The results show that the general knowledge of 80% (n = 160) of the study population was poor, contradicting results from previous studies.[10]

Furthermore, despite the fact that the study revealed that most ART recipients obtained their HIV and ART knowledge from the HIV nursing 'sister', the overall knowledge of HIV and ART amongst the recipients of ART was poor, contradicting the government's plan to decrease the incidence of HIV by promoting HIV education and counselling.

Basic terms and principles of HIV and ART were not understood by the respondents in this study and serious misconceptions regarding the disease were revealed, corresponding with results from previous studies.[2] Men and women differed on occasion in the way they answered questions, however, demographic factors such as race and gender did not prove to have a significant influence on the overall knowledge of the respondents.

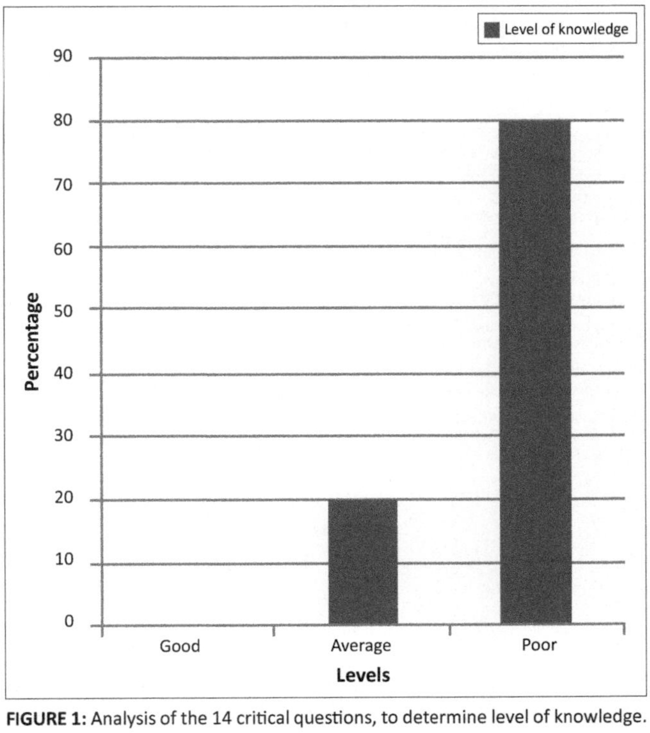

FIGURE 1: Analysis of the 14 critical questions, to determine level of knowledge.

Despite the presence of HIV counsellors who function to give adherence counselling[1] in the CHC under study, many (n = 78; 39%) respondents reported that they had not received any education on the side effects of ART and did not know that ART can potentially have dangerous side effects. This result makes one question whether or not patients were well informed and were part of the clinical decision to commence ART.[14]

A limitation identified was that the study was conducted in only one community and did not include any other communities. It was limited to the Cape Metropole area, therefore the results cannot be generalised. All respondents were able to speak and understand English, so language did not result in any bias.

Patient education is vital, as patients are enabled to take the information, carry the knowledge with them and make decisions based on what they know and have learnt. However, from this study it is clear that the HIV knowledge of ART patients at this particular CHC is poor.

Healthcare workers and HIV counsellors need to take up the role as a supportive-educative medium for the patient, by educating the patients and equipping them to make informed decisions based on what they know and understand. They, however, need to be informed, motivated and prepared to convey information and to make time for patient education using the resources available to them.

By identifying the deficit in patient knowledge, healthcare workers and HIV counsellors may decide which support modality is needed in order to educate and to promote knowledge and adherence. In addition, leaders in the community also need to be equipped with the knowledge and skills required to support and motivate members of the community with regard to HIV.

Education and health promotion empower people to take control of their own lives and their own health. This creates an environment which supports healthier lifestyles and informed decision making based on knowledge and understanding. Ultimately, this may contribute to an improvement in the quality of life of HIV-infected patients.

Based on the findings from this study, the following recommendations have been made:

1. Attention needs to be given to patient education in the clinical setting. Measures to improve patient education in this CHC need to be developed and implemented as soon as possible, especially since the research shows that patient knowledge is poor.
2. Education is essential with regard to facilitating patients to become mature individuals who are able to make informed decisions regarding their health and wellbeing.
3. Health workers and counsellors need to take note of who they are educating and what role each individual plays. Thus, they need to educate patients appropriately, as well as giving them any support necessary.
4. As the data revealed that most of the respondents' knowledge was obtained from the HIV nursing 'sister',

it is suggested that further research be conducted in order to implement an in-service training programme to further educate nurses on HIV and ART, followed by an evaluation process including monitoring of patient adherence statistics.

5. More research needs to be conducted in this clinical facility to determine the possible reasons for the poor knowledge of these particular patients.
6. The study revealed that there are gaps in research and it is thus suggested that:
   a. further research should be done in other communities to determine if there are any similarities to the results found in this study and, should more poor knowledge trends be found in other sites, the current strategy for ART patient education should be revised
   b. research also needs to be conducted to evaluate nursing staff's knowledge of HIV and ART
   c. research should also be done to determine the factors that influence patient education in the primary healthcare setting.

Conclusion

The results of this study revealed that of the respondents on ART at this CHC, 80% had poor knowledge of HIV and ART.

Despite the government's endeavours to increase awareness of HIV and ART in communities through patient education and counselling, as well as to implement patient education policies within the healthcare setting, it is disheartening to note that the majority of patients in this particular ART clinic had poor knowledge about HIV and ART, which indicates that health education is not a priority in this clinical setting. Higher priority needs to be placed on patient education and time needs to be set aside by all healthcare providers to educate patients at every visit and answer impending questions. Cost-effective treatment is reliant on the adherence of patients to their treatment, so by not educating patients about HIV and ART the cost for the government in treating these patients increases because of the occurrence of co-infections and drug resistance.

It is also imperative that health workers and counsellors dealing with HIV-infected patients, with support from the government, have up-to-date knowledge regarding all aspects of the disease and treatment so that they are able to convey the correct information to the patients they are treating.

Acknowledgments

We would like to thank all the respondents who agreed to participate in the study, as well as the staff at the CHC who accommodated us to collect the data.

Competing interests

The authors declare that they have no financial or personal relationship(s) that may have inappropriately influenced them in writing this article.

Authors contributions

L.T. (Stellenbosch University) conducted the research, analysed and interpreted the data and wrote the manuscript. E.L.S. (Stellenbosch University) supervised the research and reviewed and edited the manuscript.

References

1. Department of Health. HIV & AIDS and STI strategic plan for South Africa 2007–2011 [homepage on the Internet]. c2007 [cited 2013 Dec 22]. Available from: http://www.info.gov.za/otherdocs/2007/aidsplan2007/
2. Johnson LF. Access to antiretroviral treatment in South Africa, 2004–2011. SAJHIVMED. 2012;13(1):1–19.
3. South Africa. Department of Health: Provincial Government of the Western Cape. Clinical Guidelines of the Western Cape: Primary Care Management of Adults HIV/AIDS, TB, Asthma/COPD & STIs 2013/14 2013. Western Cape: Republic of South Africa; 2013.
4. Racey CS, Zhang W, Brandson EK, et al. HIV antiviral drug resistance: patient comprehension. AIDS Care. 2010;22(7):816–826. http://dx.doi.org/10.1080/09540120903431355
5. Bangsberg DR. Less than 95% adherence to nonnucleoside reverse-transcriptase inhibitor therapy can lead to viral suppression. Clin Infect Dis. 2006;43(7):939–941. http://dx.doi.org/10.1086/507526
6. Evian C. Primary HIV/AIDS care. Melville: Jacana Media; 2008.
7. Battaglioli-DeNero AM. Strategies for improving patient adherence to therapy and long-term patient outcomes. J Assoc Nurses AIDS Care. 2007;18(1 Suppl):S17–S22. http://dx.doi.org/10.1016/j.jana.2006.11.020
8. Bhat VG, Ramburuth M, Singh M, et al. Factors associated with poor adherence to anti-retroviral therapy in patients attending a rural health centre in South Africa. Eur J Clin Microbiol Infect Dis. 2010;29(8):947–953. http://dx.doi.org/10.1007/s10096-010-0949-4
9. Nachega JB, Lehman DA, Hlatshwayo D, et al. HIV/AIDS and antiretroviral treatment knowledge, attitudes, beliefs, and practices in HIV-infected adults in Soweto, South Africa. J Acquir Immune Defic Syndr. 2005;38(2):196–201. http://dx.doi.org/10.1097/00126334-200502010-00011
10. Kip E, Ehlers VJ, Van der Wal DM. Patients' adherence to anti- retroviral therapy in Botswana. J Nurs Scholarsh. 2009;41(2):149–157. http://dx.doi.org/10.1111/j.1547-5069.2009.01266.x
11. Orisakwe EE, Ross AJ, Ocholla PO. Correlation between knowledge of HIV, attitudes and perceptions of HIV and a willingness to test for HIV at a regional hospital in KwaZulu-Natal, South Africa. Afr J Prm Health Care Fam Med. 2012;4(1), Art. #376, 8 pages. http://dx.doi.org/10.4102/phcfm.v4i1.376
12. Smith Fawzi MC, Jagannathan P, Cabral J, et al. Limitations in knowledge of HIV transmission among HIV-positive patients accessing case management services in a resource-poor setting. AIDS Care. 2006;18(6):764-–771. http://dx.doi.org/10.1080/09540120500373844
13. Denison J. Behaviour change – a summary of four major theories. Family Health International; 2004.
14. Mukona D, Charumbira APG, Nyamakura R, et al. ART knowledge and adherence. HIV Nursing Matters. 2011;2(2):16–19.
15. Neyhart CD. Education of patients pre and post-transplant: improving outcomes by overcoming the barriers. Nephrol Nurs J. 2008;35(4):409–410.
16. Statistics South Africa. City of Cape Town – Census 2001 – Delft [data table online]. c2001 [cited 2012 Sep 10]. Available from: http://www.capetown.gov.za/en/stats/2001census/Documents/Delft.htm

17

What keeps health professionals working in rural district hospitals in South Africa?

Authors:
Louis S. Jenkins[1,2]
Colette Gunst[1,2]
Julia Blitz[1]
Johan F. Coetzee[1]

Affiliations:
[1]Division of Family Medicine and Primary Care, Faculty of Medicine and Health Sciences, Stellenbosch University, South Africa

[2]Western Cape Department of Health, South Africa

Correspondence to:
Louis Jenkins

Email:
louis.jenkins@westerncape.gov.za

Postal address:
PO Box 241, Cape Town 8000, South Africa

Background: The theme of the 2014 Southern African Rural Health Conference was 'Building resilience in facing rural realities'. Retaining health professionals in South Africa is critical for sustainable health services. Only 12% of doctors and 19% of nurses have been retained in the rural areas. The aim of the workshop was to understand from health practitioners why they continued working in their rural settings.

Conference workshop: The workshop consisted of 29 doctors, managers, academic family physicians, nurses and clinical associates from Southern Africa, with work experience from three weeks to 13 years, often in deep rural districts. Using the nominal group technique, the following question was explored, 'What is it that keeps you going to work every day?' Participants reflected on their work situation and listed and rated the important reasons for continuing to work.

Results: Five main themes emerged. A shared purpose, emanating from a deep sense of meaning, was the strongest reason for staying and working in a rural setting. Working in a team was second most important, with teamwork being related to attitudes and relationships, support from visiting specialists and opportunities to implement individual clinical skills. A culture of support was third, followed by opportunities for growth and continuing professional development, including teaching by outreaching specialists. The fifth theme was a healthy work-life balance.

Conclusion: Health practitioners continue to work in rural settings for often deeper reasons relating to a sense of meaning, being part of a team that closely relate to each other and feeling supported.

Qu'est-ce qui encourage les professionnels de la santé à travailler dans les hôpitaux de districts ruraux en Afrique du Sud?

Contexte: Le thème de la Conférence sur la Santé rurale en Afrique australe en 2014 était "Développer la Résilience pour faire face aux réalités rurales'. Il est crucial de retenir les professionnels de la santé en Afrique du Sud pour avoir des services de santé durables. Seuls 12% des médecins et 19% des infirmiers ont été retenus dans les zones rurales. Le but des ateliers était de demander aux professionnels de santé pourquoi ils continuaient à travailler dans les zones rurales.

Atelier-conférence: L'atelier comprenait 29 médecins, gestionnaires, médecins de famille académiques, infirmières et collaborateurs cliniques d'Afrique du Sud, avec une expérience de travail de trois semaines à 13 ans, souvent dans des zones rurales reculées. Au moyen de la technique du groupe nominal, la question suivante a été examinée, 'Qu'est-ce qui vous fait aller au travail chaque jour? '. Les participants ont réfléchi sur leur situation de travail et ont fait une liste et évalué les raisons importantes pour continuer de travailler.

Résultats: Cinq thèmes principaux sont apparus. La raison la plus forte pour rester travailler à la campagne était un objectif commun, provenant d'un sens profond. La seconde était de travailler en équipe, où le travail d'équipe était lié aux attitudes et relations, au soutien des spécialistes itinérants et à la possibilité de mettre en œuvre les compétences cliniques individuelles. La troisième était une culture de soutien, suivie par des opportunités de croissance et de développement professionnel continu, telles que la formation par des spécialistes de sensibilisation. Le troisième thème était un bon équilibre entre la vie familiale et professionnelle.

Conclusion: Les professionnels de santé continuent à travailler dans les zones rurales pour des raisons souvent plus profondes liées à leur raison d'être, leur appartenance à une équipe dont les membres sont étroitement liés et au sentiment d'être soutenus.

Introduction

Background

The theme of the Southern African Rural Health Conference held at the Worcester Rural Clinical School in South Africa in September 2014 was 'Building resilience in facing rural realities'. It was co-hosted by the Rural Doctors' Association of Southern Africa (RUDASA), Rural Rehab of Southern Africa (RURESA), and the Professional Association of Clinical Associates in South Africa (PACASA). Retaining health professionals in the district hospitals in the 52 health districts in South Africa is critical for sustainable health services.[1] South Africa joins many countries in Africa and other parts of the world where the number of doctors is below 1/1000 population, with the 'ratio of physicians per 1000 population essentially unchanged between 2004 (0.77) and 2011 (0.76)'.[2] Whilst the number of graduating doctors in South Africa increased by 18% between 2000 and 2012, with many doctors leaving the country, the absolute numbers have not increased. In addition there has been a shift in gender parity to more women; and in racial parity to 'more black Africans and persons of mixed ancestry, and fewer whites and Indians'.[2]

Various strategies for recruitment and especially retention of health staff have been described, but the question was what local health professionals in South Africa thought and believed about retaining staff in a district hospital: what keeps them working there, despite the many challenges. In other words: What pull factors override all the push factors of working in low-resourced rural environments? Some of the challenges/push factors include: the quadruple burden of disease found in the HIV and tuberculosis epidemic; a high rate of violence and road accidents; high maternal and child mortality; and a large non-communicable disease epidemic resulting from a Western lifestyle.[3] Other challenges include: an absolute shortage of doctors and other health professions; high turnover of junior doctors; and inequity between urban and rural, private and public practice, with only 12% of doctors and 19% of nurses being retained in the rural areas and an overall 30% of doctors caring for 85% of the uninsured population in the country.[4] The necessity of ensuring good leadership and health management to address issues like supply shortages, corruption, accommodation and infrastructure, as well as continuing medical education and 'career pathing' opportunities for health professionals, has been recognised as a compounding factor in retention.[5] South Africa has the highest Gini coefficient (0.7) in the world, with poverty, unemployment and poor education in communities often providing the background in which health challenges are embedded.[2]

Strategies to retain health professionals have been developed internationally by the World Health Organization, Australia, Canada, and South Africa.[6,7,8] Examples of the strategies employed in South Africa include: the introduction of a compulsory community service year for doctors and allied health professionals and, more recently, also for nurses; the initiation of the midlevel clinical associate programme; the start of the National Health Insurance project; and the upgrading of health infrastructure in the country. Non-government organisations, for example African Health placement (AHP) and local academic institutions, for example, the Rural Health Advocacy Project of the University of Witwatersrand, have also played a role.[9,10] However, these changes do not translate to improved retention of staff overnight and many of the challenges are still a painful daily reality for health workers at the coalface. So the question remains, why do doctors, allied healthcare workers and nurses remain in rural areas in South Africa?

Conference workshop

A workshop was conducted and consisted of 29 doctors, managers, academic family physicians, nurses and clinical associates from all over South Africa, with work experience ranging from three weeks to 13 years, often in deep rural districts. Using the nominal group technique,[11] the following question was explored, 'What is it that keeps you going to work every day?' Participants reflected on their own work situation, then listed and rated the most important reasons for continuing to work in the challenging health system as mentioned above. The focus was on 'retention in work' rather than what drives healthcare workers to apply for work in a rural area. After clarification and prioritisation of emerging themes in small groups, all participants reached consensus on the five most important reasons for continuing to work in a small rural district hospital.

Results

The five main themes that emerged are now discussed in more detail.

Shared purpose

A shared purpose, emanating from a deep sense of meaning, was the strongest reason for staying and working in a rural setting. 'I am making a difference' and 'I know that I am called to do this' were typical comments. People felt that they were making, or wanted to make, a difference to the health of the local community. Some spoke about 'going back home', having been recruited from that rural area. These health practitioners had a very particular identity within their communities of practice which were being formed all the time whilst immersed in the rural realities, a process well described by Wenger.[12]

Working in a team

Working in a team featured as second most important. It was more than just having a team, but also related to attitudes and relationships, the wider team of support coming from the visiting specialists, support to implement clinical skills within that team and even how the team fits into one's personal and community life. Visiting specialists are general specialist doctors in the various clinical disciplines who are usually based in the regional referral hospital and who reach out to the surrounding district hospitals in the periphery on a regular basis, to provide clinical service and teaching to the medical officers and family physicians. One recently-qualified family physician emphasised the fact that 'they [*visiting general specialists*] knew me' as being one of the keys to successful completion of her family medicine registrar training in a rural area. 'Teamness' involves much more than a general team spirit, but relates to a transformation in people's minds around understanding team members' passion, using the 'we' language and celebrating and rewarding people and events for mutual benefits.[13,14] Being part of a team allows a person the space to celebrate successes and to debrief from stressful encounters. It relates to becoming part of the community that the health practitioner envisioned initially and attracted him or her toward the actual community – a process that Wenger described as a healthy tension between reification (translating the abstract concept of teamwork in the brain into a visible reality) and participation (being a team player) playing itself out in everyday rural living and working.[12] This sense of belonging, or cohesion, being the 'social glue' that binds people together, with opportunities to develop, not just professionally, but also personally, came out strongly.

Culture of support

A culture of support, closely related to 'teamness', was the third dominant theme. Interpersonal work relationships, such as 'sometimes we just share our frustrations or joys around a cup of coffee', were highly valued. Receiving feedback from managers, colleagues and patients were specifically mentioned as one powerful means of support. Giving feedback does not have a financial cost, but it does imply a personal time commitment, care about team members and a leadership style that embraces vulnerability toward colleagues. Giving honest feedback with a view to developing people and considering their self-esteem, whilst also maintaining high clinical standards, is a very specific skill that needs some training and coaching.[15] These characteristics of prioritising social relationships and seeing the work community as an extension of one's personal community, together with a need for feedback, flexibility and structure, are all strong features of the millennial generation, which refers to people who turned 18 years of age in the year 2000, reflecting the age group of the majority of participants in the workshop.[16]

Opportunities for growth

Professionally, with opportunities for growth (the fourth theme), people wanted a challenging and stimulating work environment, with continuing professional development, specific teaching by outreaching specialists and having the opportunity to use their clinical skills. There was a discussion in one group about the fact that working in rural areas affords one the benefit of being able to apply all the skills one has acquired during training as a doctor.

Work-life balance

Discussions regarding a healthy work-life balance (the fifth theme) revolved around balancing a sense of structure (what needs to be done) and flexibility (what can be adapted to allow more time with family). Work does not occur outside life; people live as they work and, in rural areas, often *where* they work. So it may be more appropriate to refer to a work-family balance, or even talk about a work-family border theory, as Clark described, where people are border-crossers who make daily transitions between the two worlds of work and family, determining those boundaries, shaping their environment and being shaped *by* the environment.[17]

Discussion

The main themes emerging from the workshop paint a picture of a healthcare practitioner with a shared purpose, working in a supportive team, having personal and professional opportunities for growth, within a healthy work-life balance. These themes reflect closely the literature on retention and should inform future planning for attracting and keeping health workers.[18] These are also established key components of building resilience, which was the main theme of the conference. Close relationships, facilitative leadership, support from outreaching specialists, teamwork, work environment and a culture of learning have all been cited as dominant attributes of the workplace that increase retention.[18]

These themes could also be linked to the empowerment theory which Zimmerman presents as:

> ... both a value orientation for working in the community and a theoretical model for understanding the process and consequences of efforts to exert control and influence over decisions that affect one's life, organizational functioning, and the quality of community life.[19,20]

This model of psychological empowerment includes intrapersonal, interactional and behavioural components.[20] Figure 1 illustrates how the themes can be linked with these components of the empowerment theory as a potential framework to explain why health workers stay in rural district hospitals. It may help to inform retention strategies and even be applied to similar rural contexts elsewhere, where it has been shown that it is the total personal and professional experience, not salary alone, which impacts retention.[21]

District managers and healthcare practitioners should include these themes in their discussions of retention strategies in order to create awareness and make these themes explicit, within the challenges of working in rural areas.

IMPORTANCE	What keeps you working in the district hospital in a rural area?		
I	Intrapersonal (Identity)	Theme 1 Shared purpose	Sense of calling/purpose
			Desire to make a difference in community you serve
			Sense of belonging
M	Interactional (relationship)	Theme 2 Working in a team	Interpersonal work relationships
P			Better workplace attitude – good shared work ethic amongst the team
O		Theme 3 Culture of support	Work-related support
R			Outreach and support from specialists
T			Feedback from patients, colleagues, managers
A	Behavioural	Theme 4 Opportunities for growth	Opportunity for personal and professional growth
N			Challenge and stimulation at work
			Implement skills learnt
C		Theme 5 Work–life balance	Home/life environmental comforts
E			Family compatibility – spouse, children are happy; access to outdoor activities
			Functional health system

FIGURE 1: The main themes that keep health workers working in rural district hospitals, in order of most important to least important, as voted by the workshop participants

Conclusion

The aim of the workshop was to determine what keeps health practitioners working in rural health districts. Five main themes were identified, which included having a sense of shared purpose, working in a team, within a culture of support, having opportunities for growth and maintaining a healthy work-life balance. These should serve to inform future retention strategies of health practitioners in rural health settings.

Acknowledgements

Thanks to the 29 participants in the workshop, who shared honestly and freely from their personal and professional lives. Also thank you to the district manager of the Cape Winelands District, Dr L. Phillips, for her input and ideas during the discussions of the themes. Dr P. Kapp was very instrumental during the conceptual phase of the workshop development.

Competing interests

The authors declare that they have no financial or personal relationship(s) that may have inappropriately influenced them in writing this article.

Authors' contributions

All four authors (Stellenbosch University) participated in the conference workshop, data collection, analysis and writing up of the article. L.S.J. drafted the initial article and all authors contributed to the final article.

References

1. Government of South Africa. Chapter Ten: Promoting health. In: The National Development Plan – 2030; p. 330–351 [document on the Internet]. c2013 [cited 2014 Nov 17]. Available from: www.gov.za/sites/www.gov.za/files/ndp2030_chap10.pdf
2. Mayosi BM, Benatar SR. Health and health care in South Africa – 20 years after Mandela. N Engl J Med. 2014;371(14);1344–1353.
3. World Health Organization. Increasing access to health workers in remote and rural areas through improved retention [document on the Internet]. c2009 [cited 2014 Nov 17]. Available from: www.who.int/hrh/migration/background_paper.pdf?ua=1
4. Burch V, Reid S. Fit for purpose? The appropriate education of health professionals in South Africa. S Afr Med J. 2011;101(1):25–26.
5. Gilson L, Judith D. Leadership and Governance within the South African Health System. In: Padarath A, Enlish R, editors. South African Health Review 2011; p. 69–80 [document on the Internet]. c2011 [cited 2014 Nov 17]. Available from: www.hst.org.za/publications/south-african-health-review-2011
6. Buchan J, Couper ID, Tangcharoensathien V, et al. Early implementation of WHO recommendations for the retention of health workers in remote and rural areas. Bull World Health Organ. 2013;91:834–840.
7. Department of Health, Australian Government. Executive summary: Australian Government health workforce programs [page on the Internet]. c2013 [cited 2014 Nov 17]. Available from: http://www.health.gov.au/internet/publications/publishing.nsf/Content/work-review-australian-government-health-workforce-programs-toc~executive-summary
8. Ministry of Health, British Columbia. Rural retention program (RRP): Political framework for health authorities (Revised June 2012) [document on the Internet]. c2012 [cited 2014 Nov 17]. Available from: www.health.gov.bc.ca/pcb/pdf/retentionprogram.pdf
9. African Health Placements. Retention [page on the Internet]. No date [cited 2014 Nov 17]. Available from: http://www.ahp.org.za/retention
10. Rural Health Advocacy Project. National Department of Health human resources for health strategy 2012/13–2016/17 [page on the Internet]. No date [cited 2014 Nov 17]. Available from: http://www.rhap.org.za/read-up-on-the-national-hrh-strategys-strategic-priority-area-8-access-in-rural-and-remote-areas/
11. Lloyd-Jones G, Fowell S, Bligh JG. The use of the nominal group technique as an evaluative tool in medical undergraduate education. Med Educ. 1999;33(1):8–13.
12. Wenger E. Communities of practice: Learning, meaning, and identity. New York, NY: Cambridge University Press; 1998.
13. Patient Centred Primary Care Institute. Teamness [webinar presentation on the Internet]. c2013 [cited 2014 Oct 01]. Available from: http://www.pcpci.org/sites/default/files/webinar-related/PCPCI-Teamness%20Webinar%20Slides-04-30-13.pdf
14. Crabtree BF, Nutting PA, Miller WL, et al. Summary of the National Demonstration Project and recommendations for the patient-centered medical home. Ann Fam Med. 2010;8(Suppl 1):S80–S90.
15. Archer JC. State of the science in health professional education: Effective feedback. Med Educ. 2010;44(1):101–108.
16. Roberts DH, Newman LR, Schwartzstein RM. Twelve tips for facilitating Millennials' learning. Med Teach. 2012;34(4):274–278.
17. Clark SC. Work/family border theory: A new theory of work/family balance. Hum Relat. 2000;53(6):747–770.
18. Kotzee T, Couper ID. What interventions do South African qualified doctors think will retain them in rural hospitals of the Limpopo province of South Africa? Rural Remote Health. 2006;6(3):581.
19. Rappaport J, Seidman E. Handbook of community psychology. New York, NY: Kluwer Academic/Plenum Publisher; 2000.
20. Zimmerman MA, Israel BA, Schulz A, et al. Further explorations in empowerment theory: An empirical analysis of psychological empowerment. Am J Community Psychol. 1992;20(6):707–726.
21. Humphreys J, Wakerman J, Kuipers P, et al. Improving workforce retention: Developing an integrated logic model to maximise sustainability of small rural & remote health care services document on the Internet]. c2009 [cited 2014 Nov 17]. Available from: http://files.aphcri.anu.edu.au/research/full_report_10797.pdf

Profile and correlates of functional status in elderly patients presenting at a primary care clinic in Nigeria

Authors:
Samuel A. Ajayi[1]
Lawrence A. Adebusoye[1]
Adetola M. Ogunbode[1]
Joshua O. Akinyemi[2]
Ayodeji M. Adebayo[3]

Affiliations:
[1]Family Medicine Department, University College Hospital, Ibadan, Nigeria

[2]Department of Epidemiology and Medical Statistics, College of Medicine, University of Ibadan, Nigeria

[3]Department of Preventive Medicine and Primary Care, College of Medicine, University of Ibadan, Nigeria

Correspondence to:
Samuel Ajayi

Email:
ayosina86@yahoo.com

Postal address:
Family Medicine Department, University College Hospital, PMB 5116, Ibadan, Nigeria

Background: Assessing the functional status of elderly patients is central in measuring their health outcome. Little is known about the functional status of elderly patients attending our primary care clinic in Nigeria.

Objective: To assess the correlates of functional status in elderly patients presenting at the General Outpatient Clinic of the University College Hospital, Ibadan, Nigeria.

Method: A cross-sectional study of 360 randomly selected patients aged 60 years and above was undertaken to assess their functional status by scoring their basic activities of daily living (BADL) using the Modified Bathel Index. An interviewer-administered questionnaire was used to obtain the socio-demographic data, anthropometric measurements and morbidities of each patient.

Results: The mean age was 69.1 ± 6.6 years with a female-to-male ratio of 1.9: 1. The prevalence of overall functional disability (defined as when assistance was sought in the performance of at least one of the components of BADL) was 88.3%. The highest prevalence of functional disability was experienced in the area of personal hygiene and grooming (95.3%) and transferring from bed to chair (95.3%). Overall functional disability significantly increased with increasing age (χ^2 for trend=14.004, $p < 0.0001$), living in a polygamous family unit ($p = 0.025$), and lack of formal education ($p = 0.020$).

Conclusion: Functional disability was high amongst the elderly in this setting. Age, education, and living in a polygamous type of family unit had significant influence on the functional status. High premium should, therefore, be placed on considering these factors in reducing functional disability in the elderly.

Profil et correspondances du statut fonctionnel des personnes âgées qui se présentent à une clinique de soins primaires au Nigéria.

Contexte: L'évaluation de la situation fonctionnelle des personnes âgées est essentielle pour mesurer leurs résultats en matière de santé. On ne sait pas grand-chose sur la situation fonctionnelle des patients âgés qui fréquentent notre clinique de soins primaires au Nigéria.

Objectif: Evaluer les correspondances du statut fonctionnel des patients âgés qui fréquentent la policlinique générale de l'Hôpital académique (UCH), Ibadan, Nigeria.

Méthode: Une étude transversale de 360 patients sélectionnés au hasard, âgés de 60 ans et plus, a été faite de septembre à novembre 2011. On a évalué le statut fonctionnel en mesurant leurs activités courantes de leur vie quotidienne (ACVQ) au moyen de l'Indice Bathel Modifié(MBI). On a utilisé un questionnaire administré par un interviewer pour obtenir les données sociodémographiques, les mesures anthropométriques et les morbidités de chaque patient.

Résultats: L'âge moyen était de 69.1 ± 6.6 ans avec une proportion femme-homme de 1.9: 1. La prédominance d'incapacité fonctionnelle générale (définie comme le moment où on a besoin d'aide pour effectuer au moins l'une des composantes d'ACVQ) était de 88.3%. La prédominance d'incapacité fonctionnelle se ressentait dans le domaine de l'hygiène personnelle et de la toilette (95.3%) et dans le transfert du lit à la chaise (95.3%). L'incapacité fonctionnelle générale augmentait considérablement avec l'âge (χ^2 pour la tendance = 14.004, $p < 0.0001$), la vie dans une famille de type polygame ($p = 0.025$) et le manque d'éducation formelle ($p = 0.020$). Dans cette étude les morbidités détectées n'étaient pas vraiment liées au statut fonctionnel.

Conclusion: L'incapacité fonctionnelle était élevée chez les personnes âgées dans ce contexte. Les facteurs sociodémographiques, particulièrement l'âge, l'éducation, et la vie dans un type de famille polygame avaient plus d'influence sur le statut fonctionnel que les comorbidités. Il faudra donc mettre plus l'accent sur ces facteurs pour diminuer l'incapacité fonctionnelle chez les personnes âgées.

Introduction

The global demographic transition has caused an unprecedented increase in the elderly population with a higher rate of increase in the developing countries like Nigeria.[1,2] The United Nations General Assembly defines an elderly person as a person aged 60 years and above, whilst the World Health Organization (WHO) puts the age cut-off at 65 years and above.[3] Most developing countries use 60 years and above due to lower life expectancies and proportions of older persons within the population.

Population ageing is associated with increased morbidity and demand on healthcare services.[4]

Multi-morbidities, illness chronicity, non-specific presentations, and deranged social factors characterise the health profiles of the elderly. Therefore, assessment of functional status is critical as it provides more holistic evaluation and care for these older patients

Since 1959, the WHO asserted that health in the elderly is best measured in terms of function.[5] This is a better indicator of health in the elderly than the traditional diagnostic categories. Traditionally, health and the outcomes of treatment have been measured with regard to morbidity, mortality, incidence, or prevalence of disease. For chronic diseases, however, and particularly in the elderly, functional health status as measured by Activities of Daily Living (ADL) is now an important measure, especially in primary care.[6] Functional status is defined as the individual ability to perform normal daily activities required to meet basic needs, fulfil usual roles and maintain health and well-being.[7] ADL is used in rehabilitation as an umbrella term relating to self-care, and comprises those activities or tasks that people undertake routinely in their everyday lives. Basic activities of daily living (BADL), which is often used synonymously as ADL, refer to the basic tasks of everyday life, such as eating, bathing, dressing, toileting, and transferring.

Geriatrics as a medical specialty is yet to fully emerge in Nigeria. For this reason there is a paucity of information on the morbidity pattern, functional status and its determinants in the elderly.[8,9] Most of the previous studies were carried out in developed populations, but these may not be applicable in a developing country like Nigeria. A few available local studies were community-based; however, this hospital-based study provides baseline data that will be useful for effective planning in a primary care setting with a growing elderly population.

Ethical consideration

Ethical clearance for the study was obtained from the joint University of Ibadan and University College Hospital Ethical Review Board and the Head of the Department. The respondents either signed or thumb-printed the informed consent form before being studied. They were assured of confidentiality. The questionnaires were serially coded and the data entered on the computer. The data were protected and accessible only to the researcher, data entry clerk and statistician.

Method

Study Setting and participants

This study was conducted at the General Outpatients (GOP) Clinic, Family Medicine Department, University College Hospital (UCH), Ibadan. Ibadan is the capital city of Oyo State, southwest Nigeria, with an estimated population of 2.55 million according to the 2006 National Population Census. UCH is a 1000-bed tertiary academic institution that was founded in 1957. Patients from across Nigeria and the west-African subregion are referred to the hospital. The General Outpatients Clinic serves as a primary care clinic within a tertiary hospital setting, as most patients seen at UCH are managed at first contact, and few are subsequently referred to specialty units and other medical services like physiotherapy and clinical psychology. Elderly patients constitute about 16% of the 1200 new adult patients seen every month in this clinic.

The study population comprised 360 elderly male and female patients aged 60 years and above attending the GOPD clinic, UCH, between 08 September and 30 November 2011. The age of the respondents was determined by direct recall, use of historical events, marital age, and age of their first child.

Study design

This was a cross-sectional descriptive study which assessed the functional status of 360 elderly respondents. A simple random sampling technique was used by means of a computer-generated table of random numbers to select a sample of 360 elderly persons 60 years and over presenting at the GOP clinic. To recruit the total sample size of 360 respondents over 60 working days, six respondents who met the inclusion criteria were selected daily. From the Health Record Section of the GOP, a total of 1187 elderly patients were seen both as newly-presenting and follow-up patients over the same study period in the previous year, from September to November 2010. This gave an average of 20 elderly patients seen per working day. Random numbers were then generated using the Microsoft Excel package of the Windows XP programme; six randomly selected numbers were generated daily. These were the numbers of the patients recruited daily. All non-consenting elderly and critically ill patients were excluded from the study.

Procedure

The study involved administration of a structured interviewer-administered questionnaire and a general medical examination. The functional assessment was carried out by scoring the respondents' BADL using the Modified Barthel Index (MBI) incorporated into the questionnaire. The

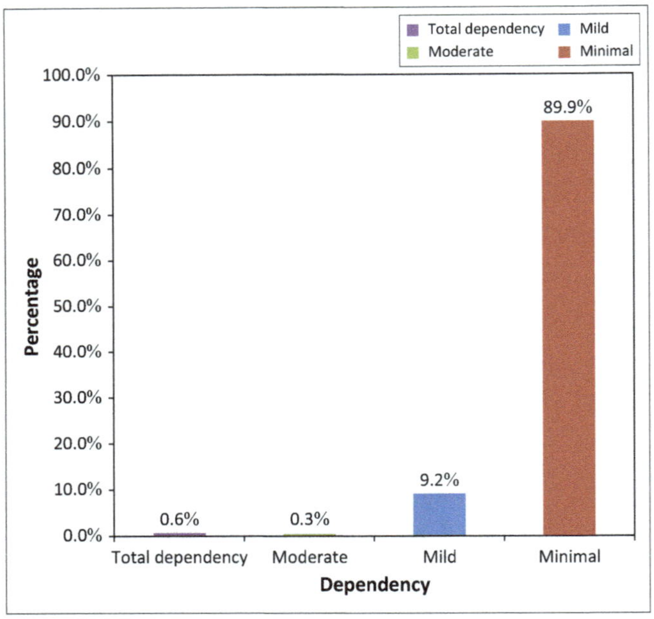

FIGURE 1: Level of Dependency amongst the respondents with functional disability.

maximum obtainable score was 100. The higher the score, the more 'independent' the individual. The score for each patient was used to predict his or her dependency needs.[10,11] Scores between 0–24 were classified as total dependency; 25–49 as severe dependency; 50–74 as moderate dependency; 75–90 and 91–99 as mild and minimal dependency respectively according to the MBI instrument. For the purpose of comparison of the results of this study with other studies, BADL performance scores were dichotomised into functional independence and functional disability. In this study, functional independence was defined as ability to fully perform all the components of the BADL using MBI without any assistance, whilst functional disability was defined as when assistance was sought in the performance of at least one of the components of BADL[12,13,14] (see Figure 1).

Thereafter, the respondents were examined, and urine chemistry and packed cell volumes were measured. Some of the respondents were referred to other specialty units within UCH for further assessment and management.

Statistical analysis

Administered questionnaires were checked, sorted and coded serially after each study day. SSPS (version 17) was used for data entering, cleaning and analysis. Descriptive statistics were used to describe the socio-demographic characteristics of the respondents. The chi-square test was used to evaluate the association between categorical variables at 5% level of significance.

Results

The mean age was 69.1 ± 6.6 years. The majority of the respondents (65%) were females, with a female-to-male ratio of 1.9:1. The modal age group was 70–74 years for the men and 60–64years for the women.

TABLE 1: Socio-demographic characteristics of the respondents.

Socio-demographic Characteristics	Male = 126 *n* (%)	Female = 234 *n* (%)	*N* = 360 Total (%)
Age group (years)			
60–64	29 (23.0)	72 (30.8)	101 (28.1)
65–69	28 (22.2)	65 (27.8)	93 (25.8)
70–74	36 (28.6)	46 (19.7)	82 (22.8)
75–79	18 (14.3)	31 (13.2)	49 (13.6)
80 and above	15 (11.9)	20 (8.5)	35 (9.7)
Marital status			
Married	116 (92.1)	100 (42.8)	216 (60.0)
Separated/Divorced	7 (5.5)	12 (5.1)	19 (5.3)
Widowed	3 (2.4)	122 (52.1)	125 (34.7)
Family type			
Monogamous	86 (68.3)	87 (37.3)	173 (48.1)
Polygamous	40 (31.7)	147 (62.7)	187 (51.9)
No. of children			
< 5 children	27 (21.4)	94 (40.2)	121 (33.6)
≥ 5 children	99 (78.6)	140 (59.8)	239 (66.4)
Ethnicity			
Yoruba	119 (94.4)	225 (96.2)	344 (95.6)
Ibo	1 (0.8)	4 (1.7)	5 (1.4)
Others**	6 (4.8)	5 (2.1)	11 (3.0)
Religion			
Christianity	70 (55.5)	130 (55.6)	200 (55.6)
Islam	55 (43.7)	103 (44.0)	158 (43.8)
Others	1 (0.8)	1 (0.4)	2 (0.6)
Education			
Number formal education	39 (31.0)	133 (56.8)	172 (47.8)
Primary education	38 (30.1)	60 (25.7)	98 (27.2)
Secondary education	15 (11.9)	22 (9.4)	37 (10.3)
Tertiary education	34 (27.0)	19 (8.1)	53 (14.7)
Occupational status			
Currently engaged	85 (67.5)	208 (88.9)	293 (81.4)
Currently unengaged	41 (32.5)	26 (11.1)	67 (18.6)
Income			
< $1.25/day	53 (42.1)	174 (74.4)	227 (63.1)
≥ $1.25/day	73 (57.9)	60 (25.6)	133 (36.9)

Only 42 (11.7%) of the respondents were functionally independent, whilst the rest had functional disability. Amongst the latter, the majority (89.9%) were minimally dependent, with only two respondents (0.6%) having total dependency (see Table 1).

The functional status of the respondents was further assessed based on the components of BADL by gender (Table 2). Overall, functional disability was most prevalent in the performance of personal hygiene, grooming and transferring from the bed to the chair, with 95.3% of the respondents having functional disability in each activity. The men were found to have more disability with bowel control than the women, although this was not statistically significant.

The association between socio-demographic characteristics and respondents' functional status is shown in Table 3. Extended Mantel-Haensel chi-square for trend showed that functional disability increased significantly with increasing age from 78.2% in the age group 60–64 years, to 100.0% at age 80 years and above ($p < 0.0001$). Significantly, a higher proportion of respondents in polygamous family settings

TABLE 2: Functional status in each components of BADL by gender.

Functional status	Male = 126 *n* (%)	Female = 234 *n* (%)	*N* = 360 Total (%)	χ^2, *p*-value
Personal hygiene/grooming				
Functionally independent	8 (6.3)	9 (3.8)	17 (4.7)	$\chi^2 = 1.140$,
Functional disability	118 (93.7)	225 (96.2)	343 (95.3)	$p = 0.286$
Bathing self				
Functionally independent	110 (87.3)	193 (82.5)	303 (84.2)	$\chi^2 = 1.430$,
Functional disability	16 (12.7)	41 (17.5)	57 (15.8)	$p = 0.232$
Feeding				
Functionally independent	109 (86.5)	157 (67.1)	266 (73.9)	$\chi^2 = 15.999$,
Functional disability	17 (13.5)	77 (32.9)	94 (26.1)	$p < 0.0001$*
Toilet use				
Functionally independent	12 (9.5)	15 (6.4)	27 (7.5)	$\chi^2 = 1.144$,
Functional disability	114 (90.5)	219 (93.6)	333 (92.5)	$p = 0.285$
Stair climbing				
Functionally independent	17 (13.5)	19 (8.1)	36 (10.0)	$\chi^2 = 2.627$,
Functional disability	109 (86.5)	215 (91.9)	324 (90.0)	$p = 1.105$
Dressing				
Functionally independent	21 (16.7)	30 (12.8)	51 (14.2)	$\chi^2 = 0.996$,
Functional disability	105 (83.3)	204 (87.2)	309 (85.8)	$p = 0.316$
Bowel control				
Functionally independent	8 (6.3)	16 (6.8)	24 (6.7)	$\chi^2 = 0.031$,
Functional disability	118 (93.7)	218 (93.2)	336 (93.3)	p = 0.859
Bladder control				
Functional independent	10 (7.9)	18 (7.7)	28 (7.8)	$\chi^2 = 0.007$,
Functional disability	116 (92.1)	216 (92.3)	332 (92.2)	p = 0.934
Mobility				
Functionally independent	12 (9.5)	19 (8.1)	31 (8.6)	$\chi^2 = 0.205$,
Functional disability	114 (90.5)	215 (91.9)	329 (91.4)	$p = 0.651$
Chair/bed transfer				
Functionally independent	7 (5.6)	10 (4.3)	17 (4.7)	$\chi^2 = 0.299$,
Functional disability	119 (94.4)	224 (95.7)	343 (95.3)	$p = 0.584$

BADL, basic activities of daily living.
*, Significant at 5% level of significance

TABLE 3: Association between socio-demographic factors and respondents' functional status.

Variable	Functional Disability (%) *n* = 318	Functionally Independent (%) *n* = 42	Total (%) (*n* = 360)	χ^2, *p*-value
Age (Years)				
60-64	79 (78.2)	22 (21.8)	101 (100.0)	$\chi^2 = 14.004$
65-69	84 (90.3)	9 (9.7)	93 (100.0)	$p < 0.0001$*
70-74	74 (90.2)	8 (9.8)	82 (100.0)	
75-79	46 (93.9)	3 (6.1)	49 (100.0)	
≥ 80	35 (100.0)	0 (0.0)	35 (100.0)	
Gender				
Male	114 (90.5)	12 (9.5)	126 (100.0)	$\chi^2 = 0.864$
Female	204 (87.2)	30 (12.8)	234 (100.0)	$p = 0.353$
Marital Status				
Currently Married	192 (88.9)	24 (11.1)	216 (100.0)	$\chi^2 = 0.162$
Not married	126 (87.5)	18 (12.5)	144 (100.0)	$p = 0.688$
Family type				
Monogamous	146 (84.4)	27 (15.6)	173 (100.0)	$\chi^2 = 5.018$
Polygamous	172 (92.0)	15 (8.0)	187 (100.0)	$p = 0.025$*
No of children				
< 5 children	102 (84.3)	19 (15.7)	121 (100.0)	$\chi^2 = 2.881$
≥ 5 children	216 (90.4)	23 (9.6)	239 (100.0)	$p = 0.090$
Education				
No formal Education	159 (92.4)	13 (7.6)	172 (100.0)	$\chi^2 = 5.395$
Formal Education	159(84.6)	29 (15.4)	188(100.0)	$p = 0.020$*
Occupation				
Currently unengaged	60 (89.6)	7 (10.4)	67 (100.0)	$\chi^2 = 0.119$
Currently engaged	258 (88.1)	35 (11.9)	293 (100.0)	$p = 0.730$
Income				
Below poverty level	204 (89.9)	23 (10.1)	227 (100.0)	$\chi^2 = 1.404$
Above poverty level	114 (85.7)	19 (14.3)	133 (100.0)	$p = 0.236$

*, Significant at 5% level of significance

TABLE 4: Association between common morbidities and respondents' functional status.

Common morbidities	Functional disability (%) n = 318	Functionally independent (%) n = 42	Total (%) (N = 360)	χ^2, p-value
Hypertension				
Yes	211 (86.5)	33 (13.5)	244 (100.0)	χ^2= 2.536,
No	107 (92.2)	9 (7.8)	116 (100.0)	p = 0.111
Cataract				
Yes	83 (93.3)	6 (6.7)	89 (100.0)	χ^2= 2.783,
No	235 (86.7)	36 (13.3)	271 (100.0)	p = 0.095
Osteoarthritis				
Yes	98 (89.9)	11 (10.1)	109 (100.0)	χ^2= 0.376,
No	220 (87.6)	31 (12.4)	251 (100.0)	p = 0.540
Diabetes Mellitus				
Yes	48 (94.1)	3 (5.9)	51 (100.0)	χ^2 = 1.929,
No	270 (87.4)	39 (12.6)	309 (100.0)	p = 0.165
Glaucoma				
Yes	17 (89.5)	2 (10.5)	19 (100.0)	p = 1.000+
No	301 (88.3)	40 (11.7)	341 (100.0)	
Malaria				
Yes	13 (86.7)	2 (13.3)	15 (100.0)	p = 0.690*
No	305 (88.4)	40 (11.6)	345 (100.0)	
Urinary Tract Infection				
Yes	9 (90.0)	1 (10.0)	10 (100.0)	p = 1.000*
No	309 (88.3)	41 (11.7)	350 (100.0)	
Refractive error				
Yes	6 (66.7)	3 (33.3)	9 (100.0)	p = 0.075*
No	312 (88.9)	39 (11.1)	351 (100.0)	
Respiratory Tract Infection				
Yes	8 (88.9)	1 (11.1)	51 (100.0)	p = 1.000*
No	310 (88.3)	41 (11.7)	309 (100.0)	
Erectile Dysfunction†	n = 114	n = 12	n = 126	p = 0.070*
Yes	24 (100.0)	0 (0.0)	24 (100.0)	
No	90 (88.2)	12(11.8)	102 (100.0)	

†, Male only, + Fishers Exact Test.
*, Significant at 5% level of significance

(92.0%) had functional disability compared with those in the monogamous families (84.4%) (p = 0.025). The prevalence of functional disability (84.6%) was less amongst respondents with some formal education compared to those without formal education (92.4%) (p = 0.020).

Table 4 depicts the association between the commonest morbidities diagnosed and the functional status of the respondents. Functional disability was higher in those visually impaired with cataracts and glaucoma, osteoarthritis, diabetes mellitus, urinary tract infection and men with erectile dysfunction. There was no significant association between co-morbidities and functional status.

Discussion

The profile and correlates of functional status are critical in ensuring holistic care for the elderly. These measurements have been found to be better indicators of health in the elderly than the traditional diagnostic categories. In this study, estimates of functional disability amongst elderly attendees at a primary care clinic were reported. Information on the socio-demographic and morbidity correlates was also provided.

The prevalence of functional disability in this study was very high (88.3%). Functional disability prevalence varies worldwide due to differences in definition criteria, measurement, and sample characteristics.[15] The prevalence is expected to be high in studies in which functional disability is based on any level of assistance in the performance of daily activities as it applied in this study.[9] Such high prevalence as found in this hospital-based study could also be expected if performed in an institutionalised setting such as an old persons' nursing home. This prevalence was much higher than what was reported in a study using the same instrument in Northern Nigeria (28.3%).[13] The reason for a higher prevalence in our study might be because it was hospital-based, whilst the northern Nigerian study was community-based. The cultural perception of the performance of BADL could also influence the respondents' scores. Requesting for assistance is a common and acceptable practice amongst the elderly in African culture, irrespective of his or her ability to carry out an activity or task. This high level of functional disability does not translate to high level of physical handicap, as was corroborated by the fact that well over three-quarters of the respondents were minimally dependent in carrying out the basic activities of daily living (BADL), which translated to needing less than ten hours of help per week.[10]

Given the definition, study setting, and cultural caveats, the prevalence of functional disability was much higher than reported in a few similar community-based studies done previously in this environment, Europe and Asia.[9,13,16,17,18]

For performance in the individual components of BADL however, the women were found to have an increased level of disability, except for bowel control. The higher prevalence of physical disability for the BADL components amongst elderly women compared to elderly men in this study have been reported in previous studies.[19,20] Whilst women, globally, live longer, functional disabilities are more prevalent amongst them.[21,22] The cumulative effect of pregnancy and childbearing, lower level of education, and poor health care may be responsible for these higher physical dependencies and functional limitations seen in elderly women. This study also showed that the majority of the respondents were still able to carry out activities that are largely dependent on the strength of the upper extremities, such as feeding and bathing, without any assistance. In the loss of independence in BADL activities, studies have shown that this is the last set of activities to be lost.[5,23]

As with most of the previous reports, advanced age and polygamy were significantly associated with functional disability in the performance of BADL, with the oldest of the old clearly having the poorest functional status.[9,13,24] All the respondents (100%) above 80 years had functional disability, which was comparable with a prevalence of 98.9% found in a community-based study in Northern Nigeria, but well above 50% recorded by the elderly Europeans.[13] Availability of better health delivery and assisting devices in the performance of BADL may be responsible for lower prevalence amongst the Europeans. The increasing trend of functional disability with increasing age has, however, been reported in all previous studies and corroborated by the WHO.[9,13,25] This, Chappell and Cooke opined, might be due to the increasing prevalence of chronic illnesses as ageing sets in.[12]

Expectedly, this study further revealed that functional disability was more prevalent amongst respondents living below poverty level and those who lack formal education. The same trend has been observed in the studies reviewed.[15,25] Poverty, ignorance, diseases and consequent disability is a vicious cycle, which Mont asserted are inseparable.[15] Poverty leads to malnutrition, poor health services and sanitation, as well as unsafe living and working conditions, which are all associated with disability.

None of the common morbidities were significantly related to functional status. The failure to find significant elevated risk of functional disability amongst those with a medical condition was also reported in the Ibadan Study of Ageing.[9] This may reflect a reporting bias: poor access to medical service as well as a high level of illiteracy, which would limit the number of elderly persons who might be aware of having a medical condition, especially asymptomatic diseases such as hypertension.[9,26] Some of the morbidities were associated with a higher prevalence of functional disability, although this was not statistically significant. These include cataract, osteoarthritis, diabetes mellitus, glaucoma, UTI and RTI. Cataract and glaucoma are the major causes of visual impairment, which will obviously affect the ability to carry out BADL. Osteoarthritis reduces joint mobility and inflicts pain, which may explain why its occurrence in this study was associated with a higher prevalence of functional disability.

Limitations of the study

This was a cross-sectional study. As such, causal relationships between functional status and the variables implicated cannot be strongly drawn. It was a hospital-based study, therefore the likely generalisability of the findings is limited.

Conclusion and recommendations

The prevalence of functional disability in the overall performance of BADL was very high amongst the study population, whilst increasing age, polygamy, illiteracy, and poverty were associated factors. These factors had more influence than co-morbidities on functional status. Therefore, a high premium should be placed on considering these factors in caring for the elderly to reduce functional disability.

In practice, the primary care physician's role in the care of the elderly must move beyond the therapeutics of the single disease-oriented models to a holistic, patient-centred care. This paradigm shift, which functional status assessment promotes, must be emphasised in the training of medical students.

A well-coordinated care for these complicated and functionally impaired patients should be the goal of all health practitioners caring for the elderly. A short, but comprehensive functional assessment tool should be routinely used in consultations of the elderly to achieve this.

Further research to validate the various functional assessment tools to make them more culturally sensitive, thereby limiting the reporting bias, is needed. Studies assessing the IADL and AADL, which encompass a range of activities performed by a person living independently in a community, will also be useful. The impact of interventions on the functional status of an elderly population in this environment needs to be explored in prospective future studies.

The relevance of functional assessment with regard to prognostication and medical cost evaluation has not been explored in this environment. Studies along these lines would be of benefit to the clients, clinicians and policy makers.

Acknowledgements

Appreciation goes to the joint University of Ibadan/ University College Hospital Ethical Review Board and the Head of Family Medicine Department for the permission granted to conduct this research.

Competing interests

The authors declare that they have no financial or personal relationship(s) that may have inappropriately influenced them in writing this article.

Authors' contributions

S.A.A. (University College Hospital, Ibadan) was the researcher and wrote most of the manuscript, L.A.A. (University College Hospital, Ibadan), A.M.O. (University College Hospital, Ibadan) and A.M.A. (University of Ibadan) supervised and edited the manuscript. J.O.A. (University of Ibadan) assisted in the statistical analysis and interpretation.

References

1. United Nations. Department of Economic and Social Affairs. Population Division. World population prospects: The 2004 Revision [homepage on the Internet]. New York: United Nations; 2005. [cited 2011 Jun 8]. Available from: http:// www.un.org/esa/population
2. Adebusoye L, Ajayi I, Dairo M, et al. Factors associated with undernutrition and overweight in elderly patients presenting at a primary care clinic in Nigeria. SA Fam Pract. 2011;53(4).
3. World Health Organization. Definition of an older or elderly person. Proposed working definition of an older person in Africa for the MDS Project [homepage on the Internet]. Brazzaville, Congo: African Regional Office; 2012. [cited on 2011 Dec 8]. Available from: http://www.who.int/healthinfo/survey/ageingdefnolder/en/.
4. Payne G, Laporte A, Deber R, et al. Counting backward to health care's future: Using time-to death modeling to identify changes in end-of-life morbidity and the impact of ageing on health care expenditure. Milibank Q. 2007;85(2):213–257. http://dx.doi.org/10.1111/j.1468-0009.2007.00485.x
5. Daly M, Taler G. Care of the elderly. In: Rakel R, Principles of family practice. 7th ed. Philadelphia: WB Saunders; 2007. p. 69–70.
6. Md Aris M, Draman S, Abdul Rahman J, et al. Functional disabilities and its associated factors among elderly patients in primary care clinics. Int Med J Malaysia. 2009;16(4):251–256.
7. Elsawy B, Higgins K. The geriatric assessment. Am Fam Physician. 2011;83(1):48–56.
8. Adebusoye L, Ladipo M, Owoaje E, et al. Morbidity pattern amongst elderly patients presenting at a primary care clinic in Nigeria. Afr J Prm Health Care Fam Med. 2011;3(1).
9. Gureje O, Ogunniyi A, Kola L, et al. Functional disability among elderly Nigerians: Results from the Ibadan study of ageing. J Am Geriatric Soc. 2006;54(11):1784. http://dx.doi.org/10.1111/j.1532-5415.2006.00944.x
10. Shah S, Vanclay F, Cooper B. Improving the sensitivity of the Barthel Index for stroke rehabilitation. J Clin Epidemiol. 1989;42(8):703-709. http://dx.doi.org/10.1016/0895-4356(89)90065-6
11. Shah S, Salek S. Modified Barthel Index or Barthel Index (Expanded). Compendium of quality of life instruments. Part II. Chichester: Wiley; 1998.
12. Chappell N, Cooke H. Age related disabilities: aging and quality of life [homepage on the Internet]. No date [cited on 2011 Aug 12]. In: J Stone, M Blouin, editors. International encyclopedia of rehabilitation. Available from: http://cirriebuffaloedu/encyclopedia/en/article/189.
13. Abdulraheem I, Oladipo A, Amodu M. Prevalence and correlates of physical disability and functional limitation among elderly rural population in Nigeria. J. Aging Res. 2011;2011:369894.
14. World Health Organization. What are the main risk factors for disability in old age and how can disability be prevented? [homepage on the Internet]. 2003 [cited on 2011 Aug 12]. Available from: http://www.euro.who.int/document/E82970.pdf.
15. Mont D. Measuring disability prevalence. Disability & Development Team HDNSP. The World Bank; 2007 [cited on 2011 Dec 8]. Available from: http://www.siteresources.worldbank.org/DISABILITY/resources.
16. Lindholt J, Ventegodt S, Hanneberg E. Development and validation of QOL5 for clinical databases. Eur J Surg. 2002;168:107-113. http://dx.doi.org/10.1080/11024150252884331
17. Burden of disease network project. Disability in old age final report. Conclusions and recommendations. Jyvaskyla: Jyvaskyla University Press; 2004.
18. Siop S, Lois M, Verbrugge L, et al. Disability and quality of life among older Malaysians [homepage on the Internet]. Population Association of America. 2008 Annual Meeting Program; New Orleans, LA; April 17–19; 2008 [cited on 2011 Nov 24]. Available from: http://www.paa2008.princeton.edu/papers/80962.
19. Tas U, Verhagen A, Bierma-Zeinstra S. Incidence and risk factors of disability in the elderly: The Rotterdam study. 2007;44(3):272–278.
20. Tas U, Verhagen A, Bierma-Zeinstra S, et al. Prognostic factors of disability in older people: A systematic review. Br J Gen Pract. 2007;57(537):319–323.
21. Jagger C, Matthews R, Matthews F, et al. The burden of diseases on disability-free life expectancy in later life. J Gerontology Ser A Biol Sci Med Sci. 2007;62:408–414. http://dx.doi.org/10.1093/gerona/62.4.408
22. Chappell N, Dujela C. Caregiving: predicting at-risk status. Can J Aging. 2008;27(2):169–179. http://dx.doi.org/10.3138/cja.27.2.169
23. Gallo J, Bogner H, Fulner T, et al. Activities of daily living and instrumental activities of daily living assessment. Handb Geriatric Assess. 2006;4:193–240.
24. Sulander T, Tuija P, Rahkonen O, et al. Trends in BADL difficulties by age and education among people aged 65-84 years. Int J Epidemiol. 2006;35:1255–1261. http://dx.doi.org/10.1093/ije/dyl183
25. World Health Organization. Disability and rehabilitation. WHO Action Plan 2006-2011 [homepage on the Internet]. 2006 [cited on 2014 Aug 12]. Available from: www.who.int/disabilities/publications/action_plan/en/.
26. Goldman N, Lin I, Weinstein M, et al. Evaluating the quality of self-reports of hypertension and diabetes. J Clin Epidemiol. 2003;56:148–154. http://dx.doi.org/10.1016/S0895-4356(02)00580-2

19

Pain management in patients with long-bone fractures in a district hospital in KwaZulu-Natal, South Africa

Authors:
Adeleye M. Awolola[1]
Laura Campbell[1]
Andrew Ross[1]

Affiliations:
[1]Department of Family Medicine, University of KwaZulu-Natal, South Africa

Correspondence to:
Adeleye Awolola

Email:
awoleye2004@yahoo.co.uk

Postal address:
6A Knightsbridge, 141 Alexandra Road, Scottsville 3201, South Africa

Background: This study reviewed pain severity and assessment as recalled by patients with long-bone fractures. The focus was on the intervals between admission, pain assessment and analgesic provision, as delay of analgesia for acute pain can result in complex chronic pain syndromes.

Aim: The aims were to explore patients' recollection of pain severity and assessment in an emergency department (ED) and whether analgesia prescribed in the ED correlated with pain severity.

Setting: The study site was a district hospital ED in KwaZulu-Natal, South Africa.

Methods: This exploratory study considered aspects of pain in adults with long-bone fracture who were admitted to an ED and later referred to an orthopaedic unit. Data collection took place in the orthopaedic unit where participants were requested to recall their pain severity (using a visual analogue scale) whilst in the ED.

Results: Ninety-three patients participated, most of whom were African males. Over 60% recalled their pain severity in the ED as 5 or greater on a visual analogue perception scale. No formal tool was used to assess or record pain in the ED, and there was no association between recalled pain severity and type of analgesia prescribed.

Conclusion: The majority of patients were assessed for pain in the ED. Analgesia given to most patients was inadequate for the degree of pain they experienced. A pain assessment protocol should be developed for doctors and nurses to serve as a guideline in assessing patients with long-bone fractures and prescribing appropriate analgesia.

Analyse de la gestion de la douleur chez les patients atteints de fractures des os longs dans un hôpital de district dans le KwaZulu-Natal en Afrique du Sud.

Contexte : Cette étude a examiné la sévérité et l'évaluation de la douleur telles que rapportées a posteriori par des patients atteints de fractures des os longs. L'accent était mis sur les intervalles entre l'admission, l'évaluation de la douleur et l'administration d'analgésique, le retard de l'analgésie en cas de douleur aiguë pouvant entrainer des syndromes complexes de douleur chronique.

But : Les objectifs étaient d'analyser le souvenir de la sévérité et de l'évaluation de la douleur des patients dans un service d'urgence (SU), et si l'analgésie prescrite dans le SU correspondait à la sévérité de la douleur.

Cadre : Le site d'étude était le SU d'un hôpital de district dans le KwaZulu-Natal en Afrique du Sud.

Méthodes : Cette étude exploratoire a examiné les aspects de la douleur chez les adultes atteints de fracture des os longs admis dans un SU et plus tard envoyés vers une unité orthopédique. La collecte des données s'est faite au sein de l'unité orthopédique, où les participants ont été invités à se remémorer la sévérité de la douleur (en utilisant une échelle visuelle analogique - VAS) lors de leur passage au SU.

Résultats : Quatre-vingt treize patients ont participé, dont la plupart étaient des hommes africains. Plus de 60% se sont rappelé d'une sévérité de la douleur au service d'urgence de 5 ou plus sur une échelle de perception de type EVA. Aucun outil formel n'a été utilisé pour évaluer ou enregistrer la douleur au SU, et il n'existait aucun lien entre le souvenir de la sévérité de la douleur et le type d'analgésie prescrit.

Conclusion : La majorité des patients ont été évalués quant à la gestion de la douleur au sein du SU. L'analgésie administrée à la plupart des patients était insuffisante par rapport au degré de douleur qu'ils avaient subi. Un protocole d'évaluation de la douleur doit être développé pour les médecins et les infirmières afin de servir de ligne directrice en termes d'évaluation de l'état des patients atteints de fractures des os longs et de prescription d'une analgésie appropriée.

Introduction

Internationally many patients with acute pain following trauma do not receive any form of analgesia on admission to a hospital emergency department (ED).[1] As an example, research carried out in the United States of America assessed analgesia administered to patients with acute trauma in an ED and reported that half received no analgesia at discharge.[1] Two-thirds waited for up to one hour before receiving any analgesia, and a third received inappropriate analgesia in relation to pain severity. It is particularly concerning that analgesia was not administered in the ED, even to patients with clearly documented evidence of moderate to severe pain.[1]

It is pertinent to review pain in patients with bone fractures in South Africa, as the incidence of bone fractures is high. It has been estimated that a road traffic collision occurs every four seconds in South Africa, and the resultant trauma leads to multiple injuries, including fractures.[2] EDs in South Africa are generally underprepared for their workload, and improvements could be made, including management of pain.[3] This study grew from a concern that patients in KwaZulu-Natal, South Africa who were referred to an orthopaedic unit from an ED appeared to have unmanaged pain.

With regard to pain following a fracture, a large study of patients with extremities fractures reported that only 64% received any analgesia, and analgesic management did not form part of ED protocols.[4] A paediatric ED study indicated that only a third of children with acute, severe pain due to long-bone fractures received any analgesia.[5]

Under-treatment of acute pain is of concern, because if pain remains untreated a patient may develop a complex pattern of chronic pain and disability.[6] This chronic pain results from 'central sensitisation' where the nervous system develops a process of 'wind-up' and becomes regulated to a persistent state of high reactivity.[6] This persistent state maintains pain, even after the initial injury might be healed. Acute pain following acute trauma such as bone fractures has been demonstrated to induce central sensitisation.[7] Although the time between fracture pain and central sensitisation has not been determined, it would seem necessary to treat any acute pain as soon as possible. Most importantly, prompt and appropriate pain management is essential as a fundamental human right.[8]

An extensive literature search found no literature on pain management of patients with long-bone fracture in a South African ED setting, and hence this study will add to the information available on this important topic. The aim of this study was to assess patients' perceptions of pain severity following a long-bone fracture and to review their perceptions of how this pain was assessed in an ED. Associations between recalled pain severity and analgesia that was prescribed were explored. An ED presents a unique opportunity for prompt and appropriate management of any acute pain.

Research methods and design

The design was an exploratory cross-sectional study, and the setting was a district hospital (DH) in KwaZulu-Natal which serves a large community of over 220 000 people. Approximately 50 patients with long-bone fractures are reviewed every month in the ED. For the purpose of this study long-bone fractures were considered to be fractures of the humerus, ulna, radius, femur, tibia and fibula. All patients with long-bone fractures are assessed and stabilised in the ED, and only those requiring admission with multiple open, severely displaced and severely painful fractures are referred onwards for specialist care in an orthopaedic unit. Approximately 40 patients with long-bone fractures are referred from the ED to the orthopaedic unit each month. This study population was chosen because pain in this group of patients is usually severe, and there is a need for prompt, appropriate management in the ED to prevent long-term complications.

As this was an exploratory study, a sample size of 100 was chosen as expedient. Inclusion criteria included adult patients with acute long-bone fractures who were referred from an ED to the orthopaedic unit. The following patients were excluded: those with associated pain which may not be related to long-bone fracture (for example, bone cancer), those who presented to the ED more than one week post-fracture, and those who were unable to give consent.

Every third patient admitted to the orthopaedic unit who met the inclusion criteria was recruited over the study period. Data were collected using two methods: an interview between the patient and the researcher, which was carried out in the orthopaedic unit, and a hospital chart review. The interviews took place at various times after admission to the orthopaedic unit, and patients were requested to recall their stay in the ED. They were asked to recall the following: their maximum pain severity in the ED, whether someone assessed their pain in the ED, and their estimations of intervals between admission and pain assessment and analgesia administration.

Pain management is recognised as a fundamental human right, and at the time of interview the researcher (A.M.A.), who is a medical doctor, assessed pain using a visual analogue scale (VAS) in the orthopaedic unit and immediately prescribed appropriate analgesia if required.

Participants were requested to score the severity of their recalled pain in the ED on the VAS. The VAS was considered to be easy to use in a clinical setting and has been validated in diverse cultural and linguistic settings.[9] The VAS has been found to be useful in measuring pain in bone fractures in a range of injuries, including spinal fractures.[10]

Data on analgesia prescribed in the ED were obtained from patients and patient chart review. Data were captured on a Microsoft Excel spreadsheet and analysed descriptively.

Associations between recalled pain severity and analgesia prescribed in the ED were explored using the Chi-square test and analysis of variance (ANOVA).

Ethical considerations

Permission to conduct the study was obtained from the Research Ethics Committee at the University of KwaZulu-Natal (Ref. BE 023/13), the Provincial Department of Health and hospital managers.

Results

Two hundred and seventy-five patients were admitted to the orthopaedic unit over an eight-month period from January to August 2014, and 93 patients were interviewed as part of this study. Ages of the participants ranged from 18 to over 60 years, and over half (56.0%) were in the 30–50-years age group. The majority were male (84.0%) and most were black African (94.0%), with 3.0% of participants being white and 3.0% from other racial groups. The age distribution is represented diagrammatically in Figure 1.

Half of the fractures occurred in the leg (51.6%). Some patients had more than one type of fracture; for instance, 31.2% had both tibia and fibula fractures. The fracture sites are represented in Figure 2.

Most participants (62.4%) were interviewed by the researcher more than 48 hours following admission to the ED. The majority (96.0%) perceived that they had some form of pain assessment in the ED, and these participants recalled being only verbally questioned about pain with no formal pain evaluation scale used. Two per cent of the participants recalled that they were not asked about pain intensity. Most (82.0%) recalled receiving an initial pain assessment from a doctor only and 18.0% received an initial pain assessment from a nurse only. The perceived intervals between ED admission and pain assessment are summarised in Figure 3.

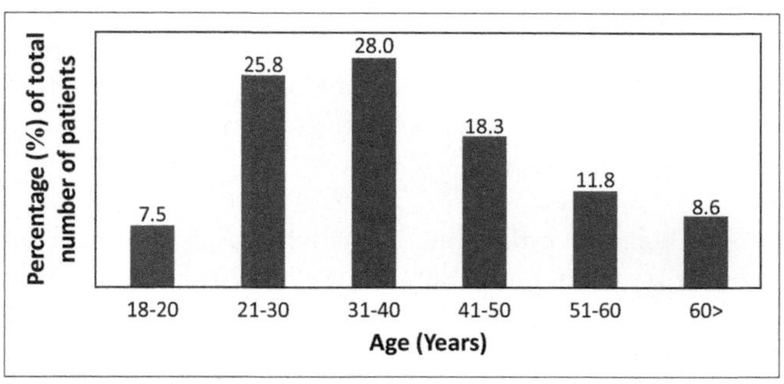

FIGURE 1: Age distribution of participants.

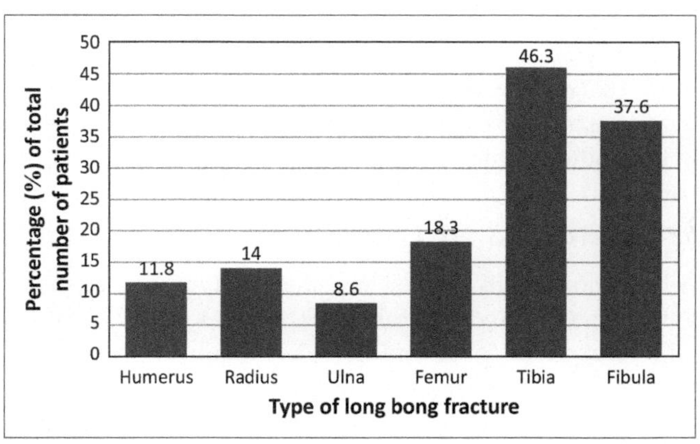

FIGURE 2: Site of long-bone fracture.

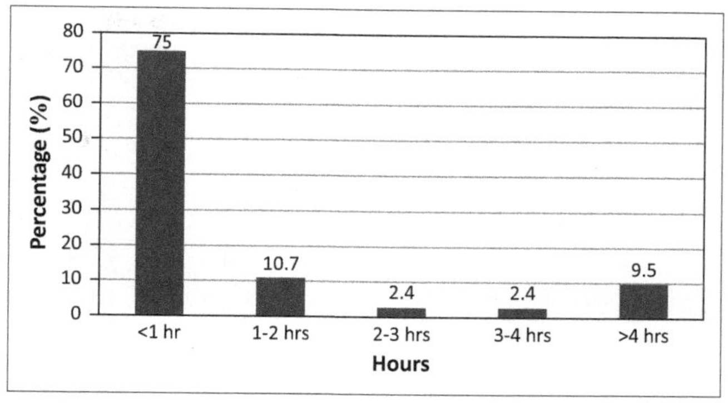

FIGURE 3: Perceived intervals between emergency department admission and pain assessment.

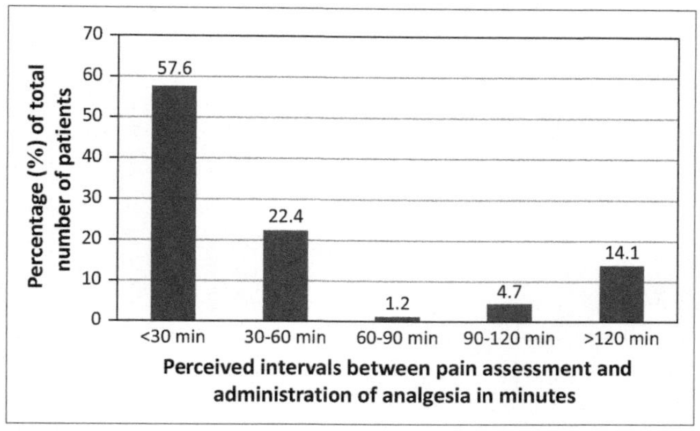

FIGURE 4: Perceptions of interval between pain assessment and administration of analgesia.

Participants' reports concerning the interval between pain assessment and administration of analgesia are illustrated in Figure 4.

A chart record review of the time spent in the ED revealed that half of the analgesia prescribed was administered orally (46.0%) and half via injection (54.0%). The analgesia varied from a weak class to a strong class (as described by the World Health Organization).[11] Some patients received more than one class of analgesia. Some patients (4.3%) reported receiving analgesia but information on the specific type was not recorded in the patient's chart (information not available). Some patients (33.3%) received opioid-like agents such as tramadol and/or paracetamol with codeine (classified by the researcher as 'other analgesia' in Figure 5). Paracetamol was administered orally whilst nonsteroidal anti-inflammatory agents (NSAIDs) were administered either orally or via intramuscular (IM) injections. Opioids used for analgesia were given via IM or intravenous injection. The types of analgesia recorded during ED stay are shown in Figure 5.

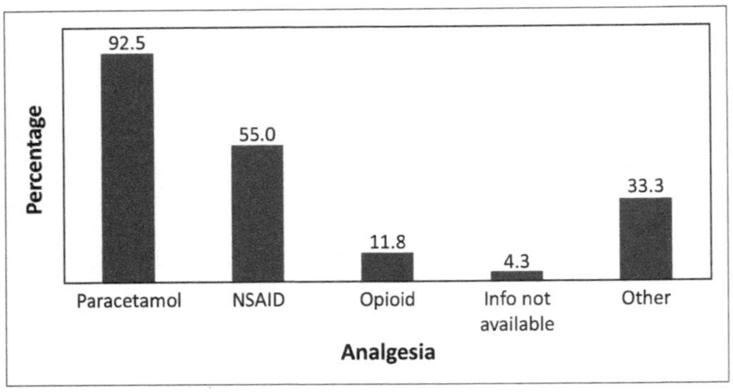

FIGURE 5: Types of analgesia recorded during emergency department stay.

TABLE 1: Recalled pain score on the visual analogue scale.

Recalled pain score reported on VAS	% respondents
1	4.3
2	7.5
3	10.8
4	10.8
5	32.3
6	10.8
7	11.6
8	7.3
9	2.2
10	2.2

Most of the participants (64.0%) recalled their pain as being at level 5 or greater. The range of recalled VAS pain scores is summarised in Table 1.

ANOVA showed no association between type of analgesia provided in the ED and participants' recalled pain score on the VAS ($F = 1.001$, and $p = 0.396$).

Discussion

The aim of the study was to explore participants' recall of pain they experienced whilst in the ED and to assess intervals between admission, assessment and receipt of analgesia. Importantly the study also considered whether ED analgesia correlated with pain severity. Participants had severe or complex fractures, and review of pain assessment and treatment is vital as a lack of early pain management intervention can lead to complications such as chronic pain syndromes.

Results indicated that more males that females were referred to the orthopaedic unit and participants reported significant levels of pain whilst in the ED. Participants were mainly reviewed by doctors in the ED and the intervals between admission, assessment and receipt of analgesia varied between participants. This suggests that no standardised systems were in place for assessment of pain and delivery of analgesia.

The study methods were primarily descriptive, however analysis using ANOVA was found to be useful to hone in on the lack of correlation between reported pain severity and type/World Health Organization class of analgesia prescribed. Each of the findings will be discussed in more detail below.

More men were admitted than women. Although chronic pain syndromes tend to be more common in women, it is important not to neglect the prompt management of acute pain in men.[6] Most participants were in the age group 30–50 years, and a relatively young population may have a higher predisposition to central sensitisation resulting in chronic pain.[12] Further study could consider other demographic features which could predispose to central sensitisation, including not being employed, low educational status and smoking.[6]

In this study the majority of participants were assessed for pain by a doctor rather than by a nurse. This is an interesting finding, as in South Africa there are generally more nurses than doctors available in an ED setting. South African literature advocates that nurses should become more involved with triage of patients in EDs.[13] The potential assessment of pain by nurses requires further exploration in this context.

Although most participants recalled that their pain was assessed within an hour of admission to the ED, the time between assessment and analgesia availability varied and was prolonged (over two hours) in some instances. This finding has major implications in terms of human rights issues, and can also potentially induce chronic pain syndrome. The literature supports that if nurses became more involved, gaps between admission, assessment and analgesia administration may be shortened.[14]

It was of concern that no tool was used to measure or record pain in the ED. This is similar to findings of a Tanzanian study on pain in an ED setting.[15] The introduction of a nurse-initiated triage of pain could potentially improve assessment of pain, using a standardised, validated pain assessment tool. Such an assessment tool could be supported by a pain assessment protocol to serve as a guideline in prescribing appropriate analgesia.

Despite patients rating their pain score as 5 or more, the two most commonly prescribed analgesics were oral paracetamol and an NSAID, which according to the World Health Organization are not adequate for moderate to severe pain.[11] This finding is similar to that of another ED-based study, which showed that an NSAID was the commonest analgesia used for patients with fractures, and was usually administered as a once-off IM dose.[15] Reasons why relatively mild analgesia was prescribed despite patients reporting moderate to severe pain, and how effective mild analgesia is in this setting require further investigation.

Limitations of the study

A limitation to this study is that the recall of data was used. Patients were asked to recall events such as severity of pain, who assessed the pain, and the interval between admission, assessment and analgesic administration, and their recall may have been impaired or distorted as they were in an acutely stressful situation. An alternative data collection method using a point prevalence of pain in an ED or continuous assessment of patients from admission to discharge may permit the gathering of more reliable data.

Conclusion and recommendations

It was encouraging that the majority of patients were assessed for pain and given analgesia in the ED. However, it was of concern that the majority was assessed by doctors, and the potential role of the ED nurse in pain management requires further exploration. As an example, ensuring cooperation and collaboration between nurses and doctors may require attention; a complication may arise if a nurse assesses a pain as significant and a doctor prescribes a mild analgesia.

There appeared to be no standardised methods to assess and record pain, and analgesia prescriptions did not seem to be appropriate for the severity of the pain. In addition, there were prolonged periods between pain assessment and analgesia provision.

A pain assessment protocol should be developed for doctors and nurses to serve as a guideline in assessing patients with long-bone fractures and prescribing appropriate analgesia. This protocol could also provide an opportunity for continuous re-evaluation and assessment of patients in a bid to ensure that no opportunity is missed to provide adequate analgesia. Further research is required in this important area to guide the training and practice of healthcare professionals.

Acknowledgements

The authors would like to thank the management of Northdale Hospital, Pietermaritzburg for providing us with an opportunity to conduct the study there. Special thanks go to the staff in the ED and the orthopaedic departments for their assistance.

Competing interests

The authors declare that they have no financial or personal relationship(s) that may have inappropriately influenced them in writing this article.

Authors' contributions

A.M.A. (University of KwaZulu-Natal) was responsible for protocol development, data collection and analysis, and writing up the manuscript, whilst L.C. (University of KwaZulu-Natal) was involved in conceptualisation of the research, data review and writing up the manuscript and A.R. (University of KwaZulu-Natal) assisted with data review and writing up the manuscript.

References

1. Lewis LM, Lasater LC, Brooks CB. Are emergency physicians too stingy with analgesics? South Med J. 1994;87(1):7–9. http://dx.doi.org/10.1097/00007611-199401000-00002
2. Brysiewicz P, Bruce J. Emergency nursing in South Africa. Int Emerg Nurs. 2008;16(2):127–131. http://dx.doi.org/10.1016/j.ienj.2008.01.001
3. Hardcastle T, Samuels C, Muckart D. An assessment of the hospital disease burden and the facilities for the in-hospital care of trauma in KwaZulu-Natal, **South Africa**. World J Surg. 2013;37(7):1550–1556. http://dx.doi.org/10.1007/s00268-012-1889-1
4. Brown JC, Klein EJ, Lewis CW, Johnston BD, Cummings P. Emergency department analgesia for fracture pain. Ann Emerg Med. 2003;42(2):197–205. http://dx.doi.org/10.1067/mem.2003.275
5. Jone JS, Johnson K, McNich N. Age as a risk factor for emergency medicine analgesia. Am J Emerg Med. 1996;14:157–160. http://dx.doi.org/10.1016/S0735-6757(96)90123-0
6. Phillips K, Clauw DJ. Central pain mechanisms in chronic pain states – Maybe it is all in their head. *Best Pract Res Clin Rheumatol. 2011;25:*141–154. http://dx.doi.org/10.1016/j.berh.2011.02.005
7. Woolf CJ. Central sensitization: Implications for the diagnosis and treatment of pain. Pain. 2011;152(3):s2–15. http://dx.doi.org/10.1016/j.pain.2010.09.030
8. Hall JK, Boswell MV. Ethics, law, and pain management as a patient right. Pain Physician. 2009;12(3):499–506.
9. Kopf A, Patel NB, editors. Guide to pain management in low-resource settings. Seattle, WA: International Association for the Study of Pain; 2010, Chapter 10: p. 67–78.
10. Haonga BT, Makupa JE, Muhina RI, et al. Pain management among adult patients with fractures of long bones at Muhimbili Orthopaedic Institute in Dar es Salaam, Tanzania. J Health Res. 2011;13(4):1–8. http://dx.doi.org/10.4314/thrb.v13i4.56959
11. Vargas-Scaffer G. Is the WHO Analgesic ladder still valid? Twenty-four years of experience. Can Fam Physician. 2010;56(6):514–517.
12. Lottrup Petersen K. Gender differences in pain and secondary hyperalgesia after heat/capsaicin sensitization in healthy volunteers. J Pain. 2006;7(3):211–217. http://dx.doi.org/10.1016/j.jpain.2005.10.013
13. Bruijns L, Wallis A, Burch VC. Effect of introduction of nurse triage on waiting times in a South African emergency department. Emerg Med J. 2008;25:395–397. http://dx.doi.org/10.1136/emj.2007.049411
14. Wong EML. The effect of a triage pain management protocol for minor musculoskeletal injury patients in a Hong Kong emergency department. Australas Emerg Nurs J. 2007;10(2):64–72. http://dx.doi.org/10.1016/j.aenj.2007.02.003
15. Casey ER, Muro F, Thielman NM, *et al.* Analysis of traumatic injuries presenting to a referral hospital emergency department in Moshi, Tanzania. *Int J Emerg Med.* 2012;5:28–32. http://dx.doi.org/10.1186/1865-1380-5-28

Medicines availability at a Swaziland hospital and impact on patients

Authors:
Kholiwe Shabangu[1]
Fatima Suleman[2]

Affiliations:
[1]Discipline of Pharmaceutical Sciences, School of Health Sciences, University of KwaZulu-Natal, Durban, South Africa

[2]Discipline of Pharmaceutical Sciences, School of Health Sciences, Westville Campus, University of KwaZulu-Natal, South Africa

Correspondence to:
Fatima Suleman

Email:
sulemanf@ukzn.ac.za

Postal address:
Private Bag X54001, Durban, 4000, South Africa

Background: The burden of non-communicable diseases (NCDs) in low- and middle-income countries is increasing. Where patients are expected to make increased out-of-pocket payments this can lead to treatment interruptions or non-adherence. Swaziland is no exception in this regard.

Aim: The aim of the study was to investigate the availability of medicines for NCDs in a hospital and the impact of out-of-pocket spending by patients for medicines not available at the hospital.

Setting: The study was conducted at Raleigh Fitkin Memorial Hospital in Manzini, Swaziland.

Methods: Exit interviews to assess availability of a selected basket of medicines were conducted with 300 patients diagnosed with diabetes, hypertension or asthma. The stock status record of a basket of medicines for these conditions in 2012 was assessed at the Central Medical Stores. Results were analysed using the Statistical Package for Social Sciences version 20.0.

Results: Most of the patients (n = 213; 71%) confirmed not receiving all of their prescribed medicines at each visit to the hospital in the past six months. On average patients spent 10–50 times more on their medicines at private pharmacies compared to user fees in the health facility. Stock-outs at the Central Medical Stores ranging from 30 days to over 180 days were recorded during the course of the assessment period (12 months), and were found to contribute to inconsistent availability of medicines in the health facility.

Conclusion: Out-of-pocket expenditure is common for patients with chronic conditions using this health facility, which suggests the possibility of patients defaulting on treatment due to lack of affordability.

Disponibilité des médicaments dans un hôpital du Swaziland et son impact sur les malades.

Contexte: Le fardeau des maladies non transmissibles (MNT) dans les pays à revenus faibles et moyens est en augmentation. Quand les patients doivent débourser des sommes importantes il en résulte des interruptions ou la non-adhésion au traitement. Le Swaziland ne fait pas exception à la règle.

Objectif: Le but de l'étude était d'examiner la disponibilité des médicaments pour les MNT dans un hôpital et l'impact des frais à la charge des patients pour les médicaments non disponibles à l'hôpital.

Lieu: L'étude a été faite au Raleigh Fitkin Memorial Hospital de Manzini, au Swaziland.

Méthodes: Des entretiens de sortie ont eu lieu avec 300 patients souffrant de diabète, pour évaluer la disponibilité d'un panier sélectionné de médicaments. L'état des stocks d'un panier de médicaments pour ces maladies en 2012 a été évalué au Dépôt médical central. Les résultats ont été analysés en utilisant le logiciel « Statistical Package for Social Sciences », version 20.0.

Résultats: La plupart des patients (n = 213; 71%) ont admis qu'ils n'avaient pas reçu tous les médicaments prescrits à chaque visite à l'hôpital au cours des six derniers mois. En moyenne les patients ont dépensé de 10 à 50 fois plus pour leurs médicaments dans les pharmacies privées, comparé aux frais d'utilisation dans les services de santé. Au cours de la période d'évaluation (12 mois) on a constaté des ruptures de stock de 30 à 180 jours dans le Dépôt médical central, ce qui a contribué à la disponibilité irrégulière des médicaments dans le service de santé.

Conclusion: Les frais à la charge des patients sont courants pour les patients souffrant de maladies chroniques utilisant ce service de santé, ce qui peut amener ceux-ci à interrompre le traitement en raison de son coût élevé.

Introduction

Non-communicable diseases (NCDs) have emerged as a clear threat not only to human health but also to development and economic growth globally. The World Economic Forum estimated that 63% of all deaths occurring globally are caused by NCDs.[1] Moreover, NCDs are no longer considered only to be diseases of the affluent, but also affect large number of patients in developing countries. Eighty percent of deaths from NCDs are said to be occurring in low- and middle-income countries, which poses a real challenge to health systems in these countries.[1] Furthermore, globally NCDs are increasingly becoming common amongst all age groups, with a quarter of all related deaths occurring amongst people below the age of 60 years.[2] In addition NCDs account for over 48% of healthy life-years lost globally, compared to 40% for communicable diseases and 1% for injuries.[3]

In Swaziland both communicable diseases and NCDs continue to be a major challenge.[4] The death rate due to NCDs stood at 4.9/1000 in 2008.[5] NCDs have received inadequate attention in Swaziland, given the serious double burden of disease that prevails in the country: communicable diseases and HIV infection and AIDS.[6]

The Swaziland Government is solely responsible for procurement and storage of essential medicines for the country's public health facilities. This has not been without challenges. The Swaziland National Pharmaceutical Policy states that the current warehouse can hold six months' supply of medicines and medical supplies that it procures, stores and distributes to all Government hospitals, mission hospitals, parastatals, clinics and health centres. It is further claimed that this restricted capacity places a burden on the logistics system, with repeated ordering of inventory, and contributes to frequent stock-outs of prescription medicines at health facilities.[7]

User fees of 10 Swazi Lilangeni (SZL) (US $1.13) for hospitals and SZL 5 (US $0.56) (Central Bank of Swaziland Exchange rate: US $1 = SZL10 as at 15 November 2013) are applied at clinics, which includes consultation and the supply of medicines (when available).[7] When medicines for the treatment of NCDs are out of stock at health facilities and patients are required to purchase them from private pharmacies this would constitute a major barrier to access.

The aim of the study was to investigate the availability of a basket of medicines for selected NCD conditions in a health facility in Swaziland and the impact of out-of-pocket spending by patients for medicines that are not available at this hospital.

Research methods and design

Study design

The study was a prospective cross-sectional survey that evaluated the impact on patients on chronic medication in the event that their prescribed medicines for asthma, diabetes or hypertension were out of stock at Raleigh Fitkin Memorial Hospital (RFMH) in Manzini, Swaziland.

Setting

The study took place at RFMH, a 350-bed regional referral hospital situated in Manzini, the hub of Swaziland. The hospital attends to an average of approximately 200 000 patients per year (in- and outpatients). Approximately 40% of patients seen at RFMH have asthma, diabetes or hypertension. The number of outpatients that receive medications from the pharmacy averages 750 patients a day, as not all outpatients visit the hospital pharmacy. An average of 200 patients is admitted into the hospital wards per day, which accounts for an average of 57% bed occupancy at any given time (Human Resources Offices of RFMH 2013, personal communication, March).

Study population and sampling strategy

The study population comprised all patients seen for the three NCDs (diabetes, asthma and hypertension) in the facility, and who had a single diagnosis of one of these three conditions. On average a total of 1111 patients attended RFMH every month for consultations for asthma, diabetes orhypertension (Human Resources Offices of RFMH 2013, personal communication, March).

A statistical formula was used to calculate the number of patients to be interviewed based on the monthly statistics of the hospital,[8] with a 5% margin of error, a 95% confidence interval and a 50% response distribution. Setting the response distribution at 50% is the most conservative assumption when one is not sure what to expect the results for each question to be. By using 50% the largest sample size is calculated.

Based on the calculation a sample of 300 patients with the chronic conditions of diabetes, hypertension or asthma were selected at their point of exit from the pharmacy and interviewed using a questionnaire. A quantitative coded structured questionnaire with some open-ended questions on patients' perception of costs of medicines that were not available at the hospital was used for exit interviews with patients that fulfilled the inclusion criterion. The questionnaire was divided into three sections: the demographics section, including patients' employment status; a section on patients' experiences of stock-outs of medicines; and a section on out-of-pocket costs of buying the medicines. Both SiSwati and English versions of the questionnaires were available to allow patients to choose their preferred language of interview.

At Central Medical Stores (CMS) stock status data for the ten selected medicines making up the chosen basket, based on the current treatment for these conditions in the existing national Standard Treatment Guidelines and the Essential Medicines List at the time of the study, were used to check availability of the medicines and the time it took for them to become available at RFMH after receipt for the period July 2012 to June 2013.

Data collection

Data were collected from patients who had come to fetch their medicines from the pharmacy through exit interviews. The interviews were done after patients had collected their prescribed medicines at the pharmacy, and were conducted by two second-year pharmacy students from the Southern Africa Nazarene University after the prescriptions had been pre-selected by the dispensing personnel (i.e. pharmacy technicians and pharmacists). The selection of medical files was conducted by the professional staff based on the diagnosis of the patient (those having any of the three NCDs under study, with a diagnosis as presented in the clinical notes for more than six months, were eligible). The data collectors then randomly selected adult patients (18 years of age and over) from these files. The data collection was carried out over a period of six weeks, from 23 August 2013 to 4 October 2013. Only patients who were refilling their medications at RFMH during the study period were eligible.

The questionnaire was used to: (1) determine if patients had been exposed to out-of-stock of medicines for their chronic conditions in this facility; (2) establish the coping strategies they were using in order to access their medicines in the event that they were out of stock in the facility; (3) identify the consequences of the unavailability of medicines in the facility to patients and their immediate families; and (4) establish the affordability or otherwise of purchasing medicines out of pocket and any complications experienced due to medicines not being available in the facility.

Data collection at CMS was done through the Senior Pharmacist, who provided the stock status records for the selected medicines from July 2012 to June 2013 to the principal researcher. The records were used to calculate the number of days each medicine was out of stock at the CMS (from the date it was recorded as stock-out) and how soon it was made available to RFMH after the date of receipt (time between getting the stock and processing the stock to RFMH).

Data analysis

Data were categorised, coded and entered first into an Excel spreadsheet and later imported into the Statistical Package for Social Sciences (version 20.0), where descriptive statistical analysis was conducted. The open-ended questions were coded and categorised into themes.

Ethical considerations

Ethical clearance to perform the study was obtained from the University of KwaZulu-Natal Humanities and Social Sciences Research Ethics Committee (HSS/0620/013M) and the Ministry of Heath Ethics Committee in Swaziland (MH/599C/FWA00015267). Patients provided informed consent and participation was voluntary.

Results

Demographic information

The largest age group in the sample was that aged 50–64 years (n = 128; 42.7%), and most of the patients with chronic conditions were females (n = 215; 71.7%). The results showed that whilst the majority of patients (n = 249; 83%) had received some form of education, only a few (n = 51; 17%) had reached tertiary education. The rest (n = 51; 17%) had never been to school. Most of the patients were married (n = 154; 51.3%).

The rate of unemployment amongst these patients was very high (n = 118; 39.3%); only 25% (n = 75) were employed, with those who were self-employed accounting for 22.7% (n = 68).

Results on income distribution (see Table 1) showed that 44.3% (n = 133) of the interviewed patients had a monthly income of less than SZL 500 (US $50). Only 9.7% ($n$ = 29) of the patients had an income above SZL 5000 (US $500) per month.

Health status and health-seeking behaviour

Of the participants in the study, most were hypertensive (41%; n = 123) and diabetic (39.3%; n = 118). Fifty nine (19.7%) of these patients were asthmatic. Most of the patients had been diagnosed with their conditions for more than two years (n = 205; 68.3%). Although most of the patients (n = 243; 81%) reported returning on a monthly basis to refill prescriptions, the two other options provided were reported by 3% (once every 2 months, n = 9) and 16% (only when feeling sick, n = 48). Patients who failed to come for their refills on a monthly basis were asked why they failed to adhere to their appointments. In response, 38.2% (n = 21) said they did not have money for transport to the facility, 29.1% (n = 16) said they did not find it necessary to do refills on a monthly basis, 20% (n = 11) said they were not informed that they were supposed to come to the hospital on a monthly basis, and 12.7% (n = 7) said they did not have money to pay for a consultation (user fees). The participants' monthly income distribution is indicated in Table 1.

Medicine availability and coping strategies of patients

Results showed that only 24.7% (n = 74) of interviewed patients said they always got all their prescribed medicines at the hospital's dispensary, as indicated in Table 2. Further analysis of these patients showed that 13.5% (n = 10) of them

TABLE 1: Patients' monthly income distribution (SZL).

Monthly income (SZL)	Number of patients	%
≤500	133	44.3
501–1000	67	22.3
1001–2000	48	16
2001–5000	23	7.7
> 5000	29	9.7

SZL, Swazi Lilangeni.
Central Bank of Swaziland Exchange rate: US $1 = SZL10 as at 15 November 2013.

TABLE 2: Medicine availability and coping strategy of patients (*n* = 300).

Variables	Frequencies	%
Always received prescribed medicines in the facility		
Yes	74	24.7
No	213	71
Don't know	13	4.3
Frequency of not receiving prescribed medicines in the past six months		
Once	94	31.3
Twice	29	9.7
More than three times	29	9.7
Not sure	148	49.3
Received all prescribed medicines on the day of interview		
Yes	237	79
No	50	16.7
Not sure	13	4.3
Proportion of prescribed medicines received		
None (0% – 50%)	25	8.3
Partly (51% – 80%)	12	4
Mostly (81% – 99%)	26	8.7
Completely (100%)	237	79
Instruction conveyed by dispensing personnel for medicines not available in the facility		
Returned to the doctor	18	6
Referred to private community pharmacy	282	94
Turnaround time for buying medicines at the chemist		
As soon as I leave the facility	119	39.7
Whenever, after getting money	152	50.7
When I go to town as there is no chemist in the community	8	2.7
When I get paid	11	3.7
When I feel sick	10	3.3
Out-of-pocket expenditure by patients in private pharmacies		
< SZL 100	191	63.9
SZL 100–SZL 300	86	28.8
SZL 301–SZL 500	7	2.3
> SZL 500	15	5
Health insurance cover		
Yes	15	5
No	285	95
Health insurance cost incurred		
< SZL 1000	5	1.7
> SZL 1000	4	1.3
Not sure, paid by spouse	6	2
Number of family members supported		
1	82	27.3
2	37	12.3
3	18	6
> 5	27	9
None	136	45.3

had asthma, 48.6% (*n* = 36) had diabetes and 37.8% (*n* = 28) had hypertension. Seventy-nine per cent (*n* = 237) of the patients reported having received all their prescribed medication on the day they were interviewed; 13% (*n* = 30) of these were asthma patients, 48% (*n* = 114) diabetic patients and 39% (*n* = 93) hypertension patients. However, 16.7% (*n* = 50) of the patients did not receive all their prescribed medicines on the day they were interviewed, and 4.3% (*n* = 13) were not sure if they had received all of their prescribed medicines or not, which could indicate either their lack of understanding of their treatment or a breakdown in communication and counselling by health professionals in the facility treating them. Most (94%) of the patients were referred to a private

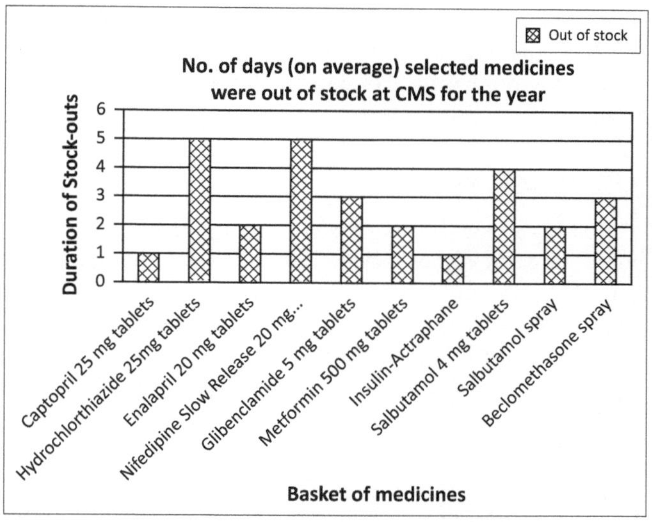

1, 0-30 days; 2, 31-60 days; 3, 61-120 days; 4, 121-180 days; 5, 181-240 days.

FIGURE 1: Availability of the selected basket of medicines at the CMS during the period June 2012 to July 2013.

pharmacy in the event of medicines stock-out at the health facility.

It is important to note that half of the patients who were interviewed (50.7%) indicated that they only bought their medicines when they had money to do so. Patients estimated what they paid for medicines at the pharmacy, with 63.7% (*n* = 191) paying less than SZL 100 (US $10) for their medication at private pharmacies. About 29% (*n* = 86) of the patients indicated that they were paying between SZL 100 and SZL 300 (US $10–US $30), whilst 2.3% (*n* = 7) said they were paying between SZL 301 and SZL 500 (US $30 – US $50) for their medication at a private pharmacy. Five per cent (*n* = 15) were paying more than SZL 500 (US $50) when buying their medication out of pocket in the event of stock-out at the facility for that month. Only 5% of the patients had health insurance cover.

Stock availability at the Central Medical Stores

It is evident from Figure 1 that on average, hypertensive medications were least available in the 12-month period when compared to the other groups, followed by asthma medication. Diabetes medication was more available when compared to the other groups of medications. The results also showed that on average medicines for the selected NCDs were out of stock at the CMS for between two and four months (31–120 days) out of the year.

In terms of turnaround time, most (70%, *n* = 7) of the medicines were issued to the health facility within less than 15 days after receipt by the CMS (based on back orders), namely beclomethasone spray, enalapril 20 mg, Actraphane insulin, captopril 25 mg, metformin 500 mg and nifedipine slow release 20 mg tablets. This is the lead time stipulated in the Pharmaceutical Standard Operational Procedures of the country for ordering of medicines by health facilities. Salbutamol spray was issued between 25 and 30 days after receipt, whilst glibenclamide was issued between 35 and

40 days after receipt at the CMS. Data on hydrochlorothiazide 25 mg tablets was unavailable at the time of data collection, hence one could not gather whether this medicine was issued to the health facility or not.

Discussion

This study showed that in the sample population NCDs were more common in those above 35 years of age and in females. This result is similar to that found in sample populations in other studies, that reported that mostly females were affected by chronic conditions compared to males.[9] This may also be due to the generally high rate of health-seeking behaviour amongst the female population.[10]

Almost half of those who were interviewed (44%) earned a monthly income of less than SZL 500 (US $50), which means that patients may have to forgo other household necessities in order to access medications or health services to manage their conditions. Although these patients were not asked how they were financing their health expenditure, a number of studies have shown that patients with chronic conditions will use a variety of ways to finance their health expenditure: some would sell their assets or borrow money.[11] Outpatient treatment costs have been implicated in catastrophic health expenditure in another setting – India.[12]

Just over half (50.7%) of the patients reported they had not received all of the medicines prescribed when presenting for a refill in the six months prior to the survey. It was notable though that the balance were 'Not sure', and no patient reported always receiving all their medicines at every refill visit. This factor could result in a number of outcomes in the care of patients, which would include complication of their conditions due to foregoing therapy (as they might be unable to afford private pharmacy prices), hospitalisation, expensive treatment for complications and loss of income due to hospitalisation.

Although some patients were able to buy the out-of-stock medicines at private pharmacies immediately after leaving the facility, a significant number (60.4%) could not because of financial constraints. Out-of-pocket amounts spent on medicines by these patients were estimated to be between 10 times and 50 times more than the user fees (SZL 10) charged to access healthcare services in any health facility in the country.

A 2004 study amongst 875 adults with diabetes in the United States of America showed that out-of-pocket medication costs posed a significant problem, affecting their adherence as well as other aspects of their life.[13] Patients' decision-making process would need to be researched further in terms of priority items that income is expended upon, and the position that medicines play in that process. Health systems may be failing these patients, and the result could be an additional burden on healthcare resources when they present with complications or in advanced stages of their conditions.

The stock availability of the selected medicines at the CMS varied. Some medicines were out of stock for a period of less than 30 days a year (captropril and Actraphane insulin), whilst others were out of stock for more than six months (hydrochlorothiazide and nifedipine slow release 20 mg). The latter two are also used in the treatment of cardiovascular conditions, and the severity of the out-of-stock situation may actually be more extreme than is reflected in this exploratory research. The turnaround time of medicines upon receipt at the CMS to the RFMH was acceptable, as it varied from one to 30 days.

This evidence demonstrates that the Ministry of Health needs to assess and improve the availability of medicines in health facilities if required, in order to negate a greater impact on healthcare resources at a later stage of the patient's condition. Access to essential health care and medicines is a basic human right, and at the least the essential medicines for primary care should be available at all times.

Limitations

The study setting is not representative, as patients were sampled from one facility in one region, and hence the results cannot be generalised to other public health facilities in the country. A study with a larger target group would need to be done in more public health facilities to see if the responses are the same and to be able to generalise results.

The cost of medicines in the private pharmacies is not based on actual costs on the day of the interview; as such, the cost of medication at the private pharmacies could not be verified, and the costs are estimates provided by patients. A pricing study should be conducted on the basket of medicines to ascertain the price and availability of these essential medicines at private pharmacies.

Costs to patients are not exhaustive. Whilst the direct out-of-pocket costs of buying the medicines could be estimated, these were a small fraction of the total costs incurred by patients and their families in their efforts to access treatment for their conditions. Inclusion of indirect costs like transport and loss of income would provide a better picture of the financial catastrophe which patients face in order to access health care.

Recommendations

Research on coping strategies for patients with NCDs should be conducted on a larger population and include more public health facilities in order to ascertain how they are coping with the burden of out-of-pocket expenditure when accessing their medicines at private pharmacies. A pricing survey should be conducted to determine actual costs to patients of essential medicines within the private sector. Models of public-private partnerships to make essential medicines available to patients in the event of stock-outs should be developed and explored. Pharmacists in the CMS should be evaluated to determine their skills in medicine supply management, and reasons for stock-outs need to be clarified.

Conclusion

NCDs have shown to be a growing threat in diseases that increase morbidity and mortality in low- and middle-income countries. Proper management of these conditions and uninterrupted availability of medicines will result in a significant reduction of complications and the need for expensive treatment and improved health outcomes in NCD patients in the country.

This exploratory study has suggested that availability of essential medicines for three NCDs at a hospital in Swaziland is problematic, and that patients face a difficult choice when required to access these medicines from the private sector. Logistic supply systems for medicines need to be examined to determine where the bottlenecks are and to overcome these in order to provide an uninterrupted supply of medicines to patients.

Acknowledgements

The authors acknowledge the valuable contributions of Raleigh Fitkin Memorial Hospital and the Central Medical Stores management team for opening its doors and allowing us to carry out this study amongst their patients and using their stock records to access information on medicine availability.

Competing interests

The authors declare that they have no financial or personal relationship(s) that may have inappropriately influenced them in writing this article.

Authors' contributions

F.S. (University of KwaZulu-Natal) and K.S. (University of KwaZulu-Natal) conceptualised and designed the study. K.S. undertook the data collection, and F.S. the data validation. Both authors were responsible for writing up all sections of the article.

References

1. Bloom DE, Cafiero ET, Jané-Llopis E, et al. The global economic burden of noncommunicable diseases. Geneva: World Economic Forum; 2011.
2. World Health Organization. Global status report on non-communicable diseases. Geneva: World Health Organization; 2010.
3. World Health Organization. Preventing chronic diseases: A vital investment. WHO global report. Geneva: World Health Organization; 2005.
4. Central Statistical Office. Swaziland Demographic and Health Survey 2006–07. Mbabane: Ministry of Health; 2008.
5. World Health Organization. Global strategy to reduce the harmful use of alcohol. Geneva: World Health Organization; 2011.
6. World Health Organization. A global brief on hypertension: Silent killer, global public health crisis. Geneva: World Health Organization; 2013.
7. Ministry of Health. Swaziland national pharmaceutical policy. Mbabane: Ministry of Health; 2011. Available from: http://apps.who.int/medicinedocs/.../s19028en.pdf
8. Machin D, Campbell MJ. Statistical tables for the design of clinical trials. Oxford: Blackwell; 1987.
9. Hannan C. Women, gender, equality and diabetes. Int J Gynecol Obstet. 2009;104:S4–S7. PMID: 19155007, http://dx.doi.org/10.1016/j.ijgo.2008.11.021
10. Juel K, Christensen K. Are men seeking medical advice too late? Contacts to general practitioners and hospital admissions in Denmark 2005. J Publ Health. 2008;30(1):111–113. PMID: 17981887, http://dx.doi.org/10.1093/pubmed/fdm072
11. Van Damme W, Van Leemput L, Por I, Hardeman W, Meessen B. Out-of-pocket health expenditure and debt in poor households: Evidence from Cambodia. Trop Med Int Health. 2004;9(2):273–280. PMID: 15040566, http://dx.doi.org/10.1046/j.1365-3156.2003.01194.x
12. Bhojani U, Thriveni BS, Devadasan R, et al. Out-of-pocket healthcare payments on chronic conditions impoverish urban poor in Bangalore, India. BMC Public Health. 2012;12:990. PMID: 23158475, http://dx.doi.org/10.1186/1471-2458-12-990
13. Piette JD, Heisler M, Wagner TH. Problems paying out-of-pocket medication costs among older adults with diabetes. Diabetes Care. 2004;27(2):384–391. PMID: 14747218, http://dx.doi.org/10.2337/diacare.27.2.384

A theoretical alternative intraosseous infusion site in severely hypovolemic children

Authors:
Nkhensani Mogale[1,2]
Albert-Neels van Schoor[2]
Marius C. Bosman[2]

Affiliations:
[1]Department of Anatomy, Sefako Makgatho Health Sciences University, South Africa

[2]Department of Anatomy, University of Pretoria, South Africa

Correspondence to:
Nkhensani Mogale

Email:
nkhensani1909@gmail.com

Postal address:
PO Box 94446, Boordfontein 0201, South Africa

Background: Studies have shown that the venous system tends to collapse during hypovolemic shock. The use of the bone marrow space for infusions is an effective alternative, with the tibial insertion site being the norm.

Objectives: This study was conducted to determine a quick intraosseous infusion method that could be an alternative to the tibial route in neonates during emergency situations.

Method: A sample of 30 neonatal cadavers was dissected to explore a possible alternative to the tibial insertion site. The needle was inserted in the superolateral aspect of the humerus. The needle infusion site was then dissected to determine possible muscular and neurovascular damage that might occur during the administration of this procedure, with the greatest concern being the posterior circumflex humeral artery and axillary nerve exiting the quadrangular space. The distance of the needle insertion site was measured in relation to the soft tissue as well as to bony landmarks.

Results: The calculated 95% confidence interval shows that the needle can be safely inserted into the intraosseous tissue at the greater tubercle of the humerus 9.5 mm – 11.1 mm from the acromion. This is about a little finger's width from the acromioclavicular joint.

Conclusion: Anatomically, the described site is suggested to offer a safe alternative access point for emergency infusion in severely hypovolemic newborns and infants, without the risk of damage to any anatomical structures.

Point de perfusion intra-osseux alternatif théorique chez les enfants gravement hypovolémiques.

Contexte : Des études ont montré que le système veineux tendait à l'effondrement lors d'un choc hypovolémique. L'utilisation de l'espace de la moelle osseuse pour des perfusions est une alternative efficace, le point d'insertion tibial étant la norme.

Objectifs : Cette étude a été menée afin d'établir une méthode de perfusion intra-osseuse rapide qui pourrait être une alternative à la voie tibiale chez les nouveau-nés lors de situations d'urgence.

Méthode : Un échantillon de 30 cadavres néonatals a été disséqué pour explorer une alternative possible au point d'insertion tibial. L'aiguille a été insérée dans la partie supéro-externe de l'humérus. Le point de perfusion de l'aiguille a ensuite été disséqué afin de déterminer d'éventuels dommages musculaires et neurovasculaires qui auraient pu se produire lors de l'administration de cette procédure, la plus grande préoccupation étant l'artère circonflexe humérale postérieure et le nerf axillaire sortant de l'espace quadrangulaire. La distance entre le point d'insertion de l'aiguille a été mesurée par rapport au tissu mou et à des repères osseux.

Résultats : L'intervalle de confiance à 95% calculé montre que l'aiguille peut être insérée en toute sécurité dans le tissu intra-osseux au niveau du tubercule majeur de l'humérus à 9.5 mm – 11.1 mm de l'acromion. Ceci représente environ la largeur d'un petit doigt à partir de l'articulation acromio-claviculaire.

Conclusion : Sur le plan anatomique, on suggère le point décrit afin d'offrir un point d'accès alternatif sûr pour la perfusion d'urgence chez les nouveau-nés et les nourrissons gravement hypovolémiques, sans risque de dommage aux structures anatomiques.

Introduction

Proper fluid resuscitation is needed in most life-threatening situations and it is of paramount importance that appropriate access is obtained as quickly as possible and without complications. Several studies[1,2,3,4,5,6] have shown that the venous system tends to collapse during life-threatening conditions, making the normal route of infusion unpredictable and unreliable. Health care workers often work under strenuous conditions and need a safe, quick and reliable method to administer fluid resuscitation. This study was conducted to determine an intraosseous (IO) infusion site different from existing access points as a possible alternative infusion route in severely hypovolemic newborns and infants.

The use of the bone marrow space as an infusion site was initially proposed by Drinker et al. when they described the sternum as a potential site for transfusions.[1,2] Later, in 1940, Tocantins[3] described the administration of fluids into the general circulation via the bone marrow using animal experiments to demonstrate this phenomenon. In the same year, Tocantins and O'Neill[4] documented 14 cases that involved the injection of blood, plasma or saline into the sternal bone marrow of adults and the marrow of the tibia or femur in infants. In 1942, Papper[5] described access to the marrow space for the use of intravenous (IV) fluids. This led to investigations into the administration of drugs and other fluids with the IO space as an access route to the central circulation. In his study, Papper also stressed the inaccessibility of veins in very young patients and that long periods of continued fluid therapy frequently produce thrombosis of veins with the associated possibility of infection or embolism.[5] These observations suggested that an alternative route, such as IO infusion, would be of great value.

IO infusion is as quick as with central lines and even faster than with peripheral lines. The use of the IO space for patient resuscitation reached its peak during World War II, when it was commonly used in soldiers experiencing haemorrhagic shock.[7] Use of IO infusion methods became rare after the war, but the practice was revived in the 1980s and the method has been in use since then. The increased use of this method over the years can be attributed to the evolution of technology that allows for easier penetration of the dense adult bone cortex.[2,7]

The speed of vascular access plays an important role in preventing death and irreversible organ damage. Central lines are often not used in children owing to the difficulty experienced when accessing the venous system compared to in adults, and health care workers need advanced skills to place central lines safely and successfully in children. Primary health care facilities in developing countries are often underequipped to handle the installation of central venous lines, which makes a simple alternative attractive.[8] In addition, the difficulty with venous access, particularly in a shocked child, necessitates the need for a quick alternative.

IO insertion can be used for administration of fluids to a haemodynamically shocked neonate in whom attempts to access the vascular system have been unsuccessful. Under these conditions, it is usually impossible to administer drugs through peripheral veins, because insufficient perfusion would most probably cause them to collapse.[9] Rapidly securing vascular access may be a considerable challenge in the presence of shock or intravascular volume depletion, causing peripheral venous shutdown.[10] This is associated with cardiopulmonary arrest, oedema and extensive burns.[8] IO insertion may also be useful in older children, as they can become dehydrated very quickly. This is especially relevant in the case of gastrointestinal infections, which occur often in South Africa. External jugular insertion is associated with high malposition rates and is particularly difficult in the very young owing to these patients' short necks. Several serious complications may also arise, including laceration of the internal jugular vein and infection.[2] The other preferred route in newborn babies is the umbilical vein, but direct drug injection into this structure has proved to be dangerous.[9] IO administration is second to that of the umbilical vein, but if the umbilical vein is not available then this route becomes a viable option.

IO vascular access permits the administration of life-saving fluids and medications in critically ill patients. Drugs administered intraosseously enter the circulation as fast and in the same concentration as those administered intravenously.[8] Current technology allows IO infusion to be considered as a preferential safe and effective route of drug administration in cardiac arrest cases, and should also be considered the first alternative to failed IV access.[2]

IO infusion has proven successful in neonates when the anteromedial surface of the tibia was used as the insertion site.[8] The technique is simple because the landmarks are easily palpable.[8] Similar methods have been explored in adults,[10] with both the proximal humerus (superolateral aspect of the greater tubercle) and the tibia being successfully infused.

It has been shown that in adults, the rate at which the infused contents enter the systemic circulation is comparable whether an IO insertion site is used on the proximal humerus or on the tibia.[7] The current study is an anatomical exploration to determine whether an easily palpable landmark can be identified on the proximal humerus as a possible alternative IO infusion site to tibial infusion in neonates. To our knowledge, this is the first study to simulate an IO infusion method on the proximal humerus of neonates. This method could prove useful during treatment of traumatic accidents where injury to the lower limbs of the neonate would prevent tibial infusion.

Research method and design

A sample of 30 neonatal cadavers (age range 0–28 days) of low to normal birth weight (1.5 kg or higher) was used in the study. A total of 60 humeri were studied. A 22-gauge Jelco IV spinal needle was inserted at the greater tubercle of the humerus. The area around the insertion site was dissected (Figure 1) to determine the possibility for muscular or neurovascular damage during administration of this procedure.

The humerus was chosen because of the large amount of vascular bone marrow that exists in the long bones of neonates

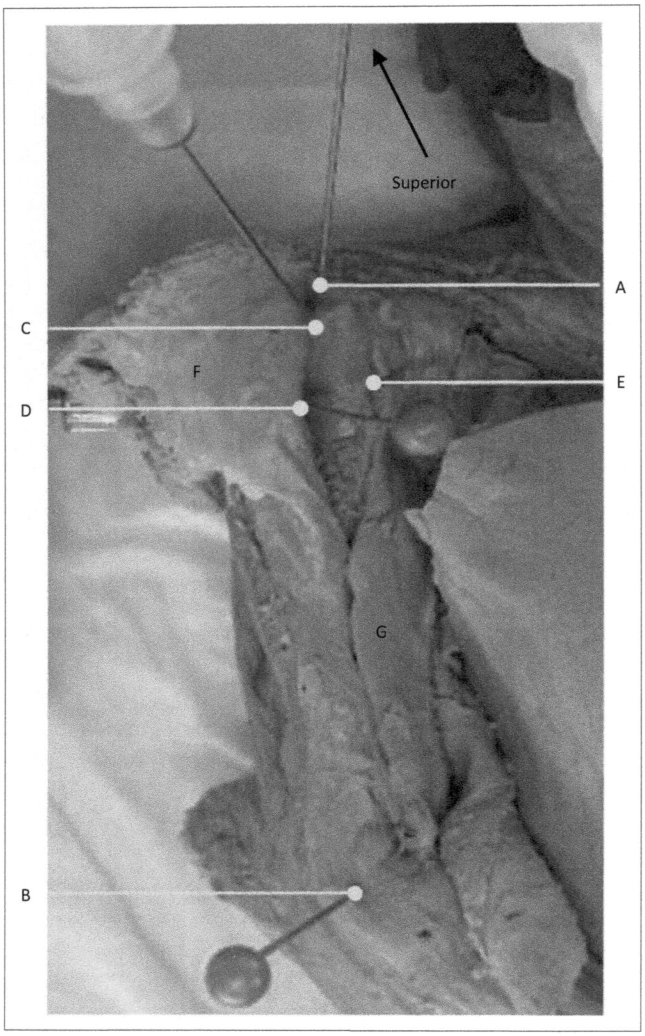

Source: Nkhensani Mogale/University of Pretoria

FIGURE 1: Anterior view of a right neonatal shoulder after the deltoid muscle (F) has been reflected. Pins were inserted into the acromion (A), lateral epicondyle of the humerus (B), the greater tubercle of the humerus (C), the axillary neurovascular bundle as it exits the quadrangular space (D) and the long head of the of the biceps brachii muscle (E). The muscular belly of the biceps brachii muscle (G) is also visible.

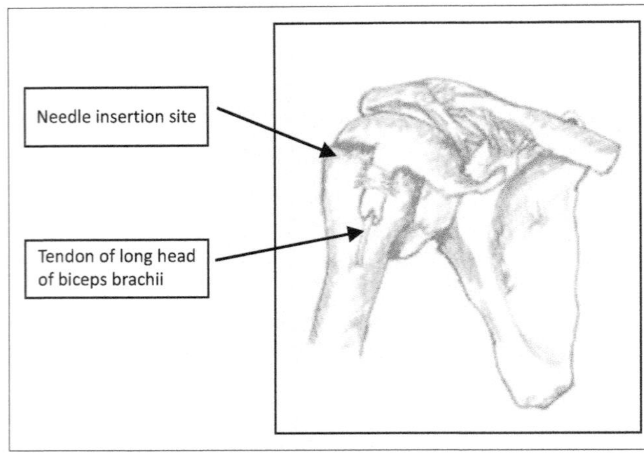

Source: Mpho Mogale

FIGURE 2: The needle insertion site and the tendon of the long head of biceps brachii muscle shown in the bicipital groove/intertubercular sulcus.

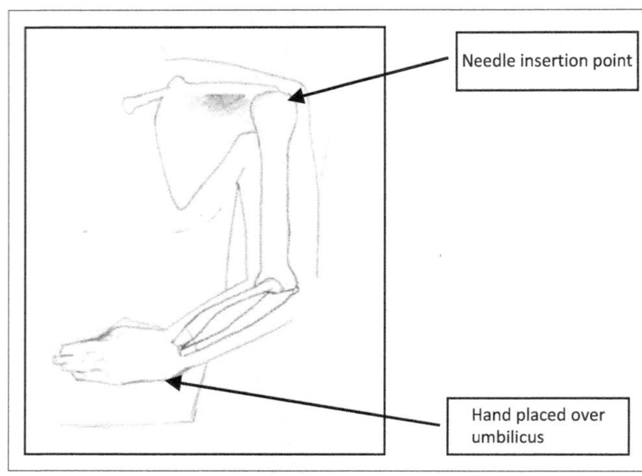

Source: Mpho Mogale

FIGURE 3: Body in supine position with the humerus adducted against the trunk.

and consequently provides access to a non-collapsible venous plexus. (Marrow sinusoids drain into large medullary venous channels, which empty into the systemic venous circulation via nutrient and emissary veins.)[2,7,9] The needle was inserted in the superolateral aspect of the humerus (as in adults), with the direction of the needle insertion observed and the measured distance between the needle and landmarks recorded (Figure 2). The needle position was then recorded whilst measuring the distance to the soft tissue (neurovascular bundle, long head of the biceps brachii muscle) as well as the relative distances between bony landmarks (acromion and lateral epicondyle of the humerus).

Certain standard placement methods were followed. This involved placing the neonatal cadaver in a supine position to present the greater tubercle of the humerus to the investigator. The humerus was adducted against the trunk, with the elbow posteriorly directed towards the table. The hand was secured on the abdomen near the umbilicus (Figure 3). This position provided a more prominent insertion site and ensured protection of the vital neurovascular structures located under the arm. This position also ensures maximal approach to the humeral head.[9,11] The lateral aspect of the acromion, in line with the acromioclavicular joint, was palpated by feeling the depression when the arm is abducted and then returning to the correct position on the abdomen with the hand near the umbilicus. This position was labelled as point A using a coloured pin. The lateral epicondyle of the humerus (point B) was identified by palpating the distal aspect of humerus and also marked with a coloured pin. The deltoid muscle was then carefully reflected (Figure 4) to expose the neurovascular bundle in the quadrangular space (between the axillary nerve and the posterior circumflex humeral artery) (point D). The long head of the biceps brachii muscle (point E) was exposed within the bicipital groove/intertubercular sulcus. The needle was inserted in the greater tubercle at the mid point of the head (between point A and the surgical neck of the humerus) and labelled as point C.

A sliding calliper of 0.02-mm accuracy was then used to measure the short distances between:

- the acromion (A) and lateral epicondyle (B)

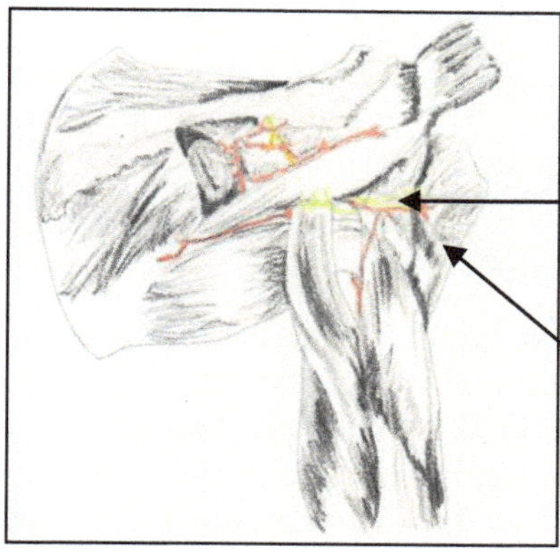

Source: Mpho Mogale

FIGURE 4: Posterior view of the reflected head of the deltoid muscle with the neurovascular bundle (posterior circumflex humeral artery and the axillary nerve) shown.

- the acromion (A) and the needle insertion point on the greater tubercle of the humerus (C)
- the needle insertion point on the greater tubercle of the humerus (C) and the lateral epicondyle (B)
- the needle insertion point on the greater tubercle of the humerus (C) and axillary neurovascular bundle (D)
- the needle insertion point on the greater tubercle of the humerus (C) and the long head of the biceps brachii muscle (E).

Data analysis

A paired *t*-test was used to compare measurements in the left and right humeri. The minimum and maximum distances were recorded and the mean, standard deviation and 95% confidence interval were calculated.

Ethical considerations

Ethical clearance was obtained from the Research Ethics Committee of the Faculty of Health Sciences, University of Pretoria (reference number S114/2011). As this study made use of human tissue, all the neonatal cadavers were obtained and dissected under the rules and regulations defined in the *South African Health Act* (Act 61 of 2003). All cadavers were donated by the family members or obtained as a result of the deceased being unclaimed by family members. The material was handled with respect and care at all times, and properly safeguarded.

Information regarding the cadaver's age, height and weight was noted and only the researchers conducting the study had access to it. No information that could reveal the identities of the cadavers was obtained.

Results

A paired *t*-test revealed no significant difference between pairwise measurements of the right and left humeri ($P > 0.05$ for all measurements). Measurements of the right and left sides of the neonatal cadavers were therefore combined to give a sample size of 60 dissected humeri. The results are summarised in Table 1.

The mean body length of the cadavers was 0.43 m ± 0.07 m (mean ± SD) and mean weight was 1.69 kg ± 0.74 kg. The calculated confidence interval shows that the ideal insertion point for the IO needle lies 9.5 mm – 11.1 mm (mean of 10.3 mm) from A on a line connecting A and B. As the described IO insertion is proposed for application in emergency procedures, the health care worker has to be able to find the site quickly. The insertion point can be determined as the distance equal to the width of the little finger (fifth distal phalanx) from the acromioclavicular joint (approximately 11 mm). The results also suggest that a health care worker should be able to perform the procedure without injury to the important neurovascular structures in that area (posterior circumflex humeral artery and axillary nerve). The results showed that the point of the needle insertion is on average 11 mm from the axillary nerve and accompanying posterior circumflex humeral vessels as they run through the quadrangular space (range: 10.5 mm – 11.6 mm; 95% confidence level), and 8 mm from the long head of the biceps brachii tendon running in the intertubercular groove (range: 7.8 mm – 8.7 mm; 95% confidence level).

Discussion

The vascular network of the long bones provides an ideal route for IO infusion. Drugs or fluids injected into the bone marrow cavity in the proximal humerus pass into the venous sinusoids to the central venous channels and move into the systemic circulation through the nutrient veins. This route is quickly accessible and does not collapse during shock, in contrast to what is often seen in the venous system. Of the drugs tested to date, none has proven unsuccessful for use by IO infusion in neonates.[11,12] This success can be attributed to neonates having a highly vascular bone marrow in their long bones, which contains a network of non-collapsible venous sinusoids in the medullary cavity of the spongy bone that drain into the venous circulation.[13] Although technological developments have made this method practically applicable, risks such as disturbance of the proximal humerus growth plate, pain during infusion and potential for infection in the affected bone[13,14] cannot be eliminated completely. However,

TABLE 1: Distances of the soft tissue and bony landmarks from the intraosseous needle insertion site on the greater tubercle of the humerus (n = 60).

Statistics	A–B (mm)	A–C (mm)	B–C (mm)	C–D (mm)	C–E (mm)
Mean	64.8	10.3	57.4	11.1	8.2
s.d.	9.1	3.1	8.0	2.2	1.7
Range of 95% confidence interval	62.5–67.1	9.5–11.1	55.4–59.4	10.5–11.6	7.8–8.7

s.d., standard deviation.

these risks have to be weighed against the benefits and the best infusion method should be explored. Therefore, this procedure should be performed once all the risk factors have been considered and it has proved to be the most beneficial method of treatment for the patient.

IO infusion is indicated for neonatal fluid resuscitation in life-threatening situations when attempts at obtaining vascular access elsewhere have been unsuccessful. The IV route of administering drugs and fluids is generally the preferred choice, but can be difficult in obese and oedematous children as well as in children experiencing cardiac arrest or circulatory shock.[8,14]

Our measurements show the upper and lower limits of the distance from C to E to be 8.7 mm and 7.8 mm, respectively. This suggests that the IO needle can be inserted about 5 mm into the bone after initial contact before care must be taken to avoid contact with the epiphyseal growth plate. The epiphyseal growth plate separates the proximal head of the humerus from the shaft and is located distal to the greater tubercle of the humerus. Care must be taken not to angle the needle inferiorly in order to avoid injury to the growth plate. The needle must also never be inserted deeper than the distance from the lateral border of the greater tubercle to the long head of biceps brachii (approximately 8 mm in the studied sample).

IO needle placement is not definitive therapy; rather, it allows for the administration of life-saving medication and fluids when intravascular access is vital. IO needles may be left in place in the marrow for up to 96 hours, but IV access is usually obtained sooner (within 6–12 hours after IO access) to reduce the risk of infection or dislodgement of the needle.[15,16]

Conclusion

This study indicated that, based on the anatomical data collected, the humeral IO site is likely to be a safe alternative to the tibial IO site in neonates. When the IO needle is inserted as per the method discussed in this study, the risk of injury to the soft tissue and epiphyseal growth plate is minimised. Although this study was limited to a neonatal sample, we suggest that the described technique may be viable and safe in older infants and children as well.

Acknowledgements

The authors wish to thank the Department of Anatomy, University of Pretoria, for the use of the neonatal cadavers for data collection. Mpho Mogale is acknowledged for the illustrations (Figures 2–4).

Competing interests

The authors declare that they have no financial or personal relationship(s) that may have inappropriately influenced them in writing this article.

Authors contributions

N.M. (Sefako Makgatho Health Sciences University) was involved in the original background research for the project and writing the thesis, contributed to the design of the project and collected the data. She wrote the first draft of the manuscript. A-N.v.S. (University of Pretoria) was the study supervisor and made considerable contributions towards the original research design and thesis. He was involved in data analysis and also made substantial additions and corrections to the draft of the manuscript in preparing the article for submission. M.C.B. (University of Pretoria) provided anatomical merit to the article and assisted with editorial input and formatting.

References

1. Drinker CK, Drinker KR, Lund CC. The circulation in the mammalian bone marrow. Am J Physiol. 1922;62:1–92.
2. Phillips L, Brown L, Campbell T, Miller J, Proehl J, Youngberg B. Recommendations for the use of intraosseous vascular access for emergent and nonemergent situations in various health care settings: a consensus paper. J Paediatr Nurs. 2011;26:85–90. http://dx.doi.org/10.1016/j.pedn.2010.10.001
3. Tocantins LM. Rapid absorption of substances injected into bone marrow. P Soc Exp Biol Med. 1940;45:292–296. http://dx.doi.org/10.3181/00379727-45-11657
4. Tocantins LM, O'Neill JF. Infusion of blood and other fluids into the general circulation via the bone marrow. Surg Gynecol Obstet. 1941;73:281–287.
5. Papper EM. Bone marrow route for injecting fluids and drugs into the general circulation. Anesthesiology 1942;3:307–313. http://dx.doi.org/10.1097/00000542-194205000-00008
6. Tocantins LM, O'Neill JF, Prince AH. Infusions of blood and other fluids via the bone marrow in traumatic shock and other forms of peripheral circulatory failure. Ann Surg. 1941;114:1085–1092. http://dx.doi.org/10.1097/00000658-194112000-00015
7. Ngo AS, Oh JJ, Chen Y, Yong D, Ong MEH. Intraosseous vascular access in adults using the EZ-IO in an emergency department. Int J Emerg Med. 2009;2:155–160. http://dx.doi.org/10.1007/s12245-009-0116-9
8. Boon JM, Gorry DL, Meiring JH. Finding an ideal site for intraosseous infusion of the tibia: an anatomical study. Clin Anat. 2003;16:15–18. http://dx.doi.org/10.1002/ca.10071
9. Ellemunter H, Simma B, Trawöger R, Maurer H. Intraosseous lines in preterm and full term neonates. Arch Dis Child Fetal Neonatal Ed. 1999;80:F74–F75. http://dx.doi.org/10.1136/fn.80.1.F74
10. Ong ME, Chan YH, Oh JJ, Ngo AS. An observational, prospective study comparing tibial and humeral intraosseous access using the EZ-IO. Am J Emerg Med. 2009;27:8–15. http://dx.doi.org/10.1016/j.ajem.2008.01.025
11. Tay ET, Hafeez W. Intraosseous access [document on the Internet]. c2015 [updated: 2015 Apr 09; cited 2015 Jun 10]. Available from: http://reference.medscape.com/article/80431-overview
12. De Sá RA, Melo CL, Dantas RB, Delfim LVV. Vascular access through the intraosseous route in pediatric emergencies. Rev Bras Ter Intensiva. 2012;24(4):407–414.
13. Sunde GA, Heradstveit BE, Vikenes BH, Heltne JK. Emergency intraosseous access in a helicopter emergency medical service: a retrospective study. Scand J Trauma Resusc Emerg Med. 2010;18:52–56. http://dx.doi.org/10.1186/1757-7241-18-52
14. Peutrell JM. Intraosseous cannulation. Anaesth Intens Care. 2006;7:28–30. http://dx.doi.org/10.1383/anes.2006.7.1.28
15. Eslami P, Reynolds M. Pediatric intraosseous access [document on the Internet]. c2010 [updated 2014 Feb 13; cited 2015 Jun 10]. Available from: http://emedicine.medscape.com/article/940993-overview
16. Tyagi A, Drake J, Midha R, Kestle J. Axillary nerve injuries in children. Pediatr Neurosurg. 2000;32:226–229. http://dx.doi.org/10.1159/000028942

22

Quality of care for patients with non-communicable diseases in the Dedza District, Malawi

Authors:
Rachel Wood[1]
Vanessa Viljoen[1]
Lisa Van Der Merwe[1]
Robert Mash[1]

Affiliations:
[1]Family Medicine and Primary Care, Stellenbosch University, South Africa

Correspondence to:
Robert Mash

Email:
rm@sun.aca

Postal address:
PO Box 241, Cape Town 8000, South Africa

Introduction: In Malawi, non-communicable diseases (NCDs) are thought to cause 28% of deaths in adults. The aim of this study was to establish the extent of primary care morbidity related to NCDs, as well as to audit the quality of care, in the primary care setting of Dedza District, central Malawi.

Methods: This study was a baseline audit using clinic registers and a questionnaire survey of senior health workers at 5 clinics, focusing on care for hypertension, diabetes, asthma and epilepsy

Results: A total of 82 581 consultations were recorded, of which 2489 (3.0%) were for the selected NCDs. Only 5 out of 32 structural criteria were met at all 5 clinics and 9 out of 29 process criteria were never performed at any clinic. The only process criteria performed at all five clinics was measurement of blood pressure. The staff's knowledge on NCDs was basic and the main barriers to providing quality care were lack of medication and essential equipment, inadequate knowledge and guidelines, fee-for-service at two clinics, geographic inaccessibility and lack of confidence in the primary health care system by patients.

Conclusion: Primary care morbidity from NCDs is currently low, although other studies suggest a significant burden of disease. This most likely represents a lack of utilisation, recognition, diagnosis and ability to manage patients with NCDs. Quality of care is poor due to a lack of essential resources, guidelines, and training.

Qualité des soins des patients atteints de Maladies non transmissibles dans le district de Dedza au Malawi.

Introduction: Au Malawi, les maladies non transmissibles (MNT) sont responsables pour 28% des décès chez les adultes. Le but de cette étude était de déterminer l'ampleur de la morbidité due aux MNT dans les soins primaires, et de vérifier la qualité des soins dans le cadre des soins primaires dans le district de Dedza au centre du Malawi.

Méthodes: Cette étude était une première vérification basée sur les registres cliniques et une enquête par questionnaire des personnels de santé qualifiés à 5 cliniques, se concentrant sur l'hypertension, le diabète, l'asthme et l'épilepsie.

Résultats: On a enregistré 82581 consultations, dont 2489 (3.0%) étaient pour les MNT sélectionnées. Seuls cinq des 32 critères structurels ont été remplis aux cinq cliniques et neuf des 29 critères du processus n'ont jamais été mis en œuvre à aucune des cliniques. Les seuls critères de processus accomplis aux cinq cliniques étaient la prise de la tension artérielle. Les connaissances du personnel sur les MNT étaient basiques et l'obstacle principal à la prestation de soins de qualité était le manque de médicaments et d'équipement essentiel, des connaissances et des directives insuffisantes, le paiement pour les services à deux cliniques, l'inaccessibilité géographique et le manque de confiance des patients dans le système de santé primaire.

Conclusion: A l'heure actuelle, la morbidité due aux MNT dans les soins primaires est faible, bien que d'autres études suggèrent une charge morbide significative. Cela indique probablement l'absence d'utilisation, de reconnaissance, de diagnostic et de capacité de gérer les patients atteints de MNT. La qualité des soins est mauvaise due au manque de ressources essentielles, de directives et de formation.

Introduction

According to the United Nations 'the global burden and threat of non-communicable diseases constitutes one of the major challenges for development in the 21st century, which undermines social and economic development throughout the world, and threatens the achievement of internationally agreed development goals'.[1] The challenge of non-communicable diseases (NCDs) is seen in Sub-Saharan Africa (SSA), where health systems are already struggling to cope with HIV and AIDS and other infectious diseases, maternal and child health as well as trauma. Most of the premature deaths from NCDs occur in low and middle income countries.[2] The prevalence of NCDs and their complications have been found to already be high in some SSA settings and may also be underreported.[3] Studies in SSA show that the prevalence of diabetes mellitus may be as high as 16% in some settings, whilst hypertension ranges from 6% to 48%.[3] The lack of resources and effective health services for NCDs in many areas leads to late diagnosis and poor management, which impacts on mortality and morbidity.[3] Epilepsy is also common, with a prevalence of up to 3.7% and is also inadequately managed, with 80% – 90% of patients receiving no treatment. It has been predicted that by 2030, NCD's will cause 46% of all deaths in SSA.

Chronic care for patients with NCDs, such as type 2 diabetes, hypertension, asthma, chronic obstructive pulmonary disease and epilepsy, is usually situated in primary care.[1] Primary care providers, facilities and services however are often poorly prepared to offer quality chronic care.[1] High quality primary care for NCDs requires attention to the provision of essential medication and equipment, training of primary care providers, and organisation of the health services to offer care that is patient-centred, timely and efficient, co-ordinated, continuous, comprehensive, integrated and which includes self-management support.[6]

The Malawi government included NCDs in the Malawi Health Sector Strategic Plan for 2011–2016, which indicates their awareness of the issue. According to the plan, 'the level of hypertension is higher in Malawi (35% of adults) than in the United States of America and the United Kingdom (27%)'. Additionally, it states that NCDs are thought to be a leading cause of deaths in adults, second only to HIV and AIDS. In collaboration with the Ministry of Health, the Malawi Health Sector Strategic Plan focuses on opportunistic screening and treatment of NCDs with cheap, but effective medications.

The motivation for this study came from the healthcare workers at Nkoma Hospital in central Malawi, who wanted to understand more about the morbidity related to NCDs in their hospital and associated primary care platform. A small unpublished survey was performed at the out-patient department and suggested that 40% of patients with NCDs could have been seen at their local primary care clinic, but preferred to travel to the hospital for care. The lack of capacity to care for NCDs in primary care was thought to be placing an additional burden on the hospital and patients. The four main NCDs, as identified by clinicians at Nkhoma Hospital, were hypertension, diabetes mellitus, asthma and epilepsy.

The aim of this study therefore was to establish the extent of primary care morbidity related to NCDs and to audit the quality of care for NCDs (specifically hypertension, diabetes mellitus, asthma and epilepsy) in the primary care setting in the Dedza District of central Malawi. No previous similar studies were identified in the literature from Malawi, and this study should help managers and policy makers to plan better health services for patients.

Methods

Study design

This was a baseline audit of primary care morbidity related to NCDs and the quality of primary care. The study included a retrospective survey of the five clinic registers to evaluate the extent of primary care morbidity related to NCDs, and questionnaire-based interviews to obtain qualitative and quantitative data on the quality of care.

Study setting

Nkhoma Hospital is a mission hospital in the rural Lilongwe region that acts as a referral centre for Lilongwe and Dedza districts. Dedza district was selected as the study setting as another research study was being conducted in the Lilongwe district. Dedza district has 5 clinics: Kalulu, Kasina, Mayani, St. Joseph's and Tsoyo. This platform serves a total population of 98 693. Kasina and St. Joseph's clinics were missionary funded, whilst the others were funded by the government. This results in the need for patients to pay a small fee-for-service at Kasina and St Joseph, but also meant the clinics were slightly better resourced. All of the clinics, except one, had both reliable water and electricity supplies.

None of the clinics had a doctor, whilst in four of the clinics care was provided by a medical assistant, who was a mid-level doctor. At the remaining clinic, care was offered by a nurse. Medical records were patient-retained and only basic information regarding attendance was recorded in the clinic register: date, patient name, age, gender, suspected diagnosis and medications provided.

Prior to the study the hospital had conducted training for the primary care clinics on locally developed protocols for the management of NCDs. The health workers at the hospital had also requested the researchers, who were three medical students attending for a four-week elective period, to conduct this baseline audit of the quality of care on their behalf. The intention was that the results would guide the local health services in how to improve the quality of care in the future.

Study population

The study included all five of the primary care clinics in the Dedza district, their clinic registers and the most senior clinician involved in NCD care at each clinic.

Data collection

Data were extracted using a standardised data collection tool from the clinic registers for the previous 14 months

(September 2013 to October 2014) on patient consultations for NCDs, their age and gender.

A questionnaire was constructed to obtain information on the structure (e.g. availability of equipment, medication, educational material and human resources) and process of care (e.g. screening, examining, patient counselling and education, management and follow-up). Likert scales were used to evaluate the process of care with a four point scale that ranged from never to every visit. Two sources were used in determining the content of the questionnaire, the integrated audit tool for NCDs developed by the Department of Health in the Western Cape, South Africa[1] and the local NCD clinical management protocols developed by Nkhoma Hospital. The questionnaire also included open questions to document the health workers perspective on the strengths and weaknesses of NCD care.

The interviews with the senior health worker at each clinic enabled the completion of the questionnaire, which was based on their self-reported quality of care. Data could not be extracted from patient records as these were retained by the patients.

Data analysis

Data was captured on a Microsoft Excel spreadsheet and descriptive statistics were used to determine the frequency of consultations for NCDs out of all consultations conducted at the clinics as well as to determine a mean score or frequency for the criteria used to assess quality of care. The limited qualitative data in response to the open questions was collated and key themes extracted.

Ethical considerations

Ethical approval for the study was obtained from the Health Research Ethics Committee of Stellenbosch University (S14/08/171) and permission from the local hospital chief medical officer.

Results

Primary care morbidity

A total of 82 581 consultations were recorded for the Dedza District primary care platform over the previous 14 months, which included 2489 (3.0%) visits for the designated NCDs. Out of the 2489 visits 891 (35.8%) were for epilepsy, 865 (34.7%) for asthma, 717 (28.8%) for hypertension and 16 (0.6%) were for diabetes. The two clinics (Kasina and St Josephs) run by faith-based organisations had a higher proportion of the visits (1416/2489 [56.9%]) than the three government clinics (1073/2489 [43.1%]).

Quality of care

This next section presents the results of the audit of clinical care based on interviews with the senior health workers at the clinics.

TABLE 1: Results of structural criteria for primary care clinics (N = 5).

Structural criteria	n
Diabetes mellitus	
Protocol on diabetes	0
Scale for weight	1
Height measure	5
Glucometer	2
Blood pressure machine	5
Adult size BP cuff – medium	5
Ault size BP cuff – obese	1
Ophthalmoscope	1
Snellen chart	2
Nylon monofilament	0
Equipment for taking HbA1c blood test	0
Patient education materials	1
Metformin in stock	1
Glibenclamide in stock	1
Insulin in stock	0
Epilepsy	
Protocol on epilepsy	0
Patient education materials	1
Phenobarbitone in stock	3
Phenytoin in stock	0
Carbamezapine in stock	1
Asthma	
Protocol on asthma	0
Peak expiratory flow meter	0
Patient education materials	2
Salbutamol inhalers	5
Aminophylline tablets	5
Beclomethasone inhalers	1
Hypertension	
Protocol on hypertension	0
Urine dipsticks for proteinuria	0
Patient education materials	1
Hydrochlorothiazide	4
Propranolol	1
Atenolol	1

Structural criteria

The results of the structural criteria, such as clinical guidelines, basic equipment, self-management resources and medication in stock on the day of the audit are presented in Table 1.

Table 1 gives a clear indication of the limited and often absent structural criteria (protocols, educational material, equipment, medication) at the clinics. None had protocols for any of the NCDs. Most of the clinics had no patient education materials and only one of the five had resources available for every disease.

Only the most basic forms of diagnostic and screening equipment were available, in limited supply, or there was a complete absence thereof. All five clinics had a measuring tape and blood pressure machine, but only one had an additional obese size cuff. Only one clinic had a proper functioning weighing scale and only two had a glucometer with which to diagnose diabetes mellitus. No equipment for taking an HbA1c blood test was available in the whole district. There were no peak expiratory flow meters or urine dipsticks.

TABLE 2: Results of process criteria for primary care clinics (N = 5).

Process criteria	Frequency			
	Never	Once a year	More than once per year	Every visit
Diabetes mellitus				
Measure the patient's weight	3	0	1	1
Test the urine for protein	5	0	0	0
Measure the blood glucose	4	0	0	1
Measure the HbA1C	5	0	0	0
Measure the blood pressure	3	0	0	2
Measure the cholesterol	5	0	0	0
Examine the fundi	5	0	0	0
Check the red reflex	5	0	0	0
Test visual acuity	5	0	0	0
Examine the feet	4	0	0	1
Provide patient education	2	1	2	0
Asthma				
Counsel about smoking	0	1	0	4
Counsel about inhaler technique	1	2	0	2
Inquiry about number of exacerbations	1	0	0	4
Provide patient education	0	0	2	3
Hypertension				
Measure the patient's weight	4	0	0	1
Test the urine for protein	5	0	0	0
Measure the blood glucose	4	0	0	1
Measure the blood pressure	0	0	0	5
Measure the cholesterol	5	0	0	0
Measure the creatinine	5	0	0	0
Counselling on lifestyle changes	0	1	0	4
Provide patient education	0	1	0	4
Epilepsy				
Inquiry about frequency of seizures	0	0	1	4
Inquiry about medication side effects	2	1	0	2
Counselling on medication	0	1	0	4
Counselling on lifestyle changes	1	2	1	1
Counselling on alcohol use/ abuse	2	0	2	1
Provide patient education	0	1	3	1

Regarding medication, only one of the clinics had a supply of oral medication for diabetes and none had insulin. The supply of medication for epilepsy was also limited and no clinics had phenytoin. All five clinics had a supply of reliever asthma medication (salbutamol and aminophyline), but only one had a supply of controller medication (inhaled corticosteroids). Most clinics had access to a thiazide diuretic, but no other medication for hypertension was readily available.

Process criteria

Table 2 presents the results of the audit on the process of care in terms of the clinic's self-reported frequency of performing key clinical processes.

Only basic forms of NCD screening and follow-up monitoring were said to be a part of consultations. In most cases, however, these processes did not occur as frequently as optimal standards of care require.

The only process criteria performed at all five clinics was measurement of blood pressure in those with hypertension. Only two clinics stated that they performed any of the process criteria for people with diabetes and only one could actually measure glucose. None of the clinics were able to perform blood tests and even urinalysis or weighing patients was difficult.

Patient counselling and education was variable as some issues were tackled at every visit, such as counselling on medication for people with epilepsy, whilst other issues were less frequently dealt with, such as inhaler technique.

Qualitative findings

The knowledge on NCD care, with regard to diagnosis and management, of staff members was found to be very basic. This was especially true for diabetes mellitus, where only one interviewee had sufficient knowledge in order to make a diagnosis of the disease.

The main barrier to NCD care was identified as medication shortages. Other prevalent barriers noted were accessibility to the clinics, and affordability of transport costs, fee-for-service and medication at the faith-based organisation's clinics. Other considerations were equipment and staff shortages, lack of training and clinicians' lack of confidence in their own skills levels.

The barriers acknowledged to play a role in hindering patients' ability to attend to their medical needs were poverty, lack of NCD knowledge and lack of confidence in the health system. Additionally, health-seeking behaviour was also influenced by patients resorting to care provided by traditional healers.

Discussion

The quality of primary care for NCDs in the Dedza District of central Malawi is generally poor. In this part of Malawi the commonest NCDs seen in primary care were asthma and epilepsy, and NCDs made up only 3% of primary care visits, in contrast to South Africa, where hypertension and diabetes are the commonest conditions and NCDs make up 14% of visits.[8]

The reported prevalence of NCDs in the region suggest that NCDs are under-represented in Malawian primary care morbidity compared to the expected burden of disease (16% diabetes mellitus; 6% – 48% hypertension and 3.7% epilepsy).[9] The WHO reports that 28% of deaths in Malawi are due to NCDs (cardiovascular diseases 12%, cancers 5%, chronic respiratory diseases 2% and diabetes 1%) and 36.4% of adults have raised blood pressure.[10] Previous studies have reported that NCDs and their risk factors are major public health problems in Malawi.[10] The low primary care morbidity from NCDs may therefore represent a lack of ability to diagnose and treat NCDs in primary care or low utilisation of primary care for this purpose.

Prevalence rates in rural areas may be lower than in more urban settings, but the findings of this study support the argument that primary care services are unprepared to recognise and manage NCDs.

By international and even regional standards the quality of care in Malawi is sub-optimal, with fundamental gaps in structural criteria such as the availability of basic equipment, supply of medications, implementation of guidelines and capability of primary care providers. The gaps in structural criteria suggest that the resources needed to support the process criteria are largely absent and therefore it is not surprising that the process of care is also reported as poor. It is likely that the actual process of care is worse than the findings of this study as they are self-reported, due to a lack of access to actual patient records. Although patient outcomes could not be measured in this audit they are also likely to be poor.

Many countries in the region are recognising that NCDs are an important part of their burden of disease. For example, Uganda has recognised NCDs as a priority, especially at primary care level, and has developed a department to address research, delivery of interventions and policies.[11] This includes the development and testing of standard guidelines for NCD prevention and care. Networks, such as the Chronic Disease Initiative for Africa, have been researching and developing African responses to the growing prevalence of NCDs.[12]

In several countries researchers have been reporting on quality improvement initiatives and demonstrating that significant increases in the quality of care are possible with simple interventions and minimal resource allocation.[13,14] Interventions that may make an immediate difference to Malawian primary NCD care include:

- Development and implementation of national management guidelines for the commonest NCDs.
- Training and upskilling of primary care providers to diagnose and manage NCDs.
- Supply of essential medication and equipment for management of NCDs at the primary care level.
- Attention should also be given to continuous quality improvement cycles to monitor progress and better informational continuity in the medical record for patients requiring chronic care.

Limitations of this study include the inability to differentiate between new or follow-up visits for patients with NCDs in the clinic registers. It was not possible therefore to determine the actual number of patients with these conditions attending primary care. Data in the clinic registers were sometimes missing, incomplete or illegible. Development of the criteria was strongly based on South African guidelines and audit tools and although evidence-based may not have been entirely appropriate for the Malawian context. Interviews to assess the process criteria were conducted in English, which may have limited the complexity of responses in some cases and were held with the most senior person available at the time of the visit. Clinics were remote and access difficult so that visits had to be undertaken when transport was available.

Conclusion

Primary care morbidity from NCDs is currently very low in the primary care services of Dedza District in central Malawi, although other studies suggest a significant burden of disease. This most likely represents a lack of utilisation, recognition, diagnosis and ability to manage patients with diabetes, hypertension, asthma or epilepsy. The quality of care is very low with basic structural criteria not met and an inability to deliver on the process criteria. The health system needs to provide guidelines, training, medication and basic equipment to tackle NCDs.

Acknowledgements

The researchers would like to acknowledge the clinical staff at Nkhoma Hospital, as well as at the Dedza District Clinics, for their assistance with this research. Special thanks should be made to Dr Ter Haar (Medical director of Nkhoma Hospital) for his invaluable assistance. The researchers are grateful to the Chronic Diseases Initiative for Africa for covering the publication fees.

Competing interests

The authors declare that they have no financial or personal relationship(s) that may have inappropriately influenced them in writing this article.

Authors' contributions

L.H.v.d.M., V.L.V. and R.T.W. (University of Stellenbosch) performed the study as undergraduate MBChB students, and were supervised by Prof. R.M. (University of Stellenbosch). All authors conceptualised the study, data collection and analysis was performed by the students, and all authors interpreted the findings and contributed to the final manuscript.

References

1. United Nations General Assembly. Political declaration of the high-level meeting of the General Assembly on the prevention and control of non-communicable diseases [homepage on the Internet]. 66th session of the United Nations General Assembly, 16th September 2011 [cited 2015 Feb 21]. Available from: http://www.un.org/en/ga/ncdmeeting2011/
2. WHO Global status report on non-communicable diseases [homepage on the Internet]. Geneva: World Health organization, 2014 [cited 2015 Apr 2]. Available from: http://www.who.int/nmh/publications/ncd-status-report-2014/en/
3. Dalal S, Beunza JJ, Volmink J, et al. Non-communicable diseases in sub-Saharan Africa: What we know now. Int J Epidemiol. 2011;40(4):885–901. http://dx.doi.org/10.1093/ije/dyr050
4. Unwin N, Mugusi F, Aspray T, et al. Tackling the emerging pandemic of non-communicable diseases in sub-Saharan Africa: The essential NCD health intervention project. Public Health. 1999;113(2):141–146. http://dx.doi.org/10.1016/s0033-3506(99)00139-0
5. World Health Organization. Global status report on non-communicable diseases 2010 [homepage on the Internet]. 2010 No date [cited 2014 Dec]. Available from: http://www.who.int/nmh/publications/ncd_report_full_en.pdf
6. World Health Organization. Innovative care for chronic conditions: Building blocks for action [homepage on the Internet]. No date [cited 2015 Feb 21]. Available from: http://www.who.int/chp/knowledge/publications/icccreport/en/

7. Government of Malawi, Ministry of health. Malawi health sector strategic plan 2011–2016 [homepage on the Internet]. No date [cited 2014 Sep]. Available from: http://www.medcol.mw/commhealth/publications/3%20Malawi%20HSSP%20Final%20Document%20(3).pdf

8. Mash B, Fairall L, Adejayan O, et al. A morbidity survey of South African primary care. PLoS ONE [document on the Internet]. 2012;7(3):e32358. http://dx.doi.org/10.1371/journal.pone.0032358

9. Msyamboza KP, Ngwira B, Dzowela T, et al. The burden of selected chronic non-communicable diseases and their risk factors in Malawi: Nationwide STEPS survey. PloS ONE [document on the Internet]. 2011;6(5):e20316. Available from: http://dx.doi.org/10.1371/journal.pone.0020316

10. World Health Organization. Malawi statistics: Non-communicable diseases [homepage on the Internet]. No date [cited 2015 Feb 1]. Available from: http://www.who.int/countries/mwi/en/

11. Schwartz JI, Guwatudde D, Nugent R, Kiiza CM. Looking at non-communicable diseases in Uganda through a local lens: An analysis using locally derived data [document on the Internet]. 2014. Available from: http://dx.doi.org/10.1186/s12992-014-0077-5

12. Chronic disease initiative for Africa [homepage on the Internet]. No date [cited 2015 Feb. 21]. Available from: http://www.health.uct.ac.za/fhs/research/groupings/cdia/about

13. Kande C, Mash R. Improving the quality of care for patients with hypertension in Moshupa District, Botswana: Quality improvement cycle. Afr J Prm Health Care Fam Med [serial on the Internet]. 2014;6(1). Available from: http://dx.doi.org/10.4102/phcfm.v6i1.578

14. Govender I, Ehrlich R, Van Vuuren U, et al. Clinical audit of diabetes management can improve the quality of care in a resource-limited primary care setting. Int J Qual Health Care. 2012;24(6):612–618. http://dx.doi.org/10.1093/intqhc/mzs063

Appendix starts on the next page→

Appendix 1

Non-communicable diseases research questionnaire

Use of protocols

This refers to the protocols for diabetes, asthma, hypertension and epilepsy provided by Nkhoma Hospital. Training occurred on the 10th of September at Nkhoma Hospital

Question	Yes	No
Are you aware of the protocols?		
Have you read the protocols yourself?		
Have you received training on the use of the protocols?		
Have you tried to implement the protocols at your clinic?		

How useful do you think the protocols are for the clinic?

DIABETES

Structural criteria

Which of the following equipment is available and working properly in the clinic TODAY for the management of diabetes?

Question	Yes	No
Protocol on diabetes		
Scale for weight		
Height measure		
Glucometer		
Blood pressure machine		
Adult size BP cuff – medium		
Ault size BP cuff – obese		
Opthalmoscope		
Snellen chart		
Nylon monofilament		
Equipment for taking HbA1c blood test		
Patient education materials		
Metformin		
Glibenclamide		
Insulin		

Process criteria

When you treat a patient with diabetes at your facility, how often do you perform any of the following activities?

Question	Never	Once a year	More than one visit per year	Every visit
Measure the patient's weight				
Test the urine for protein				
Measure the blood glucose				
Measure the HbA1C				
Measure the blood pressure				
Measure the cholesterol				
Examine the fundi				
Check the red reflex				
Test visual acuity				
Examine the feet				
Provide patient education				

How would you diagnose a patient with diabetes?

What treatment would you prescribe for a new patient with type 2 diabetes?

ASTHMA

Structural criteria

Which of the following equipment is available and working properly in the clinic TODAY for the management of asthma?

Question	Yes	No
Protocol on asthma		
Peak expiratory flow meter		
Patient education materials		
Salbutamol		
Aminophylline		
Beclomethasone		

Process criteria

When you treat a patient with asthma at your facility, how often do you perform any of the following activities?

Question	Never	Once a year	More than one visit per year	Every visit
Counsel about smoking				
Counsel about inhaler technique				
Inquiry about number of exacerbations (assessment of control)				
Provide patient education				

HYPERTENSION

Structural criteria

Which of the following equipment is available and working properly in the clinic TODAY for the management of hypertension?

Question	Yes	No
Protocol on hypertension		
Scale for weight		
Glucometer		
Blood pressure machine		
Adult size BP cuff – medium		
Ault size BP cuff – obese		
Urine dipstix for proteinuria		
Patient education materials		
Hydrochlorothiazide (HTCZ)		
Propanolol		
Atenolol		

Process criteria

When you treat a patient with hypertension at your facility, how often do you perform any of the following activities?

Question	Never	Once a year	More than one visit per year	Every visit
Measure the patient's weight				
Test the urine for protein				
Measure the blood glucose				
Measure the blood pressure				
Measure the cholesterol				
Measure the creatinine				
Counselling on lifestyle changes				
Provide patient education				

How useful was the protocol when you tried to use it in the clinic?
How would you diagnose a patient with hypertension?
What treatment would you prescribe for a new patient with hypertension?

EPILEPSY

Structural criteria

Which of the following equipment is available and working properly in the clinic TODAY for the management of epilepsy?

Question	Yes	No
Protocol on epilepsy		
Patient education materials		
Phenobarbitone		
Phenytoin		
Carbamazepine		

Process criteria

When you treat a patient with epilepsy at your facility, how often do you perform any of the following activities?

Question	Never	Once a year	More than one visit per year	Every visit
Inquiry about frequency of seizures				
Inquiry about medication side effects				
Counselling on medication				
Counselling on lifestyle changes				
Counselling on alcohol use/abuse				
Provide patient education				

How useful was the protocol when you tried to use it in the clinic?
How would you diagnose a patient with epilepsy?
What treatment would you prescribe for a new patient with epilepsy?

Health system performance

What are the main challenges that you experience to offer quality of care for NCDs at this clinic?
What do you think are the main challenges that patient's experience to access quality of care for NCDs at this clinic?
What do you think are the main challenges that patients experience in managing their own NCDs?

23

Causes of mortality and associated modifiable health care factors for children (< 5-years) admitted at Onandjokwe Hospital, Namibia

Authors:
Johnface F. Mdala[1]
Robert Mash[1]

Affiliations:
[1]Division of Family Medicine and Primary Care, Stellenbosch University, South Africa

Correspondence to:
Robert Mash

Email:
rm@sun.ac.za

Postal address:
PO Box 241, Cape Town 8000, South Africa

Introduction: Many countries, especially those from sub-Saharan Africa, are unlikely to reach the Millennium Development Goal for under-5 mortality reduction by 2015. This study aimed to identify the causes of mortality and associated modifiable health care factors for under-5 year-old children admitted to Onandjokwe Hospital, Namibia.

Method: A descriptive retrospective review of the medical records of all children under five years who died in the hospital for the period of 12 months during 2013, using two different structured questionnaires targeting perinatal deaths and post-perinatal deaths respectively.

Results: The top five causes of 125 perinatal deaths were prematurity 22 (17.6%), birth asphyxia 19 (15.2%), congenital anomalies 16 (12.8%), unknown 13 (10.4%) and abruptio placenta 11 (8.8%). The top five causes of 60 post-perinatal deaths were bacterial pneumonia 21 (35%), gastroenteritis 12 (20%), severe malnutrition 6 (10%), septicaemia 6 (10%), and tuberculosis 4 (6.7%). Sixty-nine (55%) perinatal deaths and 42 (70%) post-perinatal deaths were potentially avoidable. The modifiable factors were: late presentation to a health care facility, antenatal clinics not screening for danger signs, long distance referral, district hospitals not providing emergency obstetric care, poor monitoring of labour and admitted children in the wards, lack of screening for malnutrition, failure to repeat an HIV test in pregnant women in the third trimester or during breastfeeding, and a lack of review of the urgent results of critically ill children.

Conclusion: A significant number of deaths in children under 5-years of age could be avoided by paying attention to the modifiable factors identified in this study.

Causes de mortalité et facteurs de soins de santé chez les enfants (< 5 ans) admis à l'hôpital d'Onandjokwe en Namibie.

Introduction: De nombreux pays, en particulier ceux de l'Afrique sub-saharienne, n'atteindront pas les Objectifs de Développement du Millénaire de réduction de la mortalité des moins de 5 ans en 2015. Cette étude avait pour but d'identifier les causes de mortalité et les facteurs de santé modifiables associés chez les moins de 5 ans admis à l'hôpital d'Onandjokwe, en Namibie.

Méthode: Un examen descriptif rétrospectif des dossiers médicaux de tous les enfants de moins de 5 ans qui sont décédés à l'hôpital pendant la période de 12 mois en 2013, au moyen de deux questionnaires structurés différents ciblant respectivement les décès périnatals et post-périnatals.

Résultats: les cinq causes principales des 125 décès périnatals étaient la prématurité 22 (17.6%), l'asphyxie néonatale 19 (15.2%), les anomalies congénitales 16 (12.8%), les causes inconnues 13 (10.4%) et le décollement placentaire 11 (8.8%). Les cinq causes principales des 60 décès post-périnatals étaient la pneumonie bactérienne 21 (35%), la gastroentérite 12 (20%), la malnutrition grave 6 (10%), la septicémie 6 (10%), et la tuberculose 4 (6.7%). 69 (55%) décès périnatals et 42 (70%) décès post-périnatals auraient pu être évités. Les facteurs modifiables étaient: la présentation tardive à un établissement de santé, le non dépistage des signes de danger à la clinique anténatale, l'orientation à longue distance, les hôpitaux de district qui n'offrent pas de service d'obstétrique d'urgence, la surveillance médiocre de l'accouchement et des enfants admis dans les services, l'absence de dépistage de la malnutrition, la non répétition du test de VIH chez les femmes enceintes au troisième trimestre ou pendant l'allaitement, et le non examen des résultats urgents des enfants gravement malades.

Conclusion: Un nombre important de décès chez les enfants de moins de 5 ans aurait pu être évité si on avait fait attention aux facteurs modifiables identifiés dans cette étude.

Introduction

The under-five mortality rate is one of the health indicators used by the World Health Organization (WHO) to assess a country's progress with improving the health of its citizen.[1] Globally there has been an overall decrease in under-five mortality since 1990, when many countries started working towards the fourth Millennium Development Goal (MDG), which aims to decrease under-five mortality by two thirds by the year 2015.[1] However, in Sub-Saharan Africa and South Asia there has been slow progress in attaining the MDG goal, and many countries in these regions are unlikely to meet the target.[1,2,3,4]

Globally almost 40% of all under-five deaths are due to preventable or treatable infectious causes, particularly bacterial pneumonia and diarrhoea diseases, as well as birth complications and malnutrition.[1,2,3,4,5,6,7,8,9,10,11,12,13,14,15,16,17,18,19] There is also a high neonatal mortality in many poor countries due to premature birth, birth asphyxia and sepsis.[12,13,14,15,16] Many proven strategies to reduce mortality have not been implemented, such as high quality antenatal care, skilled birth attendance, and prioritising services in remote and rural communities where the most vulnerable children and pregnant women live.[11,12,13,14,15,16] The deaths in older children after the perinatal period have remained high due to low coverage of pneumococcal vaccine, poor sanitation and water supply, and poor food security in low-income countries, as well as displacement of populations in countries with war or conflict.[3]

Differences in the burden of diseases have been acknowledged as well as the need for specific countries to identify their local health challenges and priority areas.[3] Therefore, efforts should be made to identify modifiable factors which contribute to the death of children, and to develop strategies to address these challenges locally.

Namibia, over the last 43 years, has shown a progressive trend towards decreasing the under-five mortality rate from a high of 118 per 1000 live births in 1968 to 31 per 1000 live births in 2012.[18,20] However, the under-five mortality rate is still above the target of 24 deaths per 1000 live births in 2015 and therefore efforts to identify country specific causes which could be targeted, are necessary.[18,19,20] The recent introduction of pneumococcal and rotavirus vaccines in many African countries, including Namibia, should have a further impact on reducing mortality.[3]

South Africa, a neighbouring country to Namibia, has been collecting data on perinatal mortality since 2000, and has also started under-five child mortality reviews, whereby the causes of deaths and avoidable contributors are identified and priority interventions designed.[13,14,15,16,17,21,22,23] The need to monitor trends in under-five mortality is important in Namibia, although production of useful quality data that can be used in planning needs improvement.[21] The interventions that have been implemented in South Africa to improve under-five survival include: changes to the nurseries; creation of Kangaroo Mother Care areas; provision of essential equipment, including Continuous Positive Airway Pressure (CPAP) machines at hospitals; allocation of specific staff for newborn children; retention of key experienced staff in maternity and neonatal units; improved laboratory services and drug availability; change of attitude amongst health care workers that newborns need specialised care; training of large numbers of doctors and nurses; use of standardized admission forms and record charts; admission, or readmission, of older neonates to the newborn care facilities and not to normal paediatrics wards, and use of the Perinatal Problem Identification Programme (PPIP).[22]

Therefore, since no such facility-based reviews of under-5 deaths have been performed in Namibia to determine the local causes of deaths and modifiable factors, this study will be an important cornerstone in introducing such practice and designing specific interventions to decrease deaths in our settings, based on local findings.

Aims and objectives

The primary aim of this study was to identify the causes of deaths of children under the age of five years who died at Onandjokwe Hospital, Northern Namibia from 01 January 2013 to 30 December 2013. The secondary aim was to look at the management of these children in the paediatric department and to identify modifiable factors in the quality of care that might be targeted in future to reduce child mortality. The specific objectives were:

- to identify key demographic and clinical information (age, gender, and length of stay in hospital, time of death, nutritional profile, and HIV exposure and/or status);
- to identify the immediate and underlying causes of death as well as the significant conditions contributing to death, and
- to identify any modifiable causes of death, where they occurred in the health care delivery chain and who was responsible for the modifiable factor (clinical worker, care giver and/or family member or administrator).

Methods

Study design

The study was a descriptive retrospective review of the medical records of all children under five years who died in the hospital during 2013. The study population was divided into two groups that were assessed using two different questionnaires: a questionnaire collecting Perinatal Mortality Data for those who died before the first week of life and a second questionnaire collecting data for children who died between eight days and five years.

Study settings

The study was conducted at the Onandjokwe Lutheran Hospital in Northern Namibia, which is located 750 km from the capital city of Windhoek. The hospital has been providing health care services for 108 years, has a 450 bed capacity, and serves a population of about 340 000 people. Children are admitted in five difference wards, namely: neonatal ward (neonates delivered in hospital), ward 1 (neonates delivered at home and/or discharged and readmitted from home), ward 7 (general medicine, malnutrition and surgical cases), ward 9 (children who need isolation and are suffering from diarrhoea) and the Intensive Care Unit (ICU). The department has one specialist paediatrician and three medical officers allocated to the department at all times. The hospital operates as a referral hospital and receives referrals from four district hospitals. The hospital has a Perinatal and Maternal Mortality Audit Committee comprised of the hospital administrators, paediatric, obstetrics and gynaecology departments. The members meet once per month to audit only maternal deaths and deaths during the perinatal period. Deaths of children who die after the perinatal period are not reviewed as there is no hospital committee responsible to audit them.

Study population

All children that died at the hospital in 2013, from 28 weeks gestation or a birth weight of > 1000 g to the age of five years were included in the study.

Research tools

Two separate questionnaires were used, namely the Perinatal Data Collection questionnaire and the Child Data Collection Questionnaire. The perinatal questionnaire was a validated questionnaire adopted from the PPIP of South Africa.[11,12,13,14,15] This questionnaire was used to collect data from records of neonatal deaths (28 weeks gestation and birth weight > 1000 g to seven days old). The Child Questionnaire was a validated questionnaire adopted from the Child Problem Identification Programme (Child PIP) of South Africa.[17] This questionnaire was used to collect data from the records of children who died between the ages of 8 days to five years.

Data collection

The clinical and laboratory records of all children and neonates who died were identified, as they occurred in the wards throughout the year. The investigator was made aware of the deaths through notification by the ward nurse and by regular visits to all the wards that admitted children. All pending results were also collected from the laboratory by the investigator. Data were extracted from the records by the investigator using the questionnaires.

Owing to the fact that the hospital did not have any committee in place to audit the deaths of children beyond the perinatal period, the investigator alone audited these 60 records to determine the causes of the deaths and the modifiable risk factors. The Perinatal and Maternal Mortality committee reviewed all deaths in the perinatal period, which were presented to them by the investigator, and a consensus obtained.

Data analysis

Data was captured from the questionnaires using the file numbers as identifiers and information entered into an Excel spreadsheet. The data was double-entered from the same questionnaires to clean the missing data and the wrongly copied information. The data analysis was done using Epi-info seven whereby frequencies were generated and the proportions calculated; no testing of associations was required.

Results

The research findings are divided into two sections: the first section presents the findings from the perinatal death review and the second section provides the findings related to children after the perinatal period up to five years old.

Perinatal results

During the review period there were 6171 hospital deliveries and 141 home deliveries brought to hospital within 7 days, with 6118 live births and 56 intrauterine foetal deaths (IUFD) at above 28 weeks gestation or 1000 g birth weight.

A total of 69 neonates died within seven days after delivery and therefore the total number of perinatal deaths was 125. Amongst the 125 children who died within the perinatal period, 60 (48.0%) were female and 65 (52.0%) were male. The in-hospital Perinatal Mortality Rate was therefore 20.2 per 1000 live births.

Amongst those who died during the perinatal period 56 (44.8%) were IUFDs, 28 (22.4%) died within 24 hours of delivery, 30 (24.0%) died one to three days after delivery and 11 (8.8 %) died four to seven days after delivery.

Amongst those who died during the perinatal period, half of the total population had low birth weight, as shown in Table 1.

The top five causes of perinatal deaths were prematurity, birth asphyxia, congenital anomalies, unknown and abruptio placenta, as shown in Table 2.

Obstetrics causes were found to contribute in 47 (37.6%) perinatal deaths, of which the top five causes were pre-eclampsia, abruptio placenta, poor progress of labour, chorioamnionitis and severe maternal anaemia as shown in Table 3.

TABLE 1: Birth weight by gender (*N* = 125).

Gender	Extreme Low Birth weight (< 1500 g)	Low Birth Weight (1500-2999.9 g)	Normal Birth Weight (> 2500 g)	Total
Male	11 (8.8%)	25 (20.0%)	24 (19.2%)	**60 (48.0%)**
Female	11 (8.8%)	29 (23.2%)	25 (20.0%)	**65 (52.0%)**
Total	**22 (17.6%)**	**54 (43.2%)**	**49 (39.2%)**	**125 (100%)**

TABLE 2: Causes of deaths during the perinatal period (N = 125).

Cause of death	n	%
Prematurity	22	17.6
Birth asphyxia	19	15.2
Congenital abnormality	16	12.8
Unknown cause	13	10.4
Abruption placenta	11	8.8
Cord around the neck	8	6.4
Pre-eclampsia	8	6.4
Meconium aspiration	7	5.6
Septicaemia	6	4.8
Chorioamnionitis	3	2.4
Cord prolapse	2	1.6
Intrauterine growth restriction	2	1.6
Ruptured uterus	2	1.6
Maternal trauma	1	0.8
Rubella infection	1	0.8
Hypoglycaemia	1	0.8
Necrotizing enterocolitis	1	0.8
Congenital abnormal placenta	1	0.8
Anaemia	1	0.8

TABLE 3: Obstetric causes of perinatal mortality (N = 125).

Obstetric cause	n	%
Pre-eclampsia	13	10.4
Abruptio placenta	7	5.6
Poor progress of labour	6	4.8
Chorioamnionitis	3	2.4
Severe maternal anaemia	3	2.4
Malpresentation	2	1.6
Premature labour	2	1.6
Premature rupture of membranes	2	1.6
Ruptured uterus	2	1.6
Cord around the neck	2	1.6
Foot prolapse	1	0.8
Intrauterine growth restriction	1	0.8
Umbilical cord prolapse	1	0.8
Trauma to the abdomen	1	0.8
Advanced AIDS	1	0.8

Family factors were found to contribute in 23 (18.4%) perinatal deaths, of which the top two factors were late presentation of the neonate (more than 24 hours after delivery at home) and home delivery without assistance by a trained health professional, as shown in Table 4.

In 21 (16.8%) perinatal deaths, the top four factors related to antenatal care that may have contributed to these deaths were: no maternal weight chart and no blood pressure recorded despite patients visiting the clinic, poor management of pre-eclampsia at the referral hospital, long distance referral of sick neonates (more than 200 km) and three district hospitals not performing emergency caesarean sections, as shown in Table 5.

In 74 (59.2%) perinatal deaths the top three modifiable factors related to in-patient services at Onandjokwe referral hospital were: poor labour monitoring in the labour room, lack of surfactant in severe premature neonates and lack of beds and space in ICUs for critically ill neonates, as shown in Table 6.

TABLE 4: Family modifiable factors for perinatal mortality (N = 125).

Family factor	n	%
Late presentation to health care facility	9	7.2
Home delivery	7	5.6
Poor antenatal attendance	3	2.4
Did not attend antenatal care	2	1.6
Referred, but did not go	2	1.6

TABLE 5: Clinics, health centres and referring district hospitals modifiable factors (N = 125).

Clinic factor	n	%
Substandard antenatal care services	11	8.8
Poor management of pre-eclampsia at district hospital	3	2.4
Long distance referral	2	1.6
District hospital not performing emergency Caesarean section	2	1.6
Delayed initiation of Highly Active Anti-retroviral Therapy	1	0.8
Lack of transport	1	0.8
Poor management of gestational diabetes at district hospital	1	0.8

TABLE 6: Referral hospital modifiable factors for perinatal mortality (N = 125).

Referral hospital factors	n	%
Poor labour monitoring	16	12.8
Lack of surfactant	11	8.8
Lack of Continuous Positive Airway Pressure (CPAP) machine	8	6.4
Lack of beds and space in Intensive Care Unit	5	4.0
Delayed Caesarean section	4	3.2
Few nurses in labour room	4	3.2
Few nurses in neonatal unit	4	3.2
Poor monitoring of neonates in the neonatal unit	4	3.2
Poor monitoring of labour in mothers kept at waiting area waiting to be transferred to labour room	4	3.2
Shortage of theatre nurses when emergency Caesarean section is indicated	3	2.4
Poor decision made by a doctor when consulted in case of poor progress of labour	3	2.4
No space for patient to be admitted in labour room	2	1.6
Insufficient clinic information for next person to act	2	1.6
Lack of air ambulance	2	1.6
Lack of paediatric surgeon	2	1.6

The research found that 69 (55%) of perinatal deaths might have been avoidable if the process of care had been different and, in 15 (12%) of the deaths the researcher was not sure whether better care or the same care would have helped to avoid the deaths (Figure 1).

Post-perinatal (children 8 days to 5 years) results

There were 4898 admissions of children aged eight days to five years during the review period amongst whom there were 60 deaths, 31 (51.7%) of which occurred under one year of age. A total of 6956 infants aged less than one month were admitted during the review period, of whom 132 died, giving an in-hospital Infant Mortality Rate of 19.1 per 1000 admissions.

The study population consisted of 25 (41.7%) males and 35 (58.3%) females. The HIV status of the mothers showed that 29 (48.3%) were HIV negative, 23 (38.3%) were HIV positive and 8 (13.3%) mothers did not know their HIV status and were not tested during the admission. A total of 9 (15%)

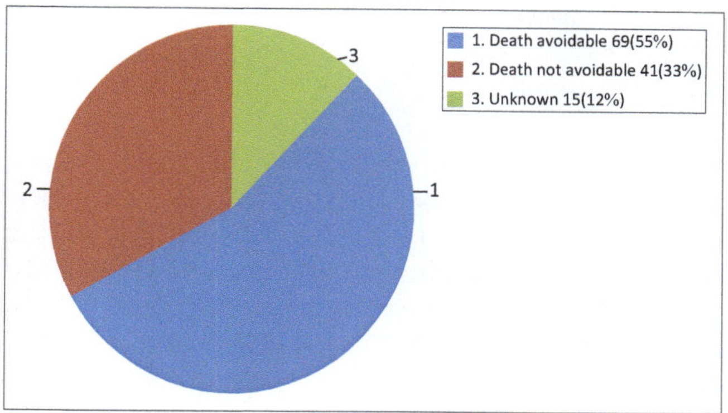

FIGURE 1: The researcher opinion whether the death was avoidable or not avoidable (N = 125).

children had confirmed HIV positive results using either DNA PCR or HIV rapid testing.

The study found that 21 (35.0%) died seven or more days after admission, 19 (31.7%) died within one to three days of admission, 12 (20%) within 24 hours of admission and eight (1.3%) four to six days after admission. The study also found that 24 (40.0%) of the deaths occurred during normal weekday working hours (07:00 – 19:00), 20 (33.3 %) during week nights and 16 (26.7%) during weekend days or public holidays.

The study found that 38 (63%) of the study population had known underlying medical conditions likely to predispose the children to poor health, amongst which 14 (23.3%) had severe malnutrition, nine (15%) HIV infection, nine (15%) congenital anomalies (mostly Down's syndrome and microcephaly due to birth asphyxia), four (6.7%) post-prematurity without catch up weight gain, one (2.6%) ischaemic foot gangrene and one (2.6%) congenital rubella infection.

The top five causes of death were bacterial pneumonia, gastroenteritis, severe malnutrition, septicaemia, and tuberculosis, as shown in Table 7.

In 24 (40.0%) deaths, family factors were found to contribute of which the top three factors were late presentation of the child to the health care facility (more than 24 hours after the start of the illness), not attending follow-up for HIV-exposed children (these children should receive Nevirapine prophylaxis and HIV PCR testing), and leaving the child in the care of the grandmother or other family members, as shown in Table 8.

In 18 (31.7%) deaths, care at the referring clinic, health care centre or district hospital was a contributing cause, of which the top three factors were failure to make a nutritional assessment and to diagnose malnutrition, not actively tracing HIV-exposed children that defaulted from follow-up, and failure to repeat the mother's initial negative HIV test later in pregnancy, as shown in Table 9.

In 27 (45.0%) deaths in-patient hospital services were found to be a contributing cause, the top three factors being poor child monitoring in the wards (e.g. no record of vital signs or no record being taken for more than 8 hours), urgent results of critically ill children not being reviewed for more than 24 hours, the admitting doctor missing the diagnosis at admission and therefore initiating inappropriate medications, and failure to identify severe malnutrition on admission, as shown in Table 10.

TABLE 7: Distribution of causes of death amongst study population (N = 60).

Cause of death	n	%
Bacterial pneumonia	15	25.0
Gastroenteritis	12	20.0
Severe malnutrition	6	10.0
Septicaemia	6	10.0
Pulmonary tuberculosis	4	6.7
Congenital anomalies e.g. malrotation of small intestines, ventricular septal defect, transposition of great vessels	3	5.0
Bacterial meningitis	2	3.3
Pneumocystis Jirovecii pneumonia	2	3.3
Aspiration pneumonia	2	3.3
Burn wound	1	1.7
Carbamazepine intoxication (accidental)	1	1.7
Food poisoning	1	1.7
Cytomegalovirus hepatitis	1	1.7
Head injury due to fall from tree	1	1.7
Post-prematurity respiratory failure	1	1.7
Alcohol intoxication	1	1.7
Unknown cause	1	1.7

TABLE 8: Family modifiable factors for child deaths (N = 60).

Family factor	n	%
Late presentation for treatment	8	13.3
Not bringing HIV-exposed child for follow up	7	11.7
Child left with relatives by the mother	3	5.0
Poor ARV adherence	1	1.7
Poor food security	1	1.7
Early mixed feeding	1	1.7
Mother culturally cannot consent for operation	1	1.7
Kept medication at places easily accessible by child	1	1.7
Defaulted scheduled operation for adenotonsillectomy	1	1.7

TABLE 9: Referring clinic, health centre and district hospital modifiable factors (N = 60).

District health services factor	n	%
Nutritional assessment not done	5	8.3
No follow-up of HIV-exposed children	4	6.7
Negative HIV test in early pregnancy was not rechecked later	4	6.7
Initial treatment not started at clinic during referral process	3	5
Late referral from district hospital to Onandjokwe Hospital	2	3.3

Findings revealed that 42 (70%) of the deaths would have been avoidable if the process of care had been different, as shown in Figure 2.

Discussion

Key perinatal mortality findings

The perinatal data found that more than half of perinatal deaths might have been avoidable if the process of care and quality of health care provided had been better. The high proportions of avoidable perinatal deaths have been

TABLE 10: Referral hospital modifiable factors (N = 60).

Referral hospital factors	n	%
Poor child monitoring in the ward	8	13.3
Urgent results not reviewed more than 24 hrs	5	8.3
Missed diagnosis at admission	4	6.7
Nutrition assessment not done	4	6.7
Not started on antibiotics early	4	6.7
Lack of ICU bed	1	1.7
Lack of teamwork	1	1.7

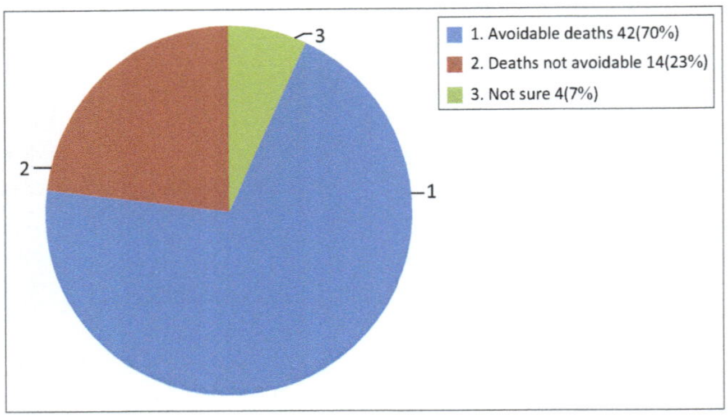

FIGURE 2: The review opinion whether the death was avoidable (N = 60).

observed in neighbouring South Africa, whereby close to half of the deaths were avoidable.[12,13,14,15,16] The similarity in the identified challenges might be explained by their shared colonial history, whereby Namibia was part of South Africa until independence in 1990, with closely related social, cultural and geographical challenges.

The avoidable factors related to family, health care providers and health system performance identified in this study correlate closely with the factors identified in South Africa. For example, common factors include family and/or patient delay in seeking medical attention during labour, never attending antenatal care and inadequate equipment and supplies, such as the availability of CPAP.[12,13,14,15,16] However, in some provinces of South Africa the zonal health teams have been implementing corrective actions and infrastructure to tackle the identified modifiable factors.[22]

Prematurity and birth asphyxia were the top two challenges which were identified to be neonatal related cause of deaths. These two challenges are the most common factors leading to deaths in many parts of the world, especially in developing countries, and including South Africa.[2,3,4,5,6,7,8,9,10,11,12,13,14,15,16] The proportion of unexplained deaths was high in this study, providing challenges to the need for increased perinatal deaths investigation to prevent deaths in future pregnancies. This can be explained by the limited diagnostic resources in developing countries that do not always allow for a definitive diagnosis to be reached.

Key child eight days to five years mortality findings

The proportion of avoidable deaths was found to be slightly higher compared to South Africa, which reported that 37% of their deaths were avoidable.[16,23] This might be due to the efforts of South African health care facilities to improve the quality of care as a result of the Child Problem Identification Programme reports since 2004.

Children who become sick with underlying medical conditions appeared more likely to have a poor outcome, and the study found a significant number of children with underlying severe malnutrition, HIV infection and congenital anomalies. Several studies have shown that the Mother To Child Transmission (PMTCT) for HIV and malnutrition have an important influence on childhood mortality.[5,6,7,8,9] The recent success of PMTCT programmes in South Africa and Namibia have reduced rates of HIV infections and subsequent childhood deaths, however the prevalence of malnutrition in Namibia is still high: 16.5% compared to South Africa's 10.2%.[17]

Community-acquired pneumonia and gastroenteritis contributed to more than half of the deaths in this study. This finding is consistent with findings in most settings in the world.[1,5,6,7,8,9,19,21,22,23] This can probably be explained, not only by avoidable factors in the health services, but also by low immunisation coverage and by developmental issues such as a lack of access to adequate sanitation and clean water.

The modifiable factors identified in the study, such as late presentation of the child to the health care facility, lack of follow-up of HIV-exposed babies, lack of nutritional assessment and poor monitoring of admitted children, have also been pointed out in studies from other African countries.[1,2,3,4,5,6,7,8,9]

Limitations of the study

The results were dependent on the quality of record keeping and, in some cases, the medical record contained only a few notes written by the admitting doctor. However, additional information obtained from patients' health passports helped to identify some of the missing gaps in the record of care for these children.

Recommendations and/or implications

The audit of childhood deaths for risk identification and management, in order to avoid further deaths, should be part of the routine activities in all hospitals which admit children. This will help them to identify the modifiable factors in their local settings and to plan the locally applicable interventions.

The findings of this study should be shared amongst the role players from the community level and across the health care system, involving the individual health care workers, primary care facilities, hospitals, regional health administration authorities and the ministry of health. The following recommendations were generated:

Community level: People at the community level should be educated on the importance of early attendance of the primary health care facility as soon as an illness begins in children under five years of age. The community counsellors and health extension workers who visit the community, should, when someone has a sick child, emphasise early clinic and/or hospital visits within 24 hours.

At the clinic: Staff should be reminded of the implementation of, and adherence to the Integrated Management of Childhood Illness (IMCI) guidelines. These include: early management of sick children whilst waiting for the ambulance; regular growth monitoring and assessment of nutritional status; interventions for malnutrition, and education of mothers who visit clinics for immunisation on the preparation of the Oral Rehydration Solution (ORS). At least three packets of ORS should be supplied to all mothers with children at home under five years old.

District hospital: The doctors should be provided with refresher training on the identified gaps in clinical care and be motivated to attend the Continuous Medical Education presentations on paediatric care organised at Onandjokwe Hospital and Ondangwa doctors' journal club. All four district hospitals should be able to provide emergency caesarean sections services by sending staff for training on emergency obstetric care, supplying them with the relevant guidelines and necessary resources. The doctors and nurses from these four district hospitals may be sent to Onandjokwe Hospital for upskilling.

At the referral hospital: All medical officers should rotate through the paediatric department as part of their first year orientation to the hospital. The hospital should budget for the ongoing training of medical doctors and nurses working in the paediatric department, for the purchase of necessary equipment and resources, and for distributing nurses, with consideration, to the special needs of intrapartum care and the neonatal unit.

Government: The posts for nurses should be increased to cope with the volume of patients in labour and paediatrics wards. Budgets should be provided for purchasing necessary equipment, supplies and medicine such as surfactant for premature neonates, and for supplying CPAP machines to the district hospitals. The capacity of all district hospitals should be strengthened to provide obstetric emergency care services.

By the nurse: Regular nutritional assessment of children and the application of IMCI principles should be implemented.

The doctor: Doctors should make personal effort to update themselves on the latest guidelines and standard operating procedures and to attend CME, especially in areas related to management of pre-eclampsia, gestational diabetes and common childhood illnesses. Quality improvement initiatives should target the following clinical processes: blood pressure measurement in pregnant women, maternal weight monitoring and the review of urgent blood results within 24 hours.

Hospital managers: Prioritise distribution of staff amongst departments with special consideration to care of children and pregnant women, to procure essential resources such as surfactant, CPAP machines, expand the ICU bed capacity, establish a hospital committee which will be responsible for coordinating death audits and track the implementation plans to decrease deaths.

District manager: He, or she should take note of the identified modifiable factors at the clinics and health centres, and the family factors. He, or she should co-ordinate a response from the community, clinic staff, health extension workers and environmental health practitioners in collaboration with the regional health administrators. They should plan for infrastructure development that favours emergency neonatal and obstetric care.

Conclusion

The major causes of mortality at Onandjokwe during the perinatal period were prematurity, birth asphyxia, congenital anomalies, abruptio placenta and unknown causes. The major family modifiable factors were late presentation of the neonate more than 24 hours after delivery at home, home delivery without assistance by a trained health professional and poor antenatal care attendance. The antenatal care modifiable factors were clinics not monitoring maternal weight and blood pressure, poor management and follow-up of pre-eclampsia patients at the referral hospital, long distance referral of sick neonates and three district hospitals not performing emergency caesarean sections. Modifiable factors related to in-patient services at Onandjokwe referral hospital were poor labour monitoring in the labour room, lack of surfactant in severe premature neonates and lack of beds and space in the ICU for critically ill neonates

The major causes of mortality in children eight days to five years old were bacterial pneumonia, gastroenteritis, severe malnutrition, septicaemia, and tuberculosis. The underlying medical conditions identified were severe malnutrition, HIV infection, congenital anomalies (mostly Down's syndrome and microcephaly due to birth asphyxia), and post-prematurity. The major modifiable family factors were late presentation of the child to the health facility (more than 24 hours after starting of the illness), defaulting of HIV-exposed children from follow-up and sick children being cared for by grandmothers or other family members. Modifiable factors at clinics and referring hospitals were failure to make a nutritional assessment and diagnose malnutrition, lack of active recall of the HIV-exposed child and failure to repeat HIV testing in pregnant women who initially test negative. The modifiable factors during in-patient services were poor child monitoring in the ward, urgent results of critically ill children not reviewed for more than 24 hours, admitting doctor missing the diagnosis at admission and lack of nutritional assessment at admission.

Acknowledgements

My sincere appreciation goes to my lovely wife Dr Flavia Strato, who encouraged me every time to continue my study and to Dr Arina Schlemmer who gave empathic technical guidance at all times. My thanks also go to Dr Tadesse Meknon and Mr Emmanuel Magesa who provided necessary lectures on data analysis. Appreciation is extended to Onandjokwe Hospital Research Committee team members, who voted in support of the retention of death files in the paediatric wards until the researcher is informed and has completed review of the information.

Competing interests

The authors declare that they have no financial or personal relationship(s) that may have inappropriately influenced them in writing this article.

Authors' contributions

J.F.M. (Stellenbosch University) performed the research and wrote the manuscript for his MMed degree under the supervision of R.M. (Stellenbosch University). Both authors approved the final manuscript.

References

1. UNICEF. Progress for children: Achieving the MDGs with equity [homepage on the Internet]. 2010 [cited 2012 Jan 12]. Available from: http://www.unicef.org/protection/Progress_for_Children-No.9_EN_081710.pdf
2. UNICEF. Infant and under-five mortality [homepage on the Internet]. 2001 [cited 2012 Jan 13]. Available from: http://www.unicef.org/specialsession/about/sgreport-pdf/01_InfantAndUnder-FiveMortality_D7341Insert_English.pdf
3. African Union. Status reports on maternal newborn and child health [document on the Internet]. 2012 [cited 2012 Dec 12]. Available from: http://www.carmma.org/download/file/fid/470
4. United Nations Inter-agency Group for Child Mortality. Levels and trends in child mortality [homepage on the Internet]. 2013 [cited 2013 Dec 9]. Available from: http://www.childinfo.org/files/Child_Mortality_Report_2013.pdf
5. O'Connor J, Youde LS, Allen JR, Hanson RM, Baur LA. Outcomes of a nutrition audit in a tertiary paediatric hospital: Implications for service improvement in Ghana. J Paediat Child Health [serial on the Internet]. 2004 May-June [cited 2012 Jan 14]; 40(5–6):295–298. Available from: http://www.ncbi.nlm.nih.gov/pubmed/15151584
6. Venkatesh K, Bruyn G, Marinda E, et al. Morbidity and mortality among infants born to HIV-infected women in South Africa: Implications for child health in resource-limited settings. J Trop Pediatr [serial on the Internet]. 2011 Apr [cited 2013 Sep 7];57(2):109–119. Available from: http://www.ncbi.nlm.nih.gov/pmc/articles/PMC3107462/
7. Hugh R, Mwakasungura E, Chonya S, et al. Clinical assessment and treatment in paediatric wards in the north-east of the United Republic of Tanzania. Bull World Health organ [serial on the Internet]. 2008 [cited 2012 May 2];86(2):132–139. Available from: http://www.ncbi.nlm.nih.gov/pubmed/18297168
8. Nojomi M, Naserbakhat M, Ramezany M, Anbary K. Under-5 year mortality: Result of in-hospital study. Acta Medica Iranica [serial on the Internet]. 2009 [cited 2012 Jul 11];47(4):319–324. Available from: http://acta.tums.ac.ir/index.php/acta/article/viewFile/3636/3320
9. English M, Esamai F, Wasunna A, et al. Assessment of inpatient paediatric care in first referral level hospitals in 13 districts in Kenya. The Lancet [serial on the Internet]. 2004 [cited 2012 Jul 12];363(9425):1948–1953. Available from: http://www.ncbi.nlm.nih.gov/pubmed/15194254
10. Elhassan E, Hassanb A, Mirghani O, Adam I. Morbidity and mortality pattern of neonates admitted into nursery unit in Wad Medani Hospital. Sudan JMS [serial on the Internet]. 2010 March [cited 2012 Mar 7];5(1). Available from: http://www.sudjms.net/issues/5-1/pdf/
11. Lee A, Cousens S, Wall S, et al. Neonatal resuscitation and immediate newborn assessment and stimulation for the prevention of neonatal deaths: a systematic review, meta-analysis and Delphi estimation of mortality effect. BMC Public Health [serial on the Internet]. 2011 [cited 2012 Mar 7];11(Suppl.3):12. Available from: http://www.biomedcentral.com/1471-2458/11/S3/S12
12. Pattinson R. Saving babies: A perinatal care survey [homepage on the Internet]. 2000 [cited 2012 Mar 2]. Available from: http://www.hst.org.za/uploads/files/saving_babies.pdf
13. Pattinson R. Saving babies: Perinatal care survey. South Africa [homepage on the Internet]. 2001 [cited 2012 Mar 2]. Available from: http://www.ppip.co.za/downloads/Saving babies 2001.pdf
14. Pattinson R. Saving babies: South Africa: Perinatal care survey of South Africa [homepage on the Internet]. 2002 [cited 2012 Mar 3]. Available from: http://www.ppip.co.za/downloads/Saving babies 2002.pdf
15. Pattinson R. Saving babies: Perinatal care survey [homepage on the Internet]. 2003–2005 [cited 2012 Mar 3]. Available from: http://www.ppip.co.za/downloads/Saving Babies 2003-5.pdf
16. Pattinson R. Saving babies: Perinatal care survey [serial on the Internet]. 2006-2007 [cited 2012 Mar 04]. Available from: http://www.ppip.co.za/downloads/Saving babies 2006-7.pdf
17. WHO. Malnutrition prevalence, weight for age (% of children under 5), county comparison [homepage on the Internet]. 2006 [cited 2014 Jul 2]. Available from: http://www.indexmundi.com/facts/indicators/SH.STA.MALN.ZS/compare?county
18. United Nations. Infant and child mortality, Namibia Demographics [homepage on the Internet]. 2011 [cited 2014 Jul 1]. Available from: http://www.indexmundi.com/namibia/infant-and-child-mortality.html
19. Westwood A, Claaseen J. Childhood in-hospital mortality from acute gastro-enteritis. SAMJ [serial on the Internet]. 2010 [cited 2012 Mar 13];100(4):196. Available from: http://www.samj.org.za/index.php/samj/article/view/4050
20. Ministry of Health and Social Services, Namibia. Demographic and health survey [homepage on the Internet]. 2013 [cited 2014 Jul 12]. Available from: https://dhsprogram.com/pubs/pdf/FR298/FR298.pdf
21. Nannan N, Dorrington R, Laubscher R, et al. Under-5 mortality statistics in South Africa: Shedding light on trend and causes [homepage on the Internet]. 1997–2007 [cited 2014 Jul 10]. Available from: http://www.mrc.ac.za/bod/MortalityStatisticsSA.pdf
22. Pattison R. Saving children: Survey of child health care [homepage on the Internet]. 2005 [cited 2012 Mar 5]. Available from: http://www.mrc.ac.za/maternal/savingchildren.pdf
23. Stephen C, Bamford L, Patrick E. Saving children: Five years of data, sixth survey of child healthcare in South Africa [document on the Internet]. 2009 [cited 2014 July 20]. Available from: http://www.worldcat.org/title/saving-children-2009-five-years-of-data-a-sixth-survey-of-child-healthcare-in-south-africa/oclc/793512369

Risks associated with communication delays in infants from underserved South African communities

Authors:
Jeannie van der Linde[1]
De Wet Swanepoel[1,2,3]
Frances P. Glascoe[4]
E.M. Louw[5]
Jannie F.M. Hugo[6]
Bart Vinck[1,7]

Affiliations:
[1]Department of Speech-Language Pathology and Audiology, University of Pretoria, South Africa

[2]Ear Sciences Centre, School of Surgery, University of Western Australia, Nedlands, Australia

[3]Ear Science Institute Australia, Subiaco, Australia

[4]Department of Pediatrics, Vanderbilt University, United States

[5]Department of Statistics, University of Pretoria, South Africa

[6]Department of Family Medicine, University of Pretoria, South Africa

[7]Department of Speech-Language Pathology and Audiology, Ghent University, Belgium

Correspondence to:
Jeannie van der Linde

Email:
jeannie.vanderlinde@up.ac.za

Postal address:
Private Bag X20, Pretoria 0002, South Africa

Background: For optimal development young children need warm, responsive, enriched and communicative environments for learning social, language, and other skills. Infants and toddlers exposed to psychosocial risk lack enriched environments and may present with communication delays.

Aim: To investigate the relationship between psychosocial risks and communication delays in infants from underserved communities in South Africa.

Setting: Primary healthcare facilities in Tshwane district, South Africa.

Methods: A parent interview and Rossetti Infant Toddler Language Scales were used to collect data from caregivers of 201 infants aged 6–12 months, selected through convenience sampling. Associations between communication delays and risks were determined (Chi-square and Fisher's exact tests). A log-linear model analysis was used to model the simultaneous effect of significant risks on the probability of having communication delays.

Results: Communication delays were present in 13% of infants. Infants with two or more siblings, born from mothers aged 18–29 years who own their house, had a 39% chance of presenting with communication delays.

Conclusion: Developmental screening and early intervention is important in primary healthcare contexts in South Africa, as a clear relationship has been established between three risk factors and communication delays in infants.

Risques associés à des retards de communication verbale chez les nourrissons des communautés sud-africaines non desservies.

Contexte: Pour s'épanouir complètement les jeunes enfants ont besoin d'un environnement chaud, réceptif, enrichi et communicatif pour apprendre le langage social et d'autres compétences. Les nourrissons et les tout-petits exposés à des risques psychosociaux souffrent d'un manque d'environnements enrichissants et pourraient souffrir de retards de communication verbale.

Objectif: Pour étudier la relation entre les risques psychosociaux et les retards de communication verbale chez les nourrissons des communautés non desservies en Afrique du Sud.

Lieu: Services de soins primaires dans le district de Tshwane, en Afrique du Sud.

Méthodes: Une entrevue avec les parents et l'Echelle de Compétence linguistique pour les Nourrissons de Rossetti ont été utilisés pour rassembler les données de 201 nourrissons de 6 à 12 mois provenant de leurs gardiens, sélectionnés au moyen d'échantillonnages de proximité. On a remarqué un lien entre les retards et les risques de communication verbale (tests Chi carré et de Fisher). On a utilisé un modèle d'analyse log-linéaire pour modéliser l'effet simultané des risques importants sur la probabilité d'avoir des retards de communication verbale.

Résultats: On a trouvé des retards de communication verbale chez 13% des nourrissons. Les nourrissons qui vivent avec deux frères ou sœurs ou plus, nés de mères âgées de 18 à 29 ans qui ont leur propre maison, avaient 39% plus de chance d'avoir des retards de communication verbale.

Introduction

For optimal development young children need a warm, responsive, enriched and communicative environment for learning social, language and other skills.[1] Infants and young children exposed to risk conditions may present with developmental delays or disorders that may ultimately impact socio-emotional, educational and vocational outcomes.[2] These risks include any potential factors that affect a child's ability to interact with his or her environment,[3,4] which in turn results in developmental delays or disorders.

Communication delays are most prevalent in children under the age of three years.[4] If communication delays remain undetected, this negatively impacts later educational and social performance, has long-term financial implications, and results in future delays or disorders.[5,6] As a result of environmental factors such as unemployment, limited medical resources, lack of educational services, violence, crime and HIV infection and AIDS,[2] the prevalence of communication delays or disorders is increasing.

In the United Kingdom an incidence of speech and language disability of 5.6% has been reported in children aged 0–2 years.[7] Similar findings reported in a systematic review which included several countries indicated a median prevalence of 5% for speech and language delays in children of two years of age.[8] In developing countries such as South Africa the prevalence of communication delays will probably be higher, due to more biological and psychosocial risks such as poverty, violence, nutritional deficiencies, HIV infection and substance abuse.[9] Advanced or very young maternal age,[10] lack of parent-child interaction,[11] low parental educational levels, poor parental mental and physical health, insufficient parental coping strategies and confidence[12] are pervasive risk factors characteristic of South Africa.[9] These risks are likely to predispose infants to developmental delay.

Limited parental education negatively impacts communication acquisition in infants and young children due to a lack of parental knowledge and stimulation during the infants' early years.[13] Approximately 16% of adults (20 years or older) in South Africa are functionally illiterate, 34% have completed secondary levels of education only and 29% have completed Grade 12.[14] Almost half of South Africans are deemed poor (45.5%), with 20% living in extreme poverty.[15] Living in poor conditions restricts the quality and quantity of prenatal care, placing the unborn infant at risk of low birthweight and prematurity.[16] Risk factors such as poverty and low parental education can occur in isolation or in combination, and it is generally accepted that an increase in the number of risk factors results in an increase in developmental risk to the infant.[3]

The impact of risk factors such as parental education at a level less than high school, limited social support, poverty and more than three children in the home is difficult to establish in infants before the ages of 2 to 3 years.[17] Still, the most important phase of communication acquisition and development occurs between 8 and 24 months.[5,18,19] Wide-ranging prevalence of language delay with high rates of spontaneous resolution have been reported.[5,8,20] This illustrates the variability in the emergence of language skills, which in turn complicates the evaluation of infants' and young children's communication development.[5]

The first two years of life are crucial in communication acquisition and development, and since the emergence of communication skills reportedly varies between individuals,[5,8,20] the link between early risk factors and communication delays may provide reliable indicators to improve early detection. This might be especially informative in underserved or disadvantaged communities in countries like South Africa, where infants are exposed to multiple psychosocial risks along with health risks such as poverty, limited healthcare services and HIV infection and AIDS.[9]

In a previous study conducted across a spectrum of disadvantaged and advantaged urban communities in Melbourne, Australia, early risk factors could only explain 7% of the variation in language skills at the age of two years.[20] A few South African studies have reported on risks and communication delays, but only in specific target populations such as infants with cleft lip and palate and babies with dysphagia.[21,22] However, the relationships between risk factors and communication delays still need to be explored for infants in South Africa. More specifically, the relationships between risks and communication delays should be explored in underserved communities, which are deemed the poorest, most disadvantaged in the country, lack adequate public healthcare services and represent almost 50% of the population.[15,23]

Preventative strategies such as developmental screening or surveillance and intervention can be implemented from birth onwards to compensate for the risks, to eliminate or reduce the resultant communication delays. Early intervention in underserved communities is, however, hindered by financial constraints and a lack of resources to implement family-centred services.[24] Identifying risk factors that may predispose to communication delays or disorders in infants in underserved communities is an important priority to strengthen primary prevention strategies. The objective of the current study was therefore to investigate the relationship of certain environmental risks in an underserved South African community with delays in early communication development.

The research question was 'What is the relationship between certain environmental risks and communication delays in infants from an underserved community?'

Research methods and design

A cross-sectional research design was used to explore the relationship between risks and communication delays in infants.

Setting

Three clinics situated in underserved communities of the Tshwane district in the Gauteng province of South Africa (Olievenhoutbosch, Salvokop and Daspoort clinic) were utilised for data collection. Olievenhoutbosch clinic serves a population of 70 863 individuals residing in an area of 11.39 km^2.[14] Both Salvokop and Daspoort form part of the Pretoria subdistrict. The clinic situated in Salvokop area serves a population of 7123 and Daspoortclinic a population of 6355 individuals.[14]

Participants

Convenience sampling was used as all of the parents or caregivers who visited the primary healthcare clinics for immunisation and health-related reasons over a three-month period were approached. The following inclusion and exclusion criteria were used: Only caregivers of infants aged between 6 and 12 months, who were proficient in Afrikaans or English, were asked to participate.

Two hundred and one infants were recruited (45% female), with similar age distributions for male (mean 8.68 months; standard deviation (SD) 1.86) and female infants (mean 8.73 months; SD 1.94). Ninety-four per cent of the participants resided in Olievenhoutbosch, whereas the remainder were from other areas such as Salvokop (2%), Daspoort (0.05%) and Mamelodi (0.5%). The majority of participants (98.5%) were black persons, with 1.5% of other ethnicities. Home language distribution in the study sample was as follows: Sepedi (33%), isiZulu (16%), Shona (11%), isiNdebele (10%), isiXhosa (6%), Southern Sotho (5%), Setswana (5%) and other (14%).

One-third (33%, n = 66) of mothers exited the educational system at Grade 10 or less, and 40% earned a monthly household income of less than R1500 ($150). One-third of the infants (33%, n = 66) had two or more siblings. Both parents were unemployed in 14% (n = 28) of cases and 77% (n = 154) lived in informal housing or stayed with others.

Data collection tools and procedures

Data collection material included a structured interview schedule used to gain information from parents/caregivers, and a diagnostic communication assessment used to identify communication delays in infants. A structured interview schedule that consisted of closed-ended questions was developed to obtain participant background information, i.e. date of birth, duration of pregnancy, and gender, as well as the risk factors. Environmental risk factors that were investigated in the study were: level of education,[2,4,13,17] housing status,[2,4,9] age of mother at birth of infant,[3,4,9,10,17] number of children,[1,4,17] unemployment,[9,16,17] average household income[9,16,17] and gender of the infant.[4,5,20]

The Rossetti Infant Toddler Language Scale (RITLS) was used for the diagnostic communication assessment. The RITLS is a comprehensive, easy-to-administer and relevant tool to assess preverbal and verbal communicative abilities and interaction in infants and young children.[25] Although this is a criterion-referenced tool, it has been widely used and validated in the past.[21,26,27,28,29,30] The tool is designed to assess the following domains: pragmatics, gesture, play, language comprehension, language expression and interaction attachment.

The RITLS classifies infant development into three-month intervals, for instance 0–3 months and 3–6 months. At each interval developmental milestones under each of the domains are presented. When an infant at a specific age interval has one or more unmet milestone(s) in a specific developmental domain (such as language expression), the milestones of the previous interval are evaluated until the infant has met all the milestones at that age interval. The infant's developmental level is therefore the interval at which he or she obtained all the milestones within a developmental domain. It is therefore possible that the infant's developmental level is different for each of the evaluated domains; for example, an infant may present with a delay in expressive language and pragmatics, whilst the receptive language, interaction attachment and play skills are age-appropriate. An infant's progress is classified as delayed when one or more of the communication domains' specific developmental levels differ by six months or more from the chronological age (for instance, when a 12-month-old infant's language expression scores on a 3–6-month developmental level, the infant presents with a communication delay).[25]

The first items in the 'gesture' subdomain only start at 9–12 months. Hence infants can only present with delays when they are 15 months or older. Since participants in the current study were all between six and 12 months of age and their development of gestures could not be classified as delayed, this subdomain was excluded from the results.

Prior to data collection ethical clearance was obtained from the Tshwane district research committee, Department of Health and the Faculty of Health Sciences and Humanities at the University of Pretoria. Parental and/or caregiver informed consent was obtained before data collection commenced. Both the interview and RITLS were carried out by the same speech-language pathologist, who has more than 10 years' experience in the field. The structured interview with the parents/caregivers was conducted first. After the background information was obtained and the risks were identified by means of the interview schedule, the RITLS was completed by observing the infant during interaction with the parent and free play. If aspects of communication behaviour under investigation were not observed, the behaviour was elicited by the speech-language pathologist or the parent and/or caregiver's report on their infant's communicative behaviours was utilised to complete the RITLS.

Since the RITLS is a validated tool administration and scoring of the assessment was done by the same experienced speech-language pathologist to ensure reliability of data.

Inter-rater reliability was also established, as independent raters observed 14% of the assessments and the outcomes of the tests were deemed similar to what the researcher obtained.

Data analysis

To determine the existence of a significant association between risk factors and the outcome of the RITLS (indicating a communication delay or not) the Chi-square and Fisher's exact test statistics were used, with a significance level of $p \leq 0.05$.

Only risk factors significantly associated with communication delays ($p \leq 0.05$) were included in the second phase of the statistical analysis. Here a log-linear model analysis was used to model the probabilities of developing communication delays, taking into account both single and simultaneous effects of relevant risk factors. As the data (age of mother) were too limited to be added into the model in the categories < 18 years ($n = 7$), 19–34 years ($n = 165$) and < 35 years ($n = 27$), they were recategorised into two groups, namely 18–29 years and 35 years and older. Although a maternal age of 18–29 years is not an environmental risk, the effect of the age of the mother still needed to be explored.

For ease of interpretation the outcomes of the model were expressed as indices and converted into odds of communication delays for this specific combination of categories. Based on the odds the estimated probability of having a communication delay for a specific set of risk factors was calculated using the following formula:

$$\text{prob} = \frac{\text{odds}}{1+\text{odds}}. \quad \text{[Eqn 1]}$$

Results

A communication delay, as determined by the outcome of the RITLS, was present in 13% ($n = 26/201$) of the infants. The association of communication delay with each of the six risk factors constituted the first phase of the statistical analysis (Table 1). Three risk factors were found to be significantly associated with the prevalence of communication delays in the study population: (1) infants of mothers having three or more children showed a significantly higher prevalence of delays (sample percentage of 20%) than those of mothers having less than three children (10%) (Chi-square, $p = 0.046$); (2) having an informal housing status or staying with others was related to a marginally significantly lower prevalence in communication delays (10%) compared to when mothers have their own house (21%) (Chi-square, $p = 0.052$); and (3) the prevalence of communication delays in infants born of mothers aged 18 years or younger (43%) and 35 years or older (19%) was significantly higher than amongst those born of mothers between the ages of 19 and 34 years (11%) (Fisher's exact test, $p = 0.04$).

The outcome of the log-linear analysis in terms of indices and odds is shown in Table 2, with the three significant risk factors presented as combined factors. The indices were used to calculate the probabilities of both individual and combined risk factors by multiplying the overall main effect (index of the intercept) with one or more indices of the individual categories.

There was a probability of 39% of having a communication delay for infants with two or more siblings, born of a mother aged 18–29 years who owns her own house. In contrast, when infants have none or only one sibling, and their caregivers own their house, irrespective of the age of the mother at birth, those infants had only a 14% risk of

TABLE 1: Association of communication delay with psychosocial risk factors.

Risk factors	Delayed (%)	Significance (*p* value)	Test statistic
Gender (*n* = 201)			
Male (*n* = 111)	13	0.8797	Chi-square
Female (*n* = 90)	13		
Level of education (*n* = 200)**			
Grade 10 or less (*n* = 66)	18	0.1262	Chi-square
Grade 11–12, and/or tertiary (*n* = 134)	10		
Number of children (*n* = 201)			
2 or less (*n* = 135)	10	0.0458*	Chi-square
3 or more (*n* = 66)	20		
Employment (*n* = 201)			
Yes (*n* = 173)	12	0.2187	Fisher's exact
No (*n* = 28)	21		
Housing status (*n* = 201)			
Home owners (*n* = 47)	21		
nformal housing or staying with others (*n* = 154)	10	0.0516*	Chi-square
Average household income (*n* = 199)**			
Less than R1500 (*n* = 80)	11	0.6468	Chi-square
R1500 or more (*n* = 119)	13		
Age of mother at birth of youngest infant (*n* = 199)**			
18 yrs or less (*n* = 7)	43*		
19–34 yrs (*n* = 165)	11*	0.0397*	Fisher's exact
35 yrs and older (*n* = 27)	19*		

*, Statistically significant association ($p \leq 0.05$); **, Numbers differ due to missing data

TABLE 2: Associated probability of single and combined risk factors predisposing to communication delay.

Parameter	Categories	Index	Odds	Probability *n* (%)
Housing status	Home owners	1.55	0.341	0.25 (25)
	Informal housing/staying with others	0.64	0.140	0.12 (12)
Age of mother and number of children	18–29 yrs, ≧ 3 children	1.90	0.418	0.30 (30)
	≧ 18 yrs, < 3 children	0.49	0.107	0.097 (10)
	≧ 30 yrs, ≧ 3 children	1.07	0.235	0.19 (19)
Age of mother and number of children and housing status	18–29 yrs, ≧ 3 children Home owners	1.90 1.55	0.647	0.39 (39)
	18–29 yrs, ≧ 3 children Informal housing/staying with others	1.90 0.64	0.267	0.21 (21)
	≧ 18 yrs, < 3 children Home owners	0.49 1.55	0.167	0.14 (14)
	≧ 18 yrs, < 3 children Informal housing/staying with others	0.49 0.64	0.068	0.06 (6)
	≧ 30 yrs, ≧ 3 children Home owners	1.07 1.55	0.364	0.267 (27)
	≧ 30 yrs, ≧ 3 children Informal housing/staying with others	1.07 0.64	0.150	0.13 (13)
Overall effect	-	0.22	-	-

presenting with a communication delay (see Table 2). Table 2 summarises the associated probability for single and combined risk factors.

Discussion

Prevalence of communication delay for infants aged 6–12 months (13%) in this study was high in comparison to the incidence of reported speech and language disability (5.6%) in children aged 0–2 years in the United Kingdom.[7] The median prevalence of speech and language delays in children of two years of age reported in a systematic review was 5%.[8] Variability in prevalence studies may be attributed to methodological differences and confounding factors such as risk exposure in study populations.[8,31]

The adverse impact of risks, specifically the number of siblings, on communication development in infants was demonstrated in the current study. This finding is in accordance with previous research that also confirmed that children with two or more siblings are at risk of communication delays.[12,32,33] One of the possible reasons for younger siblings having delayed communication may be the fact that the older siblings are more verbal and may be speaking on behalf of the younger siblings.[12] Also, larger families imply that parental interaction and attention is divided between the children, which may result in less attention and interaction than when there are only one or two children in the home. In 2006 the average fertility rate of black South African women was 2.9; as a result an average household will have approximately three children.[34] In the current study one-third of the infants had two siblings or more, and it may be expected that these mothers will have another child in future, as 85% were 34 years of age or younger. This is in line with the fertility rate of 1.4 for 35–39-year-old black South African women.[34] Developmental surveillance of infants who have two or more siblings may therefore be warranted in underserved communities.

Interestingly, infants living in homes owned by their parents had a higher probability (25%) of communication delay than those who lived in informal housing or with others (12%). Recent findings have demonstrated that the diversity of neighbourhoods in which infants live shapes their social learning independently of their caregiver and/or family interaction.[35] The diverse neighbourhood of informal settlements or living in close proximity to others seemingly may aid social and communication development in infants. Consequently what was deemed a risk factor in the past[9] may facilitate more opportunities for communication interactions and be conducive to social learning.

The impact of combined risk factors on communication development revealed that an infant was at greatest risk (39% probability) of developing a communication delay when: (1) mothers were between the ages of 18 and 29 years; (2) the parents own their own home; and (3) there are three or more children in the household. This information might allow primary healthcare workers, on the platform of community-oriented primary care,[36] to identify infants at highest risk of communication delays in underserved communities in South Africa.

Considering that one in three infants were at risk of communication delay, the need for early communication intervention services, including developmental screening and comprehensive assessment and intervention, is evident. Completing a risk profile and conducting communication screening for infants could enable healthcare workers to identify at-risk infants and refer them for the required services. Such services may include creating awareness amongst parents on communication development and stimulation, and/or clinic and/or home-based early intervention. Internationally early intervention is becoming more prevention-orientated, encouraging individualising of children's learning experiences using evidence-based practices.[37] Therefore implementing preventative strategies in at-risk populations in South Africa is well in line with the international focus of prevention-orientated early intervention services.

A study in the United States of America reported that 13% of infants were identified with developmental delays, but that only 10% of these infants received services by 24 months of age.[38] Furthermore, black children were less likely to receive services than those from other ethnic and racial groups.[38] It therefore appears that service delivery to at-risk infants is not only a local but also an international quandary, where disparities in service delivery to different ethnic and racial groups exist. Eradicating the gap in service delivery to improve availability of services to *all* infants at risk of communication delay should be advocated for in South Africa.

Limitations

A limitation in the current study was that only caregivers or parents who were proficient in Afrikaans or English were included in the study. However, increased use of English in public administration, business and schools demonstrates the prominence of English in a variety of multilingual settings.[39] Even though it is the first language of only 8.6% of South Africans, its wide demographic dispersal has resulted in English being the preferred medium for use within economic and social spheres.[39] Still, since participants with limited or no verbal English or Afrikaans proficiency were excluded, the sample might not be entirely representative of the population sampled. It is therefore recommended that future research should be conducted on a randomised sample including all languages in underserved communities in South Africa.

Conclusion

A clear relationship has been established in the current study between communication delay and three risk factors – age of the mother, number of children and housing status –

in infants aged 6–12 months from these underserved communities. Furthermore, a combined effect of these risks accounted for a 39% probability of communication delay. As 13% of infants had a communication delay and more than one-third are at risk of developing communication delays in future, preventative strategies such as the implementation of a risk profile and a communication development screen should be implemented. This may ensure early identification of at-risk infants and assist healthcare workers in decision-making with regard to referral and preventative parental counselling.

Acknowledgements

The authors would like to acknowledge the Mellon Foundation for funding the vulnerable children programme of the Faculty of Humanities, University of Pretoria, the Vice-Chancellor's Academic Development Grant of the University of Pretoria, the University of Pretoria Community Oriented Primary Care living laboratory, the National Research Foundation and Department of Statistics, University of Pretoria for their assistance in the data processing and analysis.

Competing interests

The authors declare that they have no financial or personal relationship(s) that may have inappropriately influenced them in writing this article.

Authors' contributions

J.v.d.L. conducted the data collection, D.S. and B.V. supervised the research, and E.M.L. conducted the data analysis. J.v.d.L., D.S., F.P.G., E.M.L., J.F.M.H. and B.V. contributed to the writing of the article.

References

1. Glascoe FP, Leew S. Parenting behaviors, perceptions, and psychososial risk: Impacts on young children's development. Pediatrics. 2010;125:313–319. PMID: 20100743, http://dx.doi.org/10.1542/peds.2008-3129
2. Guralnick MJ. Developmental science and preventive interventions for children at environmental risk. Infants Young Child. 2013;26(4):270–285. PMID: 26213447, http://dx.doi.org/10.1097/IYC.0b013e3182a6832f
3. Paul R, Roth FP. Characterizing and predicting outcomes of communication delays in infants and toddlers: Implications for clinical practice. Lang Speech Hear Serv Sch. 2010;42(3):331–340. http://dx.doi.org/10.1044/0161-1461(2010/09-0067)
4. Rossetti L. Communication intervention birth to three. New York: Delmar, Cengage Learning; 2001.
5. Eadie PA, Ukoumunne O, Skeat J, et al. Assessing early communication behaviours: Structure and validity of the Communication and Symbolic Behaviour Scales-Developmental Profile (CSBS-DP) in 12-month-old infants. Int J Lang Commun Disord R Coll Speech Lang Ther. 2010;45(5):572–585. PMID: 19886849, http://dx.doi.org/10.3109/13682820903277944
6. Wankoff LS. Warning signs in the development of speech, language, and communication: When to refer to a speech-language pathologist. J Child Adolesc Psychiatr Nurs. 2011;24(3):175–184. PMID: 21810134, http://dx.doi.org/10.1111/j.1744-6171.2011.00292.x
7. Broomfield J, Dodd B. Children with speech and language disability: Caseload characteristics. Int J Lang Commun Disord. 2004;39(3):303–324. PMID: 15204443, http://dx.doi.org/10.1080/13682820310001625589
8. Law J, Boyle J, Harris F, Harkness A, Nye C. Prevalence and natural history of primary speech and language delay: Findings from a systematic review of the literature. Int J Lang Commun Disord. 2000;35(2):165–188. PMID: 10912250, http://dx.doi.org/10.1080/136828200247133
9. Samuels A, Slemming W, Balton S. Early childhood intervention in South Africa in relation to the developmental systems model. Infants Young Child. 2012;25(4):334–345. http://dx.doi.org/10.1097/IYC.0b013e3182673e12
10. Beitchman JH, Jiang H, Koyama E, et al. Models and determinants of vocabulary growth from kindergarten to adulthood. J Child Psychol Psychiatry. 2008;49(6):626–634. PMID: 18341544, http://dx.doi.org/10.1111/j.1469-7610.2008.01878.x
11. Barwick MA, Cohen NJ, Horodezky NB. Infant commmunication and the mother-infant relationship: The importance of level of risk and construct measurement. Infant Ment Health J. 2004;25(3):240–266. http://dx.doi.org/10.1002/imhj.20000
12. Harrison LJ, McLeod S. Risk and protective factors associated with speech and language impairment in a nationally representative sample of 4- to 5-year-old children. J Speech Lang Hear Res. 2010;53(2):508–529. PMID: 19786704, http://dx.doi.org/10.1044/1092-4388(2009/08-0086)
13. Hoff E, Johnston J, Pakulak E, et al. Language development and literacy. In: Rvachew S, editor. Encyclopedia on Early Childhood Development [book online]. 2013 [cited 2014 Aug 9]: 1–94. Available from: http://www.child-encyclopedia.com/sites/default/files/dossiers-complets/en/language-development-and-literacy.pdf
14. Statistics South Africa. Census 2011 [Internet]. Statistics South Africa; 2011 [cited 2014 Feb 20]. Available from: https://www.statssa.gov.za/Census2011/default.asp
15. Statistics South Africa. Poverty trends in South Africa. An examination of absolute poverty between 2006 and 2011 [Internet]. 2011 [cited 2014 May 5]. Report No.: 03-10-06. Available from: http://beta2.statssa.gov.za/publications/Report-03-10-06/Report-03`0-06March2014.pdf
16. Cone-Wesson B. Prenatal alcohol and cocaine exposure: Influences on cognition, speech, language, and hearing. J Commun Disord. 2005;38(4):279–302. PMID: 15862811, http://dx.doi.org/10.1016/j.jcomdis.2005.02.004
17. Glascoe FP. Early detection of developmental and behavioral problems. Pediatr Rev. 2000;21(8):272–280. PMID: 10922024, http://dx.doi.org/10.1542/pir.21-8-272
18. Reilly S, Eadie P, Bavin EL, et al. Growth of infant communication between 8 and 12 months: A population study. J Paediatr Child Health. 2006;42(12):764–770. PMID: 17096710, http://dx.doi.org/10.1111/j.1440-1754.2006.00974.x
19. Tomasello M. Constructing a Language: A usage-based theory of language acquisition. Cambridge, MA: Harvard University Press; 2003.
20. Reilly S, Wake M, Bavin EL, et al. Predicting language at 2 years of age: a prospective community study. Pediatrics 2007;120(6):e1441–e1449. PMID: 18055662, http://dx.doi.org/10.1542/peds.2007-0045
21. Groenewald H, Kritzinger A, Viviers M. Age-specific communication functioning of young children with cleft lip and palate in a South African Database. Cleft Palate Craniofac J. 2013;50(6):717–729. PMID: 23566231, http://dx.doi.org/10.1597/12-146
22. Norman V, Louw B, Kritzinger A. Incidence and description of dysphagia in infants and toddlers with tracheostomies: A retrospective review. Int J Pediatr Otorhinolaryngol. 2007;71(7):1087–1092. PMID: 17482279, http://dx.doi.org/10.1016/j.ijporl.2007.03.018
23. Kon ZR, Lackan N. Ethnic disparities in access to care in post-apartheid South Africa. Am J Publ Health. 2008;98(12):2272–2277. PMID: 18923120, http://dx.doi.org/10.2105/AJPH.2007.127829
24. Olusanya B, Ruben R, Parving A. Reducing the burden of communication disorders in the developing world: An opportunity for the millennium development project. JAMA. 2006;296(4):441–444. PMID: 16868302, http://dx.doi.org/10.1001/jama.296.4.441
25. Rossetti L. The Rossetti Infant-Toddler Language Scale, A measure of communication and interaction: Examiner's Manual. East Moline: LinguiSystems; 2006.
26. Desmarais C, Sylvestre A, Meyer F, Bairati I, Rouleau N. Three profiles of language abilities in toddlers with an expressive vocabulary delay: Variations on a theme. J Speech Lang Hear Res. 2010;53(3):699. PMID: 20530383, http://dx.doi.org/10.1044/1092-4388(2009/07-0245)
27. Sylvestre A, Mérette C. Language delay in severely neglected children: Aacumulative or specific effect of risk factors? Child Abuse Negl. 2010;34(6):414–428. PMID: 20413156, http://dx.doi.org/10.1016/j.chiabu.2009.10.003
28. Dettman SJ, Pinder D, Briggs RJS, Dowell RC, Leigh JR. Communication development in children who receive the cochlear implant younger than 12 months: Risks versus benefits. Ear Hear. 2007;28(Suppl):11S–18S. PMID: 17496638, http://dx.doi.org/10.1097/AUD.0b013e31803153f8
29. Steiner AM, Goldsmith TR, Snow AV, Chawarska K. Practitioner's guide to assessment of autism spectrum disorders in infants and toddlers. J Autism Dev Disord. 2012;42(6):1183–1196. PMID: 22057879, http://dx.doi.org/10.1007/s10803-011-1376-9
30. Rie AV, Mupuala A, Dow A. Impact of the HIV/AIDS epidemic on the neurodevelopment of preschool-aged children in Kinshasa, Democratic Republic of Congo. Pediatrics 2008;122(1):e123–e128. PMID: 18595957, http://dx.doi.org/10.1542/peds.2007-2558
31. McLeod S, McKinnon DH. Prevalence of communication disorders compared with other learning needs in 14 500 primary and secondary school students. Int J Lang Commun Disord. 2007;42(s1):37–59. PMID: 17454236, http://dx.doi.org/10.1080/13682820601173262
32. Zubrick SR, Taylor CL, Rice ML, Slegers DW. Late language emergence at 24 months: An epidemiological study of prevalence, predictors, and covariates. J Speech Lang Hear Res. 2007;50(6):1562–1592. PMID: 18055773, http://dx.doi.org/10.1044/1092-4388(2007/106)

33. Stanton-Chapman TL, Chapman DA, Bainbridge NL, Scott KG. Identification of early risk factors for language impairment. Res Dev Disabil. 2002;23(6):390–405. PMID: 12426008, http://dx.doi.org/10.1016/S0891-4222(02)00141-5

34. Statistics South Africa. Estimation of fertility from the 2007 Community Survey of South Africa. Pretoria: Statistics South Africa; 2010.

35. Howard LH, Carrazza C, Woodward AL. Neighborhood linguistic diversity predicts infants' social learning. Cognition 2014;133(2):474–479. PMID: 25156630, http://dx.doi.org/10.1016/j.cognition.2014.08.002

36. Bam N, Marcus T, Hugo J, Kinkel H-F. Conceptualizing community oriented primary care (COPC) – The Tshwane, South Africa, health post model. Afr J Prim Health Care Fam Med. 2013;5(1):Art. #423, 3 pages. http://dx.doi.org/10.4102/phcfm.v5i1.423

37. Greenwood CR, Walker D, Buzhardt J, Howard WJ, McCune L, Anderson R. Evidence of a continuum in foundational expressive communication skills. Early Child Res Q. 2013;28(3):540–554. PMID: 24882940, http://dx.doi.org/10.1016/j.ecresq.2013.02.006

38. Rosenberg SA, Zhang D, Robinson CC. Prevalence of developmental delays and participation in early intervention services for young children. Pediatrics 2008;121(6):e1503–e1509. PMID: 18504295, http://dx.doi.org/doi: 10.1542/peds.2007-1680

39. De Klerk V. Language issues in our schools: Whose voice counts? Part 1: The parents speak: Many languages in education: Issues of implementation. Perspect Educ Many Lang Educ. Spec Issue 1. 2002;20:1.

25

Nurses' compliance with prevention of mother-to-child transmission national guidelines in selected sites in Kinshasa, Democratic Republic of Congo

Authors:
Augustin R.M. Amboko[1]
Petra Brysiewicz[1]

Affiliations:
[1]School of Nursing and Public Health, University of KwaZulu-Natal, South Africa

Correspondence to:
Augustin Rashidi Amboko

Email:
ambokoaugustin@gmail.com

Postal address:
Department of Nursing, School of Nursing and Public Health, George Campbell Building, University of Kwazulu-Natal, Howard College Campus, Durban 4041, South Africa.

Background: The Democratic Republic of Congo (DRC) implemented a prevention of mother-to-child transmission (PMTCT) of HIV infection programme in maternal, newborn and child health (MNCH) services in 2001 with nurses as key personnel. To date there is no information in the DRC and specifically in Kinshasa with respect to compliance with PMTCT national guidelines.

Aim: The study aimed at describing nurses' compliance with the PMTCT national guidelines in selected PMTCT sites of Kinshasa.

Methods: A descriptive cross-sectional study was conducted in Kinshasa with 76 nurses in 18 selected PMTCT sites. The nurses' compliance with PMTCT national guidelines was assessed using a healthcare provider self-reporting questionnaire developed by the researchers.

Results: The study showed that the mean score of nurses' compliance with PMTCT national guidelines was 74% (95% CI: 69% – 78%) which progressively decreased and was significantly different across different MNCH services (p = 0.025). With respect to categories of PMTCT recommendations, nurses were compliant with those related to education in labour and delivery, and antenatal services. Sociodemographic characteristics such as training, length of service and category of nurses did not influence nurses' compliance score.

Conclusion: These findings showed that nurses were noncompliant with PMTCT national guidelines, with the score level being 80% or more in the three MNCH services/units. Improvement of nurses' 'compliance with the PMTCT national guidelines requires effective monitoring of full integration of PMTCT as routine activities in MNCH care.

Respect des lignes directrices nationales de la prévention de la transmission mère-enfant (PTME) du VIH par les infirmères dans une sélection de sites de PTME à Kinshasa en RDC.

Contexte: La République démocratique du Congo (RDC) a mis en œuvre un programme de PTME dans des services de santé de la mère, du nouveau-né et de l'enfant en 2001 en considérant les infirmières comme les membres clés du personnel. À ce jour, il n'existe pas d'informations relatives au respect des lignes directrices nationales de PTME en RDC, et plus particulièrement à Kinshasa.

But: L'étude visait à décrire le respect des directives nationales de PTME par les infirmières dans les sites de PTME sélectionnés de Kinshasa.

Méthodes: Une étude transversale descriptive a été réalisée à Kinshasa auprès de 76 infirmières dans 18 sites de PTME sélectionnés. Le respect des directives nationales de PTME par les infirmières a été évalué à l'aide d'un questionnaire d'autodéclaration des fournisseurs de soins de santé élaboré par les chercheurs.

Résultats: L'étude a montré que le score moyen associé au respect des directives nationales de PTME par les infirmières était de 74% (IC à 95 % : 69% – 78%), qui a progressivement diminué et était significativement différent entre les différents services de SMNE ; p = 0.025). En termes de recommandations quant aux catégories de PTME, les infirmières étaient conformes à celles liées à l'enseignement relatif au travail, à l'accouchement et aux services de soins prénatals. Les caractéristiques socio-démographiques telles que la formation, la durée de service et la catégorie d'infirmières n'ont pas eu d'influence sur le score du respect des directives nationales de PTME par les infirmières.

Conclusion: Ces résultats ont montré que les infirmières ne respectaient pas les directives nationales de PTME, le niveau de score étant de 80% ou plus dans les trois services/unités de SMNE. L'amélioration du respect des directives nationales de PTME par les infirmières nécessite un suivi efficace de la pleine intégration de la PTME en tant qu'activités de routine en soins de santé de la mère, du nouveau-né et de l'enfant.

Introduction

In sub-Saharan Africa countries 230 000 children were newly infected in the perinatal period with HIV in 2013. Moreover, in 2012 210 000 children under 14 years of age died as a result of HIV infection.[1] This situation is compromising the achievement of the fourth, fifth and sixth objectives of the Millennium United Nation's Development Goals in the African region.[2] To address this challenge the World Health Organization recommended that each country implement a prevention of mother-to-child transmission (PMTCT) of HIV infection programme aimed at reducing the prevalence of HIV infection in children.[1,3,4] The PMTCT programme was operationalised through the PMTCT guidelines, and the expected outcomes were to be achieved by complying with these.[5]

In most sub-Saharan African countries, however, there has been little progress in reducing mother-to-child transmission of HIV infection.[1,6] In the Democratic Republic of Congo (DRC) a progressive increase of prevalence of HIV infection in newborns was reported, based on the UNAIDS spectrum estimate, from 23.2% in 2009[7] to 23.3% in 2010[8] and 38% in 2011,[9] despite the programme being implemented in 2001 and having a high coverage, especially in Kinshasa. A prevalence of mother-to-child transmission (MTCT) of more than 20% reveals a lack of quality in implementation of PMTCT and its guidelines.[10]

There has been much research on PMTCT in most sub-Saharan African countries, including the DRC. However, this research focused on antenatal care (ANC) or postnatal care and did not review the entire continuum of maternal, newborn and child health (MNCH) in MNCH services.[11,12,13] Whilst most studies addressed isolated PMTCT interventions, such as HIV testing, HIV testing and counselling, antiretroviral treatment (ART) and/or breastfeeding, they did not address comprehensive PMTCT interventions.[12,14,15,16,17] Furthermore, the studies reviewed the records of the health services and targeted HIV-infected women, but gave little attention to the healthcare providers' practices.[11,12,13,16,17,18,19] More attention has been focused on monitoring PMTCT coverage, accessibility and utilisation rather than on standards of how PMTCT care is performed.[11,16,18,19,20,21,22]

One of major challenges that healthcare providers are experiencing is the gap between guidelines for prevention and treatment of HIV infection and compliance with these guidelines in clinical practice.[23] It is therefore critical to investigate whether healthcare providers (especially nurses) are complying with the PMTCT national guidelines in MNCH services. With the DRC striving to move to MNCH services (which include ANC, labour and delivery, and postnatal/immunisation services) and a more effective PMTCT service, it is necessary to determine the baseline status of adherence to guidelines and identify areas of failure. This will also improve the quality of PMTCT care provided by nurses, who have become the main providers of care due to task shifting.

This article was part of a larger study undertaken by the researcher, which was aimed at describing the overall compliance with PMTCT national guidelines in selected PMTCT sites in Kinshasa, DRC.

Research methods and design

Study design

The study was conducted in Kinshasa from 15 December 2011 until April 2012 and employed a cross- sectional design.

Setting

Kinshasa is the capital of the DRC. It is divided into 24 communes (municipalities), and in 2009 the population was estimated at 10 076 099.[24] There are 154 PMTCT sites and approximately 2156 healthcare providers.[25,26] At the time of the study only 35 PMTCT sites provided a continuum of PMTCT activities across the spectrum of ANC, labour and delivery to postnatal care and immunisation, where early detection of HIV infection by polymerase chain reaction (PCR) in infants six weeks after birth is done as part of the comprehensive PMTCT programme. The PMTCT sites are health facilities where MNCH care is offered, with trained staff of at least two healthcare providers per unit on integrated PMTCT/MNCH care, and a minimum package of activities (from HIV counselling and testing for pregnant women at ANC to dried blood spots [DBS] at 6 weeks after birth), and of material and equipment.

Study population and sampling strategy

The researcher selected 50% of the 35 PMTCT sites providing the full PMTCT programme. The sample size was calculated using a conservative sample size estimate.[26] As there was no prior knowledge with regard to the proportion of those who complied, the researcher assumed maximum possible variability (p = 0.5; q = 0.5 at 95% confidence interval and a precision (d) of ± 12%). The researcher then increased the sample size by 15% to take into account incomplete information,[26] thus adjusting the sample size to 76 healthcare providers.

The stratified sampling method was used to select the sample of healthcare providers. In collaboration with the Provincial Programme to Control the HIV Epidemic and STIs, 18 PMTCT sites were randomly selected. Together with the PMTCT coordinator for Kinshasa, a list of all 35 sites was printed and each site name was put into a hat and then 18 sites were randomly selected. This selected sample had 278 healthcare providers, including 262 nurses, 7 doctors and 9 lay counsellors involved in PMTCT care at the selected PMTCT sites who worked in antenatal, labour and delivery and postnatal/immunisation services/units.

The sample population of 278 healthcare providers was divided into strata as the sample population for the stratum (PMTCT site) and then the proportion of the sample population for each stratum was determined. The sample size of each stratum was obtained by multiplying the proportion of each stratum with the sample size (76). The researchers randomly selected the overall sample of 76 healthcare providers in proportion to the size of the strata in the population, based on the unique printed list of all healthcare providers. Therefore all of the 76 healthcare providers who were selected were nurses.

Data collection

The researchers developed a healthcare provider compliance questionnaire based on the DRC PMTCT national guidelines. These were categorised into patient education, treatment, diagnosis and follow-up/referral.[27] The questionnaire consisted of 62 items, which were divided into three sections for the different areas of care. There were 26 items applicable to ANC, 19 items applicable to labour and delivery, and 17 items applicable to postnatal/immunisation care. The self-administered questionnaire used a five-point Likert scale. The instrument, developed in English, was translated into French and then back into English by a qualified translator.

The selected nurses were individually contacted by the researcher. Once they had provided written consent to participate in the study, each nurse was handed the section of the questionnaire that was relevant to their respective MNCH services. The nurses completed the questionnaires and returned them to the researcher on the same day.

Data analysis

All data were captured and analysed using the Statistical Software Package for Social Sciences® (SPSS) version 19 (IBM Corp, Armonk, New York, 2010). Descriptive statistics were used to report the findings of the study and these included mean, median and interquartile range (IQR).

The healthcare providers' compliance with the guidelines was defined as the percentage of PMTCT recommendations adhered to by healthcare providers at each level in the continuum of MNCH services according to the national guidelines as assessed by means of the self-reporting questionnaire. The study rated a score of 80% – 100% as indicating healthcare providers' compliance with the relevant (to their place of work) section of the PMTCT national guidelines, and less than 80% as noncompliance. The researchers referred to Laurin's studies on quality of care[28] and the UNAIDS international commitment[2] to obtain parameters of delivering quality of care. Laurin set average quality at 70% – 84% and excellent quality of care at ≥ 85%, whilst the target of UNAIDS international commitment was at least 80% of HIV-infected women being provided with effective PMTCT services. Point estimate at 95% confidence interval has been performed for the nurses' compliance scores.

Nonparametric statistics were performed. With nurse compliance as a dichotomous variable, a Chi-square test was used to test the association of nurses' compliance with sociodemographic characteristic categories in the three services. Due to skewed data, Kruskal-Wallis tests were performed to assess differences of nurses' compliance scores across the three services/units. A p-value of < 0.05 was deemed statistically significant.

Validity and reliability

The instrument was tested for reliability and content validity. For reliability, the test-retest reliability coefficient (kappa) was more than 0.7,[29] being 0.89, 0.78 and 0.72 for the antenatal, labour and delivery, and postnatal/immunisation questionnaires respectively.

For content validity, the questionnaire items fitted with the objectives of the study and the key concepts in the conceptual framework, including the experts' opinion.[29,30]

Ethical considerations

With the researcher being a student, ethical approval was sought and granted by the Humanities and Social Sciences Research Ethics Committee of the University of KwaZulu-Natal (reference: HSS/1265/011M). Approval and authorisation for conducting research in the DRC was granted by the Minister of Health of the Province of Kinshasa. Written informed consent in French was obtained from all respondents. Confidentiality was preserved throughout the study and data could not be traced back to individuals or sites.

Results

The response rate was 100%. The sample realisation for healthcare providers was 76 nurses.

Sociodemographic characteristics

Table 1 shows the sociodemographic characteristics of the nurses in the different MNCH services/units. The data revealed no significant differences across MNCH services/units. Most of the nurses were A2 nurses, with less than 10 years of experience ($p = 0.522$; $p = 0.578$), and were trained in the standardised PMTCT training package.

The median for years of working experience was 7 years in both ANC (IQR = 6) and postnatal/immunisation care (IQR = 15), but in labour and delivery care the median was 8 years (IQR = 9).

Overall compliance of healthcare providers with prevention of mother-to-child transmission national guidelines

Figure 1 presents the proportion of nurses who were either compliant or noncompliant with PMTCT national guidelines across the continuum of MNCH services. It shows that about 57% of nurses in the antenatal service complied with PMTCT national guidelines, as opposed to 39% in both the labour and delivery and postnatal services. In the bivariate analysis there was no significant association between nurses' compliance scores with PMTCT national guidelines in the three MNCH

TABLE 1: Sociodemographic characteristics of nurses in different MNCH services/units.

Sociodemographic characteristics of nurses	Nurses per ward			*P*-value
	Antenatal ward *n* (%)	Labour and delivery ward *n* (%)	Postnatal ward *n* (%)	
Categories of nurses				
Nurses A2	15 (50%)	17 (61%)	8 (44%)	0.522
Nurses A1 and L2	15 (50%)	11 (39%)	10 (56%)	-
Length of service				
< 10 years	23 (77 %)	18 (64%)	13 (72%)	0.578
=/> 10 years	7 (23%)	10 (36%)	5 (28%)	-
Training in PMTCT				
Yes	24 (80%)	14 (50%)	9 (50%)	0.031
No	6 (20%)	14 (50%)	9 (50%)	-

MNCH, maternal, newborn and child health; PMTCT, prevention of mother-to-child transmission.
Nurse A2, nurse with diploma (4 years of secondary school + 4 years of nursing school); Nurse A1, nurse with bachelor degree (baccalaureate + 3 years); Nurse L2, nurse with bachelor and honours degree (baccalaureate + 5 years).

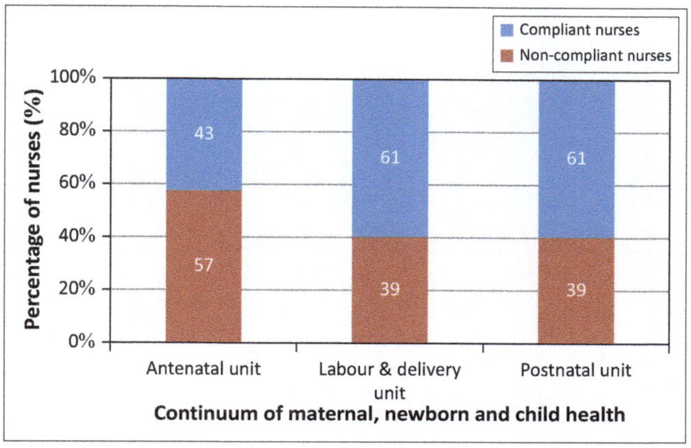

PMTCT, prevention of mother-to-child transmission; MNCH, maternal, newborn and child health.

FIGURE 1: Proportion of nurses who were compliant and noncompliant with PMTCT national guidelines across the continuum of MNCH services.

services and their sociodemographic characteristics, such as professional category ($p = 0.233$), training in PMTCT ($p = 0.821$) and working experiences ($p = 0.575$).

Table 2 shows the nurses' compliance with PMTCT national guidelines in the continuum of MNCH services. It revealed the mean score of nurses' compliance with PMTCT national guidelines to be about 74% (95% CI: 69% – 78%).

The data aggregated by service indicate that nurses in ANC were compliant with antenatal PMTCT national guidelines, but that the mean score of nurses' compliance with the section of the PMTCT national protocol relevant to the service where they worked progressively decreased from antenatal to postnatal service, respectively 80% (95% CI: 73% – 87%) in ANC; 71.3% (95% CI: 64% – 78%) in labour and delivery and 67% (95% CI: 56% – 79%) in postnatal/immunisation care. There is a significant difference in the scores of compliance in antenatal, labour and delivery, and postnatal/immunisation (continuum of MNCH) ($p = 0.025$).

Compliance with PMTCT national guidelines by nurses and recommendations in the three MNCH services/units

The data with respect to PMTCT recommendations were skewed. Table 3 reflects the findings on nurses' compliance with recommendations of PMTCT national guidelines in the three MNCH services.

For PMTCT recommendations related to education, the mean score of nurses' compliance was about 84% (95% CI: 78% – 91%) in ANC and 89% (95% CI: 79% – 99%) in labour and delivery. A very significant difference was found between the mean score of nurses' compliance with PMTCT education recommendations across the continuum of MNCH ($p = 0.000$).

For the PMTCT recommendations related to treatment, diagnosis and follow-up/referral, the mean scores of nurses' compliance were respectively 71% and 67% less than the threshold of 80% and more across the continuum of MNCH from antenatal to postnatal/immunisation services. Despite the noncompliance of nurses with PMTCT national guidelines, a significant difference was noted on compliance scores with follow-up/referral recommendations of PMTCT national guidelines across the MNCH services ($p = 0.000$).

Some sociodemographic characteristics also had a significant influence on nurses' compliance with PMTCT recommendations. It was found that the nurses' category was associated with the score of nurses' compliance with PMTCT recommendations related to education ($p = 0.034$) and diagnosis ($p = 0.043$). However, no significant association was found with other PMTCT recommendations and sociodemographic characteristics.

Discussion

The study found that the majority of nurses were trained in PMTCT and a significant proportion were noncompliant with the PMTCT national guidelines, which was much worse in the labour and postnatal care services compared to ANC. Furthermore, the treatment, diagnosis and follow-up/referral recommendations of PMTCT national guidelines on the continuum of MNCH, including the education recommendations in postnatal/immunisation services/units, constitute the weak domains of the PMTCT national guidelines in Kinshasa, DRC.

Noncompliance with healthcare standards is a common problem in developing countries,[31] with studies in Malawi, Uganda, and India having similar findings.[10,17,21] The

TABLE 2: Mean score, median score and Kruskal-Wallis test scores of nurses' compliance with PMTCT national guidelines on the continuum of MNCH services.

Categories of compliance score per ward	Mean (%)	95% CI [range (%)]	Median (%) IQR	*P*-value
Antenatal compliance with PMTCT national guidelines	80	[73–87]	85 [17]	0.025*
Labour and delivery compliance with PMTCT national guidelines	71	[64–78]	76 [27]	-
Postnatal compliance with PMTCT national guidelines	67	[56–79]	73 [34]	-
Overall compliance with PMTCT national guidelines	4	[69–78]	78 [22]	-

PMTCT, prevention of mother-to-child transmission; MNCH, maternal, newborn and child health.
*, $p \leq 0.05$

TABLE 3: Mean and median scores and Kruskal-Wallis test of nurses' compliance by categories of PMTCT recommendations and MNCH services.

Categories of recommendations of PMTCT national guidelines	Nurses per service	Mean (%)	95%CI [range, %]	Median (%) [IQR]	*P*-value
Compliance score (%) with education recommendations of PMTCT national guidelines	Antenatal service	85	[78–91]	91 [15]	0.000***
	Labour and delivery service	89	[79–99]	100 [0]	
	Postnatal service	72	[60–85]	83 [22]	
Compliance score (%) with treatment` recommendations of PMTCT national guidelines	Antenatal service	74	[62–86]	94 [50]	0.11
	Labour and delivery service	75	[67–82]	83 [25]	
	Postnatal service	63	[50–76]	67 [34]	
Compliance score (%) with diagnosis recommendations of PMTCT national guidelines	Antenatal service	64	[55–73]	66 [33]	0.29
	Labour and delivery service	72	[58–86]	94 [50]	
	Postnatal service	64	[44–83]	75 [59]	
Compliance score (%) with follow-up/referral recommendations of PMTCT national guidelines	Antenatal service	72	[55–88]	100 [100]	0.000***
	Labour and delivery service	-	-	-	
	Postnatal service	68	[47–88]	92 [75]	

PMTCT, prevention of mother-to-child transmission; MNCH, maternal, newborn and child health.
***, $p \leq 0.001$

exceptional nurses' compliance in ANC may have been influenced by context, as when the PMTCT programme was first introduced in Kinshasa more focus was placed on ANC than delivery and postnatal care. A minimum package of improved ANC services in line with PMTCT was implemented in many of the health clinics in 2003, which included staff training and supervision.[11,32] Thus the initial focus on ANC may have resulted in improved antenatal compliance.

The progressive decrease of compliance amongst nurses may express the failure in PMTCT in the DRC and shows that although the nurses receive pregnant women for delivery and mother-infant pairs in the postnatal and immunisation MNCH services, the PMTCT national programme has been poorly integrated in service support into the continuum of MNCH services.

Regarding the categories of PMTCT recommendations in the continuum of MNCH, the findings indicated that nurses were only compliant with the education recommendations in ANC and labour and delivery care, for example, providing individual post-test counselling after HIV testing (93.3%), providing information to HIV-positive women related to signs of labour and danger signs and MTCT timing (88.3%), and informing HIV-positive women regarding complete and regular immunisation according to the expanded programme on immunisation schedule for the baby with respect to clinical exceptions (88.3%) in ANC. In labour and delivery, for example, recommending early starting and follow-up of immediate exclusive breastfeeding after delivery (89.3%).

Furthermore, although in general nurses complied with the education recommendations, there were significant differences across the continuum of MNCH services. Other studies confirmed variations in this compliance, with nurses being more compliant to certain recommendations related to education than others; for example, Frizelle, Salomon and Rau underlined the noncompliance regarding breastfeeding information.[19,33] This study found that nurses providing postnatal/immunisation PMTCT care were not complying with the education recommendations. Similar results were found in studies by Mazia et al.[13] and Frizelle and Salomon[34] in Botswana, Kenya, Malawi and Uganda. The researcher agreed with these authors, who pointed out that healthcare workers in their studies were provided with deficient messages related to PMTCT. There was poor quality of counselling and information was either contradictory, with avoidance of the topic or confusing messages told to mothers by healthcare providers.

Regarding the diagnosis recommendations, nurses' compliance may be influenced by the type of strategy employed. The opt-out HIV testing strategy is more likely to influence healthcare providers' compliance to provide HIV testing than the opt-in.[17] The researchers suspected that nurses facing two ongoing HIV testing guidelines to either opt in or opt out may become confused. However, a systematic review and meta-analysis showed compliance where the CD4 count was done on the same day as HIV testing.[12,17,21] In the context of the DRC, the noncompliance may also have been influenced by the need to pay for the CD4 count, as most HIV-related interventions are free. The link between nurses' awareness about the need for the test and availability of the test might also play an important role.

However, the level of compliance with recommendations related to diagnosis in postnatal care depends, according to Grilli and Lomas,[35] on the complexity of intervention. The DNA/PCR necessitates complex activities and special supplies which are not usually available at the PMTCT sites in the DRC. In contrast, the study by Tejiokem et al.[36] in Cameroon found a high level of compliance with such interventions. The difference in these studies may be related to the location of the DNA/PCR test machine, availability of supply, the site and the health staff's roles in handling blood and infant policy- implemented diagnosis. For example, there is only one DNA/PCR test machine for early infant diagnosis in Kinshasa, challenging the transportation of DBS samples from the health districts to the capital of each of the 11 provinces in DRC and then to Kinshasa.

With respect to the treatment recommendations, the various options (nevirapine, zidovudine (AZT) and triple therapy-based regimens) available in the DRC may make it confusing for nurses recommending treatment, which may have led to their noncompliance with the guidelines.[7] Higher compliance was reported where there was only one option (Eastern Cape, South Africa).[32] Also, the poor integration of PMTCT into MNCH services may explain this reduced level of compliance. This occurs especially in labour and delivery, where invasive obstetric practices (use of forceps, rupture of membranes and suction of newborn) indicate that nurses have not been updated on MTCT progress.[37]

The study also found noncompliance with treatment recommendations in postnatal care. The study by Mazia et al. also reported low compliance with ART for newborns and HIV-positive women[13] due to the challenge of packaging of ART medication for infants. Moreover, three ongoing and overlapping guidelines based on nevirapine, AZT and triple therapy in the DRC might also influence the level of compliance of nurses with this national guideline recommendation.

Regarding the follow-up/referral recommendations, the poor integration of PMTCT in the MNCH services disadvantaged the nurses' ability to comply with the guidelines.[1,22,13] These include, for example, immunisation of HIV-exposed infants for diphtheria, tetanus and pertussis at 6 weeks after birth, and recommendation of exclusive breastfeeding or exclusive infant formula feeding; also DBS samples of exposed infants were not routinely required, and were poorly performed.

The findings also took into account the sociodemographic characteristics of nurses. Although the nurses' qualification had an influence on the score of nurses' compliance (only with education and diagnosis recommendations of PMTCT national guidelines), in general nurses' qualification, years of experience and training on PMTCT did not influence their overall level of compliance in the respective MNCH services. This confirms what has been described in the literature about factors which improve performance. A study in Armenia, Bangladesh, Bolivia, and Nigeria found that the social interactions (either formal or informal) between nurses and other professionals and experience are the most common sources of practice knowledge for nurses.[38] Thus, in the current study the homogeneity in working experience amongst nurses in the three MNCH services/units and their formal interaction in the workplace might have had an influence on their overall poor compliance with PMTCT national guidelines.

Limitations

The researchers assumed sample size estimate sampling due to no prior knowledge on healthcare providers' compliance with PMTCT national guidelines in the continuum of care, which may not have been adequate. In addition, there was a lack of representativeness of all categories of healthcare providers involved in PMTCT. Nonetheless, the random selection of healthcare providers minimised the sample bias.

Recommendations

More emphasis needs to be placed on the importance of evidence-based PMTCT guidelines in the nursing curriculum. This includes PMTCT management, nurses' self-evaluation in daily practice and the full integration of all PMTCT recommendations as routine activities in MNCH. Attention should be focused on training more nursing staff in labour, delivery and postnatal services.

The nurses' self-reported noncompliance with the diagnosis, treatment and follow-up/referral recommendations of the PMTCT guidelines requires further understanding. It is therefore recommended that further research could look at why noncompliance occurs from the nurses' perspectives to address the problem and improve nurses' compliance and implementation in order to reduce HIV infection in infants through PMTCT.

Conclusion

The results of this study found that nurses were noncompliant with PMTCT national guidelines throughout the continuum of MNCH in the 18 selected PMTCT sites in Kinshasa, particularly in the labour and postnatal phase of care. Additionally, there is failure to comply adequately with the PMTCT national guidelines in providing diagnosis, treatment and follow-up recommendations across the PMTCT cascade.

The nurses' self-reported noncompliance with the diagnosis, treatment and follow-up/referral recommendations of the PMTCT guidelines requires further understanding. In addition, more emphasis needs to be placed on the importance of evidence-based PMTCT guidelines in the nursing curriculum.

Acknowledgements

The authors acknowledge the partnership of the National AIDS Control Programme Kinshasa office team in DRC for their accompaniment in conducting this study.

Competing interests

The authors declare that they have no financial or personal relationship(s) that may have inappropriately influenced them in writing this article.

Authors' contributions

Both authors conceptualised and carried out the study and data analysis – P.B. (University of KwaZulu-Natal) as research supervisor. R.M.A. (University of KwaZulu-Natal) conceptualised and drafted the manuscript and P.B. assisted and refined the manuscript.

References

1. Joint United Nations Programme on HIV/AIDS. Global report: UNAIDS global report on HIV epidemic. Geneva: Joint United Nations Programme on HIV/AIDS; 2013.
2. Joint United Nations Programme on HIV/AIDS. Joint United Nations Programme on HIV/AIDS report on the global AIDS epidemic. Geneva: Joint United Nations Programme on HIV/AIDS; 2010.
3. Joint United Nations Programme on HIV/AIDS. Mother-to-child transmission of HIV: Technical update. Geneva: Joint United Nations Programme on HIV/AIDS; 1998.
4. Joint United Nations Programme on HIV/AIDS, World Health Organization, United Nations Children's Fund. Towards universal access: Scaling up priority HIV/AIDS interventions in the health sector. Geneva: UNAIDS; 2010.
5. Paintsil E, Andiman WA. Update on successes and challenges regarding mother-to-child transmission of HIV. Curr Opin Paediatr. 2009;21(1):94–101. http://dx.doi.org/10.1097/MOP.0b013e32831ec353
6. United Nations. Assessing progress in Africa toward the Millennium Development Goals. Addis Ababa: United Nations Development Program; 2011.
7. Programme National de Lutte contre les infections sexuellement transmissibles et le Sida. Annual Ministry of Health HIV/AIDS report 2010. Kinshasa: National Program to control HIV epidemic; 2010.
8. PNLS. Annual Ministry of Health HIV/AIDS report 2011. Kinshasa: National Program to control HIV epidemic; 2011.
9. Democratic Republic of Congo Presidency. National follow-up report of AIDS United Nations General Assembly Special Session (UNGASS). Kinshasa: Multisectoral Program to Control HIV Epidemic; 2010.
10. Ahoua L, Ayikoru H, Gnauck K, et al. Evaluation of a 5-year programme to prevent mother-to-child transmission of HIV Infection in Northern Uganda. J Trop Paed. 2010;56(1):43–52. http://dx.doi.org/10.1093/tropej/fmp054
11. Behets F, Mutombo GM, Edmonds A, et al. Reducing vertical HIV transmission in Kinshasa, Democratic Republic of Congo: Trends in HIV prevalence and service delivery. AIDS Care. 2009;21(5):583–590. http://dx.doi.org/10.1080/09540120802385595
12. Delva W, Mutunga L, Quaghebeur A, Temmerman M. Quality and quantity of antenatal HIV counselling in a PMTCT programme in Mombasa, Kenya. AIDS Care. 2006;18(3):189–193. http://dx.doi.org/10.1080/09540120500456425
13. Mazia G, Narayanan I, Warren C, et al. Integrating quality postnatal care into PMTCT in Swaziland. Global Public Health. 2009;4(3):253–270. http://dx.doi.org/10.1080/17441690902769669
14. Becquet RED, Arrive E, Stringer JS, et al. Universal antiretroviral therapy for pregnant and breastfeeding HIV-1 infected women: Towards the elimination of mother-to-child transmission of HIV-1 in resource settings. Clin Infect Dis. 2009;49:1936–1945. http://dx.doi.org/10.1086/648446
15. Mandala J, Torpey, K, Kasonde, et al. Prevention of mother-to-child transmission of HIV in Zambia: Implementing efficacious ARV regimens in primary health centers. BMC Public Health. 2009;9(314):1–9. http://dx.doi.org/10.1186/1471-2458-9-314
16. Moth IA, Ayayo ABCO, Kaseje DO. Assessment of utilisation of PMTCT services at Nyanza Provincial Hospital, Kenya. SAHARA J. 2005;2(2):244–250. http://dx.doi.org/10.1080/17290376.2005.9724847
17. Manzi M, Zachariah R, Teck R, et al. High acceptability of voluntary counselling and HIV-testing but unacceptable loss to follow up in a prevention of mother-to-child HIV transmission programme in rural Malawi: Scaling up requires a different way of acting. Trop Med Int'l Health. 2005;10(12):1242–1250. http://dx.doi.org/10.1111/j.1365-3156.2005.01526.x
18. Asiimwe A, Delvaux T, Elul B, et al. Evaluation of access to and utilization of services for the prevention of mother-to-child transmission (PMTCT) of HIV in Rwanda. Kigali: Rwanda Ministry of Health; 2007.
19. Doherty TM, McCoy D, Donohue S. Health system constraints to optimal coverage of the prevention of mother-to-child HIV transmission programme in South Africa: Lessons from the implementation of the national pilot programme. African Health Sci. 2005;5(3):213–218.
20. Hussein M, Jira C, Girma B. Assessment of effective coverage of HIV prevention of pregnant mother to child transmission services in Jimma zone, South West Ethiopia. Ethiop J Health Sci. 2011;21:1–7.
21. Chaudhuri S, Mundle M, Konar H, Das C, Talukdar A, Ghosh US. Utilization of therapeutic intervention to prevent mother to child transmission of HIV in a teaching hospital in Kolkata, India. J Obstet Gynaecol. 2010;36(3):619–625. http://dx.doi.org/10.1111/j.1447-0756.2009.01161.x
22. Both J, Roosmalen JV. The impact of Prevention of Mother to Child Transmission (PMTCT) programmes on maternal health care in resource-poor settings: Looking beyond the PMTCT programme – A systematic review. Int'l J Obstet Gynaecol. 2010;117:1444–1450. http://dx.doi.org/10.1111/j.1471-0528.2010.02692.x
23. Grover S, Lowensteyn I, Joseph L, et al. Discussing coronary risk with patients to improve blood pressure treatment: Secondary results from CHECK-UP study. J Gen Int Med. 2009;24(1):33–39. http://dx.doi.org/10.1007/s11606-008-0825-4
24. Central Intelligence Agency. Cartographer Map of Democratic Republic of Congo; 2010.
25. Programme National de Lutte contre les infections sexuellement transmissibles et le Sida. PMTCT Kinshasa province report first semester 2011. Kinshasa DRC: Provincial Program to control HIV epidemic; 2011.
26. Le CT. Introductory biostatistics. Hoboken, NJ: Wiley-Interscience John Wiley & Sons;2003. http://dx.doi.org/10.1002/0471308889
27. Burgers JS, Grol RP, Zaat JOM, Spies TH, Bij A, Mokkink, HGA. Characteristics of effective clinical guidelines for general practice. Br J Gen Pract. 2003;53:15–19.
28. Laurin J. Evaluation de la qualité des soins infirmiers. Montreal: Edisem; 1988.
29. Polit D, Beck, C. Nursing research: Generating and assessing evidence for nursing practice. Philadelphia: Lippincott Williams & Wilkins; 2008.
30. Fink A. Evaluation fundamentals: Insights into the outcomes, effectiveness, and quality of health programs. London: Sage; 2005. http://dx.doi.org/10.4135/9781412984140
31. Kelley E, Geslin C, Djibrina S, Boucar M. The impact of QA methods on compliance with integrated management of childhood illness algorithm in Niger. Bethesda: Quality Assurance Project; 2000.
32. Behets F, Matendo R, Vaz LME, et al. A. Preventing vertical transmission of HIV in Kinshasa, Democratic Republic of the Congo: A baseline survey of 18 antenatal clinics. Bull World Health Organ. 2006;84:969–975. http://dx.doi.org/10.2471/BLT.05.028217
33. Mukwato KP, Ngoma C, Maimbolwa M. Compliance with infection prevention guidelines by health care workers at Ronald Ross general hospital Mufulira District. Med J Zambia. 2009;35(3):110–116. http://dx.doi.org/10.4314/mjz.v35i3.46530
34. Frizelle K, Salomon, V. Strengthening PMTCT through communication: A review of the literature. Durban: Centre for AIDS Development Research and Evaluation; 2009.
35. Grilli R, Lomas J. Evaluating the message: The relationship between compliance rate and the subject of practice guideline. Med Care. 1994;32(3):202–213. http://dx.doi.org/10.1097/00005650-199403000-00002
36. Tejiokem MC, Faye A, Penda IC, et al. Feasibility of early infant diagnosis of HIV in resource-limited settings: The ANRS 12140-PEDIACAM Study in Cameroon. PLoS One. 2011;6(7):e21840. http://dx.doi.org/10.1371/journal.pone.0021840
37. Moore M. A behaviour change perspective on integrating PMTCT and safe motherhood programs: A discussion paper. Washington: The CHANGE Project AED/The Manoff Group; 2003.
38. Crigler L, Fort AL, Diez OD, Gearan S, Gyuzalyan H. Training alone is not enough: Factors that influence the performance of health care providers in Armenia, Bangladesh, Bolivia and Nigeria. Perf Improve Quarterly. 2005;19(1):99–116. http://dx.doi.org/10.1111/j.1937-8327.2006.tb00359.x

26

Prevalence and associated risk factors of hypertension amongst adults in a rural community of Limpopo Province, South Africa

Authors:
Sam T. Ntuli[1,2]
Eric Maimela[3]
Mariannes Alberts[4]
Solly Choma[4]
Sekgothe Dikotope[4]

Affiliations:
[1]Research Development and Administration, University of Limpopo, Polokwane Campus, South Africa

[2]Department of Public Health, University of Limpopo, Polokwane Campus, South Africa

[3]Epidemiology Services, Limpopo Department of Health, South Africa

[4]Medical Science Department, University of Limpopo, Turfloop Campus, South Africa

Correspondence to:
Sam Ntuli

Email:
tsntuli@hotmail.com

Postal address:
Private Bag X9315, Pietersburg 0700, South Africa

Background: Hypertension is problem already faced by urban populations of South Africa, but little is known about its prevalence and risk factors in rural areas.

Aim: To assess the prevalence of and risk factors associated with hypertension amongst adults in a rural community in South Africa.

Setting: Dikgale Health and Demographic Surveillance Site, Limpopo Province, South Africa.

Methods: A community-based cross-sectional survey was carried out at this site where individuals aged 15 years and older were screened using a locally adapted version of the World Health Organization STEPwise questionnaire. Demographics, anthropometry and three independent blood pressure (BP) readings were taken. The average of the three BP measurements was used in analysis, and hypertension taken as systolic and diastolic BP of ≥ 140 or ≥ 90 mmHg respectively, or at least a two-week history of antihypertensive treatment. Analysis included the Chi-square test and statistical significance was set at $p \leq 0.05$.

Results: A total of 1407 individuals were interviewed, of whom 1281 had complete BP, weight and height measurements taken. The mean age of participants was 44.2 ± 20.9 years(range 15–98 years), 63% were female, 55% were single and 90% were unemployed, whilst 13% were tobacco smokers and 20% reported drinking alcohol. Overall prevalence of hypertension was 41% and this was significantly associated with age and marital status.

Conclusion: The prevalence of hypertension was found to be high. Prevention strategies are urgently needed to address this life-threatening and important risk factor for cardiovascular disease in rural Limpopo Province.

Prévalence de l'hypertension et facteurs de risque associés chez les adultes dans une communauté rurale de la province du Limpopo en Afrique du Sud.

Objectif : Évaluer la prévalence et les facteurs de risque associés à l'hypertension chez les adultes au Site de surveillance sanitaire et démographique de Dikgale, dans la province du Limpopo.

Méthodes : Une enquête transversale à base communautaire a été réalisée au Site de surveillance sanitaire et démographique de Dikgale, dans la province du Limpopo en Afrique du Sud. Des personnes âgées de 15 ans et plus ont été sélectionnées en utilisant une version adaptée localement du questionnaire STEPwise de l'OMS. Des relevés démographiques, anthropométriques et trois relevés indépendants de pression artérielle (PA) ont été effectués lors d'une visite au domicile de chaque participant. La moyenne des trois mesures de PA été utilisée dans l'analyse. L'hypertension a été définie selon des critères du JNC 7 : pressions artérielles systolique et diastolique ≥ 140 ou ≥ 90 mmHg respectivement, ou lorsqu'un participant a eu au moins un antécédent de deux semaines de traitement antihypertenseur. L'analyse comprenait l'utilisation du test du chi deux et la signification statistique a été fixée à $p \leq 0{,}05$.

Résultats : Un total de 1407 personnes ont été interrogées, dont 1281 ont fait l'objet de mesures complètes de PA, du poids et de la taille qui ont été analysées. L'âge moyen des participants était de 44.2 ± 20.9 ans (éventail de 15 à 98 ans), 63% étaient des femmes, 55% étaient célibataires et 90% étaient au chômage. En ce qui concerne les habitudes alimentaires des participants, 89% mangeaient moins de cinq portions de fruits et légumes par jour, 13% fumaient du tabac et 20% déclaraient boire de l'alcool. La prévalence globale de l'hypertension était de 41% dans l'échantillon des participants et était associée de façon significative à l'âge et au statut matrimonial. Le sexe, la consommation d'alcool, le tabagisme, la situation professionnelle, la consommation de fruits et légumes et l'Indice de masse corporelle (IMC) n'étaient pas liés à une hypertension. La moitié des participants avaient un IMC de 25 kg/m2 ou plus et parmi ceux-ci, 27% étaient en surpoids (IMC de 25.0 – 29.9) et 23% étaient obèses (IMC ≥ 30 kg/m2).

Conclusion : La prévalence de l'hypertension a été jugée élevée dans cette étude. Des stratégies de prévention doivent urgemment être mises en œuvre pour remédier à ce facteur de risque important et potentiellement mortel en termes de maladies cardio-vasculaires dans la province rurale du Limpopo en Afrique du Sud.

Introduction

Cardiovascular disease (CVD) is now the leading cause of death worldwide, and its major impact is not only observed in developed countries but also in developing countries.[1,2] In 2008 CVD caused 30% of all global deaths, of which over 80% were recorded from developing countries.[3] Many developing countries are now in a phase of epidemiological transition and face the double burden of infectious diseases and non-communicable diseases (NCDs). Bradshaw and colleagues reported that hypertension, strokes and ischaemic heart disease are amongst the most common NCDs causing many premature adult deaths in South Africa.[4] Various studies have identified CVD as a major burden of disease in developing countries.[5,6,7]

In recent years epidemiological evidence has increasingly provided more insight into the risk factors for CVD in developing countries. These include, amongst others, obesity, alcohol intake, smoking, hypertension and diabetes mellitus.[1,8,9] Hypertension remains the most common life-threatening risk factor for CVD in developing countries.[10] This has major cost implications for low- and middle-income countries and requires urgent strategies for prevention and management of the disease. Numerous studies have been conducted worldwide to estimate the prevalence of hypertension. In sub-Saharan countries the prevalence of hypertension varies from 5% to 50%,[11,12] whilst in economically developed countries it ranges between 19% and 30%.[4,13]

In South Africa the prevalence of hypertension was estimated at 21% in the 1998 Demographic and Health Survey, and it was slightly more common in women (14%) than in men (11%).[14] Newer studies suggest a much higher prevalence of hypertension, in line with the epidemiological transition and increasing burden of chronic diseases of lifestyle in South Africa.[15,16,17,18] Despite the importance of hypertension as a risk factor for CVD and its importance as a cause of premature mortality in South Africa, few studies to date have assessed the prevalence of hypertension and its risk factors in the rural areas of the country. Therefore the aim of this study was to determine the prevalence of and associated risk factors for hypertension amongst adults in the Dikgale Health and Demographic Surveillance Site (HDSS), Limpopo Province, South Africa

Research methods and design

Study design and population

A cross-sectional community-based study was carried out in the Dikgale HDSS, Limpopo Province, South Africa. The area consists of 15 villages, 7200 householdsand a population of approximately 36 000. Unemployment within the HDSS population is high, despite high rates of literacy and education. A detailed description of the study site has been provided elsewhere.[7,19,20]

Inclusion and exclusion criteria

All individuals aged 15 years and older who permanently resided in Dikgale HDSS and had the ability to comprehend the contents of the interview were eligible to participate. Individuals who were non-cooperative or refused to provide the necessary information were excluded from the study. Pregnant women and bedridden and disabled individuals were also excluded. Members of families who were not present at the time of the assessment were excluded after three repeated visits.

Sample size and sampling technique

A minimum sample size of 1366 (approximated to 1400) was calculated based on the reported hypertension prevalence rate of 46% in South Africa,[21] a sampling error of 4%, 95% confidence, non-response rate (10%) and design effect set at 2. Each village was taken as a cluster, and all households within a cluster were visited. In a household all family members available at the time of data collection and eligible to participate were included in the study. A total of 1407 individuals gave their consent and participated in the study.

Data collection

Data collection was carried out between June 2011 and March 2012 by trained field workers. The questionnaire used for the study was a modified World Health Organization STEPwise instrument for NCD risk factor surveillance.[22] Blood pressure (BP) was measured three times using the Omron M6 Digital Automatic Blood Pressure Monitor (Kyoto, Japan), and the average of the three readings used for analysis. Height and weight were measured once using a stadiometer to the nearest 0.5 cm and the digital balance to the nearest 0.1 kg respectively. Participants were measured without shoes and wearing only light clothing. Body mass index (BMI) was calculated as weight in kg divided by height in metres squared (m^2). BMI was then categorised as underweight (< 18.5 kg/m^2), normal (18.5 kg/m^2 – 24.9 kg/m^2), overweight (25.0 kg/m^2 –29.9 kg/m^2) or obese (≥ 30 kg/m^2).

Hypertension was diagnosed when systolic BP was ≥ 140 mmHg and/or diastolic BP ≥ 90 mmHg or when a person had a history of antihypertensive treatment during the survey. Isolated diastolic hypertension was defined as diastolic BP more than 90 mmHg and systolic BP less than 140 mmHg, whilst isolated systolic hypertension referred to systolic BP of more than 140 mmHg and diastolic BP of less than 90 mmHg.[23]

Data analysis

Data entry and statistical analysis were performed using Microsoft Excel and statistical software (Stata 9.0, StataCorp, College Station, Texas, United States of America [USA]), respectively. Differences in demographic characteristics between hypertensive and normotensive groups were analysed using the Chi-square test. The student *t*-test was also used to compare the age distribution of males and females. A *p*-value of less than 5% was considered statistically significant.

Ethical considerations

Ethics approval (Ref: MREC/HS/05/2013) to conduct the study was obtained from the University of Limpopo Ethics Committee (Medunsa Campus), and the anonymity and confidentiality of individual participants and personal information was protected.

Results

Demographic characteristics

A total of 1407 individuals were interviewed during the period of the study, of whom 1281 had complete information, giving a response rate of 91%. Nine per cent (126/1407) of the participants were excluded from the study because incomplete measurements of BP, weight or height were taken. The ages of participants ranged from 15 to 98 years, with a mean of 44.2 ± 20.9 years. Of the sample 42% was aged 50 years and older and 63% was female, as indicated in Table 1. The mean age of females was significantly higher than that of males (45.9 ± 20.2 vs. 41.3 ± 21.5, $p < 0.001$). Fifty-five per cent of the participants were single and 90% were unemployed, whilst 87% were non-smokers and 80% were non-alcohol drinkers (see Table 1).

Prevalence of hypertension

The overall prevalence of hypertension was 41.4% (95% CI: 38.7% – 44.1%) with 21% (95% CI: 17.4% – 24.5%) having isolated systolic hypertension and 26% (95% CI: 22.2% – 29.8%) isolated diastolic hypertension. As displayed in Table 2, the prevalence of hypertension varied according to age group, marital status and level of education. As age increased, the prevalence of hypertension also increased ($p < 0.05$). Participants with tertiary education showed a significantly lower prevalence of hypertension compared to the other groups ($p < 0.05$). The prevalence of hypertension was found to be lower amongst single (35%) respondents compared to the other groups, the difference being statistically significant ($p < 0.05$).

The proportion of participants with hypertension was found to be higher amongst males than females (42% vs. 41%, $p > 0.05$). An insignificantly greater proportion of unemployed respondents was hypertensive compared to employed respondents (42% vs. 33%, $p > 0.05$). Other factors, such as alcohol intake ($p = 0.812$), smoking ($p = 0.516$), fruit and vegetable intake ($p = 0.752$) and BMI ($p = 0.310$), were not significantly associated with hypertension (see Table 2).

TABLE 1: Demographic characteristics of the respondents ($n = 1281$).

Characteristic	Number	%
Age (yrs)		
15–19	159	12
20–29	294	23
30–39	132	10
40–49	144	11
50–59	182	14
60+	366	28
Gender		
Male	480	37
Female	801	63
Marital status		
Single	695	55
Married	456	36
Widowed	84	7
Others	34	3

Discussion

In our study the overall prevalence of hypertension was 41%. In recent African studies the prevalence of hypertension in sub-Saharan Africa ranges between 5% and 50%.[11,12,24] Our findings are similar to those reported in rural Ghana,[25] rural Nigeria[26] and the Agincourt rural subdistrict in SouthAfrica.[27] However, the prevalence of hypertension in our study was higher than that in rural Ethiopia[28] and rural Uganda.[29,30] Our findings therefore confirm the growing concern about hypertension as a public health problem in rural South Africa.

Studies in developed countries revealed a large variation in the prevalence of hypertension, with a rate of 19.5% in

TABLE 2: Association of sociodemographics with hypertension amongst respondents in Dikgale Health and Demographic Surveillance Site

Characteristic	*n*	Normotensive *N* (%)	Hypertension *N* (%)	*p*-value
Age (yrs)				
15–19	159	105 (66)	54 (34)	< 0.001
20–29	294	202 (68)	92 (31)	
30–39	132	81 (61)	51 (39)	
40–49	144	85 (59)	59 (41)	
50–59	182	94 (52)	88 (48)	
60 +	366	181 (49)	185 (51)	
Gender				
Female	801	473 (59)	328 (41)	0.690
Male	480	278 (58)	202 (42)	
Employment status				
Unemployed	1124	651 (58)	473 (42)	0.058
Employed	126	84 (67)	42 (33)	
Marital status				
Single	699	455 (65)	244 (35)	< 0.001
Married	456	230 (50)	226 (49)	
Widowed	84	44 (52)	40 (48)	
Divorced/separated	30	16 (53)	14 (47)	
Level of education				
None	148	72 (49)	76 (51)	< 0.001
Primary	600	328 (55)	272 (45)	
Secondary	487	317 (65)	170 (35)	
Tertiary	40	30 (75)	10 (25)	
Alcohol				
No	1025	600 (58)	425 (42)	0.812
Yes	251	149 (59)	102 (41)	
Smoking				
No	1112	647 (58)	465 (41)	0.516
Yes	166	101 (61)	65 (39)	
Fruit and vegetable intake				
< 5 servings/day	1139	666 (59)	473 (41)	0.752
> 5 servings/day	142	85 (60)	57 (40)	
BMI (kg/m²)				
< 18.5	68	45 (66)	23 (34)	0.310
18.5–24.9	544	325 (60)	219 (40)	
25.0–29.9	340	190 (56)	150 (44)	
≥ 30	294	165 (56)	129 (44)	

Canada, 29% in the USA and 30% in England.[13] In South Africa the national prevalence of hypertension has increased from 21% in 1998[14] to 77.3% in 2008.[17] This might be due to rapid urbanisation, ageing of the population, an increase in psychosocial stress, diet and lifestyle changes.[31] There is evidence that the prevalence of hypertension in low- and middle-income countries is greater than in developed nations.[13] This has negative implications since in many developing countries priority is given to acute disorders and maternal and child health. In addition, the health system is inadequate because of low funds, poor infrastructure and lack of equipment.

With regard to sociodemographics, studies reported that being overweight or obese, falling within an older age group, use of alcohol, being married and level of education are associated with hypertension.[25,26,29,30,31,32,33,34] The findings of our study confirm that being married, low education level and falling within an older age group are the most common risk factors for hypertension. High BP is a multifactorial disorder, and changes with age might be due to changes in the vascular system,[35] whilst poor partner support and marital conflict were shown to increase cardiovascular reaction and BP.[36,37,38,39,40]

Earlier studies suggest that a high BMI contributes to hypertension.[41,42,43,44] Our study showed that the association between BMI and hypertension was not significant, which may partly be attributed to the declining use of dietary salt, despite the increase in obesity.[45,46]

In this study the prevalence of hypertension was slightly higher in men than in women, but the difference was not statistically significant. This finding is similar to those reported in other studies,[11,27,33] but differed from those which found the prevalence of hypertension to be higher in women than men.[7,14,29,30,47] Hypertension seems to coexist with the risk factors mentioned above, and thus may be an important clinical entity which requires medical attention. In the elderly it is well known that hypertension increases with vascular resistance. Therefore the therapeutic approach to hypertensive patients consists of a reduction in salt and caloric intake and an increase in physical activity.[48,49,51]

Limitations

The following limitations need to be considered. As the scope of this study did not include biochemical measurements, we were unable to determine the levels of blood glucose or cholesterol, which were not assessed because the participants had not fasted. Finally, as this was a cross-sectional study no causal relationship can be inferred between any of the factors and hypertension.

Conclusion

The prevalence of hypertension is relatively high in this rural community and is associated with being married, having a low education level and falling into an older age group. Given the importance of BP control in reducing the risk of CVD, there is an urgent need for strategies to promote BP screening at local health facilities as well as at community level and to promote prompt treatment initiation and follow-up of cases. In addition, salt reduction in food requires commitment at both provincial and national level.

Acknowledgements

We thank the staff of the Department of Medical Science at the University of Limpopo for their technical advice and help. Thanks also to Dr O.B. Omole and Dr P. Anguria for providing useful comments and suggestions.

Competing interests

The authors declare that they have no financial or personal relationship(s) that may have inappropriately influenced them in writing this article.

Authors' contributions

S.T.N. (University of Limpopo, Polokwane Campus) assisted in the statistical analysis and interpretation, and wrote most of the manuscript, E.M. (Epidemiology Services, Limpopo Department of Health), A.M. (University of Limpopo, Turfloop Campus), S.C. (University of Limpopo, Turfloop Campus) and S.D. (University of Limpopo, Turfloop Campus) supervised, assisted with data collection, and edited the manuscript.

References

1. Lopez AD, Mathers CD, Eszati M, Jamison DT, Murray CJL. Global burden of disease and risk factors. Washington, DC: World Bank; 2006. http://dx.doi.org/10.1596/978-0-8213-6262-4
2. Mayosi BM, Flisher AJ, Lalloo UG, Sitas F, Tollman SM, Bradshaw D. The burden of non-communicable diseases in South Africa. Lancet. 2009;374(9693):934–947. http://dx.doi.org/10.1016/S0140-6736(09)61087-4
3. World Health Organization. Cardiovascular diseases (CVDs), Fact Sheet No. 317 [updated 2015 Jan; cited 2014 Feb 3]. Available from: http://www.who.int/mediacentre/factsheets/fs317/en/index.html
4. Bradshaw D, Nannan N, Groenewald P, et al. Provincial mortality in South Africa, 2000--priority-setting for now and a benchmark for the future. S Afr Med J. 2005;95(7):496–503.
5. Mathers CD, Loncar D. Projections of global mortality and burden of disease from 2002 to 2030. PLos Med. 2006;3:e442. http://dx.doi.org/10.1371/journal.pmed.0030442
6. Kearney PM, Whelton M, Reynolds K, Muntner P, Whelton PK, He J. Global burden of hypertension: Analysis of worldwide data. Lancet. 2005;365:217–223. http://dx.doi.org/10.1016/S0140-6736(05)70151-3
7. Alberts M, Urdal P, Steyn K, et al. Prevalence of cardiovascular diseases and associated risk factors in a rural black population of South Africa. Eur J Cardiovasc Prev Rehabil. 2005;12(4):347–354. http://dx.doi.org/10.1097/01.hjr.0000174792.24188.8e
8. Steyn K, Sliwa K, Hawken S, et al. Risk factors associated with myocardial infarction in Africa: The INTERHEART Africa study. Circulation. 2005;112:3554–3561. http://dx.doi.org/10.1161/CIRCULATIONAHA.105.563452
9. O'Donnell MJ, Xavier D, Liu L, et al. Risk factors for ischaemic and intracerebral haemorrhagic stroke in 22 countries (the INTERSTROKE study): A case-control study. Lancet. 2010;376:112–123. http://dx.doi.org/10.1016/S0140-6736(10)60834-3
10. Connor M, Rheeder P, Bryer A, et al. The South African stroke risk in general practice study. S Afr Med J. 2005;95:334–339.
11. Dalal S, Beunza JJ, Volmink J, et al. Non-communicable diseases in sub-Saharan Africa: What we know now. Int J Epidemiol. 2011;40(4):885–901. http://dx.doi.org/10.1093/ije/dyr050
12. Ogah OS, Rayner BL. Recent advances in hypertension in sub-Saharan Africa. Heart. 2013;99(19):1390–1397. http://dx.doi.org/10.1136/heartjnl-2012-303227

13. Joffres M, Falaschetti E, Gillespie C, et al. Hypertension prevalence, awareness, treatment and control in national surveys from England, the USA and Canada, and correlation with stroke and ischaemic heart disease mortality: A cross sectional study. BMJ Open. 2013;3:e003423. http://dx.doi.org/10.1136/bmjopen-2013-003423

14. Steyn K, Gaziano TA, Bradshaw D, Laubscher R, Fourie J. South African Demographic and Health Coordinating Team. Hypertension in South African adults: Results from the Demographic and Health Survey, 1998. J Hypertens. 2001;19(10):1717–1725. http://dx.doi.org/10.1097/00004872-200110000-00004

15. Gómez-Olivé FX, Thorogood M, Clark B, Kahn K, Tollman S. Self-reported health and health care use in an ageing population in the Agincourt sub-district of rural South Africa. Global Health Action. 2013;6:19305. http://dx.doi.org/10.3402/gha.v6i0.19305

16. Lloyd-Sherlock P, Beard J, Minicuci N, Ebrahim S, Chatterji S. Hypertension among older adults in low- and middle-income countries: Prevalence, awareness and control. Int J Epidemiol. 2014; 43:116–128. http://dx.doi.org/10.1093/ije/dyt215

17. Peltzer K, Phaswana-Mafuya N. Hypertension and associated factors in older adults in South Africa. Cardiovasc J Afr. 2013;24(3):67–71. http://dx.doi.org/10.5830/CVJA-2013-002

18. Thorogood M, Connor M, Tollman S, Lewando Hundt G, Fowkes G, Marsh J. A cross-sectional study of vascular risk factors in a rural South African population: Data from the Southern African Stroke Prevention Initiative (SASPI). BMC Public Health. 2007;13(7):326. http://dx.doi.org/10.1186/1471-2458-7-326

19. Kanjala C, Alberts M, Byass P, Burger S. Spatial and temporal clustering of mortality in Digkale HDSS in rural northern South Africa. Global Health Action. 2010;30:3. http://dx.doi.org/10.3402/gha.v3i0.5236

20. Cook I, Alberts M, Burger S, Byass P. All-cause mortality trends in Dikgale, rural South Africa, 1996–2003. Scand J Public Health. 2008;36(7):753–760. Epub 2008 Jul 22. http://dx.doi.org/10.1177/1403494808089654

21. Gebreselassie KZ, Padyab M. Epidemiology of hypertension stages in two countries in sub-Sahara Africa: Factors associated with hypertension stages. Int J Hypertens, Article ID 959256, In press.

22. World Health Organization. WHO STEPS Surveillance manual. The WHO STEPwise approach to chronic disease risk factor surveillance. Geneva: World Health Organization; 2005.

23. Chobanian AV, Bakris GL, Black HR, et al. The Seventh Report of the joint national committee on the prevention, detection, evaluation, and treatment of high blood pressure: The JNC 7 report. JAMA. 2003;289:2560–2572.

24. De Ramirez SS, Enquobahrie DA, Nyadzi G, et al. Prevalence and correlates of hypertension: A cross-sectional study among rural populations in sub-Saharan Africa. J Hum Hypertens. 2010;24(12):786–795. http://dx.doi.org/10.1038/jhh.2010.14

25. Williams EA, Keenan KE, Ansong D, et al. The burden and correlates of hypertension in rural Ghana: A cross-sectional study. Diabetes Metab Syndr. 2013;7(3):123–128. http://dx.doi.org/10.1016/j.dsx.2013.06.015

26. Ahaneku GI, Osuji CU, Anisiuba BC, Ikeh VO, Oguejiofor OC, Ahaneku JE. Evaluation of blood pressure and indices of obesity in a typical rural community in eastern Nigeria. Ann Afr Med. 2011;10(2):120–126. http://dx.doi.org/10.4103/1596-3519.82076

27. Thorogood M, Connor M, Tollman S, Lewando Hundt G, Fowkes G, Marsh J. A cross-sectional study of vascular risk factors in a rural South African population: Data from the Southern African Stroke Prevention Initiative (SASPI). BMC Public Health. 2007;7:326. http://dx.doi.org/10.1186/1471-2458-7-326

28. Gudina EK, Michael Y, Assegid S. Prevalence of hypertension and its risk factors in southwest Ethiopia: A hospital-based cross-sectional survey. Integr Blood Press Control. 2013;6:111–117. http://dx.doi.org/10.2147/IBPC.S47298

29. Kotwani P, Kwarisiima D, Clark TD, et al. SEARCH Collaboration. Epidemiology and awareness of hypertension in a rural Ugandan community: A cross-sectional study. BMC Public Health. 2013;13(1):1151. http://dx.doi.org/10.1186/1471-2458-13-1151

30. Wamala JF, Karyabakabo Z, Ndungutse D, Guwatudde D. Prevalence factors associated with hypertension in Rukungiri district, Uganda--a community-based study. Afr Health Sci. 2009;9(3):153–160.

31. Ibrahim MM, Damasceno A. Hypertension in developing countries. Lancet. 2012;380(9841):611–619. http://dx.doi.org/10.1016/S0140-6736(12)60861-7

32. Hendriks ME, Wit FW, Roos MT, et al. Hypertension in sub-Saharan Africa: Cross-sectional surveys in four rural and urban communities. PLoS One. 2012;7(3):e32638. http://dx.doi.org/10.1371/journal.pone.0032638

33. Onwuchekwa AC, Mezie-Okoye MM, Babatunde S. Prevalence of hypertension in Kegbara-Dere, a rural community in the Niger Delta region, Nigeria. Ethn Dis. 2012;22(3):340–346.

34. Steyn K, Bradshaw D, Norman R, Laubscher R. Determinants and treatment of hypertension in South Africans: The first Demographic and Health Survey. S Afr Med J. 2008;98(5):376–380.

35. Laurent S, Cockcroft J, van Bortel L, et al. Expert consensus document on arterial stiffness: Methodological issues and clinical applications. Eur Heart J. 2006;27:2588–2605. http://dx.doi.org/10.1093/eurheartj/ehl254

36. Ewart CK, Taylor CB, Kraemer HC, Agras WS. High blood pressure and marital discord: Not being nasty matters more than being nice. Health Psychol. 1991;10(3):155–163. http://dx.doi.org/10.1037/0278-6133.10.3.155

37. Smith TW, Uchino BN, Berg CA, et al. Conflict and collaboration in middle-aged and older couples: II. Cardiovascular reactivity during marital interaction. Psychol Aging. 2009;24(2):274–286. http://dx.doi.org/10.1037/a0016067

38. Nealey-Moore JB, Smith TW, Uchino BN, Hawkins MW, Olson-Cerny C. Cardiovascular reactivity during positive and negative marital interactions. J Behav Med. 2007;30(6):505–519. http://dx.doi.org/10.1007/s10865-007-9124-5

39. Robles TF, Kiecolt-Glaser JK. The physiology of marriage: Pathways to health. Physiol Behav. 2003;79(3):409–416. http://dx.doi.org/10.1016/S0031-9384(03)00160-4

40. Holt-Lunstad J, Birmingham W, Jones BQ. Is there something unique about marriage? The relative impact of marital status, relationship quality, and network social support on ambulatory blood pressure and mental health. Ann Behav Med. 2008;35(2):239–244. http://dx.doi.org/10.1007/s12160-008-9018-y

41. Foulds HJ, Bredin SS, Warburton DE. The relationship between hypertension and obesity across different ethnicities. J Hypertens. 2012;30(2):359–367. http://dx.doi.org/10.1097/HJH.0b013e32834f0b86

42. Redón J, Cea-Calvo L, Moreno B, et al. Independent impact of obesity and fat distribution in hypertension prevalence and control in the elderly. J Hypertens. 2008;26(9):1757–1764. http://dx.doi.org/10.1097/HJH.0b013e3283077f03

43. Rudatsikira E, Muula AS, Mulenga D, Siziya S. Prevalence and correlates of obesity among Lusaka residents, Zambia: A population-based survey. Int Arch Med. 2012;5(1):14. http://dx.doi.org/10.1186/1755-7682-5-14

44. Mulenga D, Siziya S, Rudatsikira E, et al. District specific correlates for hypertension in Kaoma and Kasama rural districts of Zambia. Rural Remote Health. 2013;13(3):2345.

45. Bertram MY, Steyn K, Wentzel-Viljoen E, Tollman S, Hofman KJ. Reducing the sodium content of high-salt foods: Effect on cardiovascular disease in South Africa. S Afr Med J. 2012;102(9):743–745. http://dx.doi.org/10.7196/samj.5832

46. Charlton KE, Steyn K, Levitt NS, et al. A food-based dietary strategy lowers blood pressure in a low socio-economic setting: A randomised study in South Africa. Public Health Nutr. 2008;11(12):1397–1406. http://dx.doi.org/10.1017/S136898000800342X

47. Kokiwar PR, Gupta SS, Durge PM. Prevalence of hypertension in a rural community of central India. J Assoc Physicians India. 2012 Jun;60:26–29.

48. He FJ, Li J, Macgregor GA. Effect of longer-term modest salt reduction on blood pressure. Cochrane Database Syst Rev. 2013;4:CD004937. http://dx.doi.org/10.1002/14651858.CD004937.pub2

49. Bertram MY, Steyn K, Wentzel-Viljoen E, Tollman S, Hofman KJ. Reducing the sodium content of high-salt foods: Effect on cardiovascular disease in South Africa. S Afr Med J. 2012;102(9):743–745. http://dx.doi.org/10.7196/samj.5832

50. Lin JS, O'Connor E, Whitlock EP, Beil TL. Behavioral counseling to promote physical activity and a healthful diet to prevent cardiovascular disease in adults: A systematic review for the U.S. Preventive Services Task Force. Ann Intern Med. 2010;153(11):736–750. http://dx.doi.org/10.7326/0003-4819-153-11-201012070-00007

51. Lin JS, O'Connor EA, Evans CV, Senger CA, Rowland MG, Groom HC. Behavioral counseling to promote a healthy lifestyle for cardiovascular disease prevention in persons with cardiovascular risk factors: An updated systematic evidence review for the US Preventive Services Task Force [book on the Internet]. 2014 [cited 2014 Aug 13]. Rockville, MD: Agency for Healthcare Research and Quality (US), Report No. 13-05179-EF-1. Available from: http://www.ncbi.nlm.nih.gov/books/NBK241537/

Prevalence of and factors influencing postnatal depression in a rural community in South Africa

Authors:
Ethelwynn L. Stellenberg[1]
Johanna M. Abrahams[1]

Affiliations:
[1]Division of Nursing, Stellenbosch University, South Africa

Correspondence to:
Ethelwynn Stellenberg

Email:
elstel@sun.ac.za

Postal address:
PO Box 241, Francie van Zijl Drive, Cape Town 8000, South Africa

Background: Knowledge about postnatal depression (PND) and associated risk factors which influence the development of PND is vital for early detection, intervention and prevention.

Setting: The study was conducted in primary health care clinics (PHC) in the Witzenberg subdistrict, a rural community in South Africa.

Objectives: Objectives of this study were to determine the prevalence of PND and to identify the contributing risk factors associated with PND.

Methods: A descriptive cross sectional research design with a quantitative approach was applied. The target population was mothers, 18 years and older. A convenience sampling method was used to select a sample of 159 (10%) from a population of 1605 live births. The Edinburgh Postnatal Depression Scale (EPDS) and Beck Depression Inventory (BDI), two validated self-rating questionnaires, including a questionnaire based on demographical, psychosocial and obstetrical data, were applied. The data was analysed using various statistical tests to determine statistical associations between variables using a 95% confidence interval.

Results: PND was a serious health problem with 50.3% of the mothers who suffered from PND. A BDI analysis showed that of the participants who had PND, 28.8% was severe, 48.8% moderate and 22.5% mild. Factors influencing the development of PND included most participants (63.5%) were unmarried, 61.3% were unemployed and the majority (53.8%) had a history of a psychiatric illness. Significant associations between PND and unplanned and unwelcome babies ($p < 0.01$); partner relationship ($p < 0.01$); were identified.

Conclusion: Prevention, early detection, appropriate referral and treatment of PND are critical in managing maternal, child and family well-being.

Prévalence de, et facteurs qui influencent la dépression postnatale dans une communauté rurale d'Afrique du Sud.

Contexte: Une connaissance de la dépression postnatale (DPN) et des facteurs de risque connexes qui influencent le développement de la DPN est essentielle pour la détection précoce, l'intervention et la prévention.

Lieu: L'étude a été menée dans des cliniques de santé primaire (CSP) du sous-district de Witzenberg, une communauté rurale d'Afrique du Sud.

Objectifs: Cette étude avait pour objet de déterminer la prévalence de la DPN et d'identifier les facteurs de risques liés à la DPN.

Méthodes: On a utilisé un plan de recherche transversal descriptif avec une approche quantitative. La population visée était des mères de 18 ans et plus. On a fait appel à une méthode d'échantillonnage représentative pour sélectionner un échantillon de 159 (10%) personnes sur une population de 1605 naissances vivantes. On a appliqué l'Echelle de Dépression Postnatale d'Edinburgh (EDPE) et l'Inventaire de Dépression de Beck (IDB), deux questionnaires autoévalués et validés, comprenant un questionnaire basé sur des données démographiques, psychosociales et obstétriques. On a analysé les données au moyen de différents tests statistiques pour déterminer les associations statistiques entre les variables avec un intervalle de confiance de 95%.

Résultats: La DPN est un grave problème de santé avec 50.3% des mères qui en souffrent. Une analyse IDB a montré que parmi les participantes souffrant de DPN, 28.8% étaient sévèrement affectées, 48.8% modérément et 22.5% légèrement. Les facteurs influençant le développement de la DPN étaient que la plupart des participantes (63.5%) n'étaient pas mariées, 61.3% étaient au chômage et la majorité (53.8%) avait des antécédents de maladie psychiatrique. On a aussi remarqué des liens entre la DPN et les bébés non planifiés et non désirés ($p < 0.01$); et la relation des partenaires ($p < 0.01$).

Conclusion: La prévention, la détection précoce, l'orientation vers le service et le traitement appropriés de la DPN sont critiques pour la gestion du bien-être de la mère, de l'enfant et de la famille.

Introduction

Social value

Depression is associated with substantially reduced quality of life and functional capacity for the affected woman with PND.[1] Poor maternal mental health is especially problematic for the infants of these mothers. The investigation of the prevalence and the factors contributing to PND was fundamental in contributing to the achievement of the Millennium Development Goals, specifically in improving maternal health and reducing child mortality.[2] The lack of scientific evidence about the prevalence and factors contributing to PND in the Witzenberg subdistrict, Western Cape, South Africa made it essential that this problem was investigated scientifically. Ultimately, this study may contribute to early detection and management of PND and the improvement of the mental health services in the rural community.

Depression is the leading cause of disease burden for women in both high-income and low- and middle income countries.[3] Despite being a leading cause of disease burden for women, mental health is still the stepchild of health services and even more so in the rural areas.[4]

Postnatal depression (PND) is a severe condition, which can be described as 'a thief who steals maternity'.[5] The prevalence of PND is currently considered to be 10% – 15%, but is still increasing and becoming a serious public health problem.[6,7] In a study conducted in a South African peri-urban settlement, Khayelitsha, a prevalence rate of 34.7% of mothers at two months' postnatal suffer from PND.[8] PND affects approximately 500 000 mothers in the United States each year, and about one in five mothers may be affected by a major mental disorder in the first 12 months following childbirth.[9] The seriousness of this condition is further shown in an incident as reported in the IOL News, London, that a 35-year-old woman with PND killed her two babies, a 10-week-old son and 14-month-old daughter.[10]

Scientific value

PND is a universal and serious mood disorder that occurs within a few weeks after birth and causes considerable risks to the mother, the developing child and the entire family.[9] The derivations of PND can sometimes be visible during the postnatal period, sometimes referred to as puerperium, but are frequently only fully recognisable months later in the first year after birth. This depression may last for weeks, months or even years after origination.[11] Therefore, if PND is left untreated, it may lead to affective, cognitive, behavioural and physical problems. This may not only have an extremely negative effect on the mothering role and mother-child relationship, but on the total existence of the affected mother's family.[12]

Almost 10% of all postnatal mothers will acquire a depressive disorder.[13] It was further shown that it is most likely to occur in 16% of women during the postpartum period.[14] Mental illnesses, especially major depression, add extensively to the non-fatal burden of disease and is the second leading cause of mental disabilities. However, in South Africa the ratio between psychiatrist and patient and/or client is 1:357 142 and psychologist and patient and/or client is 1:312 500,[15] making mental illness one of the most neglected illnesses in South Africa. The Annual Health Status Report identified that in the Witzenberg subdistrict there was a marked increase in mental health cases from 347 in 2001 to 491 in 2006.[16]

Depression, anxiety, stressful life events and low levels of social support were identified as key maternal risk factors in studies conducted in Khayelitsha.[14,17] Nearly one third of employed participants (32.7%) in a study stated substantial depressive symptoms at four months postnatal.[18] Thus, it is evident that PND will influence the mother's capability to care for her baby.[19]

Maternal age is related to PND symptoms but lower socio-economic and educational levels are added risk factors.[20] Symptoms of depression are substantially higher amongst mothers with lower educational levels who are unmarried and poor.[18] PND has been found to be higher in socio-economically disadvantaged areas in SA, as shown in a study in Khayelitsha, in which the PND rate is as high as 34.7%.[8]

The levels, however, in teenage mothers have been reported to be as high as 26%.[6] The incorporation of many factors such as integration of biochemistry, hormonal functioning, genetic history and psychosocial factors such as stressful life events concede the potential for the occurrence of PND.[6]

Conceptual theoretical framework

The conceptual theoretical framework, which guided this study, is based on the clinical or medical model, bio-psychosocial model, holistic approach of nursing, and the following psychosocial theories of depression: psychoanalytic theory, object loss theory, learned helplessness theory and the cognitive theory. These models and theories were significant for this study because it is imperative for health care workers to understand depression, the origin thereof, and what the possible causes and consequences are in order to understand and manage clients most effectively.

Aim and objectives

The objectives of this study were to determine the prevalence of PND and to identify the contributing risk factors associated with PND in the Witzenberg subdistrict of the Western Cape, South Africa.

Research methods and design

Study design

A cross sectional descriptive research design with a quantitative approach was applied in this study.

Setting

The study was conducted in four of the eight clinics in the Witzenberg subdistrict, with a population of approximately 115 946 in 2011.[21] The subdistrict under study included the five towns of Ceres, Prince Alfred Hamlet, Op-Die-Berg, Wolseley and Tulbagh, with a rural predominance and a high degree of poverty.[22]

Study population sampling strategy

The target population included mothers (N = 1605) who gave birth during one calendar year and were resident in the Witzenberg subdistrict of the Western Cape. Simple random sampling was used to select four clinics (50%), two clinics in the lower socio-economic areas and two clinics in the middle socio-economic areas. Mothers (≥ 18 years old) were selected when they brought their babies to the clinics for immunisations at 6-, 10- or 14 weeks. The researcher addressed all the mothers in a group and explained the purpose of the study and requested if there were any mothers who would willingly participate. Thus, 159 mothers, approximately 10% of the target population, were selected.

Data collection

Data were collected over a period of four months, once a week at the individual postnatal clinics identified for the purpose of the study. Data collection was done by the researcher with the help of two trained field workers with a nursing background and who were fluent in Afrikaans, English and Xhosa. The field workers were trained beforehand in the interpretation of the different questionnaires and the process of data collection. Their role was to assist with interpretation. The questionnaire was self-administered and where participants had a problem understanding any question, it was explained by the researcher or the trained field worker.

The questionnaire, based on the literature and clinical experience of the PI, was designed and administered to determine the demographical data and psychosocial risk factors of the participants. The questions specifically included aspects about: maternal age, marital status, level of education, pregnancies and children, mode of delivery, psychosocial factors, psychiatric history and social support.

The Edinburgh Postnatal Depression Scale (EPDS) was used to identify postnatal depression. The questionnaire is easy to administer and takes approximately five minutes to complete and is generally accepted by mothers after birth. The questionnaire consists of ten questions specifically about the participant's feelings over the previous seven days, including the day she was interviewed.[23]

The Beck Depression Inventory (BDI) was also used in this study to determine the severity of PND. The BDI (BDI-II),[24] created by Dr Aaron T. Beck, is a 21-question multiple-choice self-report inventory and is one of the most widely used instruments for measuring the severity of depression. Each question consists of a set of at least four possible choices, with values ranging in intensity from 0–3.[25] No values were visible on the participant's copy to minimize the risk of the participant manipulating the outcome, which may lead to answers being chosen because of its specific value. The classification to determine the severity of PND was as follows:

- Score < 15: Mild Depression
- Score 15–30: Moderate Depression
- Score > 30: Severe Depression

Reliability and validity

The EPDS and BDI are two validated, self-rating questionnaires. The authors[23] of the EPDS have shown that the 10-item Postnatal Depression Scale had satisfactory validity, split-half reliability and that it is also sensitive to changes in the severity of depression over time. The BDI is a well-known screening instrument in the mental health field. It is recommended for research, as well as in the clinical setting for its reliability and validity. The reliability and validity was further ensured through the use of experts in the fields of statistics, nursing and research methodology. The pilot study also added to the validity and reliability because all three instruments were pre-tested and rectified, where required, after the pilot study.

Data analyses

All data were analysed and interpreted with the support of a qualified statistician. A computer software program, STATISTICA,[26] was used to analyse the data. Data were expressed in frequencies, tables and histograms. The relationship between continuous response variables and nominal input variables was analysed using analysis of variance (ANOVA). Statistical associations and significance between variables were determined by using a 95% confidence interval, with a significance level of ($p \leq 0.05$).

Ethical considerations

The researchers obtained written permission from the Committee for Human Science Research at the Faculty of Medicine and Health Sciences at Stellenbosch University (ref. N09/11/336). The researchers also received written consent from the Research Coordinating Committee of the Department of Health (RP16/2010), Provincial Government of Western Cape.

Potential benefits and hazards

The researcher explained the study to all the participants individually and emphasised that their participation was voluntary, and informed written consent was obtained from all participants. The risk foreseen was the sudden breakdown of participants during the interview that may then have required counselling.

Recruitment procedures

Participants were informed that participation was voluntary and that they had a choice to withdraw from the study at any stage and that their decision would not influence any further service rendered to them.

Informed consent

Voluntary written informed consent was obtained from individual participants after providing information about the research. The ethical implications, as well as the aim and objectives for the study, were explained to each participant personally.

Data protection

Data obtained from the study was coded to protect the identities of the participants and to ensure confidentiality, anonymity and privacy concerning all information. The data is stored in a secure locked cabinet providing access to the researchers only.

Results

A total of 159 participants participated in the study of which 80 (50.3%) had PND as analysed using the EPDS test (Tables 1 and 2). The BDI test showed that of the participants (80) who had PND, 23 (28.8%) had severe depression, 39 (48.8%) moderate and 18 (22.5%) mild depression (Table 3).

Demographical and obstetrical factors

Marital status

Aspects about the marital status and depression are shown in Table 1. The majority of the participants 102 (64.2%) were unmarried and 26 (16.4%) were living with a partner (Table 1). The maternal age of participants indicated that 38 (23.9%) were teenagers, age 18–19 years, of which 19 (50%) had PND. The BDI test revealed that amongst the teenagers, 21.7% had severe depression, 20.5% had moderate and 33.3% had mild depression (Table 3).

A bivariate analysis showed that 45 (56.3%) of the participants who were unmarried, 18 (22.5%) who were married and 16 (20%) who were living with a partner suffered from depression (Table 1).

BDI inventory analysis results showed that of the unmarried participants 56.5% had severe depression (Table 3).

Pregnancies

Most of the participants 71 (44.7%) had only had one (1) pregnancy followed by 39 (24.7%) who had had two (2) pregnancies. No significant results were obtained between depression and pregnancies.

TABLE 1: Summary of demographical and obstetrical factors as classified according to the Edinburgh Postnatal Depression Scale test.

Demographical and obstetrical factors	All n = 159 (%)	Not depressed n = 79 (%)	Depressed n = 80 (%)	p-value
Marital status				
Married	29 (18.2)	11 (13.9)	18 (22.5)	$p = 0.17$
Unmarried	102 (64.2)	57 (72.2)	45 (56.3)	
Living together	26 (16.4)	10 (12.7)	16 (20.0)	
Teenagers				
Mode of delivery	38 (23.9)	19 (24.1)	19 (23.8)	$p = 0.20$ $p = 0.28$
Normal births	133 (83.7)	62 (78.5%)	71 (88.7)	
Caesarean	25 (16.3)	16 (20.5%)	9 (11.3)	
Postnatal period				
Postnatal period 4	53 (33.3)	32 (40.5)	21 (39.6)	$p = 0.05$
Postnatal period: 10 weeks	52 (32.7)	22 (27.8)	30 (57.7)	
Postnatal period: 14 weeks	54 (34.0)	25 (31.6)	29 (53.7)	
Employment				
Employed	64 (40.3)	33 (41.8)	31 (38.8)	$p = 0.04$
Unemployed	95 (59.7)	46 (58.2)	49 (61.3)	
Income				
No income	40 (25.1)	21 (26.6)	19 (23.8)	$p = 0.57$
Single income	65 (40.9)	37 (46.8)	28 (35.0)	
Family income	54 (34.0)	21 (26.6)	33 (41.3)	

TABLE 2: Factors influencing the development of postnatal depression as classified according to the Edinburgh Postnatal Depression Scale test.

Factors influencing development of PND	All n = 159 (%)	Not depressed n = 79 (%)	Depressed n = 80 (%)	p-value
Psychiatric history				
Psychiatric self-history	65 (40.9)	22 (27.8)	43 (53.8)	$p < 0.01$ $p = 0.24$
Psychiatric family history	138 (86.8)	71 (89.9)	67 (83.9)	
Life events				
Major life events	67 (42.1)	28 (35.4)	39 (48.8)	$p = 0.10$
Minor life events	39 (24.5)	23 (29.1)	16 (20)	
No life events	47 (29.6)	26 (32.9)	21 (26.3)	
Major and minor	5 (3.1)	2 (2.5)	3 (3.8)	
Minor and minor	1 (0.6)	0 (0.0)	1 (1.3)	
Partnership				
Unsatisfactory partnership	65 (40.9)	21 (26.6)	44 (55.0)	$p < 0.01$
Satisfactory partnership	94 (59.1)	58 (73.4)	36 (45.0)	
Family and social support				
Have family and social support	123 (77.4)	71 (89.9)	52 (65.0)	$p < 0.01$
Have no family and social support	36 (22.6)	8 (10.1)	28 (35.0)	
Baby factors				
Unplanned babies	96 (60.4)	54 (68.4)	42 (52.5)	$p = 0.03$
Planned babies	46 (28.9)	21 (26.6)	25 (31.3)	
Unwelcome babies	13 (8.1)	3 (3.8)	10 (12.5)	
Unwelcome sex of baby	4 (2.5)	1 (1.3)	3 (3.8)	

PND, postnatal depression.

TABLE 3: Factors influencing the development of postnatal depression showing the severity of depression levels as classified according to the Beck Depression Inventory test.

Factors influencing development of PND	Depression n = 80 (50.3%)	Mild n = 18 (22.5%)	Moderate n = 39 (48.8%)	Severe n = 23 (28.8%)	p-value
Teenager					
Yes	19 (23.8)	6 (33.3)	8 (20.5)	5 (21.7)	$p = 0.56$
No	61 (76.2)	12 (66.7)	31 (79.5)	18 (78.3)	
Marital status					
Unmarried	45 (56.3)	13 (72.2)	19 (48.7)	13 (56.5)	$p = 0.03$
Married	18 (22.5)	1 (5.6)	15 (38.5)	2 (8.7)	
Living together	16 (20)	4 (22.2)	5 (12.8)	7 (30.4)	
Widow	1 (1.3)	0 (0)	0 (0)	1 (4.4)	
Mode					
Normal	71 (88.7)	17 (94.4)	33 (84.6)	21 (91.3)	$p = 0.47$
Caesarean	9 (11.3)	1 (5.6)	6 (15.4)	2 (8.7)	
Employment					
Employed	31 (38.8)	9 (50)	15 (38.5)	7 (30.4)	$p = 0.44$
Unemployed	49 (61.2)	9 (50)	24 (61.5)	16 (69.6)	
Income					
None	19 (23.8)	5 (27.8)	8 (20.5)	6 (26.1)	$p = 0.98$
Single	28 (35)	7 (38.9)	13 (33.3)	8 (34.8)	
Family	33 (41.3)	6 (33.3)	18 (46.2)	9 (39.1)	
Psychiatric history: Family					
Family: Yes	13 (16.3)	3 (16.7)	5 (12.8)	5 (21.7)	$p = 0.06$
Family: No	67 (83.7)	15 (83.3)	34 (87.2)	18 (78.3)	
Psychiatric history: Self					
Self: Yes	43 (53.8)	7 (38.9)	19 (48.7)	17 (73.9)	$p \leq 0.01$
Self: No	37 (46.2)	11 (61.1)	20 (51.3)	6 (26.1)	
Life events					
Major	39 (48.7)	4 (22.2)	23 (59)	12 (52.2)	$p = 0.01$
Minor	16 (20)	5 (27.8)	4 (10.3)	7 (30.4)	
MN and MJ	3 (3.8)	1 (5.6)	0 (0)	2 (8.7)	
MN and MN	1 (1.3)	1 (5.6)	0 (0.0)	0 (0.0)	
No life event	21 (26.2)	7 (38.9)	12 (30.8)	2 (8.7)	
Partner relationships					
Unsatisfactory	44 (55)	3 (16.7)	20 (51.3)	21 (91.3)	$p < 0.01$
Satisfactory	36 (45)	15 (83.3)	19 (48.7)	2 (8.7)	
Baby factors					
Unplanned	42 (52.3)	11 (61.1)	20 (51.3)	11 (47.8)	$p < 0.01$
Planned	25 (31.3)	5 (27.8)	14 (35.9)	6 (26.1)	
Unwelcome	10 (12.5)	1 (5.6)	4 (10.3)	5 (21.7)	
Sex of baby unwelcome	3 (3.8)	1 (5.6)	1 (2.6)	1 (4.4)	
Family and/or social support					
Yes	52 (65.0)	15 (83.3)	28 (71.8)	9 (39.1)	$p < 0.01$
No	28 (35.0)	3 (16.7)	11 (28.2)	14 (60.9)	

Mode of delivery

The results showed that of the participants ($n = 80$) with PND 88.7% had normal births (Table 1). According to the BDI test 91.3% had severe depression and 84.6% moderate depression (Table 3).

Postnatal period 6–10–14 weeks

Table 1 shows the number of participants at the various time intervals of 6–10–14 weeks. The analysis further showed that 39.6%, 57.7% and 53.7% of the participants had PND at the particular week intervals 6–10–14 weeks respectively. A significant statistical association ($p = 0.02$) was obtained between the 6-week and 10th week periods with the Bonferroni post-hoc test. A further significant association was identified between the EPDS test and postnatal period ($p = 0.05$) (Table 1).

Employment

Results showed that 95 (59.7%) of the participants were unemployed of which 49 (61.3%) of the participants with PND were unemployed. A statistical association was identified between employment and the EPDS test ($p = 0.04$) applying the Mann-Whitney U-test (Table 1). According to the BDI test 30.4% had severe and 38.5% had moderate depression (Table 3).

Income

The results showed that 119 (74.9%) of the participants have an income whilst 40 (25.1%) have no income. A further analysis showed that of the number of participants who suffered from PND 23.8% of these participants received no income (Table 1). The BDI test revealed that the participants with only a family income 46.2% had moderate depression whilst 39.1% had severe depression. No statistical significant difference was shown between the depression and income ($p = 0.98$) (Table 3).

Factors influencing the development of postnatal depression

Psychiatric history

Table 2 shows that 65 (40. 9%) had a history of a psychiatric illness, of which 53. 8% of the participants who had PND ($n = 80$) had a history of a psychiatric illness. Using the Mann-Whitney *U*-test a statistical significant association was identified between psychiatric history of the self and depression ($p < 0.01$).

The results further showed that 83.7% of the participants with PND ($n = 80$) had no family history of psychiatric illnesses. The BDI test showed that participants with no family history 78.3% had severe depression, 87.2% moderate and 83.3% mild depression (Table 3).

Life events

The results show that 67 (42.1%) of the participants had experienced a major life event which excluded the delivery of a baby, which is a natural event. In addition, results illustrated that of the 80 participants who suffered from PND, 48.7% experienced major life events, 20% a minor event and 21 (26.3%) had no life event experiences (Table 2). According to the BDI test, participants who had a major life event 59% had moderate depression and 52.2% severe depression (Table 3).

Furthermore, the study also shows a statistical significant difference between depression and life events using the Chi square test (df = 8) = 19.95, ($p = 0.01$) (Table 3).

Partner relationship

Table 2 shows that 65 (40.9%) of participants were in an unsatisfactory partner relationship, of which 55% of the 80 participants who suffered from PND, were in unsatisfactory relationships with their partners. The BDI test shows that 91.3% of the participants had severe depression and 51.3% moderate depression. A statistical significant difference between partner relationship and the EPDS test applying the Mann-Whitney *U*-test was identified ($p < 0.01$) (Table 2) and between partner relationship and depression applying the Chi square test (df = 2) = 26.25 ($p < 0.01$) (Table 3).

Family and social support

The majority of the participants 123 (77.4%) received family and social support (Table 2). However, of the participants who suffered from PND 35% received no family or social support.

The Levene's test for homogeneity of variances effect also showed a significant difference between family or social support and the EPDS test ($p < 0.01$) (Table 2).

A statistical significant difference was shown between family and social support and depression using the Mann-Whitney *U*-test ($p < 0.01$). According to the BDI test, participants who received no family or social support (60.9%) had severe depression and 11 (28.2%) had moderate depression (Table 3).

Baby factors

The baby factors are defined as those factors associated with the baby which may have contributed to PND, namely unplanned, planned, unwelcome baby or an unwelcome sex of the baby. The majority of participants 96 (60.4%), as shown in Table 2, had unplanned babies. The results further showed that of the 80 participants who suffered from PND, 52.5% were unplanned pregnancies and 31.3% were planned babies, 12.5% were unwelcome and 3.8% were unwelcome sex of the babies. The Kruskal Wallis test further showed a significant difference between baby factors and EPDS test ($p = 0.03$) (Table 2) and between baby factors and depression ($p < 0.01$) (Table 3). However to guard against Type 1 error, a post-hoc analysis was done by applying the Bonferoni test using the BDI variable specifically to determine specific statistical differences between the baby factors. The Bonferoni test revealed a statistical significant difference between unplanned and unwelcome babies ($p < 0.01$) and between planned and unwelcome babies ($p < 0.01$). The Bonferoni test was also applied using the EPDS variable to determine any statistical differences between the baby factors but no significant associations were shown.

Discussion

Key findings

The results of this study revealed that 50.3% of the participants had PND with 48.8% of the participants with moderate PND in the Witzenberg subdistrict, a rural area of South Africa. Most participants who developed PND were affected by more than one preventable risk factor. The dominant factors contributing to PND in this rural environment were that most participants 64.2% were unmarried, of which 56.3% had PND, 55% of participants with PND were in unsatisfactory relationships, and the majority 60.4% had unplanned babies, of which 52.5% of all participants with PND were unplanned. Results have shown that teenage pregnancies in this rural environment could be problematic as 23.8% of the participants with PND were teenagers. Compounded further is that more than half of the participants 53.8% who had PND had a history of a psychiatric illness and had experienced a major life event 48.7%. This rural study also showed that

59.7% of the participants were unemployed with the majority 61.3% of the participants with PND being unemployed.

Discussion of key findings

The results of this study do not correspond to the worldwide prevalence rate of 12% – 15%, as found in many of the community surveys of postnatal depression, but is similar to a study which states that some studies have identified PND up to 60%.[27] The study revealed that 55% of the participants with PND were in an unsatisfactory relationship with their partners with a statistical significant difference between partner relationship and depression ($p < 0.01$). These results between partner relationship and PND are aligned with results of a study which found that poor quality of relationships may increase PND.[9] The lack of partner support, or closeness, or partner abuse is found in nearly one in three of the women with PND.[28] Therefore, it remains important to have a spouse or partner for protection against developing PND.[29] Teenage pregnancy contributes to the development of PND.[30] This is substantiated further in a study which confirms that pregnancy at a very young age may increase the prevalence of PND.[9] It is thus a concern that in this study 38 (23.9%) of participants were teenagers, 18–19 years of age of which 19 (50%) had PND. In this particular region under study, 142 babies were born to teenagers below the age of 18 years over a period of one year, April 2014 – March 2015,[31] which increases the risk for the development of PND amongst teenagers in this region.

Most of the participants (52.5%) with PND had unplanned babies. These results are aligned with a study[8] which identified that unplanned pregnancies contribute to maternal depression.

Poor maternal mental health is especially problematic for the infants of these mothers as it reduces the caregiver's sensitivity and responsiveness at a time when a child is entirely dependent on his or her mother's well-being.[32]

Strengths and limitations

The research was conducted in a rural subdistrict of the Western Cape, South Africa, which included five towns. A quantitative study was conducted using international validated instruments, however a phenomenological qualitative research may provide in-depth experiences about specific factors that influence the development of PND. A limitation of the study was that a convenient sample was drawn of participants who were available, met the criteria and gave voluntary consent to participate in the study. The research was conducted only in the public health services and participants were predominantly of a low socio-economic level.

Implications or recommendations

The results of this study revealed that the risk factors as discussed and identified in the Witzenberg subdistrict contributed to the development of PND. In most cases, PND can be prevented and, if diagnosed early, the level of severity and consequences of the problem may be curtailed. The recommendations are thus based on the scientific evidence obtained in this study with specific reference to preventative and promotive measures.

Early assessment

Early and holistic assessment of the pregnant women during the antenatal period should be done to identify any risk factors and clinical symptoms of depression which may necessitate early referral and/or treatment.

In-service and continuous professional development

Continuous professional development and in-service training of midwives and primary health care practitioners are recommended. Nurses should be empowered to take the appropriate measures when factors or any symptoms are identified, as supported by Tammentie et al.[33]

Nutritional supplements

The nutritional status of the patient is specifically important during the antenatal visits as the midwife needs to ensure that the mother understands the importance of a balanced diet and taking her supplements, namely ferrous sulphate and folic acid tablets. There is a strong relationship between iron status and PND.[34]

Prevention of teenage pregnancies

All stakeholders of the communities, including churches, non-governmental organisations, schools, the South African Police Services and the Departments of Education and Social Development and Health should apply a unified approach in combating social pathologies such as sexual abuse and prostitution, which contribute to the high incidence of pregnancy.

Role of the department of health

Woman's health is a priority and should be addressed as a priority to ensure healthy women and babies. Standard practices should include prenatal and postnatal classes for mothers and fathers. User-friendly clinics especially designed for teenagers have become essential.

Comprehensive school health programmes must be fully implemented at all schools, such as the 'Health Promoting Schools Initiative', and should include a healthy sexuality programme.

Further research

Qualitative research is recommended in the low-income rural areas in South Africa to obtain a better understanding of the communities' understanding of mental distress and their mental health needs. In addition, as described, a phenomenological qualitative research may provide in-depth experiences about specific factors that influence the development of PND.

Conclusion

The study has shown an extremely high prevalence of risk factors for the development of PND. Prevention, early detection, appropriate referral and treatment of PND are thus critical in managing maternal, child and family well-being.

Acknowledgements

Sincere thanks to Prof. Ethelwynn L. Stellenberg for her invaluable support and guidance throughout the study. Thank you to the Directorate of Health and Nursing Management for allowing her to do the study. Furthermore, the researchers appreciate the cooperation of the staff at the clinics and the fieldworkers during this study.

Competing interests

The authors declare that they have no financial or personal relationship(s) that may have inappropriately influenced them in writing this article.

Authors' contributions

The article 'The prevalence and factors influencing postnatal depression in a rural community' is based on the research conducted by J.M.A. and supervised by E.L.S. E.L.S (Stellenbosch University) wrote the article for publication which was reviewed by J.M.A.

References

1. Sadat Z, Abedzadeh-Kalahroudi M, Kafaei Atrian M, Karimian Z, Sooki Z. The impact of postpartum depression on quality of life in women after child's birth. Iran Red Crescent Med J. 2014;16(2):e14995. PMID: 24719747, http://dx.doi.org/10.5812/ircmj.14995
2. United Nations Development Programme. The millennium development goals: Eight goals for 2015 [homepage on the Internet]. No date [cited 2015 Apr 8]. Available from: http://www.undp.org/mdg/
3. World Federation for Mental Health. DEPRESSION: A global crisis. 20th Anniversary of World Mental Health Day, October 10 2012. Available from: http://www.who.int/mental_health/management/depression/wfmh_paper_depression_wmhd_2012.pdf
4. Mkhizei N, Kometsii MJ. Community access to mental health services: Lessons and recommendations, Ch. 7 [homepage on the Internet]. No date [cited 2015 Apr 8]. Available from: http://www.hst.org.za/uploads/files/chap7_08.pdf
5. Currò V, De Rosa E, Maulucci S, et al. The use of Edinburgh Postnatal Depression Scale to identify postnatal depression symptoms at well child visit. Ital J Pediatr [serial on the Internet]. 2009;35:32. PMID: 19863812, http://dx.doi.org/1186/1824-7288-35-32
6. Robertson E, Celasun N, Stewart DE. Risk factors for postpartum depression. In: Stewart DE, Robertson E, Dennis CL, et al., editors. Postpartum depression: Literature review of risk factors and interventions. Toronto: University Health Network Women's Health Program, 2003; p. 1–63.
7. The National Audit of the Detection and Management of Postnatal Depression Jul 2006, NAPDFinalReport_FINAL030706.pdf. www.healthcareimprovementscotland.org
8. Tomlinson M, Cooper PJ, Stein A, Swartz L, Molteno C. Post-partum depression and infant growth in a South African peri-urban settlement. Child Care Health Dev. 2006;32(1):81–86. PMID: 16398794.
9. Horowitz JA, Goodman JH. Identifying and treating postpartum depression. J Obstet Gynecol Neonatal Nurs [serial on the Internet]. 2005;34(2):264–273. PMID: 15781605, http://dx.doi.org/10.1177/0884217505274583
10. Martin A. Mom with postnatal depression kills babies [homepage on the Internet]. IOL News, World News. 2012 Oct 31 [cited 2013 Jan 15]. Available from: http://www.IOL.co.za.mht
11. Sellers PM. Midwifery: A textbook and reference book for midwives in Southern Africa. 10th ed. Lansdowne: Juta; 2008.
12. Robertson R, Allwood C, Gagiano C. Textbook of psychiatry for Southern Africa. Cape Town: Oxford University Press; 2005.
13. Fraser DM, Cooper MA. Myles textbook for midwives. 15th ed. Philadelphia: Elsevier; 2009.
14. Ramchandani PG, Richter LM, Stein A, Norris SA. Predictors of postnatal depression in an urban South African cohort. J Affect Disord. 2009;113(3):279–284. PMID: 18571734, http://dx.doi.org/10.1016/j.jad.2008.05.007
15. Moultrie A, Kleintjes S. Women's mental health in South Africa. Cape Town: Department of Psychiatry, University of Cape Town, 2005; p. 347–366.
16. Groenewald P. Annual health status report. Boland/Overberg region. Worcester: Department of Health; 2006.
17. Cooper PJ, Tomlinson M, Swartz L, et al. Improving quality of mother-infant relationship and infant attachment in socio-economically deprived community in South Africa: Randomized controlled trial. BMJ. 2009;338:b974. PMID: 19366752, http://dx.doi.org/10.1136/bmj.b974
18. Darcy JM, Grzywacz JG, Stephens RL, Leng I, Clinch CR, Arcury TA. Maternal depressive symptomatology: 16-Month follow-up of infant and maternal health-related quality of life. J Am Board Fam Med. 2011;24(3):249–257. PMID: 21551396, http://dx.doi.org/10.3122/jabfm.2011.03.100201
19. Paris R, Bolton RE, Weinberg MK. Postpartum depression, suicidality, and mother-infant interactions. Arch Womens Ment Health [serial on the Internet]. 2009;12:309–321. PMID: 19728036, http://dx.doi.org/10.1007/s00737-009-0105-2
20. Milgrom J, Gemmill AW, Bilszta JL, et al. Antenatal risk factors for postnatal depression: A large prospective study. J Affect Disord. 2008;108(1–2):147–157. PMID: 18067974, http://dx.doi.org/10.1016/j.jad.2007.10.014
21. Statistics South Africa. Census 2011: Municipal factsheet. Pretoria: Statistics South Africa; 2013.
22. Witzenberg District Municipality, Cape Winelands. Witzenberg integrated development plan 2007/2011. Witzenberg; 2007.
23. Cox JL, Holden JM, Sagovsky R. Detection of postnatal depression. Development of the 10-item Edinburgh Postnatal Depression Scale. Br J Psychiatry. 1987;150(6):782–786. PMID: 3651732, http://dx.doi.org/10.1192/bjp.150.6.782
24. Beck AT, Ward CH, Mendelson M, Mock J, Erbaugh J. An inventory for measuring depression. Arch Gen Psychiatry. 1961;4:561–571. PMID: 13688369, http://dx.doi.org/10.1001/archpsyc.1961.01710120031004
25. Beck Depression Inventory [homepage on the Internet]. No date [cited 2013 Feb 8]. Available from: http://en.wikipedia.org/wiki/Beck_Depression_Inventory#Two-factor_approach_to_depression
26. StatSoft, Inc. Statistica Data Analysis Software; version 8. 2008. Available from: http://www.statsoft.com
27. Sankapithilu GJ, Nagaraj AKM, Undaru SB, Nanjegowda RB, Nagaraja V. A comparative study of frequency of postnatal depression among subjects with normal and caesarean deliveries. Online Int J Health Allied Sci. 2010;9(2):1–5.
28. Roux G, Anderson C, Roan C. Postpartum depression, marital dysfunction, and infant outcome: A longitudinal study. J Perinat Educ. 2002;11(4):25–36. PMID: 17273318, http://dx.doi.org/10.1624/105812402X88939
29. Tannous L, Gigante LP, Fuchs SC, Busnello ED. Postnatal depression in Southern Brazil: Prevalence and its demographic and socioeconomic determinants. BMC Psychiatry. 2008;3(8):1. PMID: 18173833, http://dx.doi.org/10.1186/1471-244X-8-1
30. Allen JP, Insabella G, Porter MR, Smith FD, Land D, Phillips N. A social-interactional model of the development of depressive symptoms in adolescence. J Consult Clin Psychol. 2006;74(1):55–65. PMID: 16551143, http://dx.doi.org/10.1037/0022-006X.74.1.55
31. Ceres hospital statistics: Teenage pregnancies below the age of 18 years; April 2014–March 2015.
32. Tomlinson M, Cooper P, Murray L. The mother-infant relationship and infant attachment in a South African peri-urban settlement. Child dev. 2005;76(5):1044–1054. PMID: 16150001, http://dx.doi.org/10.1111/j.1467-8624.2005.00896.x
33. Tammentie T, Tarkka MT, Astedt-Kurki F, Paavilainen E. Socio demographic factors of families related to postnatal depressive symptoms of mothers. Int J Nurs Pract. 2002;8:240–246. PMID: 12225350, http://dx.doi.org/10.1046/j.1440-172X.2002.00373.x
34. Beard JL, Hendricks MK, Perez EM, et al. Maternal iron deficiency anemia affects postpartum emotions and cognition. J. Nutr. 2005;135(2):267–272. PMID: 15671224.

Hypertension in rural communities in Delta State, Nigeria: Prevalence, risk factors and barriers to health care

Authors:
Mary I. Ofili[1]
Busisiwe P. Ncama[2]
Benn Sartorius[2]

Affiliations:
[1]Department of Nursing Science, Delta State University, Nigeria

[2]School of Nursing and Public Health, University of KwaZulu-Natal, South Africa

Correspondence to:
Mary Ofili

Email:
isiomamary@yahoo.com

Postal address:
Department of Nursing Science, College of Health Sciences, Delta State University, Abraka, Nigeria

Introduction: Hypertension is a global health challenge and its prevalence is increasing rapidly amongst adults in many African countries. Some studies on the prevalence and risk factors of hypertension have been conducted in Nigeria, but none within Delta State. We assessed the prevalence of hypertension and associated risk factors amongst adults in three villages in the Ibusa community in Delta State, Nigeria.

Method: Homesteads were randomly selected and all consenting adults (≥ 18 years of age) were recruited for this cross-sectional study (134 individuals: 48 men, 86 women). Sociodemographic data and anthropometric measurements (weight, height and abdominal circumference) were recorded. Diagnosis of hypertension was based on blood pressure ≥ 140/90 mmHg.

Result: Hypertension prevalence in this rural community was 44%. Results from one village (Ogboli: 82%) and ethnic group (Ibo: 50%) were significantly higher than in others in the same variable category. Multivariate logistic regression analysis suggested increasing age, increasing body mass index and high salt intake as prominent risk factors for hypertension. Lack of funds and equipment shortage in clinics were most often reported as barriers to health care.

Conclusion: A nutritional education programme to promote low-cholesterol and low-salt diets is recommended to specifically target people in higher-risk areas and of higher-risk ethnicity. Local barriers to accessing health care need to be addressed.

Hypertension dans les Communautés rurales du Delta State, Nigeria: Prévalence, Facteurs de Risques et Obstacles aux Soins de Santé.

Introduction: L'hypertension est un problème de santé global dont la prévalence augmente rapidement chez les adultes de nombreux pays africains. Quelques études ont été faites sur la prévalence et les facteurs de risques de l'hypertension au Nigeria, mais aucune dans le Delta State. Nous avons examiné la prévalence de l'hypertension et les facteurs de risques connexes parmi les adultes de trois villages dans la communauté Ibusa du Delta State, au Nigeria.

Méthode: Nous avons sélectionné des maisons au hasard et tous les adultes consentants (≥ 18 ans) ont été recrutés pour cette étude transversale (134 individus: 48 hommes, 86 femmes). Nous avons enregistré les données sociodémographiques et les mesures anthropométriques (poids, taille et circonférence abdominale). Le diagnostic d'hypertension a été fait en mesurant la tension artérielle ≥ 140/90 mmHg.

Résultat: Dans cette communauté rurale la prévalence d'hypertension était de 44%. Les résultats d'un village (Ogboli: 82%) et du groupe ethnique (Ibo: 50%) étaient bien plus élevés que dans les autres de la même catégorie variable. L'analyse de la régression logistique multivariée a montré que les facteurs majeurs de risque d'hypertension sont l'âge, l'augmentation de l'indice de masse corporelle et une consommation élevée de sel. Le manque de fonds et de matériel dans les dispensaires étaient le plus souvent cités comme obstacles aux soins de santé.

Conclusion: Un programme d'éducation nutritionnelle encourageant des régimes faibles en cholestérol et pauvre en sel a été recommandé pour les gens des régions et ethnicités à haut risques. Il faudra se concentrer sur les obstacles locaux d'accès aux soins de santé.

Introduction

Hypertension, also known as high blood pressure, is one of the most common non-communicable diseases affecting a large percentage of adult individuals worldwide. The World Health

Organization (WHO) estimates that more than 30 million people in Africa present with hypertension.[1] The WHO also predicts that if the condition is not curbed by 2020, three-quarters of all deaths in Africa could be attributable to hypertension.[1] More recently, studies[2,3] have revealed that hypertension (in many African countries and rural settings) is on the increase, with estimated prevalence rates ranging between 20% and 40%.

In Nigeria, depending on the study population, type of measurement and cut-off value used for defining hypertension, the prevalence of hypertension in a rural setting ranges from 13.5% to 46.4%, compared with 8.1% – 42.0% in urban settings.[4] In three rural communities of Ife North, a local government area (LGA) of Osun State in south-western Nigeria, the prevalence of hypertension was found to be 26.4%, suggesting an increasing prevalence of the disease.[5] In Abia State, hypertension was found to be high in both rural and urban settings.[6] In the Niger Delta region of Nigeria, the prevalence of hypertension in this rural community was found to be 20.2%.[7] Studies have also reported increasing age and body mass index (BMI) (i.e. obesity) as the most strongly related risk factors associated with hypertension.[5,6,8]

Despite the various efforts and initiatives in developing countries to prevent or manage hypertension, there are still some barriers limiting optimal outcomes. These barriers can exist at the level of patients, staff or health system and administration.[9] Examples of such barriers include a lack of funding, which affects basic day-to-day operation of health care facilities, scarcity of and difficult access to health care centres in a community, staff shortages in health care centres, shortage of drugs in clinics and dispensaries, limited availability of equipment and insufficient maintenance, and insufficient patient health education and communication in clinics.[9,10,11,12]

However, most of the studies regarding the prevalence and risk factors of hypertension in Nigeria focused on urban communities or rural areas in south-western and south-eastern Nigeria. To our knowledge, no studies have yet assessed prevalence of hypertension and associated predictors or risk factors in the South-South region of Nigeria (Delta State).

Research methods and design

Study area and population

Delta State is one of six states in the oil-rich South-South region of Nigeria and consists of 25 LGAs; 10 of these are urban and 15 are rural. The study was conducted in the Ibusa community in Oshimili North LGA, one of the 15 rural LGAs (Figure 1). Ten villages form part of the Ibusa community, with an overall population of 20 166.[13] All these villages have a primary school, but only four villages have a secondary school. There are three primary health care centres (only two are functional), one general hospital and one maternal and child health centre in this community. There is no formal water supply infrastructure, although some villages have functional boreholes. The villages are linked by untarred roads and the residents are predominantly farmers and hunters. The study population comprised adult residents (18 years or older) of the Idinisagba, Umuodafe and Ogboli villages.

Study design, sampling method and sample size

An epidemiological survey (homestead to homestead) was conducted. The three villages (Idinisagba, Umuodafe and Ogboli) were randomly selected as study sites. Simple random sampling were used to select homesteads for sampling, resulting in eight homesteads being sampled in Idinisagba, ten in Umuodafe and six in Ogboli. The population across the 24 homesteads was 210, of which a final sample of 134 were eligible for inclusion and willing to participate. Of the total sample, 45 participants were from Idinisagba, 67 from Umuodafe and 22 from Ogboli.

Study procedures

The questionnaire used in the survey collected various sociodemographic data on the respondents' general health care practices and their family history of hypertension. It also contained questions related to potential risk factors associated with raised blood pressure and obstacles to health care for the management of hypertension.

Blood pressure and anthropometric measurements (weight, height and abdominal circumference) were also recorded. Blood pressure was measured using a digital automatic blood pressure monitor (OMRON MX2, Omron Health Care), which has been clinically validated to provide blood pressure readings directly comparable with those of standard mercury sphygmomanometers. A portable electronic scale (Hana, Omron Health Care) was used to measure body weight and a tape measure (Sandex Powerlock-P5NE) for height and abdominal circumference measurement. All instruments were reset to zero after individual measurements.

Body weight was recorded to the nearest 0.1 kg (after removal of shoes, heavier clothing and pocket contents). Height (without shoes and head scarf) and abdominal circumference were recorded to the nearest 0.5 cm. Abdominal circumference was measured midway between the last rib and the iliac crest and measurements ≥ 102 cm and ≥ 88 cm were regarded as indicative of abdominal obesity in male and female participants, respectively. The BMI categories used in this study were based on the WHO classification:[14,15,16]

- 18.5 kg/m^2 – 24.9 kg/m^2 regarded as normal weight
- 25.0 kg/m^2 – 29.9 kg/m^2 regarded as overweight
- ≥ 30 kg/m^2 regarded as obese.

Blood pressure was measured in the left arm, with the subject in a seated position and after at least five minutes' rest. Cuffs of an appropriate size for arm circumference were used. Three blood pressure readings were taken per subject, with at least three minutes between measurements. The average

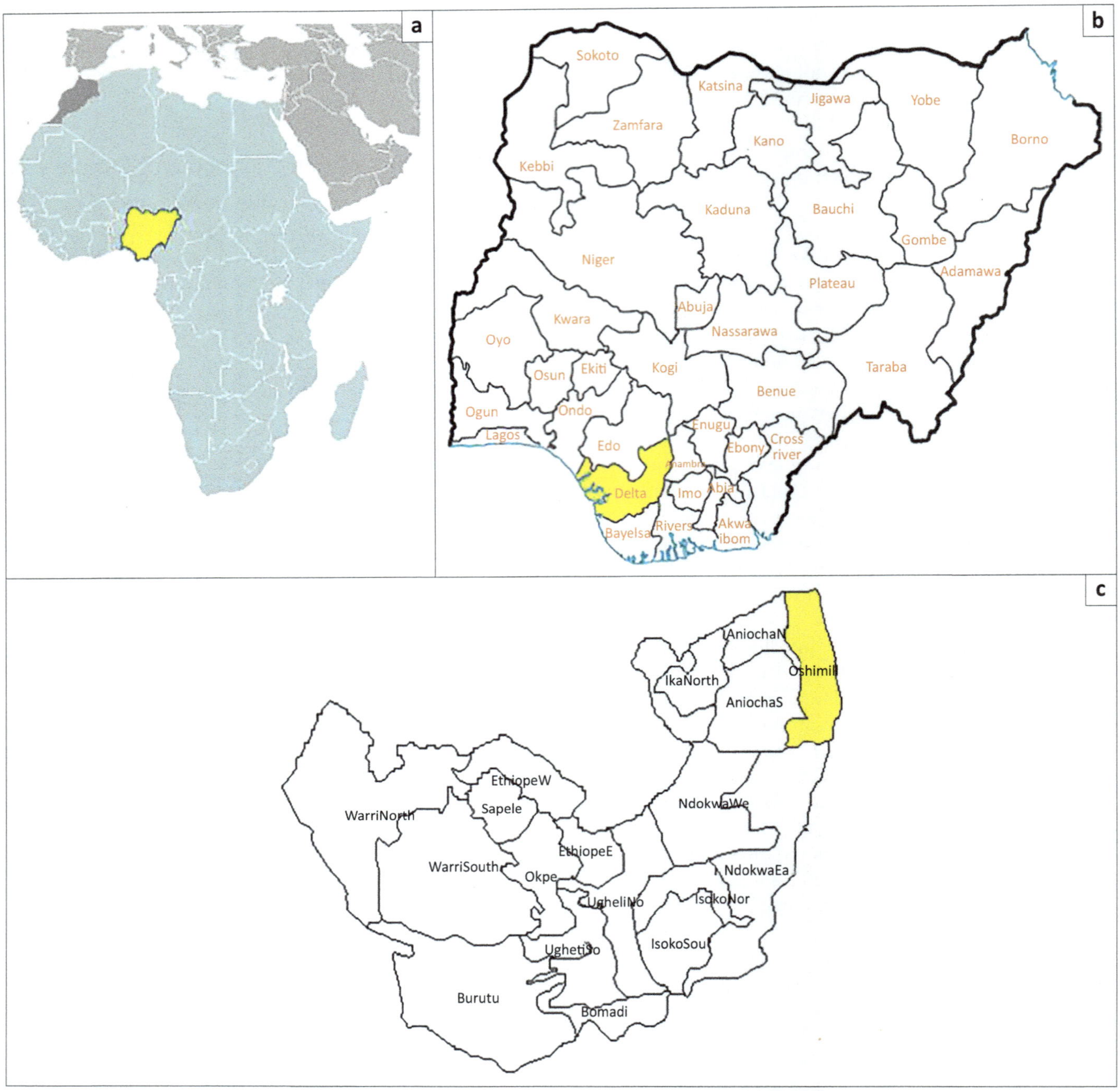

FIGURE 1: Maps of the study area and community, showing (a) location of the country (Nigeria) in West Africa, (b) the relative location of Delta State (yellow) in the southern part of Nigeria and (c) the location of the Ibusa community (yellow) in Oshimili North.

of the three readings was used in the analysis. Hypertension (stage 1) is commonly defined as a systolic pressure ≥ 140 mm Hg or diastolic pressure ≥ 90 mmHg as measured in a clinical setting,[17] together with systolic and diastolic averages exceeding 135 mmHg and 85 mmHg, respectively, during ambulatory or home blood pressure monitoring. In our study, hypertension was defined either as blood pressure measuring ≥ 140/90 mmHg or as self-reported use of anti-hypertensive medication.[18]

Data analysis

Data were processed and analysed using the statistical software package Stata (verison 13, StataCorp.). Significant associations between various explanatory variables and hypertension were assessed using the standard Pearson's chi-square (χ^2) test. If an expected cell count in the cross-tabulation had less than five observations (sparse numbers), exact methods (namely Fisher's exact test) were used instead. Bivariate and multivariate-adjusted logistic regressions were also used to assess the influence of various explanatory variables or confounders on hypertension status. Factors with a *P*-value of < 0.2 based on the bivariate associations were selected for entry into the multivariate-adjusted logistic model. An explanatory variable with an adjusted *P*-value of < 0.05 was deemed statistically significant. A goodness-of-fit test was performed to measure adequacy of the final model.

Ethical considerations

Ethical approval for this study was granted by the Humanities and Social Sciences Research Ethics Committee of the University of KwaZulu-Natal, Durban (protocol reference number: HSS/0525/013D). Gatekeeper's permission was also obtained from the ruler of Ibusa community (the Obuzor of Ibusa).

Results

Table 1 presents a summary of the characteristics of the study participants (n = 134). Half the sample (67 participants) were from Umuodafe village. The age range of respondents was between 20 and 91 years, with a mean age and standard deviation of 52.6 ± 20.6 years. The median age was 54.5 years (interquartile range: 31–72 years). More women participated in the study (86/134; 64%). The mean BMI of the sample was 25.3 kg/m^2 ± 5.9 kg/m^2 and median BMI was 24.7 kg/m^2 (interquartile range: 21.3 kg/m^2 – 27.9 kg/m^2). The majority of the participants (101/134; 75.4%) were married and all but one were Christian. Of the sample, 116 participants (87%) were from the Ibo ethnic group. More than half of the participants (78/134; 58.2%) reported secondary school or higher as their highest educational level.

TABLE 1: Characteristics of the study participants (n = 134).

Variable	Characteristic	Frequency (percentage)
Age group (years)	20–30	33 (24.6)
	31–40	10 (7.5)
	41–50	16 (11.9)
	51–60	23 (17.2)
	61–70	16 (11.9)
	71–80	30 (22.4)
	81–90	5 (3.7)
	≥91	1 (0.8)
Marital status	Single	33 (24.6)
	Married	101 (75.4)
Gender	Male	48 (35.8)
	Female	86 (64.2)
Ethnicity	Ibo	116 (86.6)
	Hausa	3 (2.2)
	Other†	15 (11.2)
Religion	Christianity	133 (99.2)
	Islam	1 (0.8)
Educational level	None or pre-school	24 (17.9)
	Primary school	32 (23.9)
	Secondary school	44 (32.8)
	Tertiary education	34 (25.4)
Village	Idinisagba	45 (33.6)
	Umuodafe	67 (50.0)
	Ogboli	22 (16.4)

†, Other ethnic groupings include Urhobo, Isoko, Ozoro, Tiv, Efik and Ibibio.

TABLE 2: Overall prevalence of hypertension in the study sample (n = 134).

Classification	Prevalence (%)
Known hypertensive patient†	34.3
Hypertension based on observed measurement‡	33.6
Hypertension based on combination of both criteria	44.0

†, Agreement between criteria (a) and (b): 79.9% or kappa score of 0.55 (moderate agreement).
‡, If hypertension was confirmed, either through self-reporting (a) or measurement during the survey (b), participants were classified as hypertensive.

The overall prevalence of hypertension in the Ibusa community was 44% (Table 2), as determined according to the reported hypertensive status or measurements during the survey.

Table 3 shows the prevalence of hypertension organised according to demographic variables. A significantly higher prevalence was seen amongst female participants than amongst male participants (52.3% vs. 29.2%; P = 0.011). Prevalence of hypertension increased significantly with age (P < 0.001), and was significantly higher in the Ogboli village (81.2%; P < 0.001) than in Idinisagba (37.8%) or Umuodafe (35.8%). Prevalence of hypertension was significantly higher amongst married individuals than amongst single participants (56.4% vs. 6.1%; P < 0.001).

In Table 4, bivariate and multivariate logistic regression analyses were used to identify risk factors associated with hypertension after adjustment for potential confounding from other variables. After multivariate adjustment, increasing age and BMI, as well as high salt intake, remained significantly associated with hypertension (P < 0.001). No significant difference in risk was found when comparing Umuodafe to Idinisagba as the reference village. However, participants from Ogboli showed markedly increased odds (risk) of hypertension compared to those from Idinisagba after multivariate adjustment (P < 0.001). Ibo ethnicity was associated with higher risk of hypertension after multivariate adjustment; however, this finding was not statistically significant at the 5% level (P = 0.062).

TABLE 3: Results of Pearson's chi-square (χ^2) analysis of prevalence of hypertension organised according to demographic variables.

Variable	Characteristic	Number of hypertensive participants (prevalence %)	P-value†
Age group (years)	20–30	0 (0.0)	< 0.001
	31–40	3 (30.0)	
	41–50	9 (56.3)	
	51–60	13 (56.5)	
	61–70	11 (68.8)	
	71–80	18 (60.0)	
	81–90	5 (100.0)	
	≥91	0 (0.0)	
Marital status	Single	2 (6.1)	< 0.001
	Married	57 (56.4)	
Gender	Male	45 (52.3)	0.011
	Female	14 (29.2)	
Ethnicity	Ibo	58 (50)	0.001
	Hausa	0 (0.0)	
	[b]Other	1 (6.7)	
Religion	Christianity	59 (44.4)	–‡
	Islam	0 (0.0)	
Educational level	None or pre-school	15 (62.5)	0.013
	Primary school	19 (59.4)	
	Secondary school	14 (31.8)	
	Tertiary education	11 (32.4)	
Village	Idinisagba	17 (37.8)	< 0.001
	Umuodafe	24 (35.8)	
	Ogboli	18 (81.8)	

†, Fisher's exact test.
‡, Not applicable, as only one individual in Islam category.

TABLE 4: Bivariate and multivariate logistic regression analyses of factors associated with hypertension.

Factor	Bivariate		Multivariate	
	OR (95% CI)	*P*	OR (95% CI)	*P*
Demographic factors				
Age	1.78 (1.43, 2.22)	< 0.001	2.03 (1.34, 3.06)	0.001
Male gender	0.38 (0.18, 0.8)	0.011	0.63 (0.19, 2.02)	0.435
Ethnicity (Ibo vs Hausa/other)	17.00 (2.19, 131.97)	0.007	19.17 (0.87, 424.17)	0.062
Educational status				
Primary school or less	1	-	1	-
Secondary school or higher	0.31 (0.15, 0.63)	0.001	0.94 (0.28, 3.24)	0.928
Marital status				
Married vs single†	20.08 (4.56, 88.48)	< 0.001	-	-
Genetic risk factors				
Hypertension in parents	0.84 (0.39, 1.8)	0.652	-	-
Family history of hypertension	1.04 (0.9, 1.21)	0.596	-	-
BMI category				
Normal	1	-	1	-
Underweight	2.10 (0.48, 9.27)	0.327	0.67 (0.07, 6.13)	0.724
Overweight	2.00 (0.89, 4.50)	0.094	4.25 (1.22, 14.83)	0.023
Obese	3.93 (1.43, 10.81)	0.008	8.17 (1.99, 33.5)	0.004
Lifestyle risk factors				
Abdominal circumference‡	1.06 (1.03, 1.09)	< 0.001	-	-
High salt intake	1.59 (0.79, 3.20)	0.193	3.43 (1.03, 11.47)	0.045
High alcohol intake	1.10 (0.55, 2.21)	0.782	-	-
Diet high in cholesterol or fat	1.78 (0.88, 3.63)	0.111	1.60 (0.54, 4.75)	0.396
Little physical activity	1.14 (0.55, 2.39)	0.72	-	-
Smoking	0.74 (0.37, 1.50)	0.406	-	-
Stress	1.24 (0.59, 2.59)	0.576	-	-
Noise	1.23 (0.61, 2.48)	0.554	-	-
Village				
Idinisagba	1	-	1	-
Umuodafe	0.92 (0.42, 2.01)	0.833	2.36 (0.74, 7.55)	0.146
Ogboli	7.41 (2.15, 25.61)	0.002	110.5 (8.74, 1397.41)	< 0.001

BMI, body mass index; CI, confidence interval; OR, odds ratio.
†, Removed from the final multivariate model owing to a high variance inflation factor (> 20).
‡, Removed from the final multivariate model owing to a high correlation (co-linearity) with BMI (Pearson correlation coefficient = 0.724; $P < 0.05$).

Table 5 shows the reported obstacles to the management of hypertension. The obstacles most frequently reported by the study participants were lack of funds (73.1%), equipment shortage in clinics (67.2%), insufficient patient health education in clinics (59.7%) and drug shortages in clinics (59.0%). Lack of public transport within the community (14.2%) was one of the least-frequently reported obstacles. Figure 2 shows the percentage of affirmative responses with regard to possible barriers to managing hypertension in descending order. Separate curves are shown for three categories of the population (overall, non-hypertensive and hypertensive).

TABLE 5: Barriers to management of hypertension reported by respondents ($n = 134$).

Barrier	Number of responses (%)
Lack of funds	98 (73.1)
Health care centres not available	30 (22.4)
Health care centres not accessible	48 (35.8)
Transport shortage within the community	19 (14.2)
Staff shortage in health care centres	31 (23.1)
Lack of communication	38 (28.4)
No social workers in clinics	20 (14.9)
Drug shortages in clinics	79 (59.0)
Equipment shortage in clinics	90 (67.2)
Late treatment supply	51 (38.1)
Equipment not in good working condition	22 (16.4)
Limited consultation rooms	20 (14.9)
Stationary shortage in clinics	18 (13.4)
Insufficient patient health education in clinics	80 (59.7)

Table 6 shows differences in the reported obstacles to the management of hypertension amongst the hypertensive patients as determined by bivariate logistic regression analysis. Equipment shortage in clinics was significantly more likely to be reported as a problem by hypertensive than non-hypertensive patients ($P < 0.001$).

Discussion

The overall prevalence of hypertension found in this study (44%) aligns with other studies in rural communities in the neighbouring West African countries.[19] However, it appears higher than the prevalence reported in rural communities in south-western Nigeria (Osun State),[5] south-eastern Nigeria (Abia State)[6] and the Niger Delta region[7] (26.4%, 22.5% and 20.2%), respectively. These differences may be attributed to the sample population used in the various studies, especially with regard to age. The higher age cut-off in this study (≥ 18 years vs. ≥ 15 years in comparative studies[4,5]) may explain the higher prevalence of hypertension, as it has been shown

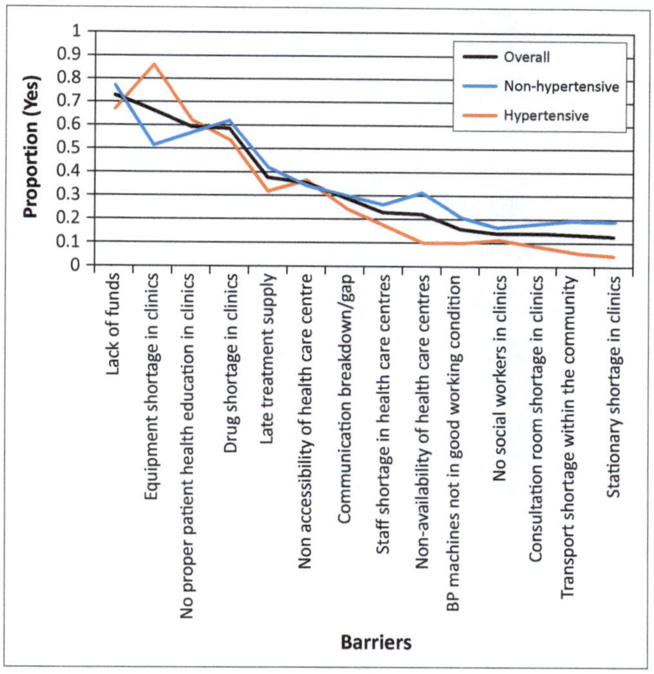

FIGURE 2: Reported barriers for management of hypertension.

TABLE 6: Differences in reported barriers to management of hypertension according to blood pressure status, as determined by bivariate regression analysis.

Barrier	OR (95% CI)	*P*-value
Lack of funds	0.62 (0.29, 1.33)	0.218
Health care centres not available	0.24 (0.09, 0.64)	0.004
Health care centres not accessible	1.12 (0.55, 2.28)	0.753
Transport shortage within the community	0.29 (0.09, 0.93)	0.037
Staff shortage in health care centres	0.63 (0.27, 1.45)	0.276
Lack of communication	0.77 (0.36, 1.66)	0.504
No social workers in clinics	0.64 (0.24, 1.73)	0.380
Drug shortages in clinics	0.71 (0.35, 1.41)	0.325
Equipment shortage in clinics	5.88 (2.46, 14.08)	< 0.001
Late treatment supply	0.64 (0.31, 1.3)	0.217
Equipment not in good working condition	0.42 (0.15, 1.14)	0.090
Limited consultation rooms in clinics	0.49 (0.18, 1.37)	0.176
Stationary shortage in clinics	0.21 (0.06, 0.78)	0.019
Insufficient patient health education in clinics	1.25 (0.62, 2.52)	0.529

CI, confidence interval; OR, odds ratio.

that blood pressure increases steadily with age, irrespective of gender.[4] There was also a markedly increased likelihood (risk) for hypertension in Ogboli village compared with other villages. This, and the overall high prevalence, may be attributed to the different cultural behaviours, for example, diets that include consumption of traditional foods such as palm kernel soup, which is a high-cholesterol food.

Beside factors that can be attributed to culture, gender, age, BMI and some lifestyle factors are well known to increase the risk for developing high blood pressure. In this study, the prevalence of hypertension was found to be higher in female participants than in male participants (29.2% vs. 52.3%), unlike findings in other studies, globally and within Nigeria, which showed a higher prevalence of hypertension in men than in women.[5,7,19] A high prevalence of hypertension in female respondents was also reported previously in a study in Abia State in south-eastern Nigeria.[6] In line with previous research,[7] our study also revealed that hypertension prevalence was significantly higher in married respondents that in unmarried individuals. The issue of family, and family burden, in relation to blood pressure cannot be over-emphasised. This may be attributed to increased responsibilities or social stresses faced by married participants.[7,20] None of the younger participants (< 30 years of age) in this study population were hypertensive. This may be because hypertension in this age demographic is biologically less common.

Multivariate logistic regression indicated a significant positive association between hypertension and increasing age, as well as BMI status (overweight or obese). In this study, age, BMI and high salt intake were the strongest predictors or risk factors for hypertension. This is consistent with findings from previous studies.[5,6,7] Increasing age, overweight and obesity are well-known risk factors for development of high blood pressure.[4,5,6,7,21,22,23,24,25,26,27] The association between high salt intake and hypertension is well established.[28] High salt intake in this study population is likely due to the local diet in these communities. Delta State is a riverine area that is rich in fish, and the main method of preservation is salting and smoking.

This study also revealed a number of obstacles to the management of hypertension. Amongst hypertensive patients, the most notable obstacle reported was equipment shortage in clinics (e.g. X-ray and echocardiography machines). These equipment shortages also place a constraint on health workers' ability to do their work properly. In comparison, studies in south-eastern Nigeria[11] and in the Limpopo province of South Africa,[9] reported financial constraints and non-compliance with treatment, lack of public transport, staff shortage, drug shortage and late treatment supply from the hospital dispensary as obstacles to managing hypertension in local health care centres.

Limitations

Determining the ages of participants was problematic as some could not remember their dates of birth or had lost their birth certificates during the Nigerian Civil War (Biafra). We used a guide sheet of important dates and historic events to estimate their ages. Given study design and sampling strategy, one should be cautious when generalising these findings (external validity) to other settings in Delta State. The findings are therefore only transferable to other settings with similar population, behavioural and economical characteristics. However, other rural settings within Delta State are likely to be similar to those in the current study, which should thus increase the external validity. Further studies should be conducted in other settings within Delta State and Nigeria to validate the findings of the current study.

Conclusion

With the overall prevalence of hypertension in rural settings ranging from 13.5% to 46.4% in Nigeria, the observed hypertension prevalence (44%) is considered high in this rural community. There was also a markedly increased risk of hypertension amongst participants from the Ogboli village compared to those from the other two villages. Our findings indicate that high blood pressure and its management are an important public health problem, even in rural African settings. In view of the scarcity of resources and facilities in many developing settings, activities aimed at controlling high blood pressure, especially in rural settings, have to compete with many other pressing health needs. However, the considerable morbidity and mortality associated with high blood pressure emphasise that measures should be taken to reduce these risk factors to improve health outcomes. This may be achieved by adopting and promoting simple and cost-effective initiatives such as body weight control and increased physical activity, reducing smoking (especially amongst rural men) and reducing salt intake. Nutritional education programmes on healthy diets (low-cholesterol and low-salt diets) organised in the community may be helpful. Health policies in community settings should give particular consideration to obstacles such as those that exist at staff and administrative levels. More intervention studies are recommended to determine the factors associated with geographical heterogeneity (higher-risk areas). This will have implications for policy makers with regard to re-directing resources for the management of hypertension in high-risk populations.

Acknowledgements

The College of Health Sciences, University of KwaZulu-Natal, Durban, and the Delta State University, Abraka (Tertiary Education Trust Fund) are acknowledged for financial support. We also thank the paramount ruler of Ibusa community (the Obuzor of Ibusa), the community leaders and the study participants who consented to participate in the survey.

Competing interests

The authors declare that they have no financial or personal relationship(s) that may have inappropriately influenced them in writing this article.

Authors' contributions

M.I.O. (Delta State University) was responsible for the conception of the study, and drafted and revised the manuscript. B.P.N. (University of KwaZulu-Natal) contributed to the conception of the study. B.S. (University of KwaZulu-Natal) performed the statistical analyses and contributed to revision of the manuscript. All authors read and approved the final manuscript.

References

1. Graziano TA. The financial burden of treating hypertension in African countries: A cost effective analysis comparing two approaches to treating hypertension in the prevention of cardiovascular disease. Yaounde: Pan African Society of Cardiology; 2005.
2. Hendriks ME, Wit FW, Roos MT, et al. Hypertension in sub-Saharan Africa: Cross-sectional surveys in four rural and urban communities. PLoS One. 2012;7(3):e32638. PMID: 22427857, http://dx.doi.org/10.1371/journal.pone.0032638
3. Ataklte F, Erqou S, Kaptoge S, Taye B, Echouffo-Tcheugui JB, Kengne AP. Burden of undiagnosed hypertension in sub-Saharan Africa: A systematic review and meta-analysis. Hypertension. 2015;65(2):291–298. PMID: 25385758, http://dx.doi.org/10.1161/HYPERTENSIONAHA.114.04394
4. Ogah OS, Okpechi I, Chukwuonye II, et al. Blood pressure, prevalence of hypertension and hypertension related complications in Nigerian Africans: A review. World J Cardiol. 2012;4(12):327–340. PMID: 23272273, http://dx.doi.org/10.4330/wjc.v4.i12.327
5. Adebayo RA, Balogun MO, Adedoyin RA, Obashoro-John OA, Bisiriyu LA, Abiodun OO. Prevalence of hypertension in three rural communities of Ife North Local Government Area of Osun State, South West Nigeria. Int J Gen Med. 2013;6:863–868. PMID: 24348064, http://dx.doi.org/10.2147/IJGM.S51906
6. Ogah OS, Madukwe OO, Chukwuonye II, et al. Prevalence and determinants of hypertension in Abia State Nigeria: Results from the Abia State non-communicable diseases and cardiovascular risk factors survey. Ethn Dis. 2013;23(2):161–167. PMID: 23530296.
7. Alikor CA, Emem-Chioma PC, Odia OJ. Hypertension in a rural community in Rivers State, Niger Delta Region of Nigeria: Prevalence, and risk factors. Nigeria Health J. 2013;13(1):18–25.
8. Spencer J, Phillips E, Ogedegbe G. Knowledge, attitudes, beliefs and blood pressure control in a community-based sample in Ghana. Ethn Dis. 2005;15(4):748–752. PMID: 16259503.
9. Sekokotla D, Steyn K, Bradshaw D, Mbananga N. Hypertension management and surveillance at primary care level: A situational analysis in the Limpopo Province. Cape Town: South African Medical Research Council; 2003.
10. Ofili MI. Prevention of high blood pressure: Nurses knowledge attitude and practice. Saarbrücken: LAMBERT Academic Publishing; 2012.
11. Okwuonu CG, Ojimadu NE, Okaka EI, Akemokwe FM. Patient-related barriers to hypertension control in a Nigerian population. Int J Gen Med. 2014;7:345–353. PMID: 25061335, http://dx.doi.org/10.2147/IJGM.S63587
12. Khatib R, Schwalm J-D, Yusuf S, et al. Patient and healthcare provider barriers to hypertension awareness, treatment and follow up: A systematic review and meta-analysis of qualitative and quantitative studies. PLoS One. 2014;9(1):e84238. PMID: 24454721, http://dx.doi.org/10.1371/journal.pone.0084238
13. National Population Commission, ICF Macro. Nigeria demographic and health survey 2008. Abuja: National Population Commission and ICF Macro; 2009.
14. World Health Organization. Physical status: The use and interpretation of anthropometry. Geneva: World Health Organization; 1995.
15. World Health Organization. Obesity: Preventing and managing the global epidemic. Geneva: World Health Organization; 2000.
16. World Health Organization. Appropriate body-mass index for Asian populations and its implications for policy and intervention strategies. Lancet. 2004;363(9403):157–163. PMID: 14726171.
17. Krause T, Lovibond K, Caulfield M, McCormack T, Williams B. Management of hypertension: Summary of NICE guidance. BMJ. 2011;343:d4891. PMID: 21868454, http://dx.doi.org/10.1136/bmj.d4891
18. National Heart, Lung and Blood Institute. Seventh report of the Joint National Committee on the prevention, detection, evaluation, and treatment of high blood pressure (JNC VII). Bethesda: National Institutes of Health; 2004.
19. Agyemang C. Rural and urban differences in blood pressure and hypertension in Ghana, West Africa. Public Health. 2006;120(6):525–533. PMID: 16684547, http://dx.doi.org/10.1016/j.puhe.2006.02.002
20. Erhun WO, Olayiwola G, Agbani EO, Omotoso NS. Prevalence of hypertension in a university community in South West Nigeria. Afr J Biomed Res. 2005;8(1):15–19. http://dx.doi.org/10.4314/ajbr.v8i1.35753
21. Kaufman J, Barkey N. Hypertension in Africa: An overview of prevalence rates and causal risk factors. Ethn Dis. 1993;3:S83–S101. PMID: 8087029.
22. Brown CD, Higgins M, Donato KA, et al. Body mass index and the prevalence of hypertension and dyslipidemia. Obes Res. 2000;8:605–619. PMID: 11225709.
23. Izzo JL, Black HR, Goodfriend TP. The essentials of high blood pressure. 2nd ed. Baltimore: Williams and Wilkins; 2001.
24. Martins D, Pan D, Karami N, Das D, Norris K. The relationship between body weight and the prevalence of isolated systolic hypertension in older subjects. J Clin Hypertens. 2000;2(4):248–252. PMID: 11416656.
25. Onwubere B. Essentials of hypertension management. Enugu: Institute for Development Studies, University of Nigeria; 2005.
26. Masaki KH, Curb JD, Chiu D, Petrovitch H, Rodriguez BL. Association of body mass index with blood pressure in elderly Japanese American men. The Honolulu Heart Program. Hypertension. 1997;29(2):673–677. PMID: 9040455, http://dx.doi.org/10.1161/01.HYP.29.2.673.
27. Tesfaye F, Nawi NG, Van Minh H, et al. Association between body mass index and blood pressure across three populations in Africa and Asia. J Hum Hypertens. 2007;21(1):28–37. PMID: 17066088, http://dx.doi.org/10.1038/sj.jhh.1002104
28. Ha SK. Dietary salt intake and hypertension. Electrolyte Blood Press. 2014;12(1):7–18. http://dx.doi.org/10.5049/EBP.2014.12.1.7

Experiences of general practitioners in the Ga-Rankuwa and Mabopane areas in dealing with patients who have sexual problems

Authors:
Benjamin Mills[1]
Indiran Govender[1]
Jannie Hugo[2]

Affiliations:
[1]Department of Family Medicine, Sefako Makgatho Health Sciences University, South Africa

[2]Department of Family Medicine, University of Pretoria, South Africa

Correspondence to:
Indiran Govender

Email:
indiran.govender@gmail.com

Postal address:
PO Box 222, Medunsa 0204, South Africa

Background: Sexual problems are common. Many patients with sexual health dysfunction use self-help literature or are often managed in general practice. However, many general practitioners (GPs) find it difficult to discuss sexual health issues because they feel uncomfortable with this and lack training in these matters. These GPs are now referring patients with sexual dysfunction to specialists.

Aim: We sought to explore how GPs working in the Mabopane and Ga-Rankuwa areas of handle sexual problems of their patients.

Setting: The setting was the Mabopane and Ga-Rankuwa areas of North-West Tshwane, in Gauteng Province.

Methods: A qualitative study comprising eight free attitude interviews with purposefully selected four male and four female GPs. All interviews were conducted in English and tape-recorded. Field notes in the form of a detailed diary was kept. The tapes were transcribed verbatim, and the transcriptions were checked against the tapes for omissions and inaccuracies.

Results: Six themes emerged from the interviews: causes of sexual problems; presentation of sexual problems to the doctor; management of sexual health problems; sex is a taboo topic; society's need for sexual health discussions, and these discussions have already begun; previous limited exposure and training, and a need for more sexual health training.

Conclusion: This study confirms earlier findings that patients could be either reluctant to discuss their problems or are open about them when presenting to doctors with sexual dysfunction. GPs were not exposed to sexual health training at medical school and, because of this shortcoming, felt that training in sexual medicine should be part of the curriculum.

Expériences des médecins généralistes dans les districts de Ga-Rankuwa et de Mabopane dans leurs rapports avec les patients qui ont des problèmes sexuels.

Contexte: Les problèmes sexuels sont courants. Beaucoup de patients souffrant de troubles sexuels utilisent des documents d'auto-thérapie ou sont souvent traités chez des généralistes. Cependant, de nombreux médecins généralistes (MG) ont du mal à discuter des problèmes de santé sexuelle car ils ne se sentent pas à l'aise pour parler de cela et n'ont pas eu de formation dans ce domaine. Ces MG envoient maintenant les patients ayant des troubles sexuels à des spécialistes.

Objectif: Nous avons essayé de déterminer comment les MG des districts de Mabopane et de Ga-Rankuwa gèrent les problèmes sexuels de leurs patients.

Lieu: Les districts de Mabopane et de Ga-Rankuwa au Nord-Ouest de Tshwane, dans la province de Gauteng.

Méthodes: Une étude qualitative comprenant huit entretiens libres avec quatre hommes et quatre femmes médecins délibérément choisis. Tous les entretiens se sont déroulés en anglais et ont été enregistrés. Des notes ont été prises sur le terrain sous forme de journal détaillé. Les bandes enregistrées ont été transcrites textuellement, et les transcriptions ont été contrôlées avec les bandes pour relever les omissions et les erreurs.

Résultats: Six thèmes sont apparus dans ces entretiens : les causes des troubles sexuels ; la présentation des problèmes sexuels au médecin; la gestion des problèmes de santé sexuelle; le sexe est un sujet tabou; la nécessité d'avoir des discussions sur la santé sexuelle dans la société et, ces discussions ont déjà commencé; exposition et formation préalables limitées, et nécessité d'avoir plus de formation en matière de santé sexuelle.

Conclusion: Cette étude confirme les résultats précédents que les patients sont soit réticents de discuter de leurs problèmes, soit en parlent librement quand ils vont chez le médecin avec des troubles sexuels. Les médecins n'ont pas eu de formation à la faculté de médecine en matière de santé sexuelle et, en raison de cette lacune, ils pensent que la médecine sexuelle devrait faire partie du programme de formation.

Introduction

In this article human sexuality refers to the integration of somatic, emotional, intellectual and social aspects of sexual being in ways that are positively enriching and that enhance personality, communication and love.[1]

Sexual problems are common at any age and in any race. The most common problems are loss of sexual drive, anorgasmia, vaginismus in women and erectile failure and premature ejaculation in men. Approximately 10% of medical outpatients experience sexual dysfunction, and this percentage is increasing.[2] In a gynaecological clinic, up to 38% of women report anxiety and inhibition during sexual activity, 16% complain of lack of pleasure and 15% have difficulties reaching orgasm.[3] Up to 40% of middle-aged men report some kind of sexual dysfunction.[4] The dysfunction may be purely psychological or physical, but is usually a combination of the two.[5] Once established, and regardless of the source, any sexual disorder is likely to induce a vicious cycle that generates anxiety, guilt, shame and fear – all of which in turn make sex even less satisfactory.

Many patients use self-help literature or are often managed in general practice.[6] An increasing number of patients are referred to urologists, gynaecologists, psychiatrists and psychologists. Specialty psychosexual services have arisen to manage sexual dysfunction.[7] This separation and specialisation sometimes deprives patients of a holistic approach to their difficulties.

Many people believe that their general practitioner (GP) is a suitable professional to whom they can confide their sexual difficulties. Attitudes towards sexuality are changing, and people expect their GP to be able to ask them about sexual problems. However, many GPs find it difficult to discuss sexual health issues because they feel uncomfortable with this and lack training in these matters.[8]

Many physical disorders and surgical procedures may lead to sexual problems.[9] Consequently, a thorough medical history and physical examination by the GP is mandatory.[2,9]

GPs have observed that, in spite of the drastic changes in public attitudes towards sexuality over recent years, many people still find it embarrassing to talk honestly about sexuality. Some sexual problems are covertly presented in the form of either emotional or psychological symptoms (such as depression or request for a change of contraceptive pill, or reporting of a vaginal discharge). There are some sexual problems that can be presented directly to the GP, such as sexually transmitted infections and fear of HIV infection.[9]

GPs report that details of the sexual values, ideas and behaviour of the client are important, but useful only if sought in a non-judgemental fashion. A thorough description of the sexual difficulty and interpersonal circumstances surrounding it is essential. The specific language chosen by the doctor to discuss the problem should reflect the patient's level of understanding. It is sometimes beneficial to reassure the reticent, anxious patient of the confidentiality of doctor-patient communication. Preferences as to activities and partners should be explored, including both homosexual and heterosexual experiences.[2]

Referral is indicated when severe underlying psychopathology is suspected, marital discord is very serious, the patient is unwilling, or unable, to cooperate, or couple-directive sexual therapy undertaken by the GP has failed.[2] Educational sessions are best conducted with both partners present because this improves mutual understanding and communication.[1]

In some countries there are institutions for research and teaching in sexology within the universities, which GPs can attend.[1] Britain's Royal Colleges view sexual medicine as an important part of training, but there is little consistency about the quality or duration of such training.[10] In South Africa there has been no substantial change in the training of GPs, although a World Health Organization report in 1975 emphasised the need for health professionals to be trained in human sexuality.[1]

In order to develop a better understanding of problems of human sexuality it is necessary for GPs to develop healthy attitudes to sexuality, marriage and contraception. In turn, he or she can transmit this assurance to those clients who seek help for what they consider to be abnormal behaviour in themselves or their partners.[1]

In order to approach the topic with confidence, the GPs must have accurate scientific knowledge regarding the facts of human reproduction and human sexuality; they must know what common sexual problems are and how to deal with them, and must know when the solution to a problem is beyond their ability and requires referral to a specialist.[1] To enhance their ability to help people with sexuality problems it is essential for GPs to develop their skills in communication.[1]

Other health professionals, besides GPs, that need to be educated and trained in this arena include undergraduate and postgraduate medical students, social workers, psychologists, teachers and marriage counsellors, because they come into contact with individuals with sexual health issues. An interdisciplinary approach is needed for training the GP to include psychology, psychiatry, gynaecology, urology, paediatrics, nursing, social work and health education.[1] Human sexuality should be developed as an autonomous discipline in the training of health professionals and become a recognised component of general health services, particularly family health.[1]

The aim of this study was to find out how GPs working in the Mabopane and Ga-Rankuwa areas of Gauteng Province, South Africa, handle sexual problems in their patients.

Research methods and design

Study design

A qualitative study using free attitude technique interviews.

Setting

The study was conducted in Ga-Rankuwa and Mabopane, two large black townships, 32 km north-west of Pretoria, South Africa. These two areas were previously part of the former Bophuthatswana and mainly Tswana speaking. Amongst these Tswana people could be found the Sotho, Shangaan, Nguni (Xhosa and Zulu) and Venda people.

Study population and sampling strategy

All 45 private GPs working in the Ga-Rankuwa and Mabopane areas constituted the population. Purposeful sampling was carried out, and eight free attitude interviews with four male and four female GPs were conducted. Purposeful sampling technique was used because the logic and power of purposeful sampling lies in selecting information-rich cases for study in depth.

All the private general practitioners (GPs) working in the Ga-Rankuwa and Mabopane areas were contacted telephonically. Three were not willing to participate in the study. The researcher interviewed doctors until data saturation was reached. The criteria for enrolment were:

- equal number of males and females;
- equal number of doctors with less than, or more than, 8 years' experience.

Data collection and analysis

The free-attitude technique was used. The technique develops the crucial attitude that Smaling refers to as 'open mindedness's'.[11] The free attitude technique was used for all the eight participants.

The interview began with the researcher giving some short information about himself and the frame of reference of the interview. The exploratory question was the only question asked which was formulated in an open-ended way so that it did not contain any suggestion. The researcher facilitated the interview by using the techniques of summarisation, reflection and clarification. The exploratory question used in the interviews was: 'How do you handle sexual health problems amongst your patients?' Each interview took between 30 to 45 min. The interviews, which were conducted by BM, were conducted in the practice of the GPs. All of the interviews were held in English.

All of the interviews were tape-recorded. Field notes in the form of a detailed diary were taken by the researchers. These were discussed daily with the other researchers. The tapes were transcribed verbatim, and the transcriptions were checked against the tapes for any omissions and inaccuracies. Each interview took an average of eight hours to transcribe. Three photocopies of each of the transcripts were made, and the master copy was kept untouched. Each transcript was reread several times by the researchers to ascertain what the interviewee said. The researchers read through all the field notes and interviews and made comments in the margins. Paper notes were attached containing the interviewers' comments about how the data could be utilised. The cut and paste technique was used to finally organise the data into the themes that emerged from the interviews so that nothing was lost. The field notes of each interview were read together with the corresponding transcript to help the researchers to organise the data into themes and sub-themes.

Trustworthiness

To aid in the trustworthiness and rigour of the research, the authors implemented various constructs as proposed by Lincoln and Guba. Although reliability and internal validity of qualitative research is often questioned, the use of trustworthiness is generally accepted as a means to remedy this issue.[12] This construct consists of credibility, transferability, dependability and conformability.

Credibility, also known as internal validity in quantitative research, refers to a study measuring what it has intended to measure.[13] For this study, the authors implemented triangulation in the process of data collection. Triangulation from two sites in Tshwane, Mabopane and Ga-Rankuwa was implemented. According to Shenton,[12] when similar results are observed from different sites the credibility of the study is increased. Also, to improve trustworthiness and triangulation of the observations purposeful sampling from an equal number of male and female GPs, and an equal number of doctors with more or less than 8 years' experience was conducted. Here the authors sought to improve credibility by having a range of demographic characteristics of participants to assist in the representativeness of the sample. Another key aspect of the credibility of this study was an intention to improve the honesty of the information provided by the participants. In order to address this, participants were allowed opportunities to withdraw from the study. Participants were informed verbally and in writing (in the informed consent document) about the research and that they could withdraw from the study at any point in time.

The authors also attempted to improve credibility by having regular discussions and debriefing sessions with the interviewer and the other researchers. The interviewer also underwent the same interview process with fellow researchers to identify flaws and potential interviewer bias. These interviews amongst fellow researchers were used to clarify interview questions, prompts and individual biases. The authors referred to this as self-clarification. The authors hoped that conducting interviews with the researchers before the interviews would sensitise the authors to possible personal bias and opinions. These could then be reduced.

Nomsa Malete (NM), previously employed by Medunsa as a research and teaching assistant, was an external expert who verified the transcription, themes, and analysis of the data. The external expert researcher checked the analysis and confirmed the accuracy of the information of the transcripts and themes obtained. The themes subsequently identified were discussed with the participants (this provided respondent validation and/or member checks), NM and co-researchers. Reflexivity, which refers to the researcher's awareness of the self as a research instrument,[13] was achieved by the researchers conducting free attitude interviews on one another to minimise, or at least become aware of, their own prejudices, viewpoints or assumptions regarding the phenomena under investigation.[13] Free attitude interviewing cannot always provide accurate responses on sensitive issues. To reduce the potential of this occurring, it was hoped that in the individual interview method (as opposed to a group discussion) participants may have felt more comfortable to discuss sensitive issues where privacy, anonymity and confidentiality may be assured. Field notes in the form of a research diary and the audio tapes, which were transcribed verbatim, were used to verify the information recorded.

Confirmability, which describes the objectivity of the study,[12,13] was addressed by providing detailed information regarding the research method used in the selection of participants, questions posed in the interviews and reasons for this research methodology. This enables other researchers to make informed decisions about this study. The study also provides a basis on which other researchers can replicate it. Along with this, the researchers have provided verbatim quotes from the participants' narratives to indicate that these were not altered in any way.

Ethical considerations

Informed written consent was obtained from all the participants, and they were assured of confidentiality and anonymity. Code names were used from the transcription phase onwards to make recognition of individual participants impossible. Ethical clearance was obtained from Medunsa Research and Ethics Committee.

Results

The characteristic profile of the eight participants are summarised in Table 1. The age group of the participating GPs ranged from 30 to 47 years.

Themes

There were six themes that emerged from the transcripts as follows: causes of sexual problems; presentation of sexual problems to the doctor; management of sexual health problems; sex is a taboo topic; society has a need for sexual health discussions, and these discussions have already begun; previous limited exposure and training, and a need for more sexual health training.

The causes of sexual problems

All doctors, except one, stated that organic or non-organic problems could cause sexual problems. The doctors mentioned sexually transmitted diseases, diabetes mellitus and some drugs can, as a side effect, result in sexual problems. Non-organic problems were related to psychological conditions. The participants stated that sexual problems affect almost everyone in one way or another. The need to take a good history to determine the cause of the sexual problem was emphasised. Quotes from participants to support this theme are:

> 'Psychological or organic problems cause sexual problems.' (NM, female, 42 years old)
>
> 'Find what could have led to the cause of the sexual dysfunction by going into the history, checking the treatment and checking for stress factors.' (MM, female, 41 years old)
>
> 'Nobody is exempted when it came to sexual problems.' (PP, male, 30 years old)
>
> 'Sexual problems could emanate from psychological problems and organic problems like diabetes and side-effects of antihypertensive and antipsychotic drugs.' (MG, female, 37 years old).

Presentation of sexual problems to the doctor

All the doctors spoke about how patients with sexual problems presented to them, but there were variations in the way patients presented them depending on the demographic characteristics (e.g. gender, age) of the doctor, the patient and the actual sexual problem. Patients were more comfortable with older and same-sex doctors. Quotes from participants to support this theme are:

> 'Patients were reluctant to talk about their sexual problems but sometimes a female would have difficulties relating the problems, but with a little bit of encouragement she may cry and then after she would pour out everything.' (PM, male, 35 years old)

TABLE 1: Profile of participants.

Participant number	Age (yrs)	Sex	Years of practice	Feels that patients are reluctant to discuss sexual problems	Personally feels that sex is a taboo subject	Never exposed to training for sexual problems	Feels there is a need for training
1	35	M	< 8	Yes	N/S*	Yes	Yes
2	37	F	< 8	N/S	Yes	Yes	Yes
3	42	F	> 8	Yes	Yes	N/S	N/S
4	41	F	> 8	Yes	N/S	N/S	Yes
5	36	M	< 8	N/S	Yes	Yes	Yes
6	30	M	< 8	Yes	Yes	N/S	Yes
7	47	M	> 8	N/S	No	Yes	Yes
8	46	F	> 8	N/S	N/S	N/S	N/S

*, N/S, Not mentioned.

'Male patients are reluctant to present to me because I am a woman doctor but I tell men to forget that I am a female doctor and just present the problem.' (MM, female, 41 years old)

'Females are more open to female doctors.' (NM, female, 42 years old)

'I see more male patients than females because there was that belief that male patients thought they were better understood as to what was happening if seen by a male doctor.' (PM, male, 35 years old)

'Patients are shy about sexual diseases and they use other terms. Older males present infection to me because they understood that I am a male. Older females do not open to me because I am a young male doctor.' (PP, male, 30 years old)

'Some patients are frank about it whilst others are shy.' (JM, female, 46 years old)

'Some females present on behalf of their partners saying that they have no interest in sex anymore.' (MM, female, 41 years old)

'A lot of patients have sexual problems and they either present directly or in an indirect way.' (MG, female, 37 years old)

The management of sexual health problems of the participants

Almost all the participants (seven out of eight) expressed difficulties in approaching and managing sexual health problems. They found it easier to manage organic problems such as sexually transmitted diseases. They were uncomfortable in managing sexual problems of a psychological nature and commonly referred patients with these problems to specialists. To satisfy the patients and to ensure that they do not lose these patients from their practice, these doctors also gave placebo vitamin injections to the patients. Quotes from participants to support this theme are:

'Sexual problems are not easy to handle.' (PP, male, 30 years old)

'Sexual problems were a big problem for me in the past but currently I sit and listen to patients and refer to books and journals when nothing seems to fit.' (MM, female, 41 years old)

'I give them injection or Vit B Co or refer them to specialists such as urologists.' (PP, Male, 30 years old)

'I do feel guilty about the way I manage these problems and all GPs are doing the same thing and I see this kind of practice as "survival of the fittest."' (PM, male, 35 years old)

'I refer some patients to the psychologist if there is a stress element involved or to the urologist if there was a surgical problem.' (JM, female, 46 years old)

'I use diplomacy to appease patients as I do not know what is happening' (TK, male 46 years old)

'I manage patients by going into the sexual pattern or habits do basic examination and educate, before considering the need for investigation.' (NM, female, 42 years old)

'When nothing seems to fit, I give them an appointment date and go look up in books and journals. Also I refer these patients to urologist and psychologists and get feedback from these specialists.' (MG, Female, 37 years old)

Sex is a taboo topic

The participants felt that sex is not a topic patients or people in general would like to talk about openly. The African culture was stated as one of the reasons why people feel sex and sexual health is taboo. It was felt that parents do not talk to their children about sex, and people do not even talk openly about sex and sexual problems with their friends. Quotes from participants to support this theme are:

'Sex is treated like a taboo among African people and these people don't talk sex just like that. And no, parents will not talk to a boy or a girl directly that you are not supposed to do that because of this and that, because it is treated like a hush subject.' (MG, female, 37 years old)

'Sex is treated like a taboo and there is no openness.' (JM, female, 46 years old)

Society has a need for sexual health discussions, and these discussions have already begun

The participants stated that the radio, sexual health talk shows on television and explicit publications on sex in magazines has made sex something nowadays to be openly talked about in a healthy way. Adolescent children are also discussing sex nowadays. This has put pressure on doctors to discuss and become comfortable with sexual health issues. Quotes from participants to support this theme are:

'A lot of open-mindedness of the whole community actually from home to schools, to churches is seen these days.' (PP, male, 30 years old)

'There was a lack of communication as far as sex was concerned and that has led to other problems like sexually transmitted diseases, pregnancies and infertilities. If many people open up it would be easy for one to detect problems and be treated accordingly.' (JM, female, 46 years old)

'Sex talk shows on radio and TV and people like Dr Ruth and Dr Paul and many others have made sex something to be openly talked about in a more healthy way.' (EK, male, 47 years old)

'Sex in the past was confined to adults but now adolescents must be included in sex education because children as young as 13 and 14 are sexually active and it has to be accepted and they have questions of their own.' (TK, male, 46 years old)

'Patients have information through TV, magazines, newspapers, radio and internet.' (MM, female, 41 years old).

Need for more sexual health training

Participants stated that they were never exposed to sexual health training at medical school and therefore expressed a need for training in this field. They suggested that training could be in the form of literature or workshops. Training should be given at the undergraduate or postgraduate levels. Also, they mentioned that a family practice journal should include 'the approach to such sexual health conditions' (MG, female, 37 years old). They felt their feeling of inadequacy and low confidence in managing these problems stems largely from a lack of training. Quotes from participants to support this theme are:

'In my clinical training, you could be told by trainers while in the wards that there was somebody with hepatomegaly or whatever but never would you be shown anybody with sexual problems.' (PM, male, 35 years old)

'I have no proper experience of how to handle sexual problems.' (PP, male, 30 years old)

'There was never a period where we were exposed to such situations, especially at medical school, and how to deal with such problems. The family practice curriculum and journal should include the approach to such conditions.' (MG, female, 37 years old)

'We are not really exposed at medical school and even outside.' (TK, male, 46 years old)

'It is a very difficult field we still need to know more about.' (MM, female, 41 years old)

'Any type of training will be needed either in the form of literature, workshops or undergraduate or postgraduate training.' (EK, male, 47 years old)

'I was not trained in counselling and stuff like that.' (TK, male, 46 years old)

'Listening, giving information and education could solve the problem but I lack the proper skills.' (NM, female, 42 years old)

'I am puzzled why the medical institutions did not look at the issue of sexual health problems.' (JM, female, 46 years old)

Integration of themes

The way in which the various themes can be integrated and related to each other is shown diagrammatically in Figure 1.

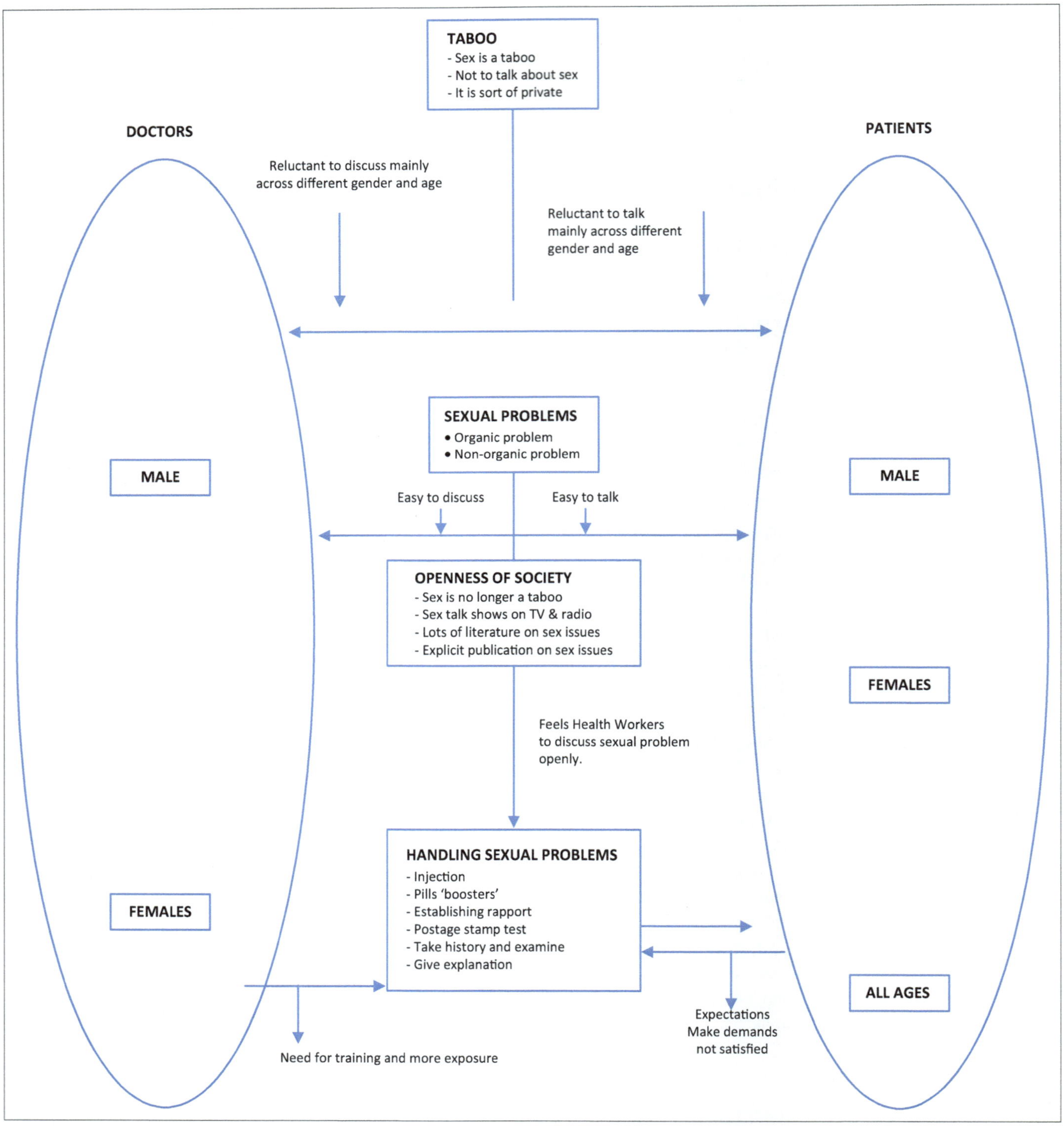

FIGURE 1: Integration of the themes between the general practitioners and their patients that emerged from the data.

The doctors perceived that patients were reluctant to consult them about their sexual problems. Most of the doctors stated that they were not exposed to sexual health problems at medical school and felt a need for more information and training in this area. Some of the doctors still felt that sex is a taboo topic.

Discussion

The results indicate that doctors did not manage their patients with sexual problems according to evidence-based guidelines. In the case of non-organic problems, the GPs prescribed vitamin tablets, vitamin B complex injections and hormones. However, vitamins are not recommended, and one would seldom prescribe hormones because giving testosterone is contra-indicated in prostatic carcinoma, which may be undetected. Assessment of serum testosterone may be a useful investigation before prescribing testosterone,[14] but none of the doctors mentioned this test. In Portugal, too, most GPs do not consult the guidelines about diagnosis and treatment of sexual dysfunction.[15]

About 90% of sexual health problems are psychological in origin, but it is essential not to overlook medical problems such as diabetes mellitus.[2,16] In the doctors' management of sexual problems with psychological causes, no mention was made about excluding diabetes mellitus.

Explicit sexual education, which is an important first step in managing sexual disorders, is not being undertaken by the doctors. Directive sexual therapy was not cited, which is indicated if a psychological basis for the dysfunction is discovered, or if adequate treatment of an underlying medical condition fails to fully alleviate the difficulty. No mention of directive sex therapy was made by the GPs as one of the ways to manage non-organic sexual problems.

No doctor said anything about making use of the 'squeeze' technique in patients with premature ejaculation. Although this technique is controversial it is still widely used by experts in the field.[17,18] The treatment of vaginismus often includes the use of graduated dilators, but none of the doctors mentioned this. The doctors also did not state how they treated orgasmic dysfunction, where particular emphasis is placed upon instructing the woman in techniques of self-stimulation. In dyspareunia, the stage of intromission is gradually negotiated in many small steps and the couple is instructed to use copious amounts of artificial lubricant, but nothing was said by the GPs with regard to this type of treatment. Doctors said sexual problems could be caused by smoking and the use of alcohol, but they never stated that they would ask these patients to stop smoking and taking alcohol.

Most of the patients with non-organic sexual problems were referred by the GPs to gynaecologists, psychiatrists, urologists or psychologists. However, the primary care physician should be able to handle most of non-organic sexual problems.[2] Referral is indicated when: (1) severe underlying psychopathology is suspected; (2) marital discord is very serious; (3) directive sexual therapy has been undertaken by the primary care physician.[2] Nobody mentioned the use of Viagra, which is effective in patients with erectile dysfunction due to diabetes mellitus or atherosclerosis, and after radical prostatectomy and spinal cord injury.[15]

It could be argued that the way in which these GPs managed sexual problems was affected by their thinking about sexual issues. The doctors who felt that sex is a taboo topic were reluctant to enquire into patients' sexual values, ideas and behaviour, which are very important.[2] There is strong evidence that GPs do not discuss sexually related issues as often as patients would like. One important enquiry that GPs need to make is to ascertain what actually happens (and what does not happen) during sexual activity. Most GPs do not address sexual health issues proactively with patients, and this needs attention.[19]

The doctors who felt that discussions about sex are out in the open could discuss sexual issues with the patients. Research has shown that taking a detailed sexual history and making a risk assessment are key skills for making a diagnosis and care plan. There are sensitive questions that the GP must ask so as to obtain a correct sexual history and determine the further management of the patient.[20]

Most of the doctors said they were never exposed to sexual problems at medical school and this could explain their difficulty in handling sexual problems. They felt they needed training in sexual problems to help them handle sexual problems in their patients. Lack of training, knowledge or education of GPs about sexual dysfunction has been reported to be the most important barrier faced by them when dealing with sexual dysfunction.[21] GPs in other countries have also stated that their training for their medical degree was inadequate when it comes to sexual health problems amongst patients.[22] Besides the United Kingdom and Portugal, research in Australia has also pointed out the need for developing, improving and evaluating strategies to improve the management of sexual health problems by GPs.[6] Some countries in Europe have identified sexual health as a priority public health area and, given the need indicated by the GPs in this study, and the country's national HIV and/or AIDS epidemic, South Africa also needs to follow this model.[23]

Limitations

All participants were black GPs working in Ga-Rankuwa and Mabopane, hence these results may not reflect findings of GPs with other race groups.

The researchers aimed, not for generalisability, but for transferability through a rich description of the experiences of GPs of patients with sexual health problems in the context of urban black townships.

Recommendations

Since doctors were not able to manage problems because of their lack of training at medical school, it is recommended that sexual medicine should become part of the curriculum at medical school. Firstly, this should include how to take a sexual history and, secondly, once a sexual problem is uncovered how to manage it. This study could be used as a pilot for a larger multicentre study.

Conclusion

The eight GPs in this study did not manage sexual problems according to recommendations in the literature. This study confirms earlier findings that patients could be either reluctant or open to discussing sexual problems when presenting to doctors. The reason for this could be either cultural or the openness of current society, as indicated by the GPs. These GPs were not exposed to sexual health training at medical school and, because of this shortcoming, the GPs felt that there is a need for training in sexual medicine, which should be part of the curriculum at medical school.

Acknowledgements

The researchers would like to acknowledge the valuable assistance of Ms Nomsa Malete (NM) in serving as an external moderator and quality assurance expert in this research.

Competing interests

The authors declare that they have no financial or personal relationship(s) that may have inappropriately influenced them in writing this article.

Authors' contributions

B.M. thought of the research question, and was involved in the protocol write up, data collection and analyses of the data. I.G. was involved in the research idea, data analysis, research article write-up, editing the final article and attending to the reviewers' comments. J.H. was involved in the protocol development, data collection and analysis.

References

1. World Health Organization. Education and treatment in human sexuality: The training of health professionals (Technical Report Series no. 572). Geneva: World Health Organization; 1975.
2. Barsky AJ. Approach to the patient with sexual dysfunction. Primary Care Medicine. Philadelphia: Lippincott Company; 1981.
3. Rosen RC, Taylor JF, Leiblum SR, Bachmann GA. Prevalence of sexual dysfunction in women: Results of a survey study of 329 women in an outpatient gynecological clinic. J Sex Marital Ther. 1993;19:171–188. PMID: 8246273, http://dx.doi.org/10.1080/00926239308404902
4. American Urological Association. Management of erectile dysfunction [homepage on the internet]. 2007 [cited 2014 Aug 21]. Available from: http://www.auanet.org/content/guidelines-and-quality-care/clinical-guidelines.cfm
5. Crowe M, Jones M. Sex therapy: The success, the failure, the future. Br J Hosp Med. 1992;48:474–482.
6. Freedman E, Britt H, Harrison CM, Mindel A. Sexual health problems managed in Australian general practice: A national, cross sectional survey. Sex Transm Infect. 2006;82:61–66. PMID: 16461607, http://dx.doi.org/10.1136/sti.2005.016931
7. Kellet J. Functions of a sexual dysfunction clinic. Int Review Psychiatry. 1995;7:183–190. http://dx.doi.org/10.3109/09540269509028325
8. Ross MW, Channon-Little LD. Discussing sexuality – A guide for health practitioners. Sydney: Mactennan & Petty; 1991.
9. Hawton K, Oppenheimer C. Sexual problems. In: McPherson A, editor The South African women's health book. Cape Town: Oxford University Press, 1996; p. 339–375
10. Lewin J, King M. Sexual medicine. Towards an integrated discipline. BMJ. 1997;314:1432. http://dx.doi.org/10.1136/bmj.314.7092.1432
11. Smaling G. Course material for the qualitative methodology. Summer school. Pretoria: HSRC; 1993 (Unpublished).
12. Shenton AK. Strategies for ensuring trustworthiness in qualitative research projects. EFI. 2004;22(2):63–75.
13. Mabuza LH, Govender I, Ogunbanjo GA, Mash B. African primary care research: Qualitative data analysis and writing results. Afr J Prm Health Care Fam Med. 2014; 6(1):Art. #640, 5 pages. PMID: 26245437, http://dx.doi.org/10.4102/phcfm.v6i1.640
14. Schmidt AC. Erectile dysfunction – Management in general practice. CME. 2000;10(3):424–428.
15. Ribeiro S, Alarcão1 V, Augusto A, Filipe LM, Mário C, Alberto G. General practitioners' knowledge, perceptions and barriers in the management of sexual dysfunction. Lisbon: Institute of Preventive Medicine, Faculty of Medicine, University of Lisbon; 2011.
16. Ellis C. Essential CME. J SA Fam Physician. 1995;16:537–553.
17. Byers, ES., Grenier, G. Premature or rapid ejaculation: Heterosexual couples' perceptions of men's ejaculatory behavior. Arch Sex Behav. 2003;32:261–270. PMID: 12807298, http://dx.doi.org/10.1023/A:1023417718557
18. *McCarthy* B, *Fucito* L. Integrating medication, realistic expectations, and therapeutic interventions in the treatment of male sexual dysfunction. J Sex Marital Ther. *2005*;31:319–328. PMID: 16020149, http://dx.doi.org/10.1080/00926230590950226
19. Gott M, Galena E, Hinchliff S, Elford H. "Opening a can of worms": GP and practice nurse barriers to talking about sexual health in primary care. Fam Pract. 2004;21(5):528–536. PMID: 15367475, http://dx.doi.org/10.1093/fampra/cmh509
20. Young F. How to take a sexual history. J Fam Health Care. 2005;15(5):149–151. PMID: 16315683.
21. Humphery S, Nazareth I. GP's views on their management of sexual dysfunction. Fam Pract. 2001;18(5):516–518. PMID: 11604374, http://dx.doi.org/10.1093/fampra/18.5.516
22. De Berardis G, Pellegrini F, Franciosi M, et al. Management of erectile dysfunction in general practice. J Sex Med. 2009;6:1127–1134. PMID: 19138378, http://dx.doi.org/10.1111/j.1743-6109.2008.01093.x
23. Lawrence M, Carey, JC. Sexual health assessment. InnovAiT. 2012;5:154–158. http://dx.doi.org/10.1093/innovait/inr135

Trends in task shifting in HIV treatment in Africa: Effectiveness, challenges and acceptability to the health professions

Authors:
Talitha Crowley[1]
Pat Mayers[2]

Affiliations:
[1]Department of Interdisciplinary Health Sciences, Stellenbosch University, South Africa

[2]Department of Health and Rehabilitation Sciences, University of Cape Town, South Africa

Correspondence to:
Talitha Crowley

Email:
tcrowley@sun.ac.za

Postal address:
PO Box 241, Cape Town 8000, South Africa

Background: Task shifting has been suggested to meet the demand for initiating and managing more patients on antiretroviral therapy. Although the idea of task shifting is not new, it acquires new relevance in the context of current healthcare delivery.

Aim: To appraise current trends in task shifting related to HIV treatment programmes in order to evaluate evidence related to the effectiveness of this strategy in addressing human resource constraints and improving patient outcomes, challenges identified in practice and the acceptability of this strategy to the health professions.

Method: Electronic databases were searched for studies published in English between January 2009 and December 2014. Keywords such as 'task shifting', 'HIV treatment', 'human resources' and 'health professions' were used.

Results: Evidence suggests that task shifting is an effective strategy for addressing human resource constraints in healthcare systems in many countries and provides a cost-effective approach without compromising patient outcomes. Challenges include inadequate supervision support and mentoring, absent regulatory frameworks, a lack of general health system strengthening and the need for monitoring and evaluation. The strategy generally seems to be accepted by the health professions although several arguments against task shifting as a long-term approach have been raised.

Conclusion: Task shifting occurs in many settings other than HIV treatment programmes and is viewed as a key strategy for governing human resources for healthcare. It may be an opportune time to review current task shifting recommendations to include a wider range of programmes and incorporate initiatives to address current challenges.

Tendances dans le transfert de tâches dans le traitement du VIH en Afrique : efficacité, défis et acceptabilité relatifs aux professions de la santé.

Contexte : On a suggéré que le transfert de tâches pouvait répondre à la demande en matière de début de traitement et de prise en charge de davantage de patients sous traitement antirétroviral. Bien que l'idée du transfert des tâches ne soit pas nouvelle, elle acquiert une nouvelle importance dans le contexte de la prestation de soins de santé actuelle.

But : Estimer les tendances actuelles en matière de transfert des tâches lié à des programmes de traitement du VIH afin d'évaluer les preuves de l'efficacité de cette stratégie dans le traitement des contraintes en termes de ressources humaines et dans l'amélioration des résultats des patients, de déterminer les défis identifiés dans la pratique et le caractère acceptable de cette stratégie pour les professions de la santé.

Méthode : Des bases de données électroniques ont été recherchées pour trouver des études publiées en anglais entre janvier 2009 et décembre 2014. Des mots-clés tels que « transfert des tâches », « traitement contre le VIH », « ressources humaines » et « professions de la santé » ont été utilisés.

Résultats : Les preuves suggèrent que le transfert de tâches est une stratégie efficace pour faire face aux contraintes en termes de ressources humaines au sein des systèmes de soins de santé dans de nombreux pays et fournit une approche peu coûteuse sans compromettre les résultats des patients. Les défis incluent un soutien en termes de supervision et un mentorat insuffisants, l'absence de cadres réglementaires, un manque de renforcement général du système de santé et la nécessité d'un suivi et d'une évaluation. La stratégie semble être généralement acceptée par les professions de la santé, bien que plusieurs arguments allant à l'encontre du transfert de tâches en tant qu'approche à long terme aient été émis.

Conclusion : Le transfert de tâches se produit dans de nombreux contextes autres que les programmes de traitement du VIH et est considéré comme une stratégie clé pour gérer les ressources humaines dans le domaine de la santé. Il est peut-être aujourd'hui opportun d'examiner les recommandations actuelles en termes de transfert de tâche pour y inclure un plus large éventail de programmes et intégrer les initiatives visant à relever les défis actuels.

Introduction

Globally the number of people living with HIV is increasing as more people are accessing life-saving antiretroviral therapy (ART), and the world is within reaching the goal of providing ART to 15 million people by 2015.[1] However, in recent years there has been a crippling shortage in well-trained healthcare workers worldwide. At least 57 countries are affected, of which 36 countries are in sub-Saharan Africa.[2] The reasons for this disparity in qualified staffing in health services in Africa include a lack of training capacity, inefficient deployment of health workers, poor remuneration and limited budgets allocated to health services.[2,3]

In 2006, the World Health Organization (WHO) recognised that decreased access to care is associated with health worker shortages, especially in sub-Saharan African countries. Task shifting was then accepted globally as a strategy to improve access to care and meet the demand for initiating and managing more patients on ART.[4,5] Consolidated guidelines proposed by the WHO in 2013 have advocated the goals of keeping HIV-infected people healthy and reducing HIV transmission, thus emphasising the importance of equitable access to ART.[6] The Fast-Track strategy of the United Nations' Joint Programme on HIV/AIDS (UNAIDS) calls for a rapid scale-up of HIV prevention and treatment strategies in order to achieve the goal of 95% of people living with HIV knowing their status, 95% ART coverage and 95% virologic suppression rates by 2030.[7] This necessitates a further scale-up of the provision of ART, whilst making sure that patients are retained in care.[8] Decentralisation and task shifting have been referred to as the two pillars of the public health approach to scale up ART in resource-limited settings.[9]

Task shifting refers to transferring tasks to healthcare workers who have not conventionally performed these tasks as part of their scope of practice.[10,11] These workers are more readily available, completed shorter training and have fewer qualifications.[12] Clearly outlined tasks are delegated to healthcare workers who have received specific skills-based training, and this approach may extend to persons specifically trained to perform a limited task only.[13] The aim is to make efficient use of human resources for health in order to minimise delays in health service delivery without compromising the standard of care,[10] with the particular aim of improving the health of extremely vulnerable populations.[13]

Task shifting is also referred to as the rational distribution of tasks amongst members within health workforce teams.[10] The four levels of task shifting (Figure 1), in which health workers of the first three levels take on tasks of senior cadres, are based on the extension of the scope of practice of:

- non-physician clinicians (NPCs)
- nurses and midwives
- lay health workers or community workers
- and people living with HIV to self-manage aspects of their care.[10]

In this article, task shifting refers primarily to the shifting of tasks from doctors to NPCs or nurses (levels 1 and 2) and the further shift of tasks to lay health workers (level 3). NPCs are a cadre of health workers who are not trained as doctors, but take on many diagnostic and clinical functions of doctors.[14] NPCs, also known as health officers, clinical officers, physician assistants, nurse practitioners or nurse clinicians, have been identified as part of the health workforce in 25 countries in sub-Saharan Africa.[14] Lay health workers have no professional or paraprofessional qualifications and perform context-specific healthcare functions for which they received informal training.[15]

The word 'substitution' has been used when referring to task shifting, especially when referring to nurses taking on the role of doctors.[16] Words such as 'task delegation' or 'task sharing' imply that the person delegating or sharing the task remains responsible for the final outcome.[17] The WHO made several recommendations for the implementation of task shifting in the context of HIV services, such as the development of

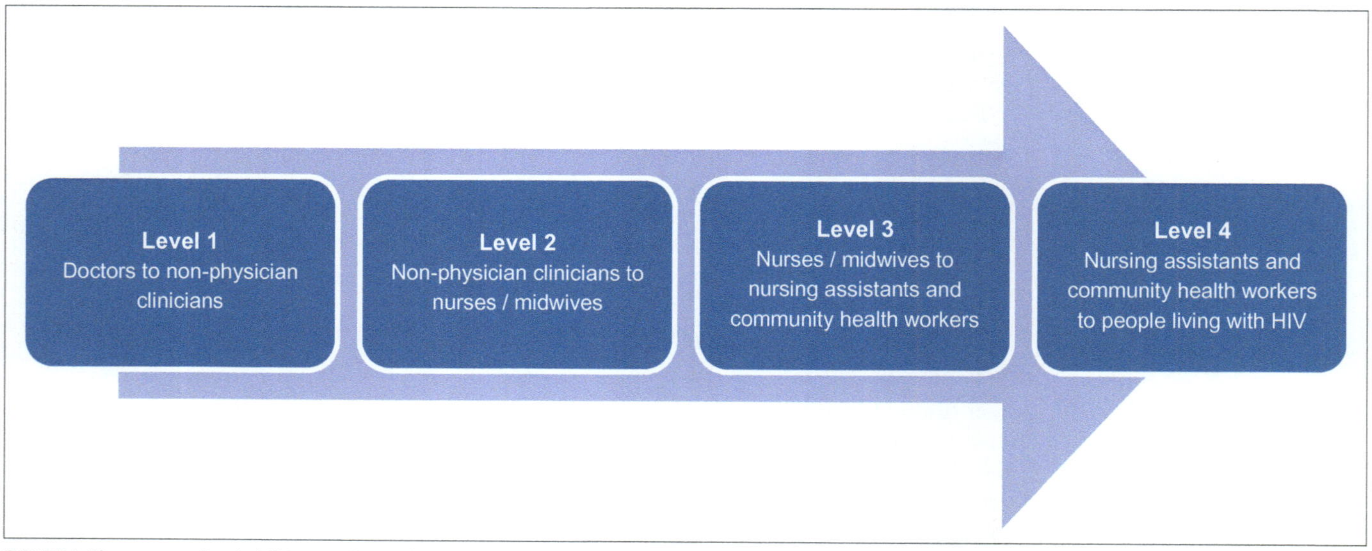

FIGURE 1: The process of task shifting as adapted from the World Health Organization global recommendations and guidelines.[10]

nationally endorsed frameworks to support the strategy, creating an enabling regulatory environment, measures to ensure quality care, maintaining stability and reorganisation of clinical care.[10]

The aim of this paper is to appraise the current trends in task shifting of HIV treatment and care to lower cadres of healthcare staff to evaluate evidence related to the effectiveness of this strategy in addressing human resource constraints and improving patient outcomes, challenges identified in practice and the acceptability of the strategy to the health professions. Attention is also drawn to the recommendations of the WHO and how countries have implemented these.

Methods

The electronic databases PubMed, CINAHL and Google Scholar were searched to identify relevant papers published between January 2009, following the publication of the WHO task shifting recommendations, and December 2014 for review. Medical subject heading (MeSH) terms included 'task shifting', 'HIV treatment', 'human resources' and 'healthcare professions'. Quantitative and qualitative studies published in English were included if they presented evidence on task shifting. We identified 395 articles of which the titles and abstracts were subsequently screened for appropriateness. The full texts of 67 articles, of which eight were systematic reviews, were assessed and 46 articles were included in this review. The majority of the reported research was conducted in Africa and sub-Saharan Africa. A critical analytical approach draws attention to current trends in task shifting and evidence related to the successes as well as the challenges of the strategy.

Review findings

Trends in task shifting: Towards community-supported care

Many countries, especially in sub-Saharan Africa, have adopted task shifting as an inevitable approach to alleviate human resource constraints and expand HIV programmes.[16,18] Task shifting seems to include more than only HIV services and is practised in almost all health facilities, either formally or informally, across a number of disciplines, including midwifery, surgery and non-communicable disease management.[3,8,19,20,21,22,23] The extent to which task shifting is implemented seems to depend on the specific discipline or service, health system capacity and health needs. In the context of HIV services, the most often reported levels of task shifting are from doctors to NPCs, nurses or midwives, and the shifting of tasks such as phlebotomy, dispensing and counselling from nurses or midwives to lay health workers.[18,24]

Lay health workers are used increasingly, especially in the context of disease prevention, health promotion, treatment support, counselling and home-based care.[2] A systematic review on the roles of community health workers in HIV care in sub-Saharan Africa reported that this group of health workers were instrumental in promoting the quality of HIV services and that their presence in clinics reduced waiting times for patients and the workload of other health workers.[24] As most community health workers live in the communities they serve, challenges of cultural and language competence are mitigated.[25]

In South Africa, a large infrastructure of lay health workers has developed in response to the HIV epidemic. In 2004, the estimated number of these workers (40 000) was almost equivalent to the number of professional nurses (43 660) working in the public sector.[26] Incorporating such an extensive lay health worker infrastructure is in line with the country's strategy for the re-engineering of primary healthcare and steps have been taken to design a formal qualification for such health workers.[27] In Malawi, lay health workers (also known as health surveillance assistants) comprise 30% of the health workforce.[28] In Malawi and Kenya, lay health workers perform mostly health prevention and promotion tasks in communities, but are increasingly performing curative tasks.[28,29]

Owing to the increasing HIV treatment burden, care has gradually moved from hospitals to decentralised healthcare facilities and has now further expanded to community-supported care for stable patients.[12,30] In Kenya, lay workers' community-based care for stable patients, supported by mobile technology, reduced clinic visits without compromising patient outcomes.[31] Other successful community-based interventions, such as adherence clubs, have also been reported.[30,32]

The task-shifting process for HIV treatment and care is well described in most contexts of care, but it is evident that it may not be the same for other, non-HIV services.[19] This may be as a result of the WHO recommendations focusing specifically on task shifting in the context of HIV. Although the potential for wider application is recognised, detailed guidelines for application to other services are not provided.

Effectiveness of task shifting in addressing human resource constraints and improving patient outcomes

The expansion of ART programmes and improved access to care in the midst of pervasive human and other resource constraints have been attributed to liberal task shifting strategies.[18,33] In most settings, task shifting has been implemented without significant increases in human resources.[4,18] The effect of task shifting has been evaluated in various countries, including South Africa, Ethiopia, Kenya, Malawi, Lesotho, Botswana, Swaziland, Nigeria, Cameroon, Zambia, Uganda, Mozambique and Rwanda.[18,34] A systematic review of the effect of task shifting found that the strategy can offer high-quality, cost-effective care to more clients than a physician-centred model.[4] The strategy also appears to be acceptable to patients.[34]

With regard to HIV treatment, care provided by non-physicians (including NPCs, professional nurses and midwives) is comparable to physician-provided care,[35] may reduce loss-to-follow-up rates and improve patient satisfaction.[36] Reduced loss to follow-up may also be attributed to decentralisation associated with task shifting as patients are receiving care closer to their homes.[12] However, neither decentralisation nor task shifting is a magic bullet for improving patient outcomes: a South African study reported that loss to follow-up is challenging whether care is decentralised or not and that rates are increasing with each calendar year since a patient started ART.[37]

Models based on decentralised HIV care do not compromise the health outcomes of patients, even when the patients are treated in the community rather than at primary care health facilities and hospitals.[12] It is also argued that task shifting may improve quality of care, as tasks such as patient education may be better delivered by nurses or lay health workers.[16,24,26] It may even lead to better retention in the healthcare workforce, especially in remote areas, by providing career opportunities for lower cadres of staff.[16,19]

Current research therefore supports the trend of adopting task shifting for HIV treatment and advocates for the expansion of task shifting policies.[24,36] However, many studies included in recent systematic reviews[12,34] were in the context of a range of support structures and investments to ensure delivery, including training and supervision. In practice, task shifting may be complex and be implemented in dissimilar forms, with substantial variation in the cadre, training and competency levels of health workers to whom tasks are shifted, for example NPCs or nurses. This makes comparisons of the success of the strategy in different countries problematic.[16,18] The generalisation of findings may not necessarily extend to wider healthcare systems and is dependent on the setting and organisation of care.[16,34,36] However, it is evident that task shifting has improved access to care for people who may not have had any access if the strategy had not been implemented. Fulton et al.[20] argue that studies should actually compare the outcomes of task shifting models with that of standard care, as many patients would not have received any treatment if not for task shifting.

Challenges identified in practice

Task shifting is not the remedy for a dysfunctional health system. For task shifting to succeed, systems and human resource support is required.[4] Although task shifting can improve access to and utilisation of services, costs of care do not necessarily decrease, as evidenced by a study in Ethiopia which reported that task shifting has not resulted in a significant decrease in the cost of ART care.[38] In South Africa, nurse-led ART has been associated with higher health service costs,[39] which may be attributed to the cost of supporting nurses through training and mentoring, limiting the potential savings.[34,39]

It is more costly to train and employ doctors and professional nurses than lay health workers, yet more skilled and experienced healthcare workers have been associated with better patient outcomes, which may partially offset cost of employing better-qualified staff.[40] Conversely, some countries may not be able to afford to employ a large number of well-trained qualified staff.[3] Task shifting is therefore a viable option for efficiently providing services that may otherwise not have been available.[19,20] Lehmann et al.,[5] and more recently also Lanktree et al.,[41] have argued that the long-term success of task shifting hinges on political and financial commitment, reorganisation of health teams, clear scopes of practice, recognition, simplified guidelines, regulatory frameworks and training, support and monitoring of infrastructure.

Several challenges to the implementation of task shifting according to WHO guidelines and recommendations have been reported. These challenges are discussed briefly.

Support, training and care reorganisation

Task shifting is complex and can be successful only when accompanied by training, reorganisation of services, mentoring, supervision and ongoing support from existing health system structures.[4,18,35] If such a strategy is implemented without sufficient clinical and managerial support, it could be less effective than the outcomes observed in clinical trials.[31,34]

When implemented in an already burdened and dysfunctional health system, task shifting alone is not enough to improve efficiency and ensure quality of care.[18] It may lead to the depletion of already limited health resources.[36] Patient outcomes may be compromised in settings where nurses are already overworked if current tasks of nurses are not shifted to lower levels of workers.[36,42] In South Africa, a high percentage of professional nursing positions remains vacant and the reality that task shifting relies heavily on nurses to take on new tasks and to supervise other, non-professional cadres of staff is therefore problematic.[11]

Adequate knowledge and skills are required for supportive supervision, but health workers capable of providing supportive supervision are also experiencing heavy workloads. Consequently, tasks may be shifted without the guarantee of supportive supervision.[3,19,28,43] Staff training is central to the implementation of task shifting, but a major limitation to this is high staff turnover.[44] Measures to limit staff turnover and increase mentoring and supervision capacity therefore need to be planned from the outset.[4]

A lack of health system resources and support, inadequate infrastructure and equipment, ineffective guidance from managers, increasing workloads and unresolved remuneration issues have been identified as barriers to the implementation and efficiency of task shifting.[3,23,43] Other barriers identified include a shortage of nurses working at primary care facilities, ongoing training in clinical skills and the expansion of clinical mentoring.[45] A number of authors have reported that there is no structured system in place or resources for supervision and mentoring after training.[19,36,42,46]

Assefa et al.[9] reported that the scale-up of ART in Ethiopia has been made possible through a range of interventions alongside task shifting. Health system strengthening, community mobilisation, case management support and patient information systems were reported as key contributory initiatives to effective scale-up. The implementation of a task shifting strategy in Malawi required regular and sustained peer-based support for health workers and their mentors. Linking training to continuous professional development credits further strengthened training uptake.[44]

Currently, there is still limited evidence about the key barriers and enablers to effect successful implementation of task shifting in resource-constrained settings with weak health systems and inadequate supervisory support.[16] Most studies to date have focused on settings with vertical programmes, which means there is minimal evidence to inform decision makers about task shifting in special risk groups and integrated health system programmes. In their systematic review, Kredo et al.[34] found moderate-quality evidence that substituting nurses for doctors to initiate and monitor ART in adults will not compromise quality of care, but that there were no studies to inform practice in special risk groups. Two examples for which there is no clear evidence are whether nurses should be allowed to prescribe both ART and other chronic medication to patients with co-morbid conditions and whether midwives can prescribe ART in the context of antenatal care. In Malawi, vertical disease-specific programmes were reported to lead to competing demands being placed on healthcare workers, which can cause role confusion and hamper the effectiveness of task shifting.[28] A recent systematic review of health system barriers and enablers for ART delivery during pregnancy and post partum identified gaps between antenatal care and HIV services that resulted in significant dropout along the maternal ART cascade. The authors suggested that this situation may be improved if tasks such as antenatal care and the provision of ART are integrated.[47] Although there is a drive towards increasing service integration, it is not clear what the ideal balance between depth and breadth of shifted tasks should be to ensure quality and efficiency.

Competency assessment and quality assurance mechanisms

A three-pronged approach to task shifting, which comprises training, on-site clinical mentoring and continuous quality assurance, has been advocated.[2,48] The WHO recommends that countries implementing task shifting should ensure that the performance of all cadres of health workers can be assessed against clearly defined roles, competency levels and standards.[10] Morris et al.[48] describe a comprehensive, continuous quality assurance programme for task shifting that was implemented in Zambia through (1) evaluation of clinical care via targeted chart reviews and monthly site reports from electronic medical records, (2) feedback and training in areas of poor site performance, and (3) an exchange programme between clinics to improve overall clinical quality. No other published studies describing specific quality assurance or clinical governance mechanisms for the wider implementation of task shifting could be found; however, routine data from a study in Khayelitsha, South Africa, showed an improvement in the quality of ART management after clinical mentoring.[49]

Some studies from South Africa, Tanzania, Uganda, Mozambique and Zambia have reported that tasks were delegated without prior training and that a 'trial-and-error' approach was followed.[3,19,23,42] A survey of 15 African countries (including the aforementioned as well as other countries) indicated that the majority of countries in which task shifting of ART was allocated to nurses follow an in-service training approach; however, such training was generally not accredited or approved by national nursing and midwifery councils.[50] In addition, there is no evidence that competencies required by task shifting are being introduced in pre-service education.[8,50]

It is also costly to develop new training programmes[36] and clarity with regard to whether training should be provided by higher education institutions or private, 'informal' training institutions is needed. Informal training may be problematic because of a lack of standardisation within and across training programmes and countries, and the quality may also be questionable.[50] In Malawi, an in-service training programme for NPCs was suspended owing to observational data indicating only 10.6% of clinical encounters were correctly managed after training.[51] In a South African study, only 60% of nurses were able to pass an open-book test after didactic in-service training, yet 62% of nurses who had failed the test also reported to initiate patients in practice following the training.[45]

Regulatory and accreditation systems

The WHO recommends accreditation and certification programmes for newly trained health workers in order to provide career paths, as well as recognition of prior learning for those who have already taken on tasks outside their scope of practice through pragmatic responses to healthcare needs.[10] Most countries use documents from their ministry of health, such as ART guidelines, to authorise ART prescription without including the long-term WHO-recommended processes such as credentialling and regulation.[50] Many nursing and midwifery councils in eastern, central and southern Africa do not have the resources or capacity to undertake changes associated with practice regulation.[52]

In South Africa, there is no formal regulatory system for nurses to prescribe ART[53] or for the scope of practice of lay health workers. Although it is reported that section 56(6) of the South *African Nursing Act* (33 of 2005) allows for nurses to be authorised to prescribe ART,[17] nurses are concerned about the lack of certification from the South African Nursing Council.[43] Although task shifting is permissible in many countries, there is no legal protection for health workers if they act outside of their scope of practice.[2,3] The scope of practice of lay health workers is constantly being expanded to enable wider service delivery. This sometimes includes curative services and tasks not in their job description.[28,29] As these health workers are unregulated, there is no control over their training or the quality of their work.[24,40] It has therefore been advocated that their training be appropriately accredited, certified and recognised.[24,29] Roles and associated competency levels should be clearly defined for existing health workers as well as for those cadres newly created by the task-shifting approach.[17]

Formal career pathways for lower cadres that have an extended scope of practice seem to be absent in most countries. Nurses and lay workers are taking on additional tasks for which they are not adequately remunerated[24,36] and no incentives or career promotion frameworks exist.[3,19,23,24,26] Investment in policy, regulation and pre-service education is needed to ensure sustainable task-shifting interventions.[8,24,50,52]

Acceptability of task shifting to the health professions

Social dynamics in healthcare teams may be affected by task shifting policies.[4] Issues such as professional boundaries, dominance and power have been identified.[11]

Professional nurses seem to embrace task shifting and feel empowered by their expanded roles.[42] They accept task shifting in relation to training and the acquisition of knowledge and skills.[53,54] Nurses have also expressed feelings of emotional reward, accomplishment, prestige and improved morale.[55] A South African study by Davies et al.[42] found that nurses experienced emotional reward through building relationships with patients and that they feel empowered by the realisation that they can also act as mentors to other nurses. They are willing and receptive to the idea as it is in the best interest of the patients, yet they acknowledge that circumstances are sometimes less than ideal.[42] The need for clear role definitions of different providers and stratification of roles at primary-care level to make task shifting more effective with respect to quality patient care and resource utilisation has been highlighted.[43]

Although task shifting seems to be generally accepted as a necessary strategy to increase access to care, there are conflicting opinions amongst doctors, in particular with respect to the perceived competency of nurses to manage HIV-infected persons.[55] A Ugandan study found that task shifting was unacceptable to most health managers and policy makers, as they considered the lower categories of health workers to be incompetent and overworked, which is exacerbated by inadequate support and supervision.[3] In Mozambique and Zambia, there has been concern that task shifting carries risks for patients, staff and management, although the concern was related mostly to insufficient support systems and workload constraints.[23] Task shifting in Tanzania was considered by respondents to be a short-term solution whilst the government worked towards more sustainable ways of addressing the health personnel crisis.[19] Lay health workers in Malawi reported confusion about their ever-expanding job description, but were willing to expand their scope of practice if appropriate training and resources were provided.[28]

Professional cadres of health workers can view task shifting either as alleviating their burden of tasks and improving access to care or as encroaching upon their profession and compromising the quality of care. As health professionals are accountable for their own practice, Scott et al.[56] argue that 'accountability implies autonomy and choice' and if there is no alternative to inadequate care, choice does not exist. For the health service to demand an extended role of nurses and other health workers, the necessary resources and an enabling environment that facilitates such accountability must be ensured.[56]

The categories of healthcare workers have become increasingly diverse over the last 20 years. This has been particularly noticeable as a result of the increased need to access chronic care and ART. The diversity of the healthcare workforce created by new cadres of health workers may give rise to complex intra- and interprofessional boundary disputes.[11] This strategy may be seen by some as de-professionalising the workforce through a loss of authority over certain aspects of work.[11] Some instances of professional protectionism have emerged, such as doctors arguing that nurses have insufficient training and skills to adequately perform tasks that were formerly only in the ambit of the medical profession, and nurses feeling that lay health workers are invading their profession. As a result, lower cadres of health workers may not feel comfortable in embracing task shifting.[2]

In South Africa, nurses were resistant to lay health workers wearing uniforms, in an attempt to maintain professional boundaries.[26] Nurses reported that they did not supervise lay health workers, despite working closely together. Some district-level informants in Tanzania were not supportive of legalising task shifting, as they feared professional conflicts between workers of different cadres.[19] A South African study, however, reported that health workers functioned well in a supportive multidisciplinary team and that the changing nature of HIV services was the driver of a team approach to care.[43]

Although the effect of role changes on professional status is still unclear, professional labels associated with a particular service, ownership of a body of knowledge, autonomy and authority remain uncontested. Lower levels of workers are unlikely to be afforded appropriate recognition and status, even if they are performing the tasks of higher-level workers.[11]

TABLE 1: Contrasting arguments for and against task shifting.

Pragmatic	Purist
Rational distribution of tasks in care teams. New cadres perform additional tasks (e.g. defaulter tracing), which will improve the quality of patient care.	Delegation of tasks to already overburdened health workers.
Expanded roles lead to empowerment.	Lowering the required level of competence promotes deprofessionalisation.
Job creation and career progression.	No job description, performance framework or increase in remuneration.
Increased community access to basic health care and improved community engagement. Efficiency of services improves patient satisfaction.	A decrease in quality of care; infringement of the rights of the community to receive care from skilled health workers.
Increased cost effectiveness (increasing the number of services provided at a given quality and cost). Alleviate skill-mix imbalances.	Decisions are based on economic and budget constraints rather than on actual health worker shortages; hidden costs associated with training and supervision.
Only a basic level of training, focused on specific skills, is needed. Some tasks require only focused training.	Comprehensive care requires advanced education, professionalism and ethics. Roles and tasks are continually evolving, requiring ongoing training.
A task-oriented approach improves efficiency of care.	A task-oriented approach causes fragmentation in care.
Ethical responsibility to adapt to the needs of the community and provide equitable access to healthcare.	Ethical responsibility to protect the community and healthcare workers from harm.

Several sound arguments both for and against the long-term implementation of task shifting have been extrapolated, categorised and presented in Table 1. Pragmatists consider the issue in a logical, practical way, arguing that task shifting is inevitable in the context of the broader health system and that the system and professionals should adapt accordingly. In contrast, purists value quality of care and the status of the health professions.

Implications and recommendations

Task shifting has been widely adopted and seems to be an effective strategy for providing services that may otherwise not be available.[20] Several challenges to the implementation of task shifting have been reported. The strategy generally seems to be well accepted by the various health professions although arguments against the strategy as a long-term approach to care have been raised.

In its current form, task shifting should not be considered as a remedy for current healthcare delivery problems. Efforts to seek long-term sustainable solutions should continue.[19,36] For most developing countries, however, task shifting is a reality in healthcare service delivery and is already moving beyond the clinic to community level. It is not likely to be a short-term measure and is seen by Margret Chan, director-general of the WHO, as an approach that offers long-term potential for all primary healthcare services.[10] Task shifting initiatives should therefore be flexible and adaptable to a specific context and ground-level needs. Research on various models of task shifting strategies in different contexts and the impact on patient outcomes should continue.

If doctors' tasks are shifted to NPCs and nurses, these latter groups' tasks should, in turn, shift to other non-professional cadres.[36] The re-engineering of primary healthcare strategies relies heavily on the use of lay health workers in communities, supervised by nurses.[11] Nurses will become increasingly responsible for overseeing the tasks of lay health workers. Tasks of lay health workers are continually expanding yet their roles are not clearly defined, and as such this cadre remains unregulated in many countries and workers experience limited regulatory protection.[3,15,24,57] Furthermore, it is not clear how supportive supervision should be defined in community-based care settings. As lay health workers take on caring roles and function autonomously, especially in rural settings, they should be appropriately trained and have clear role descriptions.

Evidence indicates that the implementation of task shifting according to WHO guidelines and recommendations is problematic, especially in resource-constrained countries. The complexity and context sensitivity of the approach make a standardised method of implementation impossible. Implementing task shifting in isolation is unlikely to address long-term sustainability of programmes. Further research is needed with regard to the interventions necessary for adequate support of personnel and effectiveness of services. Task shifting may need to form part of an interdisciplinary team approach, with patient self-management as a central focus.

Key stakeholders need to engage in discussions about whether task shifting should be programme specific or general. Programme-specific task shifting strategies may become inefficient in the near future, especially in the African context with its diverse needs and high co-morbidity rates. This is illustrated by evidence indicating that the tasks of community health workers are continually expanding. There is, however, still insufficient evidence to support task shifting for integrated care. Countries need to look beyond the immediate 'crisis management' approach to task shifting and focus on longer-term strategies that include enhanced training and monitoring of infrastructure. New models for supportive supervision, with expert clinicians as team leaders, are needed to support task shifting and ensure quality of care. Other initiatives, such those based on mobile technology, may be used to provide support to nurses and lay health workers in resource-limited settings.[31,57]

With the increasing number of patients receiving chronic treatment, triage models, in which stable patients are managed in community adherence clubs, are needed to increase service efficiency.[30,32] Public-private partnerships may be another way to share patient loads as well as clinician expertise.

Limitations

This limited review included only studies published in English since 2009, with the aim of informing benefits and challenges of the implementation of task shifting in the African context.

Conclusion

To date, research indicates that task shifting is effective in providing potentially life-saving treatment and care to a greater number of clients. It is a key strategy for managing human resources for health. A lack of implementation may therefore be considered unethical and implementation without adequate health system strengthening could lead to failure. Although task shifting has been adopted by many countries and has been implemented in many diverse settings, there is a lack of fidelity to WHO guidelines, especially concerning regulatory frameworks, supportive supervision, monitoring, and evaluation systems. Leadership and commitment from governing structures are essential to address these concerns and provide solutions. The participation of professional regulatory bodies in decision-making processes regarding task shifting is essential to ensure future success.

It has been seven years since the WHO initially introduced recommendations on task shifting. Although these recommendations did not exclude the possibility of wider application, guidelines were specific to the context of HIV-related services. It may now be an opportune time to review and modify the WHO recommendations to include a wider range of programmes and incorporate initiatives to address current challenges.

Acknowledgements

Competing interests

The authors declare that they have no financial or personal relationship(s) that may have inappropriately influenced them in writing this article.

Authors' contributions

T.C. (Stellenbosch University) was responsible for searching the databases and obtaining articles, which were critically appraised by both authors. T.C. wrote the initial manuscript and P.M. (University of Cape Town) reviewed and edited the manuscript.

References

1. United Nations Joint Programme on HIV/Aids (UNAIDS). Global report: UNAIDS report on the global AIDS epidemic 2013. Geneva: UNAIDS; 2013.
2. African Medical and Research Foundation. Position statement on task shifting [document on the Internet]. c2015 [cited 2015 Mar 30]. Available from http://amref.org/amref/en/info-hub/amrefs-position-statement-on-task-shifting-/
3. Baine SO, Kasangaki A. A scoping study on task shifting; the case of Uganda. BMC Health Serv Res. 2014;14(1):184. http://dx.doi.org/10.1186/1472-6963-14-184
4. Callaghan M, Ford N, Schneider H. A systematic review of task-shifting for HIV treatment and care in Africa. Hum Resour Health. 2010;8:8. http://dx.doi.org/10.1186/1478-4491-8-8
5. Lehmann U, Van Damme W, Barten F, Sanders D. Task shifting: The answer to the human resources crisis in Africa? Hum Resour Health. 2009;7:49. http://dx.doi.org/10.1186/1478-4491-7-49
6. World Health Organization. Consolidated guidelines on the use of antiretroviral drugs for treating and preventing HIV infection: Recommendations for a public health approach. Geneva: World Health Organization; 2013.
7. United Nations Joint Programme on HIV/Aids (UNAIDS). Fast-track: Ending the AIDS epidemic by 2030. Geneva: UNAIDS; 2014.
8. Assefa Y, Pillay Y, Van Damme W. Commentary: Operational guidance in the 2013 WHO consolidated antiretroviral guidelines. AIDS. 2014;28(Suppl 2):S171–S173. http://dx.doi.org/10.1097/QAD.0000000000000233
9. Assefa Y, Alebachew A, Lera M, Lynen L, Wouters E, Van Damme W. Scaling up antiretroviral treatment and improving patient retention in care: Lessons from Ethiopia, 2005–2013. Global Health. 2014;10:43. http://dx.doi.org/10.1186/1744-8603-10-43
10. World Health Organization. Task shifting: Global recommendations and guidelines. Geneva: World Health Organization; 2008.
11. Gilbert L. 'Re-engineering the workforce to meet service needs': Exploring 'task-shifting' in South Africa in the context of HIV/AIDS and antiretroviral therapy. S Afr Sociol Rev. 2013;44(2):54–75. http://dx.doi.org/10.1080/21528586.2013.802537
12. Kredo T, Ford N, Adeniyi FB, Garner P. Decentralising HIV treatment in lower- and middle-income countries. Cochrane Database Syst Rev. 2013;6:CD009987.
13. World Medical Association. WMA resolution on task shifting from the medical profession. Adopted by the 60th WMA General Assembly, New Delhi, India, October 2009 [document on the Internet]. c2009 [cited 2015 Mar 30]. Available from www.wma.net/en/30publications/10policies/t4/
14. Mullan F, Frehywot S. Non-physician clinicians in 47 Sub-Saharan African countries. Lancet. 2007;370:2158–2163. http://dx.doi.org/10.1016/S0140-6736(07)60785-5
15. Daniels K, Clarke M, Ringsberg KC. Developing lay health worker policy in South Africa: A qualitative study. Health Res Policy Syst. 2012;10(1):8. http://dx.doi.org/10.1186/1478-4505-10-8
16. Rashidian A, Shakibazadeh E, Karimi- Shahanjarini A, Glenton C, Noyes J, Lewin S, et al. Barriers and facilitators to the implementation of doctor-nurse substitution strategies in primary care : Qualitative evidence synthesis. Cochrane Database Syst Rev. 2013;2:CD010412. http://dx.doi.org/10.1002/14651858.CD010412
17. Armstrong S, Bhengu B, Kotze W, Nkonzo-Mtembu L, Ricks E, Stellenberg EL, et al. A new approach to professional practice. Claremont: Juta; 2013.
18. Emdin C, Millson P. A systematic review evaluating the impact of task shifting on access to antiretroviral therapy in Sub-Saharan Africa. Afr Health Sci. 2012;12(3):318–324. http://dx.doi.org/10.4314/ahs.v12i3.11
19. Munga MA, Kilima SP, Mutalemwa PP, Kisoka WJ, Malecela MN. Experiences, opportunities and challenges of implementing task shifting in underserved remote settings : The case of Kongwa district, central Tanzania. BMC Int Health Hum Rights. 2012;12:27. http://dx.doi.org/10.1186/1472-698X-12-27
20. Fulton BD, Scheffler RM, Sparkes SP, Auh EY, Vujicic M, Soucat A. Health workforce skill mix and task shifting in low income countries: A review of recent evidence. Hum Resour Health. 2011;9(1):1. http://dx.doi.org/10.1186/1478-4491-9-1
21. Lekoubou A, Awah P, Fezeu L, Sobngwi E, Kengne AP. Hypertension, diabetes mellitus and task shifting in their management in Sub-Saharan Africa. Int J Environ Res Public Health. 2010;7(2):353–363. http://dx.doi.org/10.3390/ijerph7020353
22. Joshi R, Alim M, Kengne AP, Jan S, Maulik PK, Peiris D, et al. Task shifting for non-communicable disease management in low and middle income countries – A systematic review. PLoS ONE. 2014;9(8): e103754. http://dx.doi.org/10.1371/journal.pone.0103754
23. Ferrinho P, Sidat M, Goma F, Dussault G. Task-shifting: Experiences and opinions of health workers in Mozambique and Zambia. Hum Resour Health. 2012;10(1):34. http://dx.doi.org/10.1186/1478-4491-10-34
24. Mwai GW, Mburu G, Torpey K, Frost P, Ford N, Seeley J. Role and outcomes of community health workers in HIV care in Sub-Saharan Africa: A systematic review. J Int AIDS Soc. 2013;16(1):18586. http://dx.doi.org/10.7448/IAS.16.1.18586
25. Swartz L, Kilian S, Twesigye J, Attah D, Chiliza B. Language, culture, and task shifting – an emerging challenge for global mental health. Glob Health Action. 2014;7:1–4. http://dx.doi.org/10.3402/gha.v7.23433
26. Schneider H, Hlophe H, Van Rensburg D. Community health workers and the response to HIV/AIDS in South Africa: Tensions and prospects. Health Policy Plan. 2008;23(3):179–187. http://dx.doi.org/10.1093/heapol/czn006
27. South African Department of Health. Annual Health Report 2012/13 [document available on the Internet]. c2013 [cited 2015 Mar 30]. Available from: http://Africacheck.org/wp-content/uploads/2014/02/131016dohrreport.pdf
28. Smith S, Deveridge A, Berman J, Negin J, Mwambene N, Chingaipe E, et al. Task shifting and prioritization: A situational analysis examining the role and experiences of community health workers in Malawi. Hum Resour Health. 2014;12(1):24. http://dx.doi.org/10.1186/1478-4491-12-24
29. Ochieng B, Akunja E, Edwards N, Mombo D, Marende L, Kaseje DC. Perceptions of health stakeholders on task shifting and motivation of community health workers in different socio demographic contexts in Kenya (nomadic, peri-urban and rural agrarian). BMC Health Serv Res. 2014;14(Suppl 1):S4. http://dx.doi.org/10.1186/1472-6963-14-S1-S4
30. Bemelmans M, Baert S, Goemaere E, Wilkinson L, Vandendyck M, Van Cutsem G, et al. Community-supported models of care for people on HIV treatment in sub-Saharan Africa. Trop Med Int Health. 2014;19(8):968–977. http://dx.doi.org/10.1111/tmi.12332
31. Selke HM, Kimaiyo S, Sidle JE, Vedanthan R, Tierney WM, Shen C, et al. Task-shifting of antiretroviral delivery from health care workers to persons living with HIV/AIDS: Clinical outcomes of a community-based program in Kenya. J Acquir Immune Defic Syndr. 2010;55(4):483–490. PubMed PMID: 20683336. http://dx.doi.org/10.1097/QAI.0b013e3181eb5edb
32. Wilkinson LS. ART adherence clubs : A long-term retention strategy for clinically stable patients receiving antiretroviral therapy. S Afr J HIV Med. 2013;14(2):48–50. doi:10.7196/SAJHIVMED.924 http://dx.doi.org/10.7196/sajhivmed.924

33. Munderi P, Grosskurth H, Droti B, Ross D. What are the essential components of HIV treatment and care services in low and middle-income countries: An overview by settings and levels of the health system? AIDS. 2012;26(Suppl 2):S97–S103. http://dx.doi.org/10.1097/QAD.0b013e32835bdde6

34. Kredo T, Adeniyi FB, Bateganya M, Pienaar ED. Task shifting from doctors to non-doctors for initiation and maintenance of antiretroviral therapy. Cochrane Database Syst Rev. 2014;7:CD007331. Review. PubMed PMID: 24980859. http://dx.doi.org/10.1002/14651858.CD007331.pub3

35. Fairall L, Bachmann MO, Lombard C, Timmerman V, Uebel K, Zwarenstein M, et al. Task shifting of antiretroviral treatment from doctors to primary-care nurses in South Africa (STRETCH): A pragmatic, parallel, cluster-randomised trial. Lancet. 2012;380:889–898. http://dx.doi.org/10.1016/S0140-6736(12)60730-2

36. Emdin C., Chong NJ, Millson PE. Non-physician clinician provided HIV treatment results in equivalent outcomes as physician-provided care: A meta-analysis. J Int AIDS Soc. 2013;16:18445. http://dx.doi.org/10.7448/IAS.16.1.18445

37. Grimsrud A, Kaplan R, Bekker LG, Myer L. Outcomes of a nurse-managed service for stable HIV-positive patients in a large South African public sector antiretroviral therapy programme. Trop Med Int Health. 2014;19(9):1029–1039. Epub 2014 Jul 8. PubMed PMID: 25041716. http://dx.doi.org/10.1111/tmi.12346

38. Johns B, Asfaw E, Wong W, Bekele A, Minior T, Kebede A, et al. Assessing the costs and effects of antiretroviral therapy task shifting from physicians to other health professionals in Ethiopia. J Acquir Immune Defic Syndr. 2014;65(4):e140–e147. www.jaids.com. http://dx.doi.org/10.1097/QAI.0000000000000064

39. Barton GR, Fairall L, Bachmann MO, Uebel K, Timmerman V, Lombard C, et al. Cost-effectiveness of nurse-led versus doctor-led antiretroviral treatment in South Africa: Pragmatic cluster randomised trial. Trop Med Int Health. 2013;18(6):769–777. http://dx.doi.org/10.1111/tmi.12093

40. Jacob ER, McKenna L, D'Amore A. The changing skill mix in nursing: Considerations for and against different levels of nurse. J Nurs Manag. 2015;23(4):421–426. http://dx.doi.org/10.1111/jonm.12162

41. Lanktree E, Corluka A, Cohen M, Larocque R. Addressing the human resources for health crisis through task-shifting and retention: Results from the Africa Health Systems Initiative Support to African Research Partnerships program. Hum Resour Health. 2014;12(Suppl 1):I2. http://dx.doi.org/10.1186/1478-4491-12-S1-I2

42. Davies NECG, Homfray M, Venables EC. Nurse and manager perceptions of nurse initiated and managed antiretroviral therapy (NIMART) implementation in South Africa: A qualitative study. BMJ Open. 2013;3(11):e003840. http://dx.doi.org/10.1136/bmjopen-2013-003840

43. Orner P, Cooper D, Palmer N. Investigation of health care workers' responses to HIV/AIDS care and treatment in South Africa. Cape Town: University of the Western Cape; 2011.

44. Sodhi S, Banda H, Kathyola D, Joshua M, Richardson F, Mah E, et al. Supporting middle-cadre health care workers in Malawi: Lessons learned during implementation of the PALM PLUS package. BMC Health Serv Res. 2014;14(Suppl 1):S8. doi:10.1186/1472-6963-14-S1-S8. Epub 2014 May 12. PubMed PMID: 25080192; PubMedCentral PMCID: PMC4108880. http://dx.doi.org/10.1186/1472-6963-14-S1-S8

45. Cameron D, Gerber A, Mbatha M, Mutyabule J, Swart H, West N. Nurse initiation and maintenance of patients on antiretroviral therapy : Are nurses in primary care clinics initiating ART after attending NIMART training? S Afr Med J. 2012;102(2):98–100.

46. Nyasulu JCY, Muchiri E, Mazwi S, Ratshefola M. NIMART rollout to primary healthcare facilities increases access to antiretrovirals in Johannesburg : An interrupted time series analysis. S Afr Med J. 2013;103(4):232–236. http://dx.doi.org/10.7196/samj.6380

47. Colvin CJ, Konopka S, Chalker JC, Jonas E, Albertini J, Amzel A, et al. A systematic review of health system barriers and enablers for antiretroviral therapy (ART) for HIV-infected pregnant and postpartum women. PLoS ONE. 2014;9(10):e108150. http://dx.doi.org/10.1371/journal.pone.0108150

48. Morris MB, Chapula BT, Chi BH, Mwango A, Chi HF, Mwanza J, et al. Use of task shifting to rapidly scale-up HIV treatment services: Experiences from Lusaka, Zambia. BMC Health Serv Res. 2009;9:5. http://dx.doi.org/10.1186/1472-6963-9-5

49. Green A, De Azevedo V, Patten G, Davies MA, Ibeto M, Cox V. Clinical mentorship of nurse initiated antiretroviral therapy in Khayelitsha, South Africa: A quality of care assessment. PLoS ONE. 2014;9(6):e98389. doi:10.1371/journal.pone.0098389. eCollection 2014. PubMed PMID: 24887260; PubMedCentral PMCID: PMC4041881. http://dx.doi.org/10.1371/journal.pone.0098389

50. Zuber A, McCarthy CF, Verani AR, Msidi E, Johnson C. A survey of nurse-initiated and –managed antiretroviral therapy (NIMART) in practice, education policy, and regulation in east, central and southern Africa. J Assoc Nurses AIDS Care. 2014;25:520–531. http://dx.doi.org/10.1016/j.jana.2014.02.003

51. Brentlinger PE, Assan A, Mudender F, Ghee AE, Vallejo Torres J, Martínez Martínez P, et al. Task shifting in Mozambique: Cross-sectional evaluation of non-physician clinicians' performance in HIV/AIDS care. Hum Resour Health. 2010;8:23. doi:10.1186/1478-4491-8-23. PubMed PMID: 20939909; PubMed Central PMCID:PMC2994547. http://dx.doi.org/10.1186/1478-4491-8-23

52. McCarthy CF, Kelley MA, Verani AR, St. Louis ME, Riley PL. Development of a framework to measure health profession regulation strengthening. Eval Program Plann. 2014;46:17–24. http://dx.doi.org/10.1016/j.evalprogplan.2014.04.008

53. Georgeu D, Colvin CJ, Lewin S, Fairall L, Bachmann MO, Uebel K, et al. Implementing nurse-initiated and managed antiretroviral treatment (NIMART) in South Africa: A qualitative process evaluation of the STRETCH trial. Implement Sci. 2012;7:66. http://dx.doi.org/10.1186/1748-5908-7-66

54. O'Malley G, Asrat L, Sharma A, et al. Nurse task shifting for antiretroviral treatment services in Namibia: Implementation research to move evidence into action. PLoS ONE. 2014;9(3):e92014. http://dx.doi.org/10.1371/journal.pone.0092014

55. Iwu EN, Holzemer WL. Task shifting of HIV management from doctors to nurses in Africa: Clinical outcomes and evidence on nurse self-efficacy and job satisfaction. AIDS Care. 2014;26(1):42–52. http://dx.doi.org/10.1080/09540121.2013.793278

56. Scott PA, Matthews A, Kirwan M. What is nursing in the 21st century and what does the 21st century health system require of nursing? Nurs Philos. 2013;15(1):23–34. http://dx.doi.org/10.1111/nup.12032

57. Odendaal W, Lewin S. The provision of TB and HIV/AIDS treatment support by lay health workers in South Africa: A time-and-motion study. Hum Resour Health. 2014;12(1):18. http://dx.doi.org/10.1186/1478-4491-12-18

Why are babies born before arrival at health facilities in King Sabata Dalindyebo Local Municipality, Eastern Cape, South Africa? A qualitative study

Authors:
Adeyinka A. Alabi[1]
Don O'Mahony[1]
Graham Wright[2]
Mohlomi J. Ntsaba[3]

Affiliations:
[1]Department of Family Medicine, Faculty of Health Sciences, Walter Sisulu University, South Africa

[2]School of Health Sciences, University of Fort Hare, East London, South Africa

[3]Department of Nursing, Faculty of Health Sciences, Walter Sisulu University, South Africa

Correspondence to:
Don O'Mahony

Email:
donomahony@gmail.com

Postal address:
61 Cumberland Street, Mthatha 5099, South Africa

Introduction: Babies born before arrival at a health facility have a higher risk of neonatal death and their mothers a higher risk of maternal death compared with those born in-facility. The study explored the reasons for mothers giving birth before arrival (BBA) at health facilities and their experiences of BBA.

Methods: A qualitative research design was used. Individual and focus group interviews of BBA mothers and of nurses were undertaken at a community health centre and a district hospital in King Sabata Dalindyebo Local Municipality.

Results: Reasons for BBA included a lack of transport, a lack of security at night that deterred mothers from travelling, precipitate labour, failure to identify true labour, and a lack of waiting areas at health facilities. Traditional and cultural beliefs favouring childbirth at home and nurses' negative attitudes during antenatal care and labour influenced mothers to go to health facilities when in advanced labour. Mothers were aware of possible complications associated with BBA.

Conclusion: Socio-economic, individual, cultural and health system factors influence the occurrence of BBA. Relevant parties need to address these factors to ensure that all babies in the King Sabata Dalindyebo Local Municipality are delivered within designated health facilities.

Pourquoi les bébés naissent-ils avant d'arriver aux centres médicaux de la municipalité locale de King Sabata Dalindyebo, dans l'Eastern Cape, en Afrique du Sud ? Etude qualitative.

Introduction: les bébés qui naissent avant d'arriver au centre médical ont un risque plus élevé de mort néonatale et leur mère un risque plus élevé de décès maternel que ceux qui sont nés dans l'établissement. L'étude a examiné pour quelles raisons les mères accouchent avant d'arriver à la clinique (AAA) et leur expérience d'AAA.

Méthodes: On a utilisé un modèle de recherche qualitative. On a mené des entrevues individuelles et de groupes témoins des mères AAA et des infirmières à un centre médical communautaire et à un hôpital de district de la municipalité de King Sabata Dalindyebo.

Résultats: Les raisons d'AAA étaient le manque de transport, l'insécurité la nuit qui empêchait les mères de se déplacer, l'accouchement subi, l'incapacité de reconnaitre l'accouchement véritable, and le manque de salles d'attente dans les centres médicaux. Les croyances traditionnelles t culturelles en faveur de l'accouchement à la maison et l'attitude négative des infirmières envers les soins prénatals et l'accouchement ont influencé les mères d'aller au centre médical quand elles sont prêtes à accoucher. Les mères savaient qu'il pouvait y avoir des complications dues à l'AAA.

Conclusions: des facteurs socio-économiques, individuels, culturels et du système de santé influence l'incidence de l'AAA. Les acteurs appropriés doivent remédier à ces facteurs pour faire en sorte que tous les bébés de la municipalité de King Sabata Dalindyebo naissent dans les établissements désignés de soins de santé.

Introduction

Neonatal mortality rates are highest in developing countries (22 per 1000) compared with those in developed countries (3 per 1000),[1] with the major causes of death being prematurity and birth asphyxia.[2,3] The neonatal mortality rate in South Africa is high at 15 per 1000 live births, and neonatal deaths constitute 40% of under-5 deaths, with most deaths occurring in the early neonatal period.[4] South Africa is committed to the United Nations' Millennium Development Goals (MDGs) to reduce by two-thirds the under-5 mortality rate and by three-quarters the maternal mortality ratio between 1990 and 2015. The under-5 mortality rate in 2013 was 45 per 1000 live births compared with the MDG target of 20.[5] Stillbirth rates are also highest in non-developed regions (29 per 1000 births) compared with high-income countries (3 per 1000).[6] In South Africa, the rate in 2013 was 17 per 1000.[7] Similarly, maternal mortality is high in developing countries (233 per 100 000) compared with developed countries (12 per 100 000),[8] with the major causes of death being hypertension, haemorrhage and sepsis.[9] In South Africa, the maternal mortality ratio was 140 per 100 000 in 2013, whilst the MDG-5 target was 38,[5] and HIV is an additional, major cause of maternal death.[10] Whilst South Africa is unlikely to attain the MDG targets, every effort should be made to do so. To reduce stillbirths and neonatal and maternal mortality, all births should take place in health facilities with skilled birth attendants and means of transfer for emergencies.[11,12]

Birth before arrival (BBA), defined as delivery of a baby that takes place outside healthcare facilities,[13] is associated with increased neonatal mortality and morbidity, both in developed[14,15] and developing countries.[13,16] The BBA rate in developed countries is less than 1%,[17,18] but the rate in South Africa is 10%.[19] At Mthatha General Hospital and Ngangelizwe Community Health Centre (CHC), both situated in King Sabata Dalindyebo Local Municipality, the rate was 4% and 7%, respectively, in 2012 (P Yogeswaran, personal communication, 30 January 2013). These rates are higher than 1.5%, a rate considered acceptable in South Africa by Potter et al.[20] Previous studies in South Africa have described factors influencing delivery in health facilities.[21,22,23] However, the authors found only one study that included qualitative interviews with BBA mothers in South Africa.[23] The present study explored perceptions of mothers and nurses about the contributory factors to BBA so as to inform interventions to reduce the BBA rate in King Sabata Dalindyebo Local Municipality.

Research methods and design

A qualitative approach was chosen as it would 'enable participants to speak for themselves'[24] and provide a deeper understanding of factors associated with BBA.

Setting

Both Mthatha General Hospital and Ngangelizwe CHC, with an average of 500 and 200 deliveries per month respectively, are located in the town of Mthatha, situated in the predominantly rural Oliver Reginald Tambo District, the third most deprived of 52 districts in South Africa.[25] Indicators of deprivation include the following: an estimated 59% of the population live below the poverty line; the unemployment rate is high at 44%; there is no access to piped water for 51% of households; 70% live in traditional dwellings; and 30% of households have no electricity.[26]

Sampling

Purposeful sampling was used to select BBA mothers and nurses for interview. The most senior nurse in charge selected participants after assessing that they were likely to freely and fluently express their views. BBA mothers who presented within 3 months of delivery were recruited. The sample size was determined by data saturation, namely, when no new themes or insights were obtained, recruitment was stopped.[24] The inclusion criterion for the nurses was that they must have worked at one of the study facilities for at least 1 year and must have attended to BBA mothers.

Data collection methods

For the mothers, individual in-depth interviews were conducted, whilst two focus group interviews were undertaken with the nurses, one at each site. A female research assistant trained in qualitative interviewing conducted semi-structured interviews with BBA mothers in their first language (isiXhosa), either at the hospital or at the CHC. An interview guide, based on themes identified in the literature review, was used. The guide was piloted by interviewing two mothers and minor clarifications were made to the guide. The two interviews were not included in the study. Open-ended questions were used to allow participants to freely express their views. However, probing and prompting of participants were undertaken, where necessary, to obtain clarity of information.

One author (A.A.A.) facilitated the focus group interviews, whilst the research assistant took field notes. Focus groups use group dynamics and different forms of communication such as teasing, jokes and arguing to explore views.[27] The researchers considered that focus groups would be sufficient for clarifying nurses' views. The focus groups were conducted in English. All the interviews were audiotaped and field notes were taken by the interviewer to record any emotions displayed or behavioural cues.

Data analysis

The research assistant transcribed audiotaped recordings of the interviews and field notes and translated the individual interviews into English. To ensure that transcription was accurate, an educator whose first language was isiXhosa cross-checked excerpts of the transcriptions with the recordings.

The 'framework approach' was used to inductively analyse data.[28] A 'cut and paste' using a word processor was used to group selection of data. Themes emerging from the focus group discussions and the in-depth interviews were combined, compared and triangulated using content analysis.

Trustworthiness

Four constructs were utilised to ensure the trustworthiness of the present study.[29] For credibility, triangulating of data collection methods was utilised (focus group and in-depth interviews) as well as triangulation of sources of the data by interviewing BBA mothers and nurses. The validity of data collected was ensured by having an independent translator randomly verify the accuracy and completeness of the excerpts from the transcripts with the audiotaped interviews and the translation of transcripts. For transferability, sufficient, rich and thick descriptions are given for readers to understand if the results can apply to other settings. For dependability, established research methodology was used with sufficient detail to allow a reader to judge its reliability. For confirmability, triangulation was used to reduce the effect of possible researchers' bias. The author A.A.A. is a medical practitioner trained in a predominantly biomedical paradigm, whilst the research assistant (Phelo Sithole) is a graduate in social sciences.

Ethical considerations

Ethical clearance was obtained from Walter Sisulu University Health Research Ethics and Bio-Safety Committee (Protocol No. 014/2013) and permission to carry out the study was obtained from the Department of Health, Eastern Cape Province. Informed consent was obtained from all participants. It was emphasised that they could stop participation at any time without giving a reason and without prejudicing their relationship with their healthcare providers. They were reassured that their participation was confidential as all interviews were available to researchers only and that numbers, instead of names, were to be used for analysis and publication. For one 16-year-old participant, consent was obtained from her and her grandmother.

Results

Nineteen mothers were interviewed. Six nurses participated in the CHC focus group and 9 in the hospital group.

Socio-demographic characteristics of mothers and details of BBAs: These are displayed in Table 1. The median age of mothers was 27 years with a range of 16–41 years. One had completed grade 12, 15 were single and 18 were unemployed at the time of the study. Seventeen were multiparous. One mother had all her deliveries as BBAs.

Details of delivery: Fourteen of the participants delivered at home, assisted by family or community members. Two deliveries occurred in an ambulance and one in a private car. One woman delivered in an open public space whilst walking to the clinic, whilst another delivered just outside the Mthatha General Hospital's Outpatient Department.

Birth outcomes: There were two early neonatal deaths. The mothers reported that the neonates died within minutes of birth.

Planned place of birth: Seventeen of the 19 mothers planned to deliver in either a community health centre (CHC) or hospital, whilst the remaining two wanted to deliver at home.

Qualitative findings

Five themes were identified, the first four of which were risk categories for BBA. Theme five relates to mothers' understanding of risks associated with BBA. Quotes from the participants were assigned codes as follows: each participant was assigned a number. C and H codes represent Ngangelizwe CHC and Mthatha General Hospital, respectively. For example, in the first quotation below, the number 5 indicates participant number 5, H indicates the site (Mthatha General Hospital) and the interviewee is a mother who is 27 years old.

Theme 1: Physical barriers to accessing a health facility

Accessibility to health facilities was affected by distance, bad roads, and transport and financial constraints.

TABLE 1: Socio-demographic characteristics of mothers and details of birth before arrival.

Participant	Age (years)	School level†	Marital status	Employed (Y/N)‡	Parity	Previous BBA (Y/N)	Travel time to facility (minutes)§	Time of birth
1	28	9	Married	N	3	N	50	03h00
2	22	11	Single	N	4	N	30	01h00
3	18	8	Single	N	1	N	30	04h00
4	25	4	Single	N	4	N	about 60	23h00
5	35	11	Single	N	4	N	90	15h00
6	19	5	Single	N	2	Y	30	22h00
7	20	11	Single	N	2	N	30	13h00
8	33	10	Married	Y¶	6	Y	30	10h00
9	28	3	Cohabiting	N	2	N	120	03h00
10	16	11	Single	N	1	N	20	05h00
11	41	11	Single	N	6	N	60	01h00
12	32	7	Married	N	4	N	30	01h00
13	21	9	Single	N	2	N	45	03h00
14	27	6	Married	N	3	Y	30	04h00
15	23	11	Single	N	2	N	60	06h00
16	34	9	Single	N	5	Y	30	12h20
17	29	10	Single	N	3	N	50	22h00
18	25	8	Single	N	4	N	90	02h00
19	30	3	Single	N	5	N	30	17h30

BBA, birth before arrival.
†, Highest school grade (range 1–12); ‡, Y = yes; N = no; §, A health facility designated to conduct births; ¶, Employed as a domestic worker.

Distance

About using a taxi or hired van to reach the health facility from home, one mother reported that it took her less than 30 minutes, whilst the remaining 18 reported that it took 30 or more minutes:

> 'The nearest clinic to us does not open at night. So the only option available for us was to go to Mthatha General, which would take a commercial vehicle more than one hour to reach. We called the emergency ambulance but I had already delivered by the time they came at 1 a.m.' (PH5, mother, 27)

Nurses also felt that most mothers came from locations that require transport to reach the health facility.

Poor roads

Another major issue identified was the bad state of the untarred roads, making access difficult, especially when it rained:

> 'The road to some of the locations where the mothers are staying are in a very terrible situation most especially if it is raining, this makes it very difficult for ambulances to reach those locations, even when they received emergency call from a mother in labour.' (PC2, nurse, 42)

Transport

Mothers and nurses blamed the poor response time by the public Emergency Medical Services (EMS) ambulance service for BBA. They estimated that the average response time was between 2 and 3 hours. Factors perceived as contributing to the delay were a shortage of ambulances and drivers, and drivers having difficulty in locating respondents' houses in rural areas. Nine mothers called an ambulance when in labour. One mother's experience was as follows:

> 'My mother called the ambulance at about 3 a.m. The driver could not get the description and he was lost for about two hours. By the time he arrived in our place it was 6 a.m. and I had already delivered.' (PH4, mother, 21)

Another reported that the ambulance personnel were impatient:

> 'The ambulance came some minutes after we called. We saw the ambulance parking adjacent to our house and just before we crossed to where it was, it zoomed off. I ended up delivering with the assistance of old ladies at home.' (PH1, mother, 16)

Ten mothers could not contact the EMS when they were in labour: six did not know the phone number, two did not have airtime, and two had flat batteries in their mobile phones.

Nurses identified poor EMS management and a lack of resources:

> 'We sometimes got the response from the EMS call centre that the ambulances have been taken for repair or there is no driver or the licence disks have not been renewed, so they are not working ...' (PC1, nurse, 51)

Because of delays by the EMS, one mother reported that she was advised at the clinic to save money so that she can hire a vehicle in case of emergency:

> 'They told us that we should have an arrangement for a car that can take us to the hospital when we fall in labour. The nurses told us to have money saved for transportation in case of emergency.' (PH6, mother, 23)

Only one mother was transported by a neighbour. In the absence of an ambulance, mothers stated that neighbours were usually of no help in transporting them to a health facility:

> 'The rate of crime and hijacking is the problem ... that is why people with cars refuse to take people to the hospital, especially at night.' (PH8, mother, 29)

Three mothers reported the challenges of getting a taxi at night:

> 'I did not see any taxi to take me to the hospital because it was already late and our public transport was about to stop working for the day.' (PC7, mother, 20)

Financial constraints

Nurses felt that most mothers were poor. At the time of the study, 95% were unemployed (Table 1). Four of the mothers also attributed a lack of money to hire a taxi at night as being responsible for their home birth:

> 'I delivered at home because the ambulance did not come and a cab driver charged me R400 which I did not have.' (PC8, mother, 33)

Theme 2: Traditional delivery beliefs and practices

Traditional medicines: Nurses perceived that many mothers used traditional medicines to speed up labour. One of the nurses reported that she herself had used traditional medication to hasten childbirth in the past. Nurses thought that BBA mothers were usually not willing to disclose such information until complications arose during labour:

> 'They only disclose use of traditional medicine when they are in trouble during delivery.' (PC5, nurse, 50)

However, only one mother agreed that she used traditional medicines:

> 'I took one bottle of traditional medicine 'umchamo wemfene' [*baboon's urine*] at nine months because there were no signs that I was going to deliver anytime soon and the elders believed that I was being bewitched.' (PC5, mother, 35)

Place of childbirth: Nurses perceived that Xhosa traditions and beliefs contributed to BBA:

> 'There is a belief in our tradition that if you deliver in the health facility you are not the real mother; a real mother has to deliver at home.' (PH6, nurse, 40)

Tradition also determines who takes the final decision on the place of delivery. The wish of the parturient does not count:

> 'A parturient may be educated but because of the tradition you have to give birth at home. You are not going to tell the elders on what to do.' (PH3, nurse, 56)

Traditional childbirth: Mothers reported that family members and neighbours, usually elderly women, assisted them during delivery. One mother described her labour and delivery:

> 'My grandmother gave me an empty bottle and told me to blow into it. She said this helped the baby to be active. She also used hot water to massage the tummy with the hope that this assists the baby to go down. [*During delivery*] I was on my knees and I only know now that it is not supposed to be happening like that. The right position is to lie with my back.' (PC3, mother, 18)

Nurses reported that parturients assume a squatting position during home delivery unlike in hospital where parturients lie on their backs:

> 'Some of these women are not used to hospital method of giving birth where they are requested to lie on their back, they are used to squatting, so in that case they do not like going to the hospital.' (PH1, nurse, 55)

If BBA mothers come with retained placentae, nurses discern the traditional method of delivering the placenta by tying a bottle to the umbilical cord:

> 'They usually do not tell us that a traditional birth attendant did the delivery but we can tell because we see a bottle tied up in the thigh with the placenta, in the traditional method of removing the placenta.' (PC6, nurse, 28)

Preference for female birth attendant: Four nurses reported that parturients often expressed a preference for female birth attendants:

> 'They equally do not like to be helped by a male nurse or male doctor.' (PH4, nurse, 50)

Theme 3: Health system-related issues

Antenatal care

Poor antenatal attendance: The majority (18) of mothers reported that they attended the antenatal clinic at least once during their pregnancy. However, 15 booked late (after 20 weeks) and 14 did not complete their antenatal clinic schedule. One mother felt that there was no benefit from attending antenatal care. Two gave reasons for poor attendance:

> 'It was difficult for me to attend clinic regularly because I was working as a helper and my boss would sack me if I were to be taken permission for every visit.' (PC8, mother, 33)

> 'I started attending antenatal clinic at 6 months but I could not attend regularly because I was writing examinations.' (PC3, mother, 18)

Two nurses reported that teenagers are afraid to report pregnancy for fear of being reprimanded by their parents:

> 'Some of the teenagers usually open up to their parent at a very late stage of labour leading to giving birth en-route to the hospital.' (PC3, nurse, 42)

Quality of health education: Ten mothers reported that nurses educated them about signs and symptoms of labour:

> 'The nurses told us to prepare ourselves when we are about to give birth by sorting and making ready the baby's clothes. They equally warned us not to depend on the ambulance because it is mostly used to transport sick people.' (PC2, mother, 22)

However, only 6 mothers understood the components of birth preparedness taught during antenatal care, namely when, how and where to go in labour.

Lack of resources at clinics: Two mothers saw no benefit in attending an antenatal clinic as antenatal cards were out of stock:

> 'The problem with the clinic is that they are always out of clinic cards. That is why I did not visit regularly.' (PH3, mother, 21)

Poor attitudes of nurses

Two mothers blamed the poor attitudes of nurses at the health facility for having a BBA. One mother was influenced by the perceptions of a relative:

> 'I only went to the clinic at 6 months and I did not go back again. I was afraid because my sister scared me that nurses usually assault women that started booking late.' (PC6, mother, 19)

Another mother waited until an advanced stage of labour before going to the health centre as she had personal experience of poor attitudes:

> 'I was so scared of going to the clinic when I was in early labour because I have no clinic card. Nurses are usually very angry and shout at us if we do not have a card and I did not want to be shouted at. So I decided to wait till close to the delivery time before going, but I ended up giving birth at home.' (PH2, mother, 41)

Poor quality of care

Four mothers blamed nurses for sending them back home when they presented with labour pains:

> 'After the initial examination by the nurse, she told me that I was not in labour and that I should go back home. She should have allowed me stay and observe me until she was sure about what was going on with me; rather, she sent me back home only for me to delivered at midnight at home when there was no transport.' (PC9, mother, 28)

One mother became visibly upset whilst narrating her ordeal and a counselling session was organised for her after the interview:

> 'I went to the clinic which I paid 10 Rands taxi fare, where I used to go for ANC to take my ARV/nevirapine. When I got there the nurses were in a meeting that took 3 hours. When the nurses came out of their meeting I was told that the nevirapine was out of stock and I should try another clinic which was a bit far from home, which I had to pay an extra 15 Rands to get to. It was already late in the afternoon and because of the high rate of crime I could not go back home and had to ask for a place to sleep near the clinic. I went to bed and unfortunately for me the labour pains started at 9 p.m., I could not reach the EMS because my phone battery was flat and there was no taxi to take me to

the clinic. I delivered at 3 a.m. ... The baby stopped moving after about 30 minutes of delivery.' (PC1, mother, 28)

Five CHC nurses felt that a shortage of beds (for observation) contributes to BBA:

'We discharge them when we see they are not in true labour since we do not have enough beds.' (PH5, nurse, 42)

The nurses also felt that a shortage of experienced staff at night could lead to a wrong diagnosis of false labour:

'Another problem is the low level and poor quality of experience of the nurses. I am saying this because you will find that the patient is examined by an inexperienced nurse who is supposed to be working under supervision ... and she misdiagnoses a true labour as a false labour and subsequently sends the patient home.' (PC9, nurse, 50)

Theme 4: Unanticipated events resulting in birth before arrival

Unsure of labour

Three mothers attributed their BBA to being unsure of when they were in labour:

'I started feeling abdominal pain during the day while doing laundry; however, the pain was not serious and it was on and off. My water broke around 8 p.m. and I was going to pee frequently. My grandmother suspected and as soon as she asked me to kneel down, the baby was already coming out.' (PH9, mother, 25)

Miscalculation of dates

One mother reported that being unsure of dates was the reason for BBA:

'I guess I delivered at home because I thought I was in my eight month of pregnancy not knowing I was already at the 9 month.' (PC4, mother, 25)

Precipitate labour

Eight mothers reported that they delivered at home or en route to the hospital because the labour was too fast:

'I started to feel the pains around 9 p.m. at night. I felt the pain at the lower back and I told those with me at the time. They went out to find the ambulance numbers, but by the time they came back my water broke and I had already delivered. The labour took less than an hour.' (PH10, mother, 30)

Preterm delivery

Three mothers explained that they had delivered before 8 months of pregnancy. One of these babies died and the other two were transferred to hospital. One described her experience as follows:

'I gave birth to a live baby that was covered with sac membrane, but the strange thing was that she never cried despite moving the legs. The baby stopped moving after about 30 minutes of delivery. I think the membrane that covered the head and body of baby killed her. I was clueless about how to remove the sac.' (PC1, mother, 28)

Another mother narrated her experienced as follows:

'I was 7 months pregnant when I felt the pain during the day and I told my aunt. She said we should take a walk and by the time we came back I felt like sitting down. I did that and went for a pee and the blood came out followed by a lot of water then after that the baby came. ... The nurses told me the baby was ill and has been admitted to Mandela [*Hospital*].' (PH3, mother, 21)

Theme 5: Risks associated with birth before arrival

The numbers of mothers who actually experienced complications were as follows: placenta was retained in eight, four of which were removed at a health facility; excessive blood loss was seen in seven, of whom one required a blood transfusion; perineal tears that required suturing at a health facility in five; and two neonatal deaths occurred.

Seventeen mothers perceived that a delivery outside a health facility could be dangerous. Four mothers identified that children may need suction of secretions from the mouth and nostrils:

'The child might get sick, because things that are removed at the clinic will not be removed. Things like removing thick saliva in the mouth.' (PC4, mother, 25)

Six mothers expressed a fear of injury with malpresentation or of the baby falling during home delivery:

'The child might die due to little knowledge of traditional midwives, the child might be paralyzed and maybe the child might come with a wrong position or fall during delivery.' (PH7, mother, 34)

Other risks identified were HIV transmission and the baby getting cold. One mother who experienced an early neonatal death described a complication consistent with hypothermia:

'There was delay in the arrival of the EMS and I had delivered two hours before they eventually came. Because it was winter time, the weather was very cold and we wrapped the baby in the blanket. At hospital, the nurses told me that the child had caught too much cold and he did not make it.' (PC9, mother, 28)

Discussion

Most of the mothers interviewed had intended to deliver either in a CHC or in hospital. They had a good understanding of risks associated with BBA. Some of the participants actually experienced complications such as perineal tears, retained placenta, postpartum haemorrhage and neonatal death.

Mothers and nurses identified several factors that influenced the risk of BBA. The majority of BBA mothers reported that they stayed between 30 and 120 minutes' drive from a health facility. These findings were similar to those in a mixed urban-rural setting in Nepal, where a distance of more than 1 hour to hospital was associated with an increased risk of home delivery.[30] Similarly, Blondel et al.[31] in France found that the risk of BBA was strongly associated with distance to the closest maternity unit. In contrast, Parag et al.[32] did not find any association between distance from a health facility and BBA in a peri-urban setting in South Africa.

Transportation was identified as the major source of delay in reaching a health facility. Issues identified were a poor EMS ambulance service, bad roads, a lack of safety at night and an absence of taxis especially at night. Two mothers incorrectly thought they needed to pay for airtime to call the EMS, although emergency calls are free in South Africa. Challenges were encountered in engaging the services of commercial and private vehicle owners. The difficulty of obtaining transport at night is supported by the finding that 15 of the 19 mothers delivered between 22h00 and 06h00. This finding is consistent with results from other studies,[32,33] where most BBAs occurred at night. In rural South Africa, a lack of transport contributed to BBA.[23] Similar results have been reported from Nepal[34] and Brazil.[35]

Whilst mothers were not asked directly about household income and affordability of transport, nurses reported that most BBA mothers were poor. The mothers' demographic characteristics show that only one completed grade 12, and the majority were single and unemployed. The findings were similar to those of a study of 19 states in the USA, where BBA mothers were more likely to be single and uneducated.[18] In contrast, Potter et al.[20] did not find any significant difference in educational level and marital status between mothers who had BBA and mothers who delivered in hospital in a predominantly urban area of South Africa.

Mothers blamed nurses for sending them home when they presented with labour pains. However, nurses noted that a lack of facility beds prevented them from admitting women for observation. Nurses identified a shortage of experienced nurses, leading to poor supervision of junior nurses such that they misdiagnosed true labour as false labour. Studies in Brazil[35] and Nepal[33] also identified the failure of health personnel to identify a woman in early labour as contributory to BBA.

Mothers reported that unforeseen events contributed to BBA, such as miscalculation of dates, being unsure of labour, precipitate labour and preterm labour. Fast labour was associated with BBA in South Africa[20] and Nepal,[33] whilst preterm labour was associated with BBA in South Africa.[32]

Currently, there is no maternity waiting home at Mthatha. Maternity waiting homes can be used by pregnant women to await labour if they anticipate transport difficulties, if nurses are unsure they are in labour or if there are risk factors for preterm or precipitate labour. Developing such homes is an accepted part of the policy of the Department of Health in South Africa.[36]

One woman described using traditional medicines to induce labour. However, the nurses perceived that many mothers use traditional medicines. An example is 'baboon's urine' (isiXhosa: *umchamo wemfene*) that is used to ease labour.[37] Nurses believe it can speed up labour, leading to BBA. In Africa, traditional medicines are commonly used to hasten labour and may cause adverse outcomes in pregnancy.[38,39] Nurses felt that mothers do not usually volunteer such information to health workers for fear of being reprimanded. Judgemental attitudes by healthcare workers have been noted in studies on traditional medicines.[39]

Nurses reported that Xhosa traditions can preclude a parturient from utilising a health facility for childbirth, as a parturient who delivers in hospital is not considered a real mother. Similar findings were described in Uganda.[40]

Nurses stated that, in traditional home childbirth, a woman assumes a squatting position, unlike in hospital where parturients deliver in the supine position. They suggested that this may influence mothers to choose home delivery. However, this view did not emerge during the in-depth interviews, although three mothers mentioned that they used a squatting position during delivery. A study of home deliveries in the Eastern Cape, South Africa, found that 92% of women adopted an upright position during delivery.[41] In the Lao People's Democratic Republic, one of the reasons why mothers chose home delivery was a preference for the traditional squatting position.[42] A systematic review of use of the upright position in delivery suggested several possible benefits, including a reduction in assisted deliveries and episiotomies.[43]

Nurses reported that parturients expressed a preference for female birth attendants, which implies that women should be educated on the gender composition of the healthcare workforce and the midwifery skills that are common to both.

Mothers expressed concerns about nurses' attitudes and behaviour such as shouting at parturients and a lack of prompt attention during antenatal care. This disrespectful care deters women from delivering in health facilities. Similar findings have been described in South Africa[23,44] and Sub-Saharan Africa.[45,46,47,48] Efforts are underway in South Africa[44] and internationally to improve attitudes.[49]

A lack of necessary materials such as stationery and antiretroviral drugs also contributed to the perceived poor quality of services at the health facilities. This view is consistent with the findings of Mselle et al.,[46] who found that inadequate resources contributed to low utilisation of health facilities in Tanzania.

Limitations

As the present study was qualitative, the results cannot be generalised to the whole OR Tambo District Municipality; however, they may be transferable to similar settings.

Conducting interviews in the health facilities might have restricted mothers from freely discussing issues that related to failure of the medical services. Whilst interviews conducted at their homes would be optimal, it would have been expensive and time consuming to do so.

Conclusion

The study identified that all but two BBA mothers intended to deliver in a health facility. Reasons identified as contributing to BBA were poor physical access to health facilities (transport and roads); negative attitudes by nurses; inadequate nursing skills in identifying true labour; culture and tradition favouring home delivery; inadequate recognition by mothers of labour; and preterm and precipitate labour. Mothers booked late and did not attend for the recommended number of antenatal care visits.

Recommendations

Recommendations to the Department of Health to improve the health system for mothers and babies include the following points. A maternity waiting home is needed at Mthatha for women who may encounter difficulties in accessing a health facility during labour and for women who may be in early labour. Provision of a functional, dedicated obstetric ambulance system can reduce delays in transporting parturients to health facilities.[50] A programme should be implemented to improve nurses' attitudes, based on the universal rights of childbearing women[51] and effective intervention programmes[44] to improve nurses' skills in diagnosing true labour and to allow parturients a choice of delivery position.[43] Health education for pregnant women should focus on early booking, advice on cultural practices that may be detrimental to health, the signs and symptoms of labour, and when and how to go to an appropriate health facility for delivery.

Acknowledgements

The authors thank the participating mothers and nurses and the research assistant Phelo Sithole for their contribution to this research, and the anonymous reviewers for their helpful comments.

Competing interests

The authors declare that they have no financial or personal relationship(s) that may have inappropriately influenced them in writing this article.

Authors' contributions

A.A. (Walter Sisulu University) devised the original idea for the research and collected the data. G.W. (University of Fort Hare) and M.J.N. (Walter Sisulu University) assisted with development of the protocol. G.W. (University of Fort Hare), M.J.N. and D.O.M. (Walter Sisulu University) assisted with data analysis, discussion, recommendations and writing up the final version of the manuscript.

References

1. Fund UNCs. Levels and trends in child mortality: Report 2014. New York: United Nations Children's Fund; 2014.
2. Pattinson R. Saving babies 2008–2009: Seventh report on perinatal care in South Africa. Pretoria: Tshepesa Press; 2011.
3. Lawn JE, Cousens S, Zupan J. 4 million neonatal deaths: When? where? why? Lancet. 2005;365:891–900.
4. Wang H, Liddell CA, Coates MM, et al. Global, regional, and national levels of neonatal, infant, and under-5 mortality during 1990–2013: A systematic analysis for the Global Burden of Disease Study 2013. Lancet. 2014;384:957–979.
5. Countdown to 2015. Fulfilling the health agenda for women and children. The 2014 South Africa report. Geneva: Partnership for Maternal, Newborn & Child Health, World Health Organization; 2014.
6. Lawn JE, Blencowe H, Pattinson R, et al. Stillbirths: Where? when? why? How to make the data count? Lancet. 2011;377:1448–1463.
7. Statistics South Africa. Perinatal deaths in South Africa, 2011–2013: Statistical release P0309.4. Pretoria: Statistics South Africa; 2015.
8. Kassebaum NJ, Bertozzi-Villa A, Coggeshall MS, et al. Global, regional, and national levels and causes of maternal mortality during 1990–2013: A systematic analysis for the Global Burden of Disease Study 2013. Lancet. 2014;384: 980–1004.
9. Say L, Chou D, Gemmill A, et al. Global causes of maternal death: A WHO systematic analysis. Lancet Global Health. 2014;2:e323–e333.
10. National Committee for Confidential Enquiry into Maternal Deaths. Saving mothers 208-2010. Fifth report on the confidential enquiries into maternal deaths in South Africa. Pretoria: Department of Health; 2012.
11. World Health Organization. Making pregnancy safer: The critical role of the skilled attendant. A joint statement by WHO, ICM and FIGO. Geneva: World Health Organization; 2004.
12. Department of Health. Guidelines for maternity care in South Africa. A manual for clinics, community health centres and district hospitals. 4th ed. Pretoria: Department of Health; 2015.
13. Bassingthwaighte MK, Ballot D. Outcomes of babies born before arrival at a tertiary hospital in Johannesburg, South Africa. South Afr J Child Health. 2013;7:139–145.
14. Lazić Z, Takač I. Outcomes and risk factors for unplanned delivery at home and before arrival to the hospital. Wien Klin Wochenschr. 2011;123:11–14.
15. Gunnarsson B, Smárason AK, Skogvoll E, Fasting S. Characteristics and outcome of unplanned out-of-institution births in Norway from 1999 to 2013: A cross-sectional study. Acta Obstet Gynecol Scand. 2014;93:1003–1010.
16. Orimadegun AE, Akinbami FO, Tongo OO, Okereke JO. Comparison of neonates born outside and inside hospitals in a children emergency unit, southwest of Nigeria. Pediatr Emerg Care. 2008;24:354–358.
17. McLelland G, McKenna L, Archer F. No fixed place of birth: Unplanned BBAs in Victoria, Australia. Midwifery. 2013;29:e19–e25.
18. Declercq E, MacDorman MF, Menacker F, Stotland N. Characteristics of planned and unplanned home births in 19 states. Obstet Gynecol. 2010;116:93–99.
19. National Perinatal Mortality and Morbidity Committee. National Perinatal Mortality and Morbidity Committee (NaPeMMCo) Triennial Report (2008-2010). Pretoria: Department of Health; 2011.
20. Potter P, Pelteret R, Reynolds L, Motala A, Kibel M. Born before arrival. S Afr Med J. 1984;66:397–402.
21. Peltzer K, Mosala T, Shisana O, Nqeteko A. Utilization of delivery services in the context of prevention of HIV from mother-to-child (PMTCT) in a rural community, South Africa. Curationis. 2006;29:54–61.
22. Tlebere P, Jackson D, Loveday M, et al. Community-based situation analysis of maternal and neonatal care in South Africa to explore factors that impact utilization of maternal health services. J Midwifery Womens Health. 2007;52: 342–350.
23. Silal SP, Penn-Kekana L, Harris B, Birch S, McIntyre D. Exploring inequalities in access to and use of maternal health services in South Africa. BMC Health Serv Res. 2012;12:120.
24. Kuper A, Reeves S, Levinson W. Qualitative research: An introduction to reading and appraising qualitative research. BMJ. 2008;337:404–407.
25. Day C. The district health barometer: Year 2010/11. Durban: Health Systems Trust; 2012.
26. Statistics South Africa. Census 2011 municipal report, Eastern Cape. Report No. 03-01-50. Pretoria: Statistics South Africa; 2012.
27. Kitzinger J. Qualitative research: Introducing focus groups. BMJ. 1995;311:299–302.
28. Pope C, Ziebland S, Mays N. Analysing qualitative data. BMJ. 2000;320:114–116.
29. Shenton AK. Strategies for ensuring trustworthiness in qualitative research projects. Educ Inf. 2004;22:63–75.
30. Wagle RR, Sabroe S, Nielsen BB. Socioeconomic and physical distance to the maternity hospital as predictors for place of delivery: An observation study from Nepal. BMC Pregnancy Childbirth. 2004;4:8.
31. Blondel B, Drewniak N, Pilkington H, Zeitlin J. Out-of-hospital births and the supply of maternity units in France. Health & Place. 2011;17:1170–1173.
32. Parag N, McKerrow NH, Naby F. Profile of babies born before arrival at hospital in a peri-urban setting. South Afr J Child Health. 2014;8:45–53.
33. Chaudhary P. Accidental out-of-hospital deliveries: Factors influencing delay in arrival to maternity hospital. Kathmandu Univ Med J. 2005;3:115–122.
34. Sreeramareddy CT, Joshi HS, Sreekumaran BV, Giri S, Chuni N. Home delivery and newborn care practices among urban women in western Nepal: A questionnaire survey. BMC Pregnancy Childbirth. 2006;6:27.
35. de Almeida MF, Alencar GP, Novaes MHD, et al. Accidental home deliveries in southern Sao Paulo, Brazil. Rev Saude Publica. 2005;39:366–375.

36. Pattinson RC. Reducing direct causes of maternal death. S Afr J Obstet Gynaecol. 2013;19:59–60.

37. Dold T, Cocks M. Voices from the forest: Celebrating nature and culture in Xhosaland. Johannesburg: Jacana Media; 2012.

38. Maliwichi-Nyirenda CP, Maliwichi LL. Medicinal plants used to induce labour and traditional techniques used in determination of onset of labour in pregnant women in Malawi: A case study of Mulanje district. J Med Plants Res. 2010;4:2609–2614.

39. Van der Kooi R, Theobald S. Traditional medicine in late pregnancy and labour: Perceptions of Kgaba remedies amongst the Tswana in South Africa. Afr J Tradit Complement Altern Med. 2006;3:11–22.

40. Kyomuhendo GB. Low use of rural maternity services in Uganda: Impact of women's status, traditional beliefs and limited resources. Reprod Health Matters. 2003;11:16–26.

41. O'Mahony D, Steinberg M. A population-based survey of obstetric practices among rural women in the Bizana district, Transkei. S Afr Med J. 1995;85:1168–1171.

42. Sychareun V, Hansana V, Somphet V, Xayavong S, Phengsavanh A, Popenoe R. Reasons rural Laotians choose home deliveries over delivery at health facilities: A qualitative study. BMC Pregnancy Childbirth. 2012;12:86.

43. Gupta JK, Hofmeyr GJ, Shehmar M. Position in the second stage of labour for women without epidural anaesthesia. Cochrane Database Syst Rev. 2012;5:Art. CD002006.

44. Honikman S, Fawcus S, Meintjes I. Abuse in South African maternity settings is a disgrace: Potential solutions to the problem. S Afr Med J. 2015;105:284–286.

45. Moore B, Alex-Hart B, George I. Utilization of health care services by pregnant mothers during delivery: A community based study in Nigeria. East Afr J Public Health. 2011; 8:49–51.

46. Mselle LT, Moland KM, Mvungi A, Evjen-Olsen B, Kohi TW. Why give birth in health facility? Users' and providers' accounts of poor quality of birth care in Tanzania. BMC Health Serv Res. 2013;13:174.

47. Amooti-Kaguna B, Nuwaha F. Factors influencing choice of delivery sites in Rakai district of Uganda. Soc Sci Med. 2000;50:203–213.

48. Phiri S, Moland K, Fylkesnes K. 'Born before arrival': User and provider perspectives on home deliveries and barriers to health facility childbirth in Kapiri Mposhi, Zambia. Trop Med Int Health. 2014;14:323.

49. United Nations Population Fund. The state of the world's midwifery. A universal pathway. A woman's right to health. New York: United Nations Population Fund; 2014.

50. Schoon MG. Impact of inter-facility transport on maternal mortality in the Free State Province. S Afr Med J. 2013;103:534–536.

51. White Ribbon Alliance. Respectful maternity care charter. Washington, DC: White Ribbon Alliance; 2011.

HIV and/or AIDS-related deaths and modifiable risk factors: A descriptive study of medical admissions at Oshakati Intermediate Hospital in Northern Namibia

Authors:
N.K. Mgori[1,2]
Robert Mash[1]

Affiliations:
[1]Division of Family Medicine and Primary Care, Stellenbosch University, South Africa

[2]Oshakati Intermediate Hospital, Namibia

Correspondence to:
Robert Mash

Email:
rm@sun.ac.za

Postal address:
Division of Family Medicine and Primary Care, Stellenbosch University, PO Box 241, Cape Town 8000, South Africa

Background: High rates of HIV infection have decreased life expectancy in many African countries. Regardless of worldwide efforts to escalate treatment, care and prevention strategies, the number of deaths due to AIDS-related disorders is still high. Local healthcare workers suspect that there are modifiable factors in the care of HIV and/or AIDS patients which can be identified and improved.

Aim: To describe the HIV and/or AIDS-related causes of adult mortality and identify modifiable factors amongst patients admitted to Oshakati Intermediate Hospital, northern Namibia.

Methods: Data was extracted retrospectively and coded using the modified CoDe protocol for AIDS. Modifiable factors relating to the patient, health system or clinical care were identified using a standardised data collection tool.

Results: A total of 177 HIV and/or AIDS patients were identified, 94 (53.1%) were male and 120 (68%) had a CD4 count of less than 200 cells/mL. The common HIV-related causes of death were tuberculosis (25.9%), renal failure (15.8%), *Pneumocystis jirovecii* pneumonia (11.3%), cryptococcal meningitis (9%), HIV wasting syndrome (7.9%) and AIDS-defining malignancy (7.9%). The analysis revealed 281 modifiable factors; patient-related factors were the most common (153 [54.4%]), followed by health system factors (97 [34.5%]) and healthcare personnel factors (31 [11%]).

Conclusion: Our findings have highlighted the challenges in overall HIV and/or AIDS inpatient care and surrounding primary care facilities. The identification of specific modifiable factors can be used to reduce mortality by providing training as well as rational monitoring, planning and resource allocation.

Décès liés au VIH/SIDA et facteurs de risques modifiables: Etude descriptive des admissions médicales à l'Hôpital intermédiaire d'Oshakati au nord de la Namibie.

Contexte: Le taux élevé d'infection par VIH a réduit l'espérance de vie dans de nombreux pays africains. Malgré les efforts mondiaux d'intensification des traitements, des soins et des stratégies de prévention, le nombre de décès dus aux troubles associés au SIDA est encore élevé. Le personnel de santé local pense qu'on peut identifier et améliorer certains facteurs modifiables dans les soins des malades du VIH/SIDA.

Objectif: Décrire les causes de mortalité des adultes liées au VIH/SIDA et identifier les facteurs modifiables chez les patients admis à l'Hôpital Intermédiaire d'Oshakati, au nord de la Namibie.

Méthodes: les données ont été extraites et classées rétrospectivement en utilisant le protocole modifié CoDe pour le SIDA. Les facteurs modifiables concernant le patient, le système de santé ou de soins cliniques ont été identifiés à l'aide d'un outil de collecte de données standardisé.

Résultats: On a identifié au total 177 malades du VIH/SIDA, dont 94 (53.1%) étaient des hommes et 120 (68%) avaient un taux de CD4 de moins de 200 cellules /ml. Les causes les plus fréquentes de décès lié au HIV étaient la tuberculose (25.9%), l'insuffisance rénale (15.8%), la pneumonie *Pneumocystis jirovecii* (11.3%), la méningite cryptococcique (9%), le syndrome de dépérissement lié au VIH (7.9%) et les tumeurs liées au SIDA (7.9%). L'analyse a révélé 281 facteurs modifiables; les facteurs liés au patient étaient les plus fréquents (153 [54.4%]), suivis des facteurs liés au système de santé (97 [34.5%]) et ceux liés au personnel de santé (31 [11%]).

Conclusion: Nos résultats ont mis en évidence les défis des soins en hospitalisation des malades du VIH/SIDA et dans les établissements de soins primaires avoisinants. On peut utiliser l'identification de facteurs modifiables particuliers pour réduire la mortalité en offrant des formations, des contrôles rationnels ainsi que la planification et l'allocation des ressources.

Introduction

HIV and/or AIDS is one of the major global public health problems and causes substantial morbidity, mortality, negative socio-economic impact, and human suffering.[1,2] Since the beginning of 1981, HIV and/or AIDS has become a pandemic disease, claiming some 20 million lives.[1] By the end of 2010, an estimated 34 million people of all age groups (31.6 million–35.2 million) were living with HIV worldwide.[1,2]

Sub-Saharan Africa, with only 12% of the global population, ranks top amongst the regions that are drastically affected by HIV.[3] The region contributes 68% of all HIV and/or AIDS patients in the world, whilst South-East Asia has 12%, Eastern Europe and Central Asia 4%, Latin America 4% and North America 4%. South Africa has the highest number of people living with HIV and/or AIDS (having more than 4 million patients).[2]

Namibia is amongst the countries which are significantly affected by HIV and/or AIDS. It has a relatively small population of 2.1 million and the Ministry of Health and Social Services estimates the HIV prevalence rate to be 18.2%.[4] Furthermore, in 2011–2012 it was estimated that 193 000 adults and children were living with HIV. This number is predicted to increase to 196 000 in the year 2015–2016.[5]

The HIV and/or AIDS epidemic is the largest contributor to the burden of disease in Namibia, contributing 37% to indirect causes of maternal mortality, which is an increase of 50% from 2000 to 2006. Furthermore, life expectancy has decreased from 62 years in 1996 to 44 years in 2006 due to HIV and/or AIDS.[4,5]

Over the past two decades, the government of Namibia has prioritised HIV and AIDS in its development goals for 2030. This has led to increases in universal access to antiretroviral treatment, with coverage of between 50% and 80% of eligible patients.[2]

Strategies used to curb HIV and/or AIDS morbidity and mortality in Namibia include the provision of free, highly active antiretroviral therapy (HAART); recruitment, re-training and retention of health workers; health education; screening for and ultimately treating opportunistic infections as well as sexually transmitted diseases.[3,4] The screening for opportunistic infections and preventive therapy is offered by both hospitals and clinics and includes the provision of isoniazid, co-trimoxazole, fluconazole and malaria prophylaxis in pregnancy. Ongoing adherence counselling and the retention of patients at the clinic level may also help to reduce mortality and morbidity.[4,5,6,7,8,9,10,11,12,13]

Despite the national efforts, premature deaths from HIV and/or AIDS continue and reflect deficiencies in quality of care at different levels of the health system.[4] Quality improvement projects have directed their energy at the clinic level, where most of the HIV clients are clinically stable, whilst less effort has been directed at those admitted to hospital with acute conditions.[5]

Like any other chronic condition, the management and progression of HIV and/or AIDS has both non-modifiable and modifiable factors associated with it. Modifiable factors are omissions or commissions that occur during the process of patient care and which subsequently lead to substandard care. They could be related to the patient, their caregiver, healthcare workers or the health system.[6,13]

Non-modifiable risk factors include age, race and gender. Modifiable non-HIV specific factors include smoking status, body mass index, hypertension, diabetes mellitus, and hepatitis C and B status. Other modifiable HIV-specific factors include, for example, the patient's CD4 count and viral load.[14]

There has been no formal study to assess the causes of death and modifiable factors related to inpatient mortality amongst HIV-infected patients in Namibia. Local healthcare workers suspect that there are many modifiable factors affecting patient outcomes within Oshakati Intermediate Hospital. Identification of these modifiable risk factors and prompt interventions may provide insight into how to improve the management of HIV and/or AIDS patients admitted in our hospital.[14,15]

The aim of the study, therefore, was to investigate the modifiable factors contributing to HIV and/or AIDS-related deaths amongst adults in Oshakati Intermediate Hospital.

Methods

Study design

This was a descriptive study using data extracted retrospectively from the medical records of patients who died of HIV-related disease.

Study setting

The study was undertaken at Oshakati Intermediate Hospital, which is located in Oshana region, northern Namibia. It is a 750-bed public hospital, serving approximately 750 000 Namibians and an unknown number of Angolans. The region has no district hospital; therefore, Oshakati Intermediate Hospital receives referrals from local primary care clinics as well as district hospitals in the Omusati, Kunene, Ohangwena and Oshikoto regions.

Oshakati Intermediate Hospital is also a teaching hospital; and has relatively more staff than nearby district hospitals. The internal medicine department alone has four specialist physicians, an HIV and/or AIDS clinical mentor, two medical practitioners, two interns and 14 nurses. The male and female wards have 130 beds with three high-dependency units. The HAART centre, oncology clinic and medical outpatient department are under the umbrella of the internal medicine department.

Data collection

Folders from patients who had died of HIV-related causes were selected for data collection and only patients with a confirmed HIV-positive test result were included.

An auditing team was established that consisted of the researcher, four specialist physicians, an HIV and/or AIDS clinical mentor, an intern doctor, registered nurses and one administrator. This team was responsible for reviewing patient files from medical records and determining the diagnoses, HIV-related death and likely modifiable factors.

Basic clinical and demographic information was extracted for each patient in a standardised way: age, gender, HIV status, HAART status, length of stay in the ward, CD4 count and viral load.

The diagnoses were determined after a review of the patients' medical history from the patients' health booklets, nurses' notes, clinical notes made by the admitting doctors, and progress reports from nurses and doctors at different points of care such as casualty, medical outpatients, inpatients and referral letters. The results of investigations, such as laboratory results and imaging, were reviewed. Results which were not in the files were traced manually using the available requisition numbers.

To date, no validation study exist to assess HIV-related causes of death in Namibia: The International Classification of Disease, ICD1-10, has limited value. Therefore, a protocol for determining the HIV-related cause of death, the CoDe system, was adapted from the Copenhagen HIV Programme, Centre of Global Excellence.[16] This is the standardised system for classifying and coding deaths in studies of patients with HIV infection based on detailed data collection of information on the causes of death and contributing factors. The World Health Organization's staging system was also used to categorise AIDS-specific causes of death.[2] When there were disagreements between the reviewers, a consensus agreement with the clinical HIV mentor was reached. The mentor is an employee of the International Training and Education Center for Health in Namibia, covering the northern region.

The team then considered potential modifiable factors that could be related to the patients, their caregivers, their healthcare workers or the performance of the health system. The data collection tool and process used were modelled on similar approaches in the Child Healthcare Problem Identification Programme (CHPIP system), but adapted to adults with HIV.[15] The study supervisor independently assessed the construction of the tool to improve its validity.

The causes of HIV and/or AIDS-related deaths were multi-factorial. As several factors might interact to contribute to deaths in this study, all modifiable factors were assessed per patient folder.

A pilot study was conducted to assess the quality of the clinical notes before the study. The study instrument was pre-tested a week before execution of the study on the records of patients with HIV who had recently died at the hospital. After reviewing 21 files for the pilot study, questions which were not clear were rephrased and retested; thereafter, a new questionnaire was constructed and used to capture the appropriate data for the study.

Data analysis

All the data was captured on a purpose-designed form in Microsoft Access and this programme was subsequently used to produce a data spreadsheet in Microsoft Excel. The data was cleaned and verified to minimise entry errors, outliers and missing values. Frequencies and percentages were calculated for categorical data. Statisticians at the Centre for Statistical Consultation at Stellenbosch University were consulted for inferential data analysis. Inferential data analysis was done using the Statistical Package for Social Scientists software window version 19.0 (SPSS Inc., Chicago, IL). The frequencies and Pearson Chi square test were used to analyse the association between the dependent and independent variables and $p < 0.05$ was considered statistically significant.

Ethical considerations

The proposal was approved by the Health Research Ethics Committee of Stellenbosch University (S12/11/301) and the Oshakati Intermediate Hospital ethics committee.

Results

General characteristics of HIV-infected patients

There were 2452 admissions, in both medical wards, during the period from 01 January to 31 December 2011. The overall number of deaths was 564 (23.0%), and of these deaths 201 (a case fatality rate of 35.7%) were documented as related to HIV. Out of these 201 deaths, the folders were retrieved for 177 patients.

Of 177 audited folders, 94 (53.1%) patients were on HAART and 48 (51.1%) had been initiated on HAART within the previous 90 days. Table 1 summarises the characteristics of the study population.

HIV-related deaths

Amongst the patients reviewed, 82.0% died of HIV and/or AIDS-defining conditions, whereas 18.0% had non-AIDS-defining diseases. The underlying causes of death and frequencies are shown in Table 2. Extra-pulmonary tuberculosis accounted for most deaths, followed by renal failure, *Pneumocystis jirovecii* pneumonia, cryptococcal meningitis and HIV wasting syndrome.

Modifiable factors

Three broad modifiable factors were detected: patient- and caregiver-related factors accounted for 153 (54.4%), followed by healthcare system factors 97 (34.5%) and finally healthcare

TABLE 1: General characteristics of the HIV-infected patients.

Characteristics	All (n = 177) n (%)	Males (n = 94) n (%)	Females (n = 83) n (%)
Age group (years)			
15–24	22 (12)	12 (13)	10 (12)
25–44	89 (50)	44 (47)	45 (54)
45–64	55 (31)	31 (33)	24 (29)
65	11 (6)	7 (7)	4 (5)
Duration of hospital stay (days)			
< 1	48 (27)	30 (62)	18 (37)
1–14	93 (52)	40 (43)	53 (57)
15–28	21 (12)	13(62)	8 (38)
> 28	15 (8)	11 (73)	4 (27)
CD4 counts (cells/mm³)			
< 200	120 (68)	64 (53)	56 (47)
200 +	57 (32)	30 (53)	27 (47)
HAART status			
Pre-HAART	83 (47)	40 (48)	43 (52)
On HAART < 15 days	15 (16)	10 (67)	5 (33)
On HAART 15–90 days	33 (35)	15 (45)	18 (55)
On HAART 91–365 days	15 (16)	10 (67)	5 (33)
On HAART > 365 days	31 (33)	19 (61)	12 (39)
HAART (Total)	94 (53)	54 (57)	40 (43)

TABLE 2: HIV-related deaths.

Diagnosis	n (%) (n = 177)
Extra-pulmonary tuberculosis	30 (16.9)
Renal failure	28 (15.8)
Pneumocystis pneumonia	20 (11.3)
Pulmonary tuberculosis	16 (9.0)
Cryptococcal meningitis	15 (8.5)
HIV wasting syndrome	14 (7.9)
AIDS-defining malignancies	14 (7.9)
Haematological disease	9 (5.1)
Chronic diarrhoea	8 (4.5)
CNS disease	7 (4.0)
Severe bacterial infections	5 (2.8)
Liver failure other than viral hepatitis	4 (2.3)
Alcohol abuse	3 (1.7)
Non-AIDS malignancy	2 (1.1)
Pulmonary thrombo-embolism	1 (0.6)
Cardiovascular disease	1 (0.6)

worker-related factors 31 (11.0%). Delayed presentation to a health facility was the commonest factor overall and accounted for 85.0% of patient- or caregiver-related factors. Failure to provide standard critical care services, haemodialysis or ventilator support accounted for 86.0% of health system factors whereas challenges experienced in monitoring patients was the main factor for healthcare workers (29.0%). Table 3 summarises the specific modifiable factors.

Table 4 shows the relationship between variables and HIV clinical diagnosis. More male patients died of AIDS-defining diseases compared to females, and the difference was statistically significant, (57.24% versus 42.76%; p-value < 0.05), All age groups were at the same risk of dying either from AIDS-defining conditions or a non-AIDS-defining condition (p = 0.546). Moreover, for these two groups of patients there were no differences in length of hospitalisation (p = 0.99), In addition, more patients with CD4 counts of less than 200 cell/mm³ died of AIDS-defining conditions than those with CD4 counts of more than 200 cells/mm³ (75.86% versus 31.25%; $p < 0.05$). Furthermore, more patients who were on HAART in the study group died of a non-AIDS-defining illness than

TABLE 3: Modifiable factors.

Modifiable factors	n (%)
Patient- and caregiver-related factors (N = 153)	
Delayed presentation to a health facility	130 (84.9)
Defaulted HIV treatment	21 (7.4)
Alcohol abuse	2 (1.3)
Healthcare system factors (n = 97)	
Lack of dialysis machine for HIV-positive patients	31 (31.9)
Inadequate respiratory support in the ward (oxygen supply)	26 (26.8)
Lack of ICU care for patient with HIV and/or AIDS	26 (26.8)
Inadequate blood product supply to the ward	6 (6.1)
Inadequate hospital stock of essential consumables	3 (3.1)
Basic laboratory investigations not available to ward 24 hours a day	2 (2.1)
Inadequate ward stock of essential consumables	1 (1.0)
Lack of standardised case management protocols in ward	1 (1.0)
Doctors in the ward inadequately supervised	1 (1.0)
Healthcare worker factors (n = 31)	
Essential treatment not prescribed	4 (12.9)
Inadequate monitoring of kidney disease	4 (12.9)
Inadequate monitoring/intervention of liver disease	3 (9.7)
Inadequate evaluation of treatable malignancy	1 (3.2)
Inadequate assessment of fitting or comatose patient	6 (19.3)
Inadequate fluid replacement	4 (12.9)
Insufficient case assessment and management in the ward	3 (9.7)
Inadequate switching HAART due to toxicity	2 (6.5)
Inadequate blood chemistry review	1 (3.2)
Doctor called, but did not respond	1 (3.2)
Doctor at peripheral hospital did not call referral hospital	1 (3.2)
Critical HIV patient not reviewed by doctor during weekend	1 (3.2)

TABLE 4: Association between gender and disease categorisation.

Variable	Non-AIDS	AIDS	Total	p-value
Gender				
Male	11 (34.38)	83 (57.24)	94	p = 0.019
Female	21 (65.63)	62 (42.76)	83	
Total	32	145	177	
Age grouping				
15–24	3 (9.38)	19 (13.10)	22	
25–44	15 (46.88)	74 (51.03)	89	
45–64	13 (40.63)	42 (28.97)	55	
65 +	1 (3.13)	10 (6.9)	11	
Total	32	145	177	p = 0.546
CD4				
< 200	10 (31.25)	110 (75.86)	120	
> 200	22 (68.75)	35 (24.14)	57	p < 0.01
Total	32	145	177	
Duration of stay				
< 1	39 (26.7)	9 (28.13)	48	
1–14	77 (53.10)	16 (50.0)	93	
15–28	17 (11.72)	4 (12.5)	21	p = 0.99
> 28 days	12 (8.28)	3 (9.38)	15	
Total	145	32	177	
HAART status				
HAART	24 (75.0)	70 (48.8)	94	p = 0.006
Pre-HAART	8 (25.0)	75 (51.1)	83	
Total	32	145	177	

pre-HAART patients, and the relationship is statistically significant (75.00% versus 25.00%; $p = 0.006$).

Discussion

This study demonstrated that the overall percentage of all deaths in the hospital's medical wards directly attributable to HIV was relatively high at 35.0%, although this finding was consistent with studies in similar settings.[5,6,7] As some patients died without an established HIV diagnosis, this percentage is also likely to be an underestimate.

Patient-related modifiable factors played a significant role through delayed presentation and defaulting on treatment, which led to patients' presenting with more advanced disease that was more difficult to treat successfully.[6,7,17] Other patient-related factors identified in the study were male gender, low CD4 counts of less than 200 cells/mm^3 and pre-HAART patients, which could reflect determinants or predictors of HIV-related mortality. A similar trend has also been observed in other studies.[6,7,18]

In our setup, the focus of HIV and/or AIDS prevention strategies is largely on the pregnant woman (83.0% coverage) during antenatal care and the natal and postnatal periods, which in turn capture more HIV and/or AIDS-infected woman than men. The overall HAART coverage in Namibia is estimated at 88.0% coverage and the country has adapted the updated WHO eligibility criteria to CD4 500 cell/mm^3.[3,4,5] However, the mortality rate of HIV-related death is still high. The reasons for such late presentation and poor adherence identified in other studies include barriers to accessing care, forgetfulness, socio-economic constraints, fear of discrimination or stigmatisation, drug toxicity and limited knowledge of HIV and/or AIDS.[6,7,13,15,19,20] As in our study, it is reported that early HIV diagnosis, early help-seeking behaviour, improved access to care, prompt initiation of HAART for eligible patients, and maintaining good adherence are critical to successful HIV and/or AIDS treatment.[7,19,21,17,22,23,24] Further studies are needed to identify barriers to accessing care in our setting and to understand help-seeking behaviour in local communities.

Numerous researchers have reported significant reductions in mortality in HIV and/or AIDS patients after the introduction of HAART and attention having been given to modifiable factors in the quality of care.[6,8,9,13,14,15,16,25,18,26,27]

Modifiable factors identified in this study have highlighted several areas for potential improvement in adult care, treatment and monitoring. In our study, patients who had CD4 counts of more than 200 cells/mm^3 and were on HAART died of non-AIDS-defining diseases, whereas the pre-HAART group succumbed due to AIDS-related diseases. This reflects the efficacy of HAART in preventing advanced HIV and/or AIDS disease; however, long-term use of HAART predisposes patients to metabolic complications which are also detrimental, a phenomenon being observed in developing countries.

Within the healthcare system at the hospital, there appeared to be discrimination against patients with HIV in terms of access to intensive care beds. Such discrimination might be related to a shortage of ICU beds, a lack of HIV and/or AIDS knowledge and negative attitudes towards critically ill patients. Similar findings on HIV and ICU care have been noted in some developing countries, whilst in South Africa, India and Brazil there are regulatory bodies that govern and prevent non-discriminatory practice.[28] Therefore there is a need for policy-makers, health system administrators and clinicians to devise policy frameworks or guidelines to ensure non-discriminatory access to ICU care regardless of HIV status.

A lack of dialysis for HIV-positive patients with renal failure contributed significantly to deaths, as such patients depend mainly on conservative management. The importance of dialysis and close monitoring of renal function in patients with renal impairment cannot be over-emphasised, as there has been a rapid increase in renal failure in the HIV population worldwide. The HIV virus and Tenofovir-based therapy are both associated with renal diseases.[29] There appears to be a lack of insight into and prioritisation of procurement for patients with HIV, although discussions with the management team revealed plans to construct a new dialysis unit by 2018. In the meantime, in-service training for peritoneal dialysis is being conducted as a short-term solution.

Health system managers must also ensure that essential consumables such as medication are available and should improve the turnaround time for crucial laboratory results. Blood products such as platelets take 48–72 hours to arrive from Windhoek and there is a need to construct a blood bank to serve northern Namibia.

Many patients who died were eligible for HAART, which reflects a gap in existing strategies for the screening, prevention and treatment of opportunistic infections at primary healthcare level. There is a need for our HAART centres at Oshakati and surrounding district hospitals to implement quality improvement projects that address this issue.[4,30]

The hospital relies on many foreign-trained healthcare workers who may not be familiar with HIV management. Therefore there is a need to familiarise junior colleagues with local guidelines and expose them to the HAART service with the objective of improving their HIV and/or AIDS case management skills.[30] Deficiencies in individual clinical care may be addressed by more effective continuing professional development as well as regular risk management meetings that discuss morbidity and mortality. The hospital should make attendance at educational meetings mandatory and ensure more effective interactive small-group learning as opposed to formal didactic approaches. Disciplinary measures should be taken against healthcare workers who do not follow ethical rules and continue to practise negligently. Several studies have shown that greater physician experience and expertise is associated with reduced patient morbidity and mortality.[25,31]

Not all of the medical records could be retrieved and we also faced challenges arising from, information being missing from medical records. Data on the social, demographic and economic status of the patients was often not available in the folders and therefore the effect on health-seeking practice could not be studied. The clinical notes in some files were written in poor handwriting, which made data collection difficult. The causes of death were based on clinical findings recorded in the notes and no postmortems were conducted; this was mainly due to social–cultural barriers. The findings from postmortem examinations could have better defined the causes death.

Globally there are challenges in coding HIV deaths; added to which the available tools do not reflect the common conditions affecting sub-Saharan Africa. We overcame this difficulty in our study by using both the WHO and the CoDe to capture all causes.

Conclusion

HIV and/or AIDS contributed significantly to overall inpatient mortality, and AIDS-defining diseases were the leading causes of deaths in the Oshakati Intermediate Hospital. The most common causes of death were extra-pulmonary tuberculosis, renal failure and *Pneumocystis jirovecii* pneumonia. Patient- and caregiver-related factors, particularly delays in seeking healthcare, were the most common modifiable factors. Access to critical care, dialysis and ventilator support as well as the poor monitoring of patients were the main modifiable factors in the hospital. Future studies should investigate issues related to the accessibility of healthcare and the initiation of HAART at primary care facilities. Continuing professional development, routine risk management, and better planning and procurement of essential resources will help to reduce deaths in the hospital.

Acknowledgements

We would like to express our sincere gratitude to Dr Muideen Bello, Dr Michael Pather and Dr AB Adebanjo for their continuing support. Furthermore, we would like to thank staff in the internal medicine department: Dr Ngalyuka Kioko, Dr Innocent Segamwenge, Dr William Baladron Guerra, Prof. Roberto Larrea Fabra and Dr Tadesse Teferi (HIV/AIDS ITECH-clinical mentor) for their insightful comments and participation in the mortality review process. We also thank the research assistants, Ms Mirium Bernard (MD5-Sun) and Elizabeth Nevonga (MD5-Unam), for their help with data collection. Special thanks must go to Prof. Martin Kidd and Dr Justin Harvey from the Centre for Statistical Consultation, Stellenbosch University, for their great assistance with the data analysis.

Competing interests

The authors declare that they have no financial or personal relationship(s) that may have inappropriately influenced them in writing this article.

Authors' contributions

N.M. (Stellenbosch University and Oshakati Intermediate Hospital) performed the study as a research assignment for the degree Master of Medicine in Family Medicine under the supervision of R.M. (Stellenbosch University). Both N.M. and R.M. conceptualised the study, data was collected and analysed by N.M., the final report was written by N.M. with supervision by R.M., and both authors approved the final manuscript.

References

1. Ortblad KF, Lozano R, Murray CJL. The burden of HIV: Insights from the global burden of disease study 2010. AIDS (London, England). 2013 [cited 2015 Jul 3]; 27(13):2003–2017. PMC. Web. Available from: http://www.ncbi.nlm.nih.gov/pmc/articles/PMC3748855/
2. WHO. Guidance on provider-initiated HIV testing and counselling in health facilities. [online]. 2007 [cited 2015 Jul 2]. Available from: http://whqlibdoc.who.int/publications/2007/9789241595568_eng.pdf
3. United Nations General Assembly Special Session (UNGASS). Country report. No date [cited 2014 Aug 10]. Available from: http://www.unaids.org/sites/default/files/en/dataanalysis/knowyourresponse/countryprogressreports/2010countries/namibia_2010_country_progress_report_en.pdf
4. Jonas A, Sumbi V, Mwinga S, et al. HIV drug resistance early warning indicators in Namibia with updated World Health Organization guidance. Sued O, editor. PLoS One. 2014 [cited 2015 Jul 5]; 9(7). Available from: http://www.ncbi.nlm.nih.gov/pmc/articles/PMC4079656/
5. Namibia Ministry of Health and Social Services. HIV quality management. [online]. 2010 [cited 2014 Apr 4]. Available from: http://www.healthqual.org/namibia
6. Kouanda S, Meda IB, Nikiema L, et al. Determinants and causes of mortality in HIV-infected patients receiving antiretroviral therapy in Burkina Faso: A five-year retrospective cohort study. AIDS Care. 2012;24(4):478–479. PMID: 22148973, http://dx.doi.org/10.1080/09540121.2011.630353
7. Agaba PA, Digin E, Makai R, et al. Clinical characteristics and predictors of mortality in hospitalized HIV-infected Nigerians. J Infect Dev Ctries. 2011;5(5):377–382. PMID: 21628815.
8. Francis M, Sudeshni N. Impact of HIV/AIDS on mortality among the inpatients at Motebang Hospital, Lesotho. S Afr J HIV Med. 2012;5(3):33–37. Available from: http://www.ajol.info/index.php/sajhivm/article/viewFile/34810/24873
9. Krentz HB, Kliewer G, Gill MJ. Changing mortality rates and causes of death for HIV-infected individuals living in Southern Alberta, Canada from 1984 to 2003. HIV Med. 2005;6(2):99–106. PMID: 15807715.
10. Yang CH, Huang FY, Hsiao CF, et al. Trends of mortality and causes of death among HIV-infected patients in Taiwan, 1984–2005. HIV Med. 2008;9(7):535–543. PMID: 18554309, http://dx.doi.org/10.1111/j.1468-1293.2008.00600.x
11. Chesney MA. Factors affecting adherence to antiretroviral therapy. Clin Infect Dis. 2000;30(suppl. 2):S171–176. PMID: 10860902, http://dx.doi.org/10.1086/313849
12. Palella FJ Jr, Baker RK, Moorman AC, et al. Mortality in the highly active antiretroviral therapy era: Changing causes of death and disease in the HIV outpatient study. J Acquir Immune Defic Syndr. 2006;43(1):27–34. PMID: 16878047, http://dx.doi.org/10.1097/01.qai.0000233310.90484.16
13. Lewden C, Salmon D, Morlat P, et al. Causes of death among human immunodeficiency virus (HIV)-infected adults in the era of potent antiretroviral therapy: Emerging role of hepatitis and cancers, persistent role of AIDS. Int J Epidemiol. 2005;34(1):121–130. PMID: 15561752, http://dx.doi.org/10.1093/ije/dyh307
14. Smith C, Sabin CA, Lundgren JD, et al. Factors associated with specific causes of death amongst HIV-positive individuals in the D:A:D study. AIDS. 2010;24(10):1537–1548. PMID: 20453631, http://dx.doi.org/10.1097/QAD.0b013e32833a0918
15. Krug A, Pattinson RC, Power D. Saving children – An audit system to assess under-5 health care. S Afr Med J. 2004;94:198–202. PMID: 15098280.
16. Kowalska J, Friis-Møller N, Kirk O, et al. The coding causes of death in HIV (CoDe) project: Initial results and evaluation of methodology. The CoDe working group and the D:A:D study group. Epidemiology. 2012 [cited 2015 Feb 6]; 15(4):516–523. Available from: http://www.cphiv.dk/Tools-Standards/CoDe/Publications
17. Fadare JO, Afolabi AO. The pattern of medical mortalities in a specialist hospital in North-Central Nigeria. Ann Ib Postgrad Med. 2010;8(2):101–105. PMID: 25161476, http://dx.doi.org/10.4314/aipm.v8i2.71824
18. Rins M, Meyer L, Hessol NA. Sex and the course of HIV infection in the pre- and highly active antiretroviral therapy eras. AIDS. 2005 [cited 2014 Dec 6]; 19:357–370. Available from: http://aje.oxfordjournals.org/content/168/5/532.full
19. Ghate M, Deshpande S, Tripathy S, et al. Mortality in HIV infected individuals in Pune, India. Indian J Med Res. 2011;133(4):414–420. PMID: 21537095.
20. Sani MU, Mohammed AZ, Adamu B, Yusuf S, Samaila A, Borodo M.AIDS mortality in a tertiary health institution: A four-year review. J Natl Med Assoc. 2006;98(6):862–866. PMID: 16775907.
21. Mzileni MO, Longo-Mbenza B, Chephe TJ. Mortality and causes of death in HIV positive patients receiving antiretroviral therapy at Tshepang Clinic in Doctor George Mukhari Hospital. Pol Arch Med Wewn. 2008;118(10):548–554. PMID: 19112815.

22. De Wet N, Oluwaseyi S, Odimegwu C. Youth mortality due to HIV/AIDS in South Africa, 2001–2009: An analysis of the levels of mortality using life table techniques. Afr J AIDS Res. 2014;13(1):13–20. PMID: 25174511, http://dx.doi.org/10.2989/16085906.2014.886605

23. Lucas SB, Hounnou A, Peacock C, Beaumel A, Djomand G, N'Gbichi JM, et al. The mortality and pathology of HIV infection in a West African city. AIDS. 1993;7(12):1569–1579. PMID: 7904450, http://dx.doi.org/10.1097/00002030-199312000-00005

24. Akinkuotu A, Roemer E, Richardson A, et al. In-hospital mortality rates and HIV: A medical ward review, Lilongwe, Malawi. Int J STD AIDS. 2011;22(8):465–470. PMID: 21795420, http://dx.doi.org/10.1258/ijsa.2011.011021

25. Colette S, Tim H. 16th Conference on retroviruses and opportunistic infections. Montréal, Canada; 2009 February 8–11 [cited 2014 Oct 24]. Available from: http://www.aidsmeds.com/articles/hiv_risk_factors_2297_16095.shtml

26. Smith CJ, Ryom L, Weber R, et al. Trends in underlying causes of death in people with HIV from 1999 to 2011 (D:A:D): A multicohort collaboration. Lancet. 2014;384(9939):241–248. PMID: 25042234, http://dx.doi.org/10.1016/S0140-6736(14)60604-8

27. Mocroft A, Brettle R, Kirk O, et al. Changes in the cause of death among HIV positive subjects across Europe: Results from the EuroSIDA study. AIDS. 2002; 16(12):1663–1671. PMID: 12172088, http://dx.doi.org/10.1097/00002030-200208160-00012

28. Naidoo K, Singh JA, Lalloo UG. HIV/AIDS and admission to intensive care units: A comparison of India, Brazil and South Africa. S Afr J HIV Med. 2013;14(1):15–16. http://dx.doi.org/10.7196/SAJHIVMED.887

29. Fabian J, Katz I, Gerntholtz T, et al. Chronic kidney disease in human immunodeficiency virus infection. Panminerva Med. 2007 [cited 2014 Jun 23]; 49(2):51–66. Available from: http://www.ncbi.nlm.nih.gov/pubmed/17625482

30. Maru DS, Andrews J, Schwarz D, Ramaiya A, et al. Crossing the quality chasm in resource-limited settings. Global Health. 2012 [cited 2014 May 5]; 8:41. Available from: http://www.globalizationandhealth.com/content/8/1/41

31. Kitahata MM, Van Rompaey SE, Dillingham PW, et al. Primary care delivery is associated with greater physician experience and improved survival among persons with AIDS. J Gen Intern Med. 2003 [cited 2014 May 5]; 18(2):95–103. Available from: http://www.ncbi.nlm.nih.gov/pmc/articles/PMC1494825/

Glass injuries seen in the emergency department of a South African district hospital

Authors:
Doudou Nzaumvila[1]
Indiran Govender[1]
Efraim B. Kramer[2]

Affiliations:
[1]Department of Family Medicine, Sefako Makgatho Health Sciences University, South Africa

[2]Division of Emergency Medicine, School of Medicine, University of the Witwatersrand, South Africa

Correspondence to:
Indiran Govender

Email:
indiran.govender@gmail.com

Postal address:
PO Box 222, Medunsa 0204, South Africa

Background: The emergency department of Embhuleni Hospital frequently manages patients with glass-related injuries. This study assessed these injuries and the glass that caused them in more detail.

Aim: The objectives of our study included determining the type of glass causing these injuries and describing the circumstances associated with different types of glass injuries.

Setting: The emergency department of Embhuleni Hospital in Elukwatini, Mpumalanga province, South Africa.

Methods: This was a cross-sectional study with a sample size of 104 patients. Descriptive statistics were used to assess the characteristics of the glass injuries.

Results: Five different types of glass were reported to have caused the injuries, namely car glass (7.69%), glass ampoules (3.85%), glass bottles (82.69%), glass windows (3.85%) and street glass shards (1.92%). Glass bottle injuries were mainly caused by assaults (90.47%) and most victims were mostly young males (80.23%). The assaults occurred at alcohol-licensed premises in 65.11% of cases. These injuries occurred mostly over weekends (83.72%), between 18:00 and 04:00. The face (34.23%) and the scalp (26.84%) were the sites that were injured most often.

Conclusion: Assault is the most common cause of glass injuries, usually involving young men at alcohol-licensed premises. Glass injuries generally resulted in minor lacerations, with few complications (2.68%).

Blessures causées par du verre examinées au service des urgences d'un hôpital de district sud-africain.

Contexte: Le service des urgences de l'hôpital Embhuleni traite souvent des patients blessés par des éclats de verre. Cette étude a examiné en détail ces blessures et le verre qui les a causées.

Objectif: Notre étude avait pour but de déterminer le type de verre qui avait causé ces blessures et de décrire les circonstances des différents types de blessures causées par du verre.

Lieu: Le service des urgences à l'hôpital Embhuleni à Elukwatini, dans la province du Mpumalanga, en Afrique du Sud.

Méthodes: C'est une étude transversale avec un échantillonnage de 104 patients. On a utilisé des statistiques descriptives pour évaluer les caractéristiques des blessures causées par le verre.

Résultats: Les blessures ont été causées par différents types de verre, à savoir du verre automobile (7.69%), du verre d'ampoules (3.85%), du verre de bouteille (82.69%), du verre de vitre (3.85%) et des éclats de verre dans la rue (1.92%). Les blessures causées par du verre de bouteille provenaient surtout d'agressions (90.47%) et la plupart des victimes étaient des jeunes hommes (80.23%). Les agressions avaient eu lieu dans des locaux autorisés à servir de l'alcool dans 65.11% des cas. Ces blessures ont eu lieu surtout pendant le weekend (83.72%), entre 18h00 et 04h00. Les blessures étaient le plus souvent au visage (34.23%) et au cuir chevelu (26.84%).

Conclusion: Les agressions sont la cause la plus fréquente des blessures causées par du verre et impliquent en général des jeunes hommes dans des locaux autorisés à servir de l'alcool. Les blessures causées par du verre étaient en général des lacérations mineures avec peu de complications (2.68%).

Introduction

Glass is a material commonly used for glass bottles, cookware and containers. It has the potential to be harmful. Throughout history, glass has been associated with danger, and it is a common cause of injuries warranting visits to the emergency department (ED) of hospitals.[1,2,3,4] These injuries can be accidental (non-intentional)[5,6] or intentionally inflicted;[1,2,3] the latter include 'glassing', which refers to alcohol-related violence using glass bottles.[1]

The ED of Embhuleni Hospital in Elukwatini, Mpumalanga province, South Africa, frequently manages patients with glass-related injuries. The severity of wounds varies, with most patients being discharged the same day after sutures and dressing. However, in other patients there may be far worse outcomes, such as the loss of an eye or even death.

Depending on its constitution, glass may be shattered or broken into sharp, jagged pieces or shards which can then cause harm. Glass injuries may occur at home, and this is referred to as a 'domestic glass injury' or a 'home injury'. Domestic injuries or home accidents are a public health problem worldwide.[7] In 1086 consecutive cases of injuries caused by glass, the home was reported as the most common environment in which they occurred.[8] Grieshaber and Stegmann reported that glass and other sharp objects represented almost 48% of penetrating eye injuries amongst South African children.[9] Glass tables are the commonest cause of domestic glass injuries when the victims are children.[10,11]

A 'street shard glass' is a piece of broken glass lying on the street. In some studies it was the leading cause of glass injuries for children outside the home.[12] Children are the main victims of street shard glass injuries; the feet are the most affected body part.[13,14,15]

Many types of worker are at risk of injury due to glass; they include barmen[16,17] and health workers.[18,19] Glass ampoules are potentially dangerous if not opened correctly. They account for 26% of needle-less stick and sharps injuries,[20] which may need microsurgery and extensive rehabilitation, especially when fingers are injured. Needle-less stick injuries can affect non-health workers such as cleaners if glass ampoules and vials are not disposed of in an appropriate sharps container.

Accidental glass injuries are also found amongst victims of road traffic accidents and are usually caused by the windscreen or windshield of a motor vehicle.

Intentional glass injuries are secondary to assault or intentional violence. The incidence and prevalence of violence varies between countries and is mainly associated with alcohol use.[21,22,23] South Africa has one of the highest rates of interpersonal violence injuries in the world,[24] and this is associated with alcohol use in from 27% to 47% of cases.[25] Glass bottles are used impulsively as weapons in alcohol-licensed premises (ALP), in homes or on the street.[24]

Although glass bottles can cause serious injuries, these are rarely fatal; however, such injuries do sometimes need specialist attention. They present mostly located on the scalp and the neck[1,26,27,28] and when they affect other parts of the body, such as the face and the hands, they may result in unsightly facial scars, disabling hand injuries or other physical deformities, together with post-traumatic stress.[29] Glass injuries are a common reason for visits to the ED throughout South Africa, but as yet unfortunately little research has been done in the country on this.

The aim of this study was to compile and analyse data on patients with glass injuries presenting to the ED of Embhuleni Hospital.

Methods

Design and setting

This was a descriptive prospective study undertaken at Embhuleni Hospital, which is a district hospital with 220 beds in a rural area of Mpumalanga province.

Sampling and data collection

Data was collected in the ED from 01 February to 31 July 2013 by designated and dedicated ED nurses who were not on duty. There were three nurses who were trained by the researcher; during their training, the aim and objectives of the study and how to collect the data were explained to them. Nurses in the ED were requested to call out one of the trained nurses according to a set roster displayed at the nursing station in order to collect data whenever a patient presented to the ED with a glass injury during the period of study.

Inclusion criteria:

- patients presenting to the ED of Embhuleni Hospital with glass injuries;
- who have consented to participate in the study;
- whose consent has been obtained from a family member or guardian to participate in this study, and
- whose waiver of consent has been obtained to participate in the study.

Exclusion criteria:

- patients presenting to the ED of Embhuleni Hospital with glass injuries;
- who are not under the influence of any recreational drug or alcohol, and
- who have refused to participate in this study.

The following variables were recorded from patients attending the ED:

- Gender, age, address, occupation, highest level of education.
- Persons accompanying the patient to the ED.
- Circumstances of injury.
- Type of glass.

- Type of injury (eg intentional/non-intentional).
- Geographic location of njury occurrence (eg on street, in home).
- Treatment received.
- Single or multiple injuries.
- Characteristics of injury.

Ethical clearance was obtained from Embhuleni Hospital and the ethics committee of the University of the Witwatersrand.

Results

Amongst the 113 data collection sheets of eligible participants with glass injuries who met the inclusion criteria, 9 were rejected for missing data (3 did not have the type of glass indicated, in 4 the body parts injured were not recorded, and 2 did not indicate the place where the injury occurred).This yielded a final study sample of 104.

Eight participants had injuries from car glass (7.69%), 4 from glass ampoules (3.85%), 86 from glass bottles (82.69%), 4 from glass windows (3.85%) and 2 from street shard glass (1.92%).

Injuries occurred at ALP, in the home, in road traffic accidents, on the street and at workplaces. Injuries in workplaces sometimes overlapped with injuries on ALP and road traffic accidents. Glass ampoules caused injuries at work and on the street. Glass bottle injuries (total: 86 injured patients) as a proportion of all glass injuries occurred as follows: 3 (37.50%) in workplaces (one of the injured patients was a security guard working at an ALP, hence the overlap of one injury whilst at work in an ALP), 15 (78.95%) at home, 13 (86.67%) on the street, and 56 (100.00%) on ALP. Figure 1 indicates the types of glass and places where the injuries occurred.

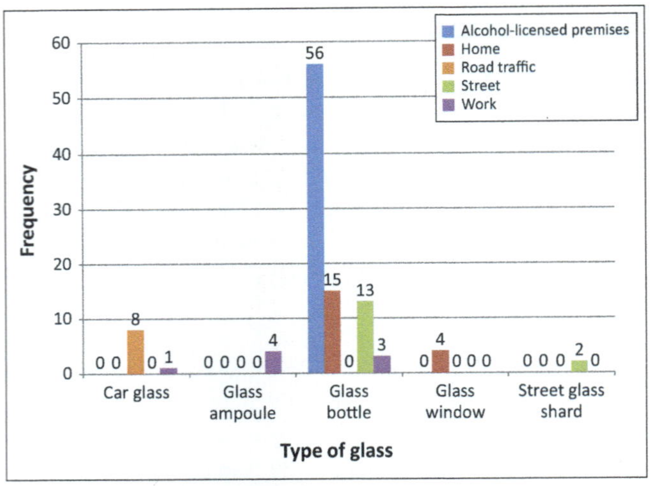

FIGURE 1: Types of glass and places where the injuries occurred.

The minimum age in cases of glass injury was 6 years and the maximum was 57 years. The mean age was 26.04 years. Sixty-seven participants (63.46%) were aged between 15 and 34 years ($p > 0.10$). Glass bottles affected almost all the age groups, whereas injuries from other types of glass were limited to certain age groups. Street shard injuries were found in those of less than 14 years of age (see Table 1).

Glass windows affected males only, whereas glass ampoules affected females only. A majority of car glass (7; 87.55%) and

TABLE 1: Demographic characteristics of patients with glass injuries.

Characteristics	Car glass *N* (%)	Glass ampoule	Glass bottle	Glass window	Street shards	Total
Gender						
Female	1 (12.50)	4 (100)	17 (19.77)	0	1 (50)	23 (22.10)
Male	7 (87.50)	0	69 (80.23)	4 (100)	1 (50)	81 (77.90)
Occupation						
Employed	4 (50)	0	29 (33.72)	2 (50)	0	35 (33.65)
Pupil	2 (25)	0	14 (16.28)	1 (25)	2 (100)	19 (18.27)
Self-employed	2 (25)	0	8 (9.30)	1 (25)	0	11 (10.58)
Student	0	4 (100)	2 (2.32)	0	0	6 (5.77)
Unemployed	0	0	33 (38.37)	0	0	33 (31.73)
Level of education						
No formal education	1 (12.50)	0	6 (6.98)	0	0	7 (6.73)
Primary school	1 (12.50)	0	3 (3.49)	1 (25)	2 (100)	7 (6.73)
Secondary school	6 (75)	0	75 (87.20)	3 (75)	0	84 (80.77)
Tertiary school	0	4 (100)	2 (2.32)	0	0	6 (5.77)
Age groups (yrs)						
5–9	1 (12.50)	0	0	0	1 (50)	2 (1.92)
10–14	0	0	0	1 (25)	1 (50)	2 (1.92)
15–19	1 (12.50)	0	20 (23.26)	0	0	21 (20.19)
20–24	0	0	26 (30.23)	0	0	26 (25)
25–29	1 (12.50)	2 (50)	15 (17.44)	1 (25)	0	19 (18.27)
30–34	3 (37.50)	1 (25)	16 (18.60)	1 (25)	0	21 (20.19)
35–39	1 (12.50)	0	5 (5.81)	1 (25)	0	7 (6.73)
40–44	0	1 (25)	2 (2.33)	0	0	3 (2.88)
45–49	1 (12.50)	0	1 (1.16)	0	0	1 (0.96)
50–54	0	0	0	0	0	1 (0.96)
55–59	0	0	1 (1.16)	0	0	1 (0.96)

TABLE 2: Characteristics of the different types of glass injury (percentages in parentheses).

Characteristics	Car glass	Glass ampoulampoule	Glass bottle	Glass window	Street shards	Total
Day of the week						
Monday	0	0	4 (4.65)	0	0	4 (3.85)
Tuesday	0	0	0	0	0	0
Wednesday	0	0	2 (2.33)	1 (25)	1 (50)	4 (3.85)
Thursday	1 (12.5)	0	7 (8.14)	0	1 (50)	9 (8.65)
Friday	3 (37.5)	0	11 (12.79)	1 (25)	0	15 (14.42)
Saturday	1 (12.5)	0	37 (43.02)	1 (25)	0	39 (37.5)
Sunday	3 (37.5)	4 (100)	25 (29.07)	1 (25)	0	33 (31.73)
Estimated time when injury happened						
08:00–12:59	0	2 (50)	5 (5.81)	1 (25)	0	8 (7.69)
13:00–17:59	1 (12.5)	1 (25)	8 (9.30)	0	1 (50)	11 (10.58)
18:00–22:59	3 (37.5)	1 (25)	22 (25.58)	3 (75)	1 (50)	30 (28.85)
23:00–03:59	2 (25)	0	42 (48.84)	0	0	44 (42.31)
04:00–07:59	2 (25)	0	9 (10.47)	0	0	11 (10.58)
Location where the injuries occurred						
ALP	0	0	56	0	0	56 (52.92)
Home	0	0	15 (65.12)	4 (100)	0	19 (17.92)
Road traffic	8 (87.5)	0	0	0	0	8 (7.55)
Street	0	0	13 (15.12)	0	2 (100)	15 (14.15)
Work	1 (12.5)	4 (100)	3 (2.32)	0	0	8 (7.55)
Escort						
EMS	7 (87.5)	0	50 (58.14)	0	2 (100)	59 (56.73)
Personnel family	1 (12.5)	0	13 (15.12)	4 (100)	0	18 (17.31)
member only	0	0	6 (6.98)	0	0	6 (5.77)
Friends only	0	4 (100)		0	0	13 (12.5)
None	0	0	9 (10.46)	0	0	8 (7.69)
SAPS officer			8 (9.30)			
Number of injuries						
Single	4 (50)	4 (100)	47 (54.65)	4 (100)	2 (100)	61 (58.65)
Multiple	4 (50)	0	39(45.35)	0	0	43 (41.35)
Injured body parts						
Abdomen	0	0	1 (1.00)	0	0	1 (1)
Arm	0	0	6 (4.80)	0	0	6 (4.03)
Back	2 (14.28)	0	0	0	0	2 (1.34)
Chest	0	0	14 (11.20)	0	0	14 (9.39)
Face	9 (64.28)	0	42 (33.60)	0	0	51 (34.23)
Foot	0	0	0	0	2 (100)	2 (1.34)
Forearm	1 (7.14)	0	12 (9.60)	1 (25)	0	14 (9.39)
Hand	0	4 (100)	10 (8.00)	3 (75)	0	17 (11.41)
Leg	1	0	0	0	0	1 (0.67)
Neck	0	0	2 (1.60)	0	0	2 (1.34)
Scalp	2 (14.28)	0	38 (30.40)	0	0	40 (26.84)

ALP, alcohol-licensed premises; EMS, emergency medical services.

glass bottle (69; 80.23%) injuries affected males. All of the unemployed participants (33; 31.73%) were injured by glass bottles.

Fifty-six of the participants (53.85%) were injured in ALP exclusively by glass bottles, as shown in Table 2, which indicates the characteristics of the different types of glass injury.

Of the 19 (16.27%) participants injured at home, glass bottles caused injury to 15 (78.95%) and the remaining 4 (21.05%) were injured by glass windows. The 8 (7.69%) occupational glass injuries were caused by car glass, glass ampoules or glass bottles. Of the 15 (14.42%) participants injured on the street, 13 (86.67%) were injured by glass bottles and 2 (13.33%) by street shard glass.

There was a trend of increasing numbers of injuries as the week progressed from Monday, with 87 (84%) occurring over the weekends, 39 of them (37.5%) on Saturdays alone. There was also an increasing number of injuries from 17:00, with more than 74 (70%) of the glass injuries occurring between 18:00 and 04:00.

Intentional glass injuries were inflicted with glass bottles. Amongst the 86 glass bottle injuries, 80 (93%) were from assaults with glass bottles; 51 (63.75%) of the victims laid criminal charges. Fifty-nine participants (56.73%) arrived escorted by emergency medical services (EMS) personnel, whereas 18 (17.31%) were accompanied by relatives, and South African Police Service (SAPS) officers escorted 8 (7.69%). Overlaps were noted, especially between EMS and relatives as escorts.

TABLE 3: Outcome of the glass injuries (percentages given in brackets).

Characteristics	Car glass	Glass ampoule	Glass bottle	Glass window	Street shards	Total
Outcome						
Discharged after treatment in ED	8 (100)	3 (75)	77 (89.53)	0	2 (100)	94 (90.38)
Admitted in short- stay room in ED	0	0	6 (6.98)	0	0	6 (5.77)
Transferred	0	1 (25)	3 (3.49)	-	0	4 (3.85)
Complications						
Anxiety disorder	0	1 (25)	0	0	0	1 (0.96)
Disembowelment	0	0	1 (1.16)	0	0	1 (0.96)
Eyeball perforation	0	0	1 (1.16)	0	0	1 (0.96)
Tendon injury	0	0	1 (1.16)	0	0	1 (0.96)

ED, emergency department.

TABLE 4: Demographic characteristics of participants with glass bottle injuries.

Characteristics	Frequency	Percentage
Gender		
Female	17	19.77
Male	69	80.23
Occupation		
Employed	29	33.78
Pupil	14	16.28
Self-employed	8	9.30
Student	2	2.33
Unemployed	33	38.37
Level of education		
No formal education	6	6.98
Primary school	3	3.49
Secondary school	75	87.21
Tertiary school	2	2.33
Age groups (yrs)		
15–19	20	23.26
20–24	26	30.23
25–29	15	17.44
30–34	16	18.61
35–39	5	5.81
40–44	2	2.33
45–49	1	1.16
50–54	0	0
55–59	1	1.16

The minimum length of an injury was 0.5 cm (121 injuries; 81.2%) and the maximum length of an injury was 16 cm. The mean length of the injuries was 3.67 cm.

Of the 149 glass injuries, 118 (79.14%) were intentional injuries, of which 71 (60.17%) were inflicted on the left side of the body. The face was the most common area involved, with 51 injuries (34.23%), followed by the injuries to the scalp (40; 26.84%).

Most patients (94; 90.38%) were discharged after treatment in the ED. The outcomes in all of the cases of glass injuries are indicated in Table 3.

The minimum total cost of managing one glass injury patient using the International Classification of Diseases (ICD 10) is estimated to be R1267.47.

There were 86 glass bottle injuries, which represented 82.69% of all glass injuries, with the majority occurring amongst male participants (80.23%) with a minimum age of 16 years and maximum age of 57 years ($p = 0.0426$) (Table 4); 26 (30.23%) of them were young adults aged between 20 and 24 years. It was also found that 3 (3.49%) were minors. It seems that age is significantly related to glass bottle injuries. Of those injured by glass bottle, 33 (38.37%) were unemployed and 75 (87.21%) had a secondary school level of education.

Amongst the 86 participants with glass bottle injuries, the majority of the injuries were due to assault (93.02%), and 56 (65.11%) reported that they were intentionally injured at ALP. Of the 3 minor participants injured by glass bottles, 2 (3.57%) were injured at ALP.

A majority of glass bottle injuries (73; 84.88%) occurred over the weekend, and there was an increasing trend towards Saturday (37; 43.02%). The glass bottle injuries were intentional in 76 (90.47%) of cases and were single injuries in 46 (54.76%) ($p \leq 0.0019$) when comparing injury and glass bottle injuries.

Out of a total of 125 glass bottle injuries, 42 (33.60%) were on the face and 38 (30.40%) on the scalp. Thus the face and the scalp were affected in almost two-thirds of glass bottle injuries.

Discussion

Glass bottles were responsible for most injuries (82.69%). Laing, Sendall and Barker also found the most common cause of glass injuries (in 75% of their patients) to be glass bottles.[1] When considering the location of the injuries, our study differed from others because although the glass bottle remained the leading cause of injuries, the percentage significantly differed from 75% in general to 45% in ALP, where other types of glass such as drinking glasses accounted for 44% of glass injuries.[1] This difference is due to the circumstances found in South Africa. The first factor has to do with local habits and customs in ALP, where beer is not served in drinking glasses but in glass bottles.[30] The second factor is that the study site is a rural area, where some glass objects are considered to be luxuries (such as glass doors, glass tables) and most of the people cannot afford these.

Male participants made up 77.90% of the participants. This is consistent with other international studies, which found that more males than females are injured with glass. A study of

1086 consecutive injuries caused by glass found a 7:3 male to female ratio,[8] and another study found that 72% of injuries affected males.[1] Some authors attributed the large proportion of glass bottle injuries in males to the consumption of alcohol, and thereafter greater risk-taking behaviour.[1] Other studies confirmed the relationship between the consumption of alcohol by males and violence using glass bottles at ALP.[30,31]

Injuries with glass ampoules were found amongst female student nurses only, which is similar to Smith's findings amongst nursing students.[20] This is because it is nurses who usually break glass ampoules in order to administer the contents.

Although glass injuries can affect any age group, some are more prone to certain types of glass injury, especially those inflicted by glass bottles and street shard glass.[32] Other studies also found the age group 20–24 years to have the highest number of glass injuries.[1] Youth violence, particularly amongst males, is exceptionally high in South Africa,[24] and our study had similar results, with intentional injuries found to be associated with glass bottles in 80 (93.02%) cases.

Street shard glass injuries (2%) in children walking barefoot were consistent with previous studies that focused on glass injuries in children, which could explain the higher percentage in these studies.[13,33,34]

Occupational glass injuries accounted for 7.55% of all injuries. Occupational injuries involved glass bottles, car glass and glass ampoules. Glass ampoule injuries accounted for 4% of glass injuries and affected the hands, which is common in this type of injury.[20] The low percentage in this study does not accurately reflect the reality of glass ampoule-related injuries at Embhuleni Hospital, since it is most likely that many health workers, especially nurses, treat these as minor injuries without any reporting or medical consultation. These underreported injuries were also highlighted by Milner,[35] who found that up to 70% of health workers failed to report them. Multiple injuries were associated with car glass (50%) compared to the other glass types, which resulted only in single injuries. Glass bottles are mainly associated with assault, causing multiple lacerations.[1,36,37] Car glass has multiple fragments, which cause multiple lesions that are minor unless they affect the eyes or become retained as foreign bodies due to their small size.[38,39]

The windscreens of cars caused 9% of glass injuries.[14] The face was the most affected body part (9; 64%), which is similar to what has been found in other studies.[40,41,42]

A glass bottle can be used as a dangerous weapon, and commonly affects the head in intentional injuries.[1,2,3,26,27,43] In our study it was found that glass bottles caused 84% of injuries and affected various body parts. The head was affected in 61.07% of glass bottle injuries. Other body parts such as the hands and forearms were also injured, but less frequently than the head and face – the hands and forearms are used by the victim as a defence mechanism. These findings are similar to those of other research regarding body parts affected by glass bottle injuries.[1,29]

Glass windows are the commonest cause of hand injuries.[5,6,16] Of the participants with this type of injury, 75% and 25% of them were injured on the hand and forearm respectively. These findings are in line with other studies.[44,45]

The foot was the only body part affected by street shard glass, as reported by other studies.[35,36,37]

There was a trend of increased glass injuries over weekends; this finding is consistent with other international and local studies which have focused on alcohol-related injuries presenting to the ED.[1,22,23,43] Intentional glass injuries were found only to have been caused by glass bottles and represented 93.02% of participants. These were used in interpersonal violence, which takes place amongst 20% – 47% of alcohol consumers in South Africa.[24] These glass bottle injuries are consistent with what is known about glass injuries,[1,2,25] but in our study all injuries occurred at places where alcohol was sold. In this respect our study differed from that conducted by some authors, who found that glass bottle assaults occurred commonly at home.[1] The pattern of days on which glass bottle injuries occurred is the same as for alcohol consumption in South Africa.[43] It was reported by some authors that alcohol consumption amongst the youth is a major contributor to crime, violence and intentional and unintentional injuries, as well as other social, health and economic problems.[43] Thus it is not unexpected that glass bottle injuries occurred during the weekend and were associated with violence.

These assaults with glass bottles were reported to the police in 61% of cases. This is in contrast to other countries, where such assaults with minor lesions and complications, as found in this study, are generally underreported.[31]

Most of these patients had minor injuries but used ambulances as transport to the hospital. Since Embhuleni Hospital is situated in a rural area, members of these poor communities do not have private transport or cannot afford transport to the hospital, so they use the ambulance as a means of accessing medical services, irrespective of whether or not it is an emergency. These injuries occurred mainly at night, when there is no public transport available, and the ambulance is their only means of travelling to hospital. Also, the most commonly injured body parts were the scalp and the face (61.07%); clinics in the area do not suture lacerations of the face and scalp, so these patients are referred to the hospital.

Factors that can explain the choice of a glass bottle in interpersonal violence are its being the only weapon available at the time, the shape of the bottle and the value of the bottle. In 86% of injuries resulting from interpersonal violence with glass bottles, these occurred on ALP. The majority of beer bottles are light, and consist of a body and a neck which is as long as any knife handle. This neck enables a person to secure an easy and comfortable grasp around it and to throw it at or strike a person with force, so that the glass bottle breaks on impact or stabs a person when broken with minimal force.[1,26,27]

The gender of the victim must also be considered as a social impact. In this study, of the 76 intentional glass bottle injuries, 59 (77.63%) were in males injured by the assailant using a glass bottle as a weapon. Although a glass bottle can be considered to be a weapon used on impulse, it causes injuries which are similar to those caused by any sharp object.[46] Glass bottles are used to take advantage of and neutralise an opponent.[30,47]

All the unemployed participants in this study were injured by glass bottles as a result of interpersonal violence, with 61% taking place on ALP. There seems to be a relationship between glass bottle injuries and unemployment: the high level of unemployment amongst young people in South Africa is a contributing factor to the high rate of liquor consumption, as alcohol is used as a means of relieving stress and is easily purchased from different types of premises.[43,48]

The age distribution for glass bottle injuries showed that the mean is 25.81 years, which is supported by the results of a similar previous study.[49] This represents the economically active age group. Unfortunately most of them were unemployed. In this age group it was found that due to their negative socio-economic situation their alcohol consumption is high[36,49] and they are prone to interpersonal violence.[48] Unemployment, poverty and abuse of alcohol are linked, and these factors are known to be generators of violence.[36,43]

Limitations

The study period was from 01 February to 31 July 2013, and the injuries over the holiday and/or Christmas period may be different due to availability of more free time and disposable income resulting from annual financial bonuses.

Conclusion

Victims of glass bottle injuries are usually young unemployed males who were injured on ALP. The injuries from assaults were mostly located on the left side of the body. The face was injured the most by car glass and glass bottle injuries, whereas the feet and hands were mostly affected by street shards and glass ampoules respectively. Glass bottle injuries were associated with assault, and most of these cases were reported to the police. The patients injured by glass mostly used ambulances to attend the hospital ED. Glass recycling can be used at or near ALP to generate income and prevent many glass injuries.

Acknowledgements

The authors wish to thank all the nurses who helped with the data collection and also the Department of Family Medicine at Sefako Makgatho Health Sciences University for its physical and financial support in getting our article published.

Competing interests

The authors declare that they have no financial or personal relationship(s) that may have inappropriately influenced them in writing this article.

Authors' contributions

D.N. (Sefako Makgatho Health Sciences University) devised the original idea for the research and collected and analysed the data. I.G. (Sefako Makgatho Health Sciences University) was involved in data analysis, writing up the research manuscript and responding to the comments from the reviewers. E.B.K. (University of the Witwatersrand) contributed to the protocol write up, data collection and data analysis.

References

1. Laing AJ, Sendall MC, Barker R. Alcohol-related violence presenting to the emergency department: Is 'glassing' the big issue? Emerg Med Australasia. 2013;25(6):550–557. PMID: 24118859, http://dx.doi.org/10.1111/1742-6723.12136
2. Emby DJ. Retained glass fragments in body tissues. S Afr Med J. 2009;99(12):858–859. PMID: 20459988, http://dx.doi.org/10.7196/samj.3570
3. Nolan G, Lawes S, Hainsworth S, Ruuty G. A study considering the force required for broken glass bottles to penetrate a skin simulant. Int J Legal Med. 2011;126(1):19–25. PMID: 21336639, http://dx.doi.org/10.1007/s00414-011-0556-7
4. Levine MR, Gorman SM, Yarnold PR. A model for teaching bedside detection of glass in wounds. Emerg Med J. 2007;24(6):413–416. PMID: 17513538, http://dx.doi.org/10.1136/emj.2007.047340
5. Rothschild MA, Karger B, Schneider V. Puncture wounds caused by glass mistaken for stab wounds with a knife. Forensic Sci Int. 2001;121(3):161–165. PMID: 11566419, http://dx.doi.org/10.1016/S0379-0738(01)00392-9
6. Karger BR, Rothschild MA, Pfeiffer H. Accidental sharp force fatalities – Beware of architectural glass, not knives. Forensic Sci Int. 2001;123(2–3):135–139. PMID: 11728738, http://dx.doi.org/10.1016/S0379-0738(01)00526-6
7. Majori S, Ricci G, Capretta F, Rocca G, Baldovin T, Buinocore F. Epidemiology of domestic injuries. A survey in an emergency department in north-east Italy. J Prev Med Hyg. 2009;50(3):164–169. PMID: 20411650.
8. Ousby J, Wilson DH. 1086 Consecutive injuries caused by glass. Injury. 1982;13(5):427–430. PMID: 7085060, http://dx.doi.org/10.1016/0020-1383(82)90099-7
9. Glassforeurope [Internet]. Main types of glass. [updated 2013 May 23; cited 2014 Aug 17]. Available from: http://www.glassforeurope.com/en/products/main-types-of-glass.php
10. Kupelian AS, Tincello DG. Penetrating glass injury to the perineum. J Obstet Gynaecol. 2004;24(6):713–714. PMID: 16147628, http://dx.doi.org/10.1080/01443610400008230
11. Kimia AA, Waltzman ML, Shannon MW, et al. et al. Glass table-related injuries in children. Pediatr Emerg Care. 2009;25(3):145–149. PMID: 19262417, http://dx.doi.org/10.1097/PEC.0b013e31819b41c8
12. Al-Khatib IA. Children's perceptions and behavior with respect to glass littering in developing countries: A case study in Palestine's Nablus district. Waste Manag. 2009;29(4):1434–1437. PMID: 19019670, http://dx.doi.org/10.1016/j.wasman.2008.08.026
13. Makary MA. Reported incidence of injuries caused by street glass among urban children in Philadelphia. Inj Prev. 1998;4(2):148–149. PMID: 9666372, http://dx.doi.org/10.1136/ip.4.2.148
14. The glass recycling company [Internet]. Why recycle [cited 2014 Aug 27]. Available from: http://www.theglassrecyclingcompany.co.za/index.php?option=com_content&view=article&id=216&Itemid=52
15. Northglen News [Internet]. Glass recycling increased [updated 2013 Mar 20; cited 2014 Aug 27]. Available from: http://www.looklocal.co.za/looklocal/content/en/north-durban-and-umhlanga/north-durban-and-umhlanga-news-general?oid=7129321&sn=detail&pid=1171318&glass-recycling-increases
16. Evans DM. Hand injuries due to glass. J Hand Surg. 1987;123(5):284. PMID: 3624998.
17. McLean W, Shepherd JP, Brann CR, Westmoreland D. Risks associated with occupational glass injury in bar staff with special consideration of Hepatitis B infection. Occup Med. 1997;47(3):147–150. PMID: 9156469, http://dx.doi.org/10.1093/occmed/47.3.147
18. Guo YL, Shiao J, Chuang YC, Huang KY. Needlestick and sharps injuries among health-care workers in Taiwan. Epidemiol Infect. 1999;122(2):259–265. PMID: 10355790.

19. Jagger J, Deitchman S. Hazards of glass capillary tubes to healthcare workers. JAMA. 1998;280(1):31. PMID: 9660356, http://dx.doi.org/10-1001/pubs.JAMA-ISSN-0098-7484-280-1-jbk0701

20. Smith DR, Leggat PA. Needlestick and sharps injuries among nursing students. J Adv Nurs. 2005;51(5):449–455. PMID: 16098161, http://dx.doi.org/10.1111/j.1365-2648.2005.03526.x

21. Humphrey G, Casswell S, Han DY. Alcohol and injury among attendees at a New Zealand emergency department. NZ Med J. 2003;116(1168):1–10. PMID: 12601422.

22. Tjipto AC, Taylor DM, Liew H. Alcohol use among young adults presenting to the emergency department. Emerg Med Australasia. 2006;18(2):125–130. PMID: 16669937, http://dx.doi.org/10.1111/j.1742-6723.2006.00819.x

23. Sivarajasingam V, Morgan P, Shepherd J, Matthews K. Vulnerability to assault injury: An emergency department perspective. Emerg Med J. 2009; 26(10):711–714. PMID: 19773489, http://dx.doi.org/10.1136/emj.2008.061580

24. Norman R, Schneider M, Bradshaw D, et al. Interpersonal violence: An important risk factor for disease and injury in South Africa. Popul Health Metr. 2010;8:32. PMID: 21118578, http://dx.doi.org/10.1186/1478-7954-8-32

25. Norman R, Bradshaw D, Schneider M, et al. Estimating the burden of disease attributable to interpersonal violence in South Africa in 2000. S Afr Med J. 2007;97(8):653–656. PMID: 17957838.

26. Madea B, Schmidt P, Lignitz E, Padosch SA. Skull injuries caused by blows with glass bottles. Forensic Path Rev. 2005;2:27–41. http://dx.doi.org/10.1385/1-59259-872-2:027

27. Madea B, Lignitz E. A response to "S.A. Bolliger, S. Ross, L. Oesterhelweg, M.J. Thali, B.P. Kneubuehl, Are full or empty beer bottles sturdier and does their fracture-threshold suffice to break the human skull?"[J Forensic Leg Med 2009 16 138–142]. J Forensic Leg Med. 2009;16(7):432. PMID: 19733339, http://dx.doi.org/10.1016/j.jflm.2009.04.001

28. Bolliger SA, Ross S, Oesterhelweg L, Thali MJ, Kneubuehl BP. Are full or empty beer bottles sturdier and does their fracture-threshold suffice to break the human skull? J Forensic Leg Med. 2009;16(3):138–142. PMID: 19239964, http://dx.doi.org/10.1016/j.jflm.2008.07.013

29. Magennis P, Shepherd JP, Hutchison I, Brown A. Trends in facial injury. BMJ. 1998;316(7128):325–326. PMID: 9487161, http://dx.doi.org/10.1136/bmj.316.7128.325a

30. Shepherd JP. The circumstances and prevention of bar-glass injury. Addiction. 1998;93(1):5–7. PMID: 9624706.

31. Hocking MA. Assaults in southeast London. J R Soc Med. 1989;82(5):281–284. PMID: 2754682.

32. Anderson ER, Grant HI, Weissman M. Penetrating glass injury to the sacral spine. Clin Med Res. 2010;8(2):114–115. PMID: 20660937, http://dx.doi.org/10.3121/cmr.2010.927

33. Baker MD, Selbst SM, Lanuti M. Lacerations in urban children. A prospective 12-month study. Am J Dis Child. 1990;144(1):87–92. PMID: 2294725.

34. Armstrong AM, Molyneux E. Glass injuries to children. BMJ. 1992;304(2):360. PMID: 1540735.

35. Milner A. Needleless intravascular access. South Afr J Anaesth Analges. 2005;11(3):97–101. http://dx.doi.org/10.1080/22201173.2005.10872407

36. Popovici I, French MT. Does unemployment lead to greater alcohol consumption? Ind Relat. 2013;52(2):444–466. PMID: 23543880, http://dx.doi.org/10.1111/irel.12019

37. Shepherd JP, Shapland M, Pearce NX, Scully C. Pattern, severity and aetiology of injuries in victims of assault. J R Soc Med. 1990;83(2):75–89. PMID: 2319550, http://dx.doi.org/10.1177/014107689008300206

38. Safeglass [Internet]. Glass history – An overview [updated 2007; cited 2014 Aug 27]. Available from: http://www.breakglass.org/glass-history.html

39. Glassforeurope [Internet]. Main types of glass [updated 2013 May 23; cited 2014 Aug 17]. Available from: http://www.glassforeurope.com/en/products/main-types-of-glass.php

40. Zhao YF, Liu Y, Jiang L, et al. A rare case of a glass fragment impacted in the parapharyngeal space associated with neurovascular compromise. Int J Oral Maxillofac Surg. 2011;40(2):209–211. PMID: 20817479, http://dx.doi.org/10.1016/j.ijom.2010.07.009

41. Cole C, Tuft S. Penetrating eye injury from rear view mirrors. Br J Ophthalmol. 2004;88(7):969–970. PMID: 15205250, http://dx.doi.org/10.1136/bjo.2003.038653

42. Ozturk K, Keles B, Cenik Z, Yaman H. Penetrating zone ii neck injury by broken windshield. Int Wound J. 2006;3(1):63–66. PMID: 16650212.

43. Parry CD, Dewing S. A public health approach to addressing alcohol related crime in South Africa. Afr J Drug Alcohol Stud. 2006;5(1):41–56.

44. Shindel AW, Rollins M, Dillon PA, Austin PF. Bladder injury from a shard of glass. J Trauma. 2006;61(6):1557. PMID: 17159710, http://dx.doi.org/10.1097/01.ta.0000235491.73456.f8

45. Baghai P, Sheptak PE. Penetrating spinal injury by a glass fragment: Case report and review. Neurosurgery. 1982;11(3):419–422. PMID: 7133359, http://dx.doi.org/10.1097/00006123-198209000-00014

46. Dawson P, Goodwill AM. A review of weapon choice in violent and sexual crime. Sci Res. 2013;4(1):20–27. http://dx.doi.org/10.4236/blr.2013.41003

47. Coomaraswamy KS, Shepherd JP. Predictors and severity of injury in assaults with bar glasses and bottles. Inj Prev. 2003;9(1):81–84. PMID: 12642566, http://dx.doi.org/10.1136/ip.9.1.81

48. Seggie J. Alcohol and South Africa's youth. S Afr Med J. 2012;102(7):587. PMID: 22748432.

49. Forcier MW. Unemployment and alcohol abuse: A review. J Occup Med. 1988;30(3):246–251. PMID: 3283302.

34

Knowledge and perceptions of risk for cardiovascular disease: Findings of a qualitative investigation from a low-income peri-urban community in the Western Cape, South Africa

Authors:
Sam Surka[1]
Krisela Steyn[1]
Katherine Everett-Murphy[1]
Thomas A. Gaziano[2]
Naomi Levitt[1,3]

Affiliations:
[1]Chronic Disease Initiative for Africa, Cape Town, South Africa

[2]Brigham and Women's Hospital, Harvard University, United States

[3]Department of Medicine, University of Cape Town, South Africa

Correspondence to:
Sam Surka

Email:
samsurka@gmail.com

Postal address:
J 47/86, Old Groote Schuur Building, Groote Schuur Hospital Observatory, Cape Town 7925, South Africa

Background: South Africa currently faces an increasing burden of cardiovascular disease. Although referred to clinics after community screening initiatives, few individuals who are identified to be at high risk for developing cardiovascular disease attend. Low health literacy and risk perception have been identified as possible causes. We investigated the knowledge and perceptions about risk for cardiovascular disease in a community.

Method: We conducted a series of focus group discussions with individuals from a low-income peri-urban community in the Western Cape, South Africa. Different methods of presenting risk were explored. The data were organised into themes and analysed to find associations between themes to provide explanations for our findings.

Results: Respondents' knowledge of cardiovascular disease and its risk factors varied, but most were familiar with the terms used to describe cardiovascular disease. In contrast, understanding of the concept of risk was poor. Risk was perceived as a binary concept and evaluation of different narrative and visual methods of presenting risk was not possible.

Conclusion: Understanding cardiovascular disease and its risk factors requires a different set of skills from that needed to understand uncertainty and risk. The former requires knowledge of facts, whereas understanding of risk requires numerical and computational skills. Without a better understanding of risk, risk assessments for cardiovascular disease may fail in this community.

Connaissance et perceptions des risques de maladies cardiovasculaires: résultats d'une étude qualitative dans une communauté périurbaine à faibles revenus du Western Cape, en Afrique du Sud.

Contexte: A l'heure actuelle, l'Afrique du Sud se trouve confrontée à une augmentation des maladies cardiovasculaires. Bien que les patients soient envoyés dans des cliniques suite à des initiatives communautaires de dépistage, peu de ceux qui sont identifiés à haut risque de contracter des maladies cardiovasculaires se présentent. La raison en est probablement les faibles connaissances en santé et en perceptions des risques. Nous avons examiné la connaissance et la perception des risques de maladies cardiovasculaires dans une communauté.

Méthode: Nous avons mené une série de discussions de groupes témoins avec des individus d'une communauté périurbaine à faibles revenus du Western Cape, en Afrique du Sud. Nous avons examiné différentes méthodes de présentation de risques. Les données ont été classées par thèmes et analysées pour trouver des rapports entre les thèmes afin d'expliquer nos résultats.

Résultats: La connaissance des personnes interrogées sur les maladies cardiovasculaires et leurs facteurs de risques différaient, mais la plupart d'entre elles connaissaient la terminologie utilisée pour décrire les maladies cardiovasculaires. Par contre, elles comprenaient mal le concept de risque. Le risque était perçu comme une idée binaire et l'évaluation des différentes méthodes narratives et visuelle de présentation des risques n'était pas possible.

Conclusion: Pour comprendre les maladies cardiovasculaires et leurs risques il faut avoir un ensemble de compétences différentes de celles requises pour comprendre l'incertitude et les risques. Le premier demande une connaissance des faits, alors que la compréhension des risques exige des compétences numériques et informatiques. Sans une meilleure connaissance des risques, l'évaluation des maladies cardiovasculaires peut échouer dans cette communauté.

Background

South Africa currently faces an increasing burden of cardiovascular disease (CVD).[1] Primary prevention of CVD, based on the early identification and treatment of high-risk individuals, is a well-established strategy aimed at reducing the rising burden of these conditions globally.[2,3,4] Identification of high-risk individuals involves screening the general population for their total CVD risk, typically using a risk assessment tool.[5,6,7,8] A non-laboratory-based risk assessment tool, in which a blood lipogram is replaced by using a body mass index value in determining a risk score, obviates the need for laboratory infrastructure and blood tests and, as a result, can lower the cost of these screening procedures.[6] This risk assessment tool has been validated in South African populations and has been found to be effective in identifying individuals at high risk of developing CVD.[6,9] In addition, community-based screening has been investigated as a means to further scale up this component of the primary prevention intervention process. In this regard, it has been found that community health workers (CHWs) are able to accurately conduct risk assessments in community settings after undergoing a training programme.[10,11]

However, when at-risk individuals are referred to the primary healthcare facility by a CHW for formal assessment and further management, the attendance level is low.[12] Numerous reasons for low attendance have been identified, including low health literacy and poor understanding of the concept of having a high risk for CVD. Although providing an individual with their CVD risk score has been found to be a useful way to motivate healthy behaviour,[13,14] it can also be challenging for patients with low health and numerical literacy.[15,16,17] Diverse demographic, socio-psychological and cultural variables also influence an individual's perception of risk and can affect health-related behaviour choices.[18]

Health literacy refers to an individual's cognitive and social skills, which determine their ability to access, understand and use information in ways that promote and maintain good health.[19] Low levels of health literacy are associated with poorer health outcomes, less use of health services and less involvement in self-management of chronic conditions.[20] In addition, according to behaviour theories such as the health belief model, the perceived severity of and susceptibility to a disease, as well as perceived benefits and barriers to changing health behaviour, can influence an individual's health-seeking behaviour.[21] Improving the primary healthcare attendance of individuals identified as being at high risk may require designing interventions that take into consideration the baseline health and numerical literacy of the target population. It will also require addressing the determinants of health-seeking behaviour as identified in known behaviour change theories.

In the context of health, risk can be defined as a measure of the chance that damage to health or loss of life will occur as a result of a particular hazard. In the context of CVD, this refers to the likelihood of events such as heart attacks or strokes, whether fatal or non-fatal. Much research in developed countries has focused on evaluating the type of visual presentation of risk (e.g. bar graphs, risk tables, heart age, etc.) that is most effective in communicating risk.[15,22,23,24,25] Understanding and being able to interpret risk is an important component of how one determines health-related behaviour and therefore ensuring that patients understand risk should be an essential component of any intervention that aims to screen individuals for CVD risk. To our knowledge, no previous study has investigated how CVD risk is understood in a low-income peri-urban setting in South Africa, nor which methods of risk presentation are most effective. This qualitative investigation aimed to deepen our understanding of knowledge and perceptions about CVD and its risk factors in this community and to explore how the concept of risk can best be presented.

Methods

Study design

A qualitative study design was used to explore the perceptions of community members in greater depth. Focus group discussions (FGDs) were chosen to encourage interaction between the respondents in order to spark further discussion and draw out latent perceptions and ideas around the topic of CVD and risk.

Setting and respondents

The study was conducted between May 2014 and July 2014 in the Nyanga township outside Cape Town in the Western Cape, South Africa. Nyanga has close to 16 000 households and a total population of about 58 000. The population is predominantly black African (99%), of which only 31% have completed secondary schooling (Grade 12). The unemployment rate is high (45%) and the average monthly income is about R3200 (approximately $320 at the time of the study) (National Census data, 2011). In recruiting community members for this study, we returned to the population in which we previously studied community-based risk assessment and in which poor CVD risk perception was identified as a reason for not attending community health centres after referral.[12] Purposive sampling was conducted by asking CHWs to recruit male and female community members (≥ 25 years) of the Nyanga township and who had no previous experience in being assessed for CVD risk. Individuals with a past history of CVD were not excluded and CHWs were allowed to recruit their existing clients. Participation was voluntary and each respondent was informed about the study objectives a week before the discussions were scheduled to take place. Prior to the FGDs, a total CVD risk score was calculated for each respondent using the non-laboratory CVD risk assessment tool and communicated to them by the CHWs. The method used to calculate these risk scores has been described previously.[11]

Data collection

We conducted three FGDs in groups consisting of between 8 and 10 respondents at a time. An experienced facilitator, fluent in the first language of the respondents but who was not from the community, conducted the discussions. Key questions were developed and respondents were asked about their knowledge, perception and understanding of various terms used to describe CVD (including heart attack, stroke, risk, risk factors and cardiovascular disease). They were also asked about causes and risk factors of CVD, modifiable risk factors, prevention, risk factors, risk factor modification, risk scores, and their preference for risk score presentation. A number of different narrative and visual methods of presenting the concept of risk were explained to the respondents. These methods included presenting risk scores, a risk chart, a pictograph and explaining the concepts of relative risk and heart age (see Table 1 for a detailed description). Respondents were asked to rate each method using a Likert scale, where 1 denoted 'easy to understand' and 5 denoted 'difficult to understand'. Respondents were also encouraged to raise other topics or issues related to cardiovascular health. At key intervals in the discussion, information was summarised by the facilitator and repeated to the respondents to ensure that it accurately reflected their intended message. The FGDs were conducted in isiXhosa and the discussions were recorded digitally. Each discussion lasted approximately 60–90 minutes. An experienced translator transcribed all the data verbatim into English.

Data analysis

The data were explored and analysed following the qualitative analysis framework described by Pope et al.[26] The transcripts were first reviewed in their entirety several times by the first author and organised into themes. All key issues and themes were examined and referenced. The transcripts were annotated and the data were indexed according to the identified themes to obtain an overall picture. The data were analysed to find associations between themes to provide explanations for the findings. Selected quotations from respondents have been included in this report to illustrate the emergent themes. These are reported without identifiers to preserve the anonymity of respondents. A post hoc analysis of the FGD findings was performed within the framework of the health belief model.

TABLE 1: The methods used to explain the concept of risk of developing cardiovascular disease.

Method of risk presentation	Explanation	Visual aid description
Five-year risk score	Your risk score is 30%. This means you have a 30% chance of having a heart attack or stroke in the next five years.	None.
Risk chart	Your risk score is 30%, which means you have moderate to high risk of having a heart attack or stroke in the next five years.	A graded, colour-coded risk chart (with low risk represented in blue, moderate risk in yellow and high risk in red) is used to show where an individual's risk lies.
Pictograph (100-face diagram)	Your risk score is 30%. In other words, in a crowd of 100 people with the same risk factors as you, 30 are likely to have a heart attack or stroke within the next five years.	A diagram depicting a hundred faces (70 smiling and coloured in yellow; 30 not smiling and coloured in blue) is used to illustrate this concept.
Relative risk	Your risk score is 30%. The score of a typical person of the same age, gender and ethnicity is 6%. Your relative risk is therefore 5. This means that you are five times more likely to have a heart attack or stroke in the next five years than a typical person of the same age, gender and ethnicity as yourself.	None.
Heart age	Although your actual age is 35 years, your 'heart age' is 40 years. This means that you have the same risk (of having a heart attack or stroke) as someone who is 40 years old. In other words, your heart is less healthy than it should be at your age.	None.

Ethical considerations

Ethical approval for this study was obtained from the Human Research Ethics committee (University of Cape Town). Written information about the study was provided and informed consent was obtained from respondents for participation and having their CVD risk scores calculated. Individuals identified as being at high risk of CVD were provided with a referral letter for follow-up at the nearest community health centre.

Results

We enrolled 30 respondents to participate in 3 FGDs; however, 2 respondents did not attend their allocated sessions. There were 4 male and 24 female respondents. Although the exact reasons for low recruitment and participation of male respondents in this study are unknown, it is in keeping with the skewed gender participation in previous CHW-led initiatives conducted in this community.[10,12]

The average age of the respondents was 53 years (± 16 years). The average level of education was nine years of schooling (grade 9).

Of the total sample, 14 respondents reported a history of hypertension, 3 reported ischaemic heart disease and 2 had a history of cerebrovascular disease. No respondents reported diabetes. A non-laboratory-based risk assessment tool was used to assess each individual's risk for having a cardiovascular event (either fatal or non-fatal) within the next five years. The following levels of risk were identified: 14 respondents were found to have low risk, 4 presented with low to moderate risk, 8 presented with moderate risk, one had moderate to high risk and one had high risk. The CVD risk profile of respondents in this study was higher than found in previous studies conducted in this population.[27,28,29] This result can likely be attributed to the purposive recruitment of existing CHW clients and the non-exclusion of individuals with a medical history of CVD.

The results of the FGDs are presented according to the three themes and respective categories shown in Table 2.

TABLE 2: Main themes and categories discussed in the focus group discussions.

Themes	Categories
Knowledge of CVD and its prevention	Cardiovascular disease. Myocardial infarction. Cerebrovascular accidents. Hypertension. Preventative measures.
Perception of risk	Concept of risk. Risk factors of CVD. Risk scores. Risk presentation.
Coping with the disease	Attitude towards making lifestyle changes. Personal, cultural and religious beliefs.

CVD, cardiovascular disease.

Knowledge of cardiovascular disease and its prevention

Cardiovascular disease

Across all FGDs respondents were hesitant and unsure when asked what they thought this term meant and were unable to provide a definition. Some respondents described CVD as conditions affecting the heart or identified specific conditions such as hypertension and diabetes. Many had heard of conditions associated with CVD but felt uninformed owing to poor communication from health care providers:

> 'We do understand this question, but we do not know these diseases because the doctor does not explain. He just tells you that you have diabetes or hypertension, but does not explain where do you get them and what are you supposed to do. They [*are*] supposed to tell us but they do not.' (Respondent 1, FGD 2)

Myocardial infarction

All respondents were familiar with the term 'heart attack', with some describing it in more general terms as 'a heart problem', whereas others provided a more detailed explanation:

> '... when blood is not circulating properly; when it [*a blood vessel*] is blocked that it can cause [*a*] heart attack, maybe when there is too much fats in the veins and blood is not flowing properly.' (Respondent 2, FGD 1)

> 'His heart is not functioning normally ... it either has irregular beats or it can stop at any time.' (Respondent 1, FGD 1)

Cerebrovascular accidents

Respondents were also familiar with the term 'stroke'. Many of the respondents personally knew people who had experienced a stroke and understood the debilitating consequences. When asked what they thought the possible causes are, some mentioned the link between having a stroke and having high blood pressure; others thought there was a progression from hypertension to asthma to having a stroke. Some respondents thought that 'thinking too much can cause strokes' as well as going into 'shock' after hearing tragic news:

> 'Thinking too much can cause [*a*] stroke because you think too much and get lost in your thoughts to the point that you can't even hear a person talking to you.' (Respondent 3, FGD 2)

Some respondents were sceptical of the diagnosis of stroke in people who were otherwise healthy and without any illnesses:

> 'The doctors diagnosed her with [*a*] stroke but that sounded creepy to me because she never complained about any pains in her body and she was not one of the people who are taking medication, and she was never diagnosed with high blood pressure. She eventually died ...' (Respondent 6, FGD 2)

Hypertension

This was also a condition many respondents were familiar with. However, none were able to provide a clear definition or explanation of what hypertension is – even those who had been diagnosed as hypertensive. One respondent explained that despite being on anti-hypertensive treatment, she did not have any real insight into her treatment and was doing only what was advised by her doctor:

> 'They say I have high blood pressure and I am taking these tablets, which I do not even know what they are for. I am just following orders. I do not have a clue about all of this.' (Respondent 7, FGD 2)

Another respondent associated her diagnosis of hypertension with stress and expressed frustration in not understanding the causative link:

> 'I was diagnosed with high blood [*pressure*] in 2002. It started with stress. I used to collapse and people would pour water to wake me up ... The doctors said my stress levels were very high. I would also have a severe headache. I have a problem of stress and the doctors recommended that I should have [*watch*] TV or play cards, just something to take my mind off things. Sometimes it feels like I am going crazy. We have these diseases and we keep asking ourselves why are we suffering from these diseases.' (Respondent 5, FGD 1)

Respondents noted that poor adherence to anti-hypertensive treatment could also put an individual at risk of a stroke:

> 'You don't take treatment for high blood pressure and you end up having [*a*] stroke. Then that means it can put you at risk, or when you were not complying with your treatment. Maybe you're mixing or confusing treatment time. Then the doctor can tell you that you are at risk because you were not taking your treatment regularly.' (Respondent 4, FGD 2)

Other causes of CVD identified by respondents included depression and 'talking too much', which refer to situations that cause emotional distress and stress:

> 'Well, when I say "talking too much" I can mention grandchildren because we have grandchildren. Our grandchildren do not listen to us; they do this today and do something else tomorrow. So when they do these things you always talk, trying to discipline the child, and the child responds negatively and that hurts you. Your heart does not relax.' (Respondent 4, FGD 2)

Preventative measures

Only modification of diet, smoking cessation and reducing alcohol consumption were identified as preventative actions that could be taken to prevent CVD. No mention was made of hereditary factors, high cholesterol, sedentary lifestyle or obesity:

> 'I understand that if you have [*a*] heart problem and high blood [*pressure*], you must not feed your body with everything. You can pretend but your blood can detect that ...' (Respondent 3, FGD 1)

Perceptions of risk

Concept of risk

The majority of respondents were unable to provide a definition or explanation of what they understood by the concept of risk. Only two respondents across the three FGDs were able to give a correct example of where the word 'risk' was used as pertaining to CVD; however, they were unable to explain what they thought it meant. In both cases, respondents explained how the term was used to convey that because of poor adherence to medication they were 'at risk' of having a stroke.

Many respondents were unclear about why some people presenting with risk factors become ill, whereas others do not:

> 'They say you [*get*] [*an*] ulcer because of alcohol. I do not know about me, because I am not drinking, and I never touched a glass of alcohol but I do have these diseases [*ulcers*].' (Respondent 4, FGD 1)

Risk factors of cardiovascular disease

Respondents understood that there were certain behaviour-related factors that contribute to developing heart disease and stroke. Tobacco smoking, excessive alcohol consumption and not being compliant with regard to medication use for hypertension were mentioned as contributing factors. Unhealthy diets were identified as a major contributing factor and respondents specifically mentioned fatty meat and salty food as being unhealthy:

> '… when you eat red meat too much [*often*], because the fat in red meat will be deposited in the arteries and block the blood flow …' (Respondent 3, FGD 1)

Many respondents also mentioned that certain methods of preparation make meat less unhealthy (trimming the fat and grilling were given as examples). Some specifically linked unhealthy diets to conditions such as hypertension and diabetes and referred to the increasing prevalence of these conditions compared to when more traditional diets, with smaller portions and prepared with less oil, were consumed:

> 'We are no longer eating traditional food … people from that era were not developing diabetes and hypertension and these diseases were not that popular … people were consuming fresh food from their gardens and they were not interested in fatty foods. They were eating indigenous food only. But here in town everything is cooked by [*in*] oil, and nobody is educating us about the portion sizes. We think we are eating health[*il*]y, but we are killing ourselves.' (Respondent 3, FGD 2)

Respondents also associated unhealthy diets with their circumstances and with poverty in general. They noted that despite being aware of having to eat more fresh fruit and vegetables and less fatty foods, they were not always able to do this owing to the cost associated with procuring leaner meats and fresh produce:

> 'Our living situation forces us to eat whatever is available. Sometimes you know you do not want to eat this, but you are forced to eat it. We do not have vegetables and we do not have land to do small gardens.' (Respondent 6, FGD 1)

All respondents were aware that tobacco smoking and excessive alcohol consumption are risk factors for heart disease:

> '… there is alcohol that kills people. Some drink excessively and they end up developing heart problems …' (Respondent 4, FGD 2)

The type of alcohol being consumed in peri-urban settings was also discussed as being more harmful than that consumed by individuals of other socio-cultural backgrounds:

> 'If I am drinking, I must drink like white people, because when they are drinking, they dilute their alcohol [*spirits*], unlike us; we just drink it raw as it is [*without the addition of a mixer*].' (Respondent 4, FGD 1)

In addition, some respondents identified cultural and religious beliefs, such as 'dark spirits' or a deity, as the cause of CVD. Most respondents, particularly in focus group 1, agreed with these attributions.

Risk scores

When asked whether they considered themselves to be at risk of developing CVD, based on their calculated risk score, respondents were unable to associate a high risk score with a higher likelihood of developing CVD. In general, respondents interpreted the risk score to have a binary outcome: they were either going to develop CVD (if they had a high score) or not (if they had a low score). Only one respondent, who was found to be at high risk, explained that because she had a high risk score, she had 'more chances of contracting these diseases'. Most respondents did not know how to interpret the risk scores, stating that 'anything is possible'. This suggests that irrespective of the risk scores calculated for each individual, there was no change in the perceived susceptibility of having a cardiovascular event.

Risk presentation

We were unable to collect any useful information with regard to comparing different methods of presenting risk scores during the FGDs. Respondents did not understand the word 'risk' and subsequently did not understand any of the methods of presenting and explaining risk. During the FGDs, we directly observed that, despite the translator explaining each method a number times, respondents remained unsure and were unable to score the different methods.

Coping with the disease

Attitude towards making lifestyle changes

Respondents felt helpless about making lifestyle changes. This was largely attributed to dire living conditions and poverty:

> '… and sometimes you do not have a cent to buy vegetables from the street vendors. I went to see a doctor and the doctor said: "Your blood pressure is high; therefore you need to eat fruit and vegetables." I asked him: "Doctor, where will I get these nutritious foods?" I have nothing. I am surviving on [*a*] child's grant of R300 [*a month*].' (Respondent 6, FGD 1)

> 'Poverty can cause these diseases. You become helpless. You do not know where to start.' (Respondent 6, FGD 2)

Personal, cultural and religious beliefs

Respondents also referred to a number of personal, cultural and religious beliefs that influenced how risk was perceived.

For example, respondents mentioned that once diagnosed with CVD, progression was beyond their control:

'It is only God who can help us ... ' (Respondent 2, FGD 1)

Discussion

Understanding diseases and their predisposing factors requires a different set of skills from that needed for understanding uncertainty and risk. The former requires knowledge of facts and that certain behaviours or biological processes can lead to specific outcomes, such as heart attacks. However, understanding risk requires abstract thinking that involves numerical literacy and computation. For example, risk scores are often numeric expressions of uncertainty about a future event. Being able to understand, interpret and work with numbers leads to improved risk comparisons and estimates,[30] whereas a lower level of numeracy skill is associated with an overestimation of risk as people tend to respond more to non-numerical aspects of the interaction, such as mood or feedback from others.[31,32]

In this study, respondents' knowledge of CVD and its risk factors varied, but most were familiar with the terminology used to describe CVD. For example, respondents were aware of some lifestyle factors that cause CVD, such as high-fat diets and excessive alcohol consumption, which suggests that there is some baseline knowledge of this topic amongst community members. Similarly, respondents were aware of a number of cardiovascular conditions, such as hypertension and stroke. However, although they were familiar with the terms, they had limited insight into the conditions. The limited insight was underscored by contrasts in the self-reported history of CVD and the calculated level of risk, which suggests low health literacy amongst respondents. An exception was respondents' awareness of the impact of living in low-income peri-urban conditions on the risk of developing CVD. This insight stemmed from the comparison with people living in more rural settings, where fewer people were perceived to develop CVD, and is in keeping with the evidence on the rising incidence of CVD associated with urbanisation.[33]

In contrast to having knowledge of CVD and its risk factors, respondents were altogether unfamiliar with the concept of risk. Risk was perceived as a binary concept, in that a cardiovascular event was either going to happen or not, depending on high or low risk, respectively. This finding is in keeping with those of other studies that explored how CVD risk is understood.[18,34,35] One of the objectives of this study was to explore different methods of conveying risk. Although the difficulty in understanding CVD risk tables and multivariable risk factors has previously been documented in the literature,[17] we underestimated the extent to which it would restrict our investigation. Consequently, we were unable to assess the effectiveness of different methods owing to respondents' lack of primary understanding of risk. Despite evidence to support the use of certain strategies to improve risk communication in general (e.g. presenting the chance of an event, presenting changes in numeric outcomes and using visual formats),[31] more research is needed with regard to developing methods for communicating risk to people with little numerical literacy.

Being able to understand risk is only one of the factors that influence how people understand and use information in their decision-making. Several theories regarding decision-making have been put forward, particularly related to risk.[18] The health belief model, developed to explain why people fail to accept screening tests for early detection of asymptomatic disease,[36] suggests that people are unlikely to take appropriate preventative action until they perceive themselves to be susceptible to developing a disease associated with serious consequences. We analysed the findings from the FGDs according to the framework of the health belief model to evaluate CVD risk assessment as a possible driver of behaviour change (Table 3 and Table 4). Although CVD risk assessment supports a number of the constructs of the proposed model (e.g. perceived susceptibility, perceived severity, perceived benefits of taking action and a cue to action), it still requires health and numerical literacy.[37]

The ability to understand risk may be further complicated by an element of fatalism. Respondents expressed a sense of helplessness ('... poverty can cause these diseases; you become helpless ...'; '... it is only God who can help us'), which suggests that they perceive an external locus of control and that they cannot control events affecting their lives.[38]

There are a number of limitations in this study. A selection bias was introduced by CHWs recruiting their existing clients, including those with a previous history of CVD. As the majority of respondents were female, a skewed distribution of gender resulted. The data were analysed by a single researcher, which may have introduced bias in interpretation. Language and cultural differences between the researcher and the respondents may also have affected understanding and interpretation of the data. In addition, respondents' numeracy skills were not determined and inferences in the discussion were based on the overall level of completed secondary schooling.

Conclusion

This study contributes to our understanding of the knowledge of and perceptions about CVD and its risk

TABLE 3: Key descriptors of the health belief model as described by Rosenstock (1974).[21]

Key descriptors	Explanation
Perceived susceptibility	The perception of the likelihood of experiencing a given disease or condition.
Perceived severity	The perception of the seriousness of the effects a given disease or condition would have on one's state of affairs, including the emotional and financial effects.
Perceived benefits of taking action	The perception of the benefits to be gained by taking an action.
Barriers to taking action	Barriers relate to the inhibitory characteristics of a treatment or preventative measure that prevent action, including, for example, the inconvenience or expense.
Cue to action	The cue to action acts as a trigger for the desired action to be taken.

TABLE 4: Analysis of the findings from focus group discussions and evaluation of the risk for cardiovascular disease within the framework of the health belief model.

Key descriptor	Findings from FGDs	Responses	Evaluation of CVD risk assessment as an intervention to drive behavioural change
Perceived susceptibility	A limited understanding exists of the causal relationship between CVD and its risk factors.	'... it [*stroke*] starts with high blood pressure and then asthma ...'	The calculation of a CVD risk score provides information that directly informs perceived susceptibility (i.e. a risk score directly communicates the likelihood of an individual having a cardiovascular event within a given period).
	The absence of external symptoms, as in the case of hypertension, negatively affects perceptions of susceptibility.	'... my blood pressure is high ever since last month ... I am at peace with it. Some things are part and parcel of our lives and you just do not know what to do and end up destroying your heart.'	
	Perceived susceptibility remained unchanged by calculation of a cardiovascular disease risk score.	'Anything is possible.'	
Perceived severity	The physical severity of consequences of CVD was perceived adequately.	'Back home in [*the*] Eastern Cape there is a woman who is suffering from stroke. She cannot even do a thing for herself ...'	The calculation of a CVD risk score provides information that indirectly informs perceived severity (i.e. the risk score communicates the likelihood of having a stroke or heart attack in the given period).
		'...she was attacked by stroke when we were at church ... She eventually died.'	
	Perceptions on the psychosocial, emotional and financial effects were not discussed.		
Perceived benefits of taking action	Awareness of the benefits of taking action was limited. Even respondents who were taking action (e.g. adhering to treatment) did not express perception of any benefits gained.	'It is also the beliefs. We believe that these tablets can cause cancer so you decide to stop taking them. And when you look at the amount [*sic*] of these pills you believe that it is true that you can develop cancer.'	The benefit of taking action (by modifying risk factors) is the reduction of risk and potential prevention of a heart attack or stroke. This is not currently quantified as part of the risk assessment (e.g. explicitly stating that smoking cessation for example, will reduce risk by 10%).
	Cultural, religious and other beliefs further detracted from the perceived benefits of taking action.		
Barriers to taking action	Poverty was identified as a barrier to making lifestyle changes.	'... our living situation forces us to eat whatever is available ...'	CVD risk assessment does not address barriers to taking action.
Cue to action	None elicited.		Once identified as being at high risk, a referral to the local clinic can be considered a cue to action.

CVD, cardiovascular disease; FGD, focus group discussion.

factors in a low-income peri-urban community in South Africa. Respondents were more knowledgeable about CVD in general than about the concept of risk. Educational initiatives focused on improving knowledge of risk and the causal relationship between predisposing factors and CVD are needed. These need to consider local cultural and religious beliefs. In addition, methods to present risk without numeracy skills being necessary for interpretation also need to be developed and tested in this community. Without a better understanding of risk, CVD risk assessments may fail in this community.

Acknowledgements

This Seed Grant has been funded in whole with Federal funds by the United States National Heart, Lung, and Blood Institute, National Institutes of Health, Department of Health and Human Services, under Purchase Order no. UCT HHSN268200900030C.

Competing interests

The authors declare that they have no financial or personal relationship(s) that may have inappropriately influenced them in writing this article.

Authors' contributions

N.L. (University of Cape Town), K.S. (Chronic Disease Initiative for Africa), S.S. (Chronic Disease Initiative for Africa) and K.E.-M. (Chronic Disease Initiative for Africa) conceived and designed the study. S.S. collected and analysed the data and drafted the paper. N.L., K.S., T.A.G. (Harvard University), S.S. and K.E.-M. contributed to revising the article. All authors gave final approval of the manuscript.

References

1. Bradshaw D, Groenewald P, Laubscher R, et al. Initial burden of disease estimates for South Africa, 2000. S Afr Med J. 2003;93(9):682–688. PMID: 14635557.
2. Conroy RM, Pyorala K, Fitzgerald AP, et al. Estimation of ten-year risk of fatal cardiovascular disease in Europe: The SCORE project. Eur Heart J. 2003;24(11):987–1003. PMID: 12788299, http://dx.doi.org/10.1016/S0195-668X(03)00114-3
3. Ferrario M, Chiodini P, Chambless LE, et al. Prediction of coronary events in a low incidence population. Assessing accuracy of the CUORE Cohort Study prediction equation. Int J Epidemiol. 2005;34(2):413–421. PMID: 15659467, http://dx.doi.org/10.1093/ije/dyh405
4. Wilson PW, D'Agostino RB, Levy D, Belanger AM, Silbershatz H, Kannel WB. Prediction of coronary heart disease using risk factor categories. Circulation. 1998;97(18):1837–1847. PMID: 9603539, http://dx.doi.org/10.1161/01.CIR.97.18.1837
5. Beswick A, Brindle P. Risk scoring in the assessment of cardiovascular risk. Curr Opin Lipidol. 2006;17(4):375–386. PMID: 16832160, http://dx.doi.org/10.1097/01.mol.0000236362.56216.44
6. Gaziano TA, Young CR, Fitzmaurice G, Atwood S, Gaziano JM. Laboratory-based versus non-laboratory-based method for assessment of cardiovascular disease risk: The NHANES I Follow-up Study cohort. Lancet. 2008;371(9616):923–931. PMID: 18342687, http://dx.doi.org/10.1016/S0140-6736(08)60418-3
7. Hippisley-Cox J, Coupland C, Vinogradova Y, Robson J, May M, Brindle P. Derivation and validation of QRISK, a new cardiovascular disease risk score for the United Kingdom: Prospective open cohort study. BMJ. 2007;335(7611):136. PMID: 17615182, http://dx.doi.org/10.1136/bmj.39261.471806.55
8. Lehmann U, Sanders, D. Community health workers: What do we know about them? Geneva: World Health Organization; 2007.
9. Gaziano TA, Pandya A, Steyn K, et al. Comparative assessment of absolute cardiovascular disease risk characterization from non-laboratory-based risk assessment in South African populations. BMC Med. 2013;11:170. PMID: 23880010, http://dx.doi.org/10.1186/1741-7015-11-170
10. Surka S, Edirippulige S, Steyn K, Gaziano T, Puoane T, Levitt N. Evaluating the use of mobile phone technology to enhance cardiovascular disease screening by community health workers. Int J Med Inform. 2014;83(9):648–654. PMID: 25002305, http://dx.doi.org/10.1016/j.ijmedinf.2014.06.008

11. Gaziano TA, Abrahams-Gessel S, Denman CA, et al. An assessment of community health workers' ability to screen for cardiovascular disease risk with a simple, non-invasive risk assessment instrument in Bangladesh, Guatemala, Mexico, and South Africa: An observational study. Lancet Glob Health. 2015;3(9):e556–e563. PMID: 26187361, http://dx.doi.org/10.1016/S2214-109X(15)00143-6

12. Levitt NS, Puoane T, Denman CA, et al. Referral outcomes of individuals identified at high risk of cardiovascular disease by community health workers in Bangladesh, Guatemala, Mexico, and South Africa. Glob Health Action. 2015;8:26318. PMID: 25854780, http://dx.doi.org/10.3402/gha.v8.26318

13. Alm-Roijer C, Fridlund B, Stagmo M, Erhardt L. Knowing your risk factors for coronary heart disease improves adherence to advice on lifestyle changes and medication. J Cardiovasc Nurs. 2006;21(5):e24–e31. PMID: 16966907.

14. Sullivan LM, Massaro JM, D'Agostino RB Sr. Presentation of multivariate data for clinical use: The Framingham Study risk score functions. Stat Med. 2004;23(10):1631–1660. PMID: 15122742, http://dx.doi.org/10.1002/sim.1742

15. Paling J. Strategies to help patients understand risks. BMJ. 2003;327(7417):745–748. PMID: 14512489, http://dx.doi.org/10.1136/bmj.327.7417.745

16. Knapp P, Raynor DK, Berry DC. Comparison of two methods of presenting risk information to patients about the side effects of medicines. Qual Saf Health Care. 2004;13(3):176–180. PMID: 15175486, http://dx.doi.org/10.1136/qshc.2003.009076

17. Van Steenkiste B, Van der Weijden T, Timmermans D, Vaes J, Stoffers J, Grol R. Patients' ideas, fears and expectations of their coronary risk: Barriers for primary prevention. Patient Educ Couns. 2004;55(2):301–307. PMID: 15530768, http://dx.doi.org/10.1016/j.pec.2003.11.005

18. Webster R, Heeley E. Perceptions of risk: Understanding cardiovascular disease. Risk Manag Healthc Policy. 2010;3:49–60. PMID: 22312218, http://dx.doi.org/10.2147/RMHP.S8288

19. Nutbeam D. Health literacy as a public health goal: A challenge for contemporary health education and communication strategies into the 21st century. Health Promot Int. 2000;15(3):259–267. http://dx.doi.org/10.1093/heapro/15.3.259

20. Schillinger D, Grumbach K, Piette J, et al. Association of health literacy with diabetes outcomes. JAMA. 2002;288(4):475–482. PMID: 12132978, http://dx.doi.org/10.1001/jama.288.4.475

21. Rosenstock IM. The health belief model and preventive health behavior. Health Educ Behav. 1974;2(4):354–386. http://dx.doi.org/10.1177/109019817400200405

22. Trevena LJ, Davey HM, Barratt A, Butow P, Caldwell P. A systematic review on communicating with patients about evidence. J Eval Clin Pract. 2006;12(1):13–23. PMID: 16422776.

23. O'Connor AM, Bennett CL, Stacey D, et al. Decision aids for people facing health treatment or screening decisions. Cochrane Database Syst Rev. 2009(3):CD001431. PMID: 19588325, http://dx.doi.org/10.1002/14651858.CD001431.pub2

24. Timmermans D, Oudhoff J. Different formats for the communication of risks: Verbal, numerical, and graphical formats. Wiley Encycl Oper Res Manage Sci. 2010. http://dx.doi.org/10.1002/9780470400531.eorms0954

25. Lopez-Gonzalez AA, Aguilo A, Frontera M, Bennasar-Veny M, Campos I, Vicente-Herrero T, et al. Effectiveness of the Heart Age tool for improving modifiable cardiovascular risk factors in a Southern European population: A randomized trial. Eur J Prev Cardiol. 2014 Mar;22(3):389-96. PubMed PMID: 24491403. http://dx.doi.org/10.1177/2047487313518479. Epub 2014/02/05. eng.

26. Pope C, Ziebland S, Mays N. Qualitative research in health care: Analysing qualitative data. BMJ. 2000;320:114–116. PMID: 10625273.

27. Alberts M, Urdal P, Steyn K, et al. Prevalence of cardiovascular diseases and associated risk factors in a rural black population of South Africa. Eur J Cardiovasc Prev Rehabil. 2005;12(4):347–354. PMID: 16079642, http://dx.doi.org/10.1097/01.hjr.0000174792.24188.8e

28. Dalal S, Beunza JJ, Volmink J, et al. Non-communicable diseases in sub-Saharan Africa: What we know now. Int J Epidemiol. 2011;40(4):885–901. PMID: 21527446, http://dx.doi.org/10.1093/ije/dyr050

29. Peer N, Steyn K, Lombard C, Gwebushe N, Levitt N. A high burden of hypertension in the urban black population of Cape Town: The cardiovascular risk in Black South Africans (CRIBSA) study. PLoS One. 2013;8(11):e78567. PMID: 24250798, http://dx.doi.org/10.1371/journal.pone.0078567

30. Trevena LJ, Zikmund-Fisher BJ, Edwards A, et al. Presenting quantitative information about decision outcomes: A risk communication primer for patient decision aid developers. BMC Med Inform Decis Mak. 2013;13(Suppl 2):S7. PMID: 24625237, http://dx.doi.org/10.1186/1472-6947-13-S2-S7

31. Weinstein ND, Atwood K, Puleo E, Fletcher R, Colditz G, Emmons K. Colon cancer: Risk perceptions and risk communication. J Health Commun. 2004;9(1):53–65. PMID: 14761833, http://dx.doi.org/10.1080/10810730490271647

32. Peters E, Vastfjall D, Slovic P, Mertz CK, Mazzocco K, Dickert S. Numeracy and decision making. Psychol Sci. 2006;17(5):407–413. PMID: 16683928, http://dx.doi.org/10.1111/j.1467-9280.2006.01720.x

33. Popkin BM, Adair LS, Ng SW. Global nutrition transition and the pandemic of obesity in developing countries. Nutr Rev. 2012;70(1):3–21. PMID: 22221213, http://dx.doi.org/ 10.1111/j.1753-4887.2011.00456.x

34. Goldman RE, Parker DR, Eaton CB, et al. Patients' perceptions of cholesterol, cardiovascular disease risk, and risk communication strategies. Ann Fam Med. 2006;4(3):205–212. PMID: 16735521, http://dx.doi.org/10.1370/afm.534

35. Van der Weijden T, Van Steenkiste B, Stoffers HE, Timmermans DR, Grol R. Primary prevention of cardiovascular diseases in general practice: Mismatch between cardiovascular risk and patients' risk perceptions. Med Decis Making. 2007;27(6):754–761. PMID: 17873263, http://dx.doi.org/10.1177/0272989X07305323

36. Janz NK, Becker MH. The health belief model: A decade later. Health Educ Q. 1984;11(1):1–47. PMID:6392204, http://dx.doi.org/10.1177/109019818401100101 4

37. Reyna VF, Nelson WL, Han PK, Dieckmann NF. How numeracy influences risk comprehension and medical decision making. Psychol Bull. 2009;135(6):943–973. PMID: 19883143, http://dx.doi.org/10.1037/a0017327

38. Fishbein M, Ajzen I. Predicting and changing behavior: The reasoned action approach. Hove: Taylor & Francis; 2011.

Knowledge of community care workers about key family practices in a rural community in South Africa

Authors:
Ethelwynn Stellenberg[1]
Marjorie van Zyl[1]
Johanna Eygelaar[1]

Affiliations:
[1]Division of Nursing, Stellenbosch University, South Africa

Correspondence to:
Ethelwynn Stellenberg

Email:
elstel@sun.ac.za

Postal address:
PO Box 241, Cape Town 8000, South Africa

Background: Interventions by community care workers within the context of community-based integrated management of childhood illness (CIMCI) may have a positive effect on child health if the health workers have adequate knowledge about key family practices.

Setting: The study was conducted in rural areas of the West Coast district in the Western Cape, South Africa.

Objectives: The objective of this study was to determine the knowledge of community care workers about five of the 16 key family practices of CIMCI.

Methods: A descriptive survey collected a self-administered questionnaire from 257 community care workers out of a possible total of 270 (95.2% response rate). Descriptive and inferential statistical analysis was applied.

Results: Only 25 of the respondents (10%) obtained a score higher than 70% on the knowledge-based items of the questionnaire. Less than 25% of respondents answered questions in these key areas correctly (pneumonia [17%], tuberculosis [13%], HIV/AIDS [9%] immunisation [3%] and recommendations for a child with fever [21%]). Statistically significant correlations were found between the total score a respondent achieved and the highest level of education obtained ($p < 0.01$), the level of in-service training ($p < 0.01$), attendance of a CIMCI five-day training course ($p < 0.01$), and completing a subsequent refresher course ($p < 0.01$).

Conclusion: The knowledge of CCWs was inadequate to provide safe, quality CIMCI. CIMCI refresher courses should be offered annually to improve CCWs' knowledge and the quality of care that they render. Regular update courses could contribute to building competence.

Les connaissances des prestataires de soins communautaires sur les pratiques familiales clés dans une communauté rurale d'Afrique du Sud.

Contexte: Les interventions par des prestataires de soins communautaires dans le contexte de la gestion intégrée communautaire des maladies de l'enfance (GICME) peuvent avoir un effet positif sur la santé des enfants si les prestataires de soins ont suffisamment de connaissances sur les pratiques familiales clés.

Lieu: L'étude a été menée dans les régions rurales de la Cote Ouest du Western Cape, en Afrique du Sud.

Objectifs: L'objectif de cette étude était de déterminer les connaissances des prestataires de soins communautaires (PSC) sur cinq des 16 pratiques familiales clés de la GICME.

Méthodes: Un plan de recherche descriptif et exploratoire avec approche quantitative a été utilisé. On a obtenu un taux de réponse de 95.2% de la population ciblée ($N = 270$). On a collecté les données au moyen d'un questionnaire auto-administré. On a utilisé une analyse statistique descriptive et différents tests statistiques.

Résultats: Seuls 25 des répondants (10%) ont obtenu un score supérieur à 70% sur les questions du questionnaire basées sur les connaissances. Les connaissances des PSC étaient très faibles dans le domaine de la morbidité élevée et des taux de mortalité des enfants. Moins de 25% des répondants ont répondu correctement aux questions dans ces domaines clés (pneumonie [17%], tuberculose [13%], VIH/SIDA [9%] immunisation [3%] et recommandations pour un enfant fiévreux [21%]). On a trouvé des corrélations statistiquement importantes entre le score total d'un répondent et le plus haut niveau d'éducation atteint ($P < 0.01$), le niveau de formation en cours d'emploi ($P < 0.01$), assistance à un cours de formation de cinq jours sur la GICME ($P < 0.01$), et l'achèvement ultérieur d'un cours de rafraichissement ($P < 0.01$).

Conclusion: Il faut offrit tous les ans des cours de rafraichissement sur la GICME pour améliorer les connaissances des PSC et la qualité des soins qu'ils donnent. Des cours de mise à jour réguliers pourraient permettre de développer les compétences.

Introduction

Social value

With an estimated 8.1 million children under the age of five years dying every year, child mortality is a worldwide problem,[1] despite the fourth Millennium Development Goal of the World Health Organization (WHO) aiming to reduce child mortality by two-thirds by 2015.[2] Almost 90% of the deaths in this age group are attributed to neonatal causes, pneumonia, diarrhoea, malaria, measles and HIV and/or AIDS.[3]

An integrated approach that focuses on the holistic well-being of the child, namely integrated management of childhood illness, aims to improve care at first-level health facilities by introducing standardised training for health workers and treatment guidelines.[4]

In 1997, the WHO and the United Nations Children's Fund (UNICEF) identified 16 key family practices that could be included in a community-based approach to integrated management of childhood illness (CIMCI).[5] Studies have shown that interventions by community care workers (CCWs) who follow the CIMCI approach reduce morbidity and mortality in children under the age of five[6,7] and may contribute to achieving the Millennium Development Goals.[5]

CCWs represent the communities that they serve and are involved in outreach in a variety of community settings.[8] However, CCW training and refresher courses are not standardised and the care workers' knowledge about CIMCI may be inadequate.

Scientific value

A study conducted in Ile-Ife in south-western Nigeria has shown that well-implemented CIMCI interventions offer an effective, low-cost approach to ensuring optimal growth, development and survival of Nigerian children.[9] CCWs use their skills to ensure that their clients receive the necessary services through capacity building and advocating the importance of a healthy lifestyle to ensure good health.[8] Explaining the importance of rehydration therapy and promoting exclusive breastfeeding are two important health-promoting interventions by CCWs that could lower the mortality of children under the age of five by 10%.[10]

The results of the Nigerian study showed that 78.5% of caregivers from CIMCI-compliant local government areas of Osun, an inland state in south-western *Nigeria*, obtained information about the home management of childhood illnesses from trained CCWs.[9] In contrast, about two-thirds (67.9%) of caregivers from non-compliant local government areas received information about the home management of childhood illnesses from relatives. The study further showed that in CIMCI-compliant local government areas, the use of an oral rehydration solution for the management of childhood diarrhoea was high (90.8%), whereas it was below 20% in non-compliant local government areas. In the CIMCI-compliant areas the recommended treatment for diarrhoea was a salt-sugar solution, together with the use of antibiotics and referral to a primary healthcare centre; in the areas that did not follow the CIMCI approach, the caregivers used home remedies such as water, garri water and salt water, and patients were not referred to a primary healthcare facility. After CIMCI implementation, the prevalence of diarrhoea was reduced from 13% to 9.5%.[9]

Training of CCWs

CCWs need to be trained appropriately to ensure that health information is disseminated effectively in their communities. A study in Kenya found that CCWs often misinterpreted signs and symptoms of common diseases, resulting in improper drug management.[11] Consequently, as one of the CIMCI interventions, CCWs were provided with specific guidelines for the treatment of pneumonia and malaria in remote areas. In a study conducted in India, poor training of CCWs revealed that only 12.8% of mothers knew that the Bacillus Calmette-Guerin vaccine is given at birth and that only 6% knew that the hepatitis B vaccine could also be given at birth. Consequently less than half (37.2%) of the mothers in the study had their children immunised according to the immunisation schedules for their children by the age of nine months.[12] The selection, retention and training of CCWs are thus critical factors for the success of India's immunisation programme.[13]

Kenyan CCWs are required to be able to read at school level (grade 9 or higher) and to volunteer in the community they live in. Women are preferred as CCWs. Candidates to be trained as CCWs are selected by health committees that are established in some communities. Remuneration for their services, recognition from the community, a feeling of self-satisfaction and appreciation expressed by the community have been cited as incentives for CCWs to adhere to their work.[11]

In the United States, 91% of CCWs are women and 37.6% are younger than 50 years. They work at private homes, community centres, clinics and hospitals. The most common health issues addressed by CCWs are HIV and/or AIDS, women's health, pre- and postnatal care, child health and cancer. CCWs assist their clients with access to both medical and nonmedical services, provide culturally appropriate health education and information, are involved in community advocacy and provide social support.[14]

Training and ongoing supervision of CCWs vary widely across the world. In ten Latin American countries where communities use training materials developed by the Red Cross, the recommended practices were adapted for local relevance.[15] This led to 29% more families recognising the warning signs of diarrhoea, 31% more families knowing the danger signs of illness in a child and the consequences of not taking action, and 12% more families being able to recognise the danger signs of pneumonia. Most notably, 6% more children with a cough accompanied with rapid breathing were taken to health services.

In the Siaya district in Kenya, CCWs received training on how to use the guideline for managing a sick child.[11] The initial training included ten days of lectures, during which case studies were reviewed and participants engaged in role-playing, and five days of clinical practice at the Siaya District Hospital. Refresher training sessions to address targeted weaknesses in clinical skills were offered for six to fifteen days. In addition to lectures and role-playing, CCWs' training involved reviewing videotaped consultations and clinical practice at local pharmacies or health facilities in groups of eight to ten. The CCWs received medicine kits to treat children diagnosed with malaria or pneumonia or who experienced diarrhoea or fever and suffered from malnutrition. Overall adherence to clinical guidelines was fairly acceptable, with, on average, 80% of all guideline-recommended procedures being performed correctly.[11]

CCWs in the USA commonly receive training on cultural awareness, knowledge of health issues and social services, interpersonal communication skills and client advocacy. The least common topic is leadership. Carers who wish to qualify as CCWs can obtain a diploma of education and training offered by a prestigious local university.[14] In contrast, no specific, formal training is offered to CCWs in Mexico, although they can attend educational workshops once or twice a month to develop their skills.[16]

In southern Asia, a study from Sylhet, Bangladesh, showed that CCWs working in rural districts received 21 days of training with regard to newborn breastfeeding and a practical session on the observation and assessment of breastfeeding.[17] Training included lectures, hands-on demonstration and practical exercises with the help of post-partum breastfeeding mothers, and video-guided lessons with support from a supervisor. In nearby Nepal, women with basic school education, as well as those who are only semi-literate or illiterate, have been trained as CCWs to diagnose and assess severity and danger signs associated with acute respiratory infection or diarrhoea in children, offer appropriate treatment and refer patients to health facilities.[18] As part of this initiative, the WHO-developed curriculum for integrated management of childhood illnesses was adapted and simplified to ensure that it met the needs of these volunteers.[18] In this rural district under study, the services of CCWs follow an integrated approach, which includes home visits to render basic nursing care, CIMCI, directly observed tuberculosis treatment, adherence support for clients on antiretroviral therapy and services for managing mental illness and chronic lifestyle diseases. According to this model, the same CCW renders the full package of care, whereas in the urban model different CCWs are responsible for the respective programmes.[19]

Aim of the study

Between 2009 and 2011, the infant mortality rate in the study area (West Coast district) was approximately 30/1000 live births, with the mortality rate amongst children younger than five years approximately 35/1000 live births. The five most common causes of death in this population were pneumonia, premature birth, diarrhoea, HIV and/or AIDS and various injuries.[20]

It was therefore deemed essential that CCWs' knowledge of key family practices be explored. Five specific practices were identified, namely breastfeeding, physical growth and development, common childhood illnesses, immunisations and danger signs for referral to a clinic or hospital. These danger signs in children include inability to drink or breastfeed, vomiting, lethargy or unconsciousness, coughing accompanied with rapid breathing (> 50 breaths per minute), coughing associated with chest indrawing, bloody diarrhoea, diarrhoea together with presentation of sunken eyes or a sunken fontanel, and sudden fever in a child younger than two months or who is not feeding properly.

Research methods and design

Study design

The study involved a descriptive, quantitative survey of CCWs' knowledge with regard to five of the 16 key family practices described for the CIMCI approach.

Setting

The study was conducted in the West Coast district, which is subdivided into five sub-districts (Swartland, Bergriver, Saldanha, Cederberg and Matzikama). At the time of the research, community-based services were rendered by 17 non-profit organisations, which employed 270 CCWs to serve a total of 12 000 clients. Table 1 shows the distribution of CCWs across the sub-districts.

Study population sampling strategy

The target population ($N = 270$) consisted of CCWs working for non-profit organisations funded by the provincial government and who provided CIMCI in the West Coast district of the Western Cape, South Africa. All CCWs were invited to participate in the study; those who refused consent or who were not available during the two weeks of data collection (owing to, for example, leave) were excluded from the study.

TABLE 1: Distribution of community care workers across the sub-districts of the West Coast district, Western Cape, South Africa.

Sub-districts in the West Coast district	Number of CCWs per sub-district
Matzikama	90
Cederberg	54
Swartland	50
Bergriver	33
Saldanha	43
Total	**270**

CCW, community care worker.

Data collection

All data were collected in 2012. One of the researchers collected the data from a self-administered questionnaire that included 25 knowledge-based items related to the five key family practices identified for this study. The questionnaire was designed to be completed within 30 minutes and was available in either English or Afrikaans. In addition to the knowledge-based section, the questionnaire also included questions related to demographic data (respondent's age; highest level of education; gender; health-related work experience; experience working with children; working hours; value of the respondent's stipend).

A variety of open- and closed-ended questions, graphs and pictures were used in the questionnaire. As the CIMCI programme has no specific score for competence, a marking schedule was designed for this study together with primary health care experts from the Division of Nursing, Stellenbosch University. The minimum score for safe, quality care was set at 70%.

Pilot study

A pilot study was conducted in the Bergriver sub-district to test the methods and the instrument to be used in the main investigation. The pilot study included 33 CCWs, representing 12.2% of the respondents of the main study.

The pilot study showed that the researcher needed to be present to give contextual structure and guide respondents during their completion of the questionnaire. This was to ensure that all the questions were completed. The questionnaire was found to be easily understood and that the allocated time was adequate for completion.

Reliability and validity

Content, construct and face validity were ensured through consultation with experts in primary health care, research methodology and statistics. Senior researchers (study supervisors), the post-graduate committee of Stellenbosch University and ethical committees of various relevant institutions approved the study design and approach. The content of the questionnaire was based on the 16 key family practices identified for inclusion in a CIMCI programme. Reliability and validity were further improved by the researcher personally collecting and capturing the data, thereby ensuring a consistent data collection process. A pilot study was also conducted.

Data analyses

Data were analysed using statistical software (STATISTICA 10, StatSoft Inc., Tulsa). Descriptive statistical tests (Spearman rank order and Mann-Whitney *U* correlation) were used to determine the level of significance between the dependent and independent variables at a 95% confidence level. The level for statistical significance was defined as $P < 0.05$.

Ethical considerations

Ethical approval was received from the Human Research Ethics Committee, Stellenbosch University, and permission from the Provincial Government of the Western Cape, and the West Coast District Department of Health.

Participation was entirely voluntary and refusal to participate was without consequence. A respondent was free to leave the study at any time, even after having agreed to take part. Informed written consent was obtained from each respondent. The purpose, procedures, risks and benefits of the research project, as well as the obligations and commitments of both the participants and the researcher, were outlined in the consent form. To ensure confidentiality and anonymity, the consent form was submitted separately from the questionnaire. The collected data were managed only by the researchers.

The right to protection from discomfort and harm is based on the ethical principle of beneficence, which dictates that participation in the study should not cause any harm to the respondent.[21] The information obtained during the study was not of sensitive nature and no known risks to the respondents were foreseen during the study. The respondents were protected from psychological harm, but would have been referred to appropriate psychological services in the event of any psychological harm.

The selection of respondents was deemed fair as all of the CCWs working in the study area were invited to take part in the study. This population of CCWs were chosen to participate in the study because they were connected to the research problem. The only participants who were excluded from the study were those not physically present during data collection and those who refused consent. Benefits derived from participating in the study were communicated to the participants and to the relevant authorities.

Results

A total of 257 CCWs completed the questionnaire (response rate, 95.2%). The most common age group amongst the respondents was 36–40 years (n = 55; 21%). The majority of respondents (n = 252; 98%) were female and close to half (n = 116; 45%) had passed grade 12 schooling. Approximately half of the respondents (n = 130; 51%) indicated that they had not received CIMCI training, despite providing services for an average of six years already; 124 respondents (48%) had received some training between 2004 and 2012, of which 58 attended a refresher course in 2012. Respondents indicated that they were expected to provide CIMCI according to a community-based model in which up to 28 clients had to be attended to per day. The mean and median number of clients attended to per day were 11 and 12, respectively.

Total scores for the 25 knowledge-based questions included in the questionnaire show that 87 of the respondents (34%) scored below 50%. The majority of the respondents scored between 50% and 69% ($n = 145$; 56%) and only 25 respondents (10%) scored between 70% and 89%. None of the participants scored 90% or more (Table 2).

Results of the Spearman's rank order test applied to the investigated variables are shown in Table 3. A positive correlation (Spearman rho = 0.1) was found between the highest school grade passed and the total knowledge score of respondents ($P < 0.01$) (Table 3). A positive correlation with a medium effect (Spearman rho = 0.3) was also found between having received training as part of the Expanded Public Works Programme (EPWP) and an individual's total scores ($P = 0.01$). A medium effect relationship ranges between $r = 0.3$ and $r = 0.49$. Additional EPWP training was associated with higher knowledge scores. The EPWP is a nationwide programme aimed at integrating the unemployed into productive work by providing learners with in-service skills training and so allows them to earn an income through a stipend.

Results of the Mann-Whitney *U*-test indicated a significant relationship between the total knowledge score obtained and attending a five-day CIMCI training course ($P < 0.01$) and later a refresher course ($P < 0.01$).

Table 4 shows the number of participants who correctly answered the questions in the key knowledge areas. Knowledge about managing conditions associated with high mortality and morbidity rates were especially poor. These included pneumonia (17%), tuberculosis (13%) and HIV and/or AIDS (9%), correct immunisation at six weeks (3%), recommendations for a child with fever (21%) and all danger signs (5%).

TABLE 2: Distribution of test scores with regard to knowledge of community-based integrated management of childhood illness ($N = 257$).

Performance category (score range)	Number of respondents *n* (%)
Poor (0%–49%)	87 (34)
Average (50%–69%)	145 (56)
Good (70%–89%)	25 (10)
Excellent (90%–100%)	0 (0)

Table 3: Relationships between the total scores and biographical data.

Variables	*N*	Test	Spearman *r*	*P*-value
Total score and EPWP	257	Spearman rho	0.3	< 0.01
Total score and age	257	Spearman rho	0.07	0.2
Total score and highest school grade passed	255	Spearman rho	0.19	< 0.01

EPWP; Expanded Public Works Programme.

TABLE 4: Number of respondents who answered questions about key family practices associated with high mortality and morbidity rates correctly ($N = 257$).

Knowledge item	Number of respondents who answered correctly *n* (%)
Only one sign to suspect pneumonia	45 (17)
Tuberculosis	34 (13)
HIV and/orAIDS	23 (9)
Correct immunisation at 6 weeks	7 (3)
Recommendations for child with fever	55 (21)
All danger signs	12 (5)

Discussion

Only 10% of the participants scored above the defined minimum score for quality care, with 34% of respondents scoring below 50%. The respondents' knowledge regarding the selected aspects of family health included in the 16 key family practices of CIMCI should be associated with scores ≥ 70%. Inadequate and incorrect knowledge may have an influence on child mortality and child morbidity in the communities where the CCWs work.

Scores on questions related to breastfeeding showed that respondents' general knowledge was only of an average standard. The most important potential advantage of exclusive breastfeeding for six months relates to the prevention of infectious diseases, especially morbidity and mortality related to gastrointestinal infections.[22] In addition, women stay in hospital only for a short period after giving birth and therefore health promotion on breastfeeding at a community level is very important.[23]

Respondents' knowledge of managing pneumonia, tuberculosis and HIV/AIDs was poor. If not diagnosed early, these conditions increase infant and child morbidity and mortality. The five most common causes of death of children under five of this region are pneumonia, prematurity, diarrhoea, HIV and/or AIDS, and injuries.[20] The respondents' knowledge was not adequate to prevent and manage diarrhoea in this region under study. If a CCW does not know how to prepare the sugar–salt solution to be administered during diarrhoea (as enquired about in the questionnaire), child morbidity and mortality could increase unnecessarily owing to dehydration. Diarrhoeal disease is the second leading cause of death in children younger than five years. This condition is both preventable and treatable.[24]

Results also showed that respondents' knowledge about immunisation and recommendations for treating a child with fever was poor. Ten danger signs (as described earlier) have been identified for referring children to a clinic or hospital and awareness of these is important for early referral to reduce or prevent child morbidity and mortality.[25]

Knowledge about immunisation is prioritised on the Road to Health card[26] that a CCW has to evaluate during a routine household visit. An Indian study showed that less than half (37.2%) of mothers completed routine immunisation schedules for their children by the age of nine months owing to poor knowledge.[12]

Studies have shown that the CIMCI approach can reduce morbidity and mortality in children under the age of five.[6,7] The literature reflects a great diversity of approaches to locations, organisation and length of training. However, if refresher training is not available, the skills and knowledge acquired in service are lost quickly.[27] The curriculum for the CIMCI course therefore needs to be standardised by the National Department of Health to ensure better quality assurance of training. In this survey, 51% of CCWs have been practising for six years without any applicable training, with refresher courses being attended at random. A large proportion of the surveyed CCWs (61%) have never attended a refresher course. It is mandatory that the community-based service model is practised in the West Coast region,[28] which requires CCWs to manage adult clients as well. Almost half of the respondents (47%) indicated that they see between 11 and 15 clients per day, with 11% indicating that they attend to more than 15 clients per day.

Strengths and limitations

Although this study was conducted in only one district (West Coast district) of the province, it reached the full population of CCWs in the five sub-districts and should be a valid and reliable picture of their knowledge of CIMCI. The findings are likely to be generalisable to the rest of the province, especially the other rural districts, which are all managed under a single chief director, have the same model of contracting CCWs and similar populations. A limitation identified was that this study specifically targeted a rural region and excluded urban areas.

Implications and recommendations

To reduce infant morbidity and mortality rates, selection criteria should be introduced to recruit suitable candidates to train as CCWs. This is supported by our results, which showed a positive correlation between advanced schooling and achieving high knowledge scores.

Knowledge should be improved, which, given the working context of CCWs, should be based on competence and practice. Training materials and activities should be developed specifically for CCWs and tailored to the literacy level of the CCWs. CIMCI refresher courses should be offered annually and these need to be standardised and implemented to strengthen CCWs' knowledge and the quality of care that they render. Regular monthly update courses could contribute to shaping competent CCWs with appropriate knowledge and skills to serve their community.

Further research

It is recommended that the training being offered to CCWs should be evaluated, including in urban settings where the model of community health work may differ. Interventions should be introduced and re-evaluated scientifically.

Conclusion

This article described an investigation into the knowledge of the CIMCI programme amongst CCWs working in a rural district in the Western Cape, South Africa. Results showed that the knowledge base of a third of the participants was poor and only 10% had sufficient knowledge to provide safe, quality care. Higher levels of basic education and all forms of training in CIMCI were associated with better knowledge scores. Standardised training is essential for delivering effective CIMCI and with the use of an appropriate curriculum CCWs could be trained and deployed within a year.[29]

Acknowledgements

Competing interests

The authors declare that they have no financial or personal relationships that may have inappropriately influenced them in writing this article.

Authors' contributions

M.v.Z. (Stellenbosch University) conducted the research under supervision of J.E. and E.S. (both Stellenbosch University). E.S. wrote the article with support from M.v.Z. The manuscript prepared for the first submission was reviewed by J.E., with E.S. and M.v.Z. managing subsequent corrections.

References

1. Rajaratnam JK, Marcus JR, Flaxman AD, et al. 2010. Neonatal, postneonatal, childhood, and under-5 mortality for 187 countries, 1970-2010: a systematic analysis of progress towards Millennium Development Goal 4. Lancet. 2010;375:1988–2008. http://dx.doi.org/10.1016/s0140-6736(10)60703-9
2. You D, Jones G, Hill K, Wardlaw T, Chopra M. Levels and trends in child mortality, 1990-2009. Lancet. 2010;376:931–933. http://dx.doi.org/10.1016/S0140-6736(10)61429-8
3. World Health Organization. MDG 4: Reduce child mortality [homepage on the Internet]. c2015 [cited 2011 February 2]. Available from http://www.who.int/topics/millennium_development_goals/child_mortality/en/index.html.
4. Ahmed HM, Mitchell M, Hedt B. National implementation of Integrated Management of Childhood Illness (IMCI): policy constraints and strategies. Health Policy. 2010;96:128–133. http://dx.doi.org/10.1016/j.healthpol.2010.01.013
5. Winch PJ, Leban K, Casazza L, Walker L, Pearcy K. An implementation framework for household and community integrated management of childhood illness. Health Policy Plan. 2002;17(4):345–353. http://dx.doi.org/10.1093/heapol/17.4.345
6. Winch PJ, Gilroy KE, Wolfheim C, et al. Intervention models for the management of children with signs of pneumonia or malaria by community health workers. Health Policy Plan. 2005;20(40):199–212. http://dx.doi.org/10.1093/heapol/czi027
7. Edward A, Ernst P, Taylor C, Becker S, Masive E, Perry H. Examining the evidence of under-five mortality reduction in a community-based programme in Gaza, Mozambique. Trans R Soc Trop Med Hygiene. 2007;101(8):814–822. http://dx.doi.org/10.1016/j.trstmh.2007.02.025
8. Ingram M, Reinschmidt KM, Schachter KA, et al. Establishing a professional profile of community health workers: results from a national study of roles, activities and training. J Community Health. 2012;33:417–424. http://dx.doi.org/10.1007/s10900-008-9111-y
9. Ebuehi OM, Adebajo S. Improving caregivers' home management of common childhood illnesses through community level interventions. J Child Health Care. 2010;124(3):S237–S245. http://dx.doi.org/10.1177/1367493510364167
10. Boschi-Pinto C, Bahl R, Martines J. Limited progress in increasing coverage of neonatal and child health interventions in Africa and Asia. J Health Popul Nutr. 2009;27(6):755–762.
11. Rowe SY, Kelly JM, Olewe MA, et al. Effect of multiple interventions on community health workers' adherence to clinical guidelines in Siaya district, Kenya. Trans R Soc Trop Med Hyg. 2007;101:188–202. http://dx.doi.org/10.1016/j.trstmh.2006.02.023
12. Abdulraheem IS, Onajole AT, Jimoh AAG, Oladipo AR. Reasons for incomplete vaccination and factors for missed opportunities among rural Nigerian children. JPHE 2011;3(4):194–203.
13. Patel AR, Nowalk MP. Expanding immunization coverage in rural India: a review of evidence for the role of community health workers. Vaccine. 2010;28:604–613. http://dx.doi.org/10.1016/j.vaccine.2009.10.108
14. Rosenthal EL, Wiggins N, Ingram M, Mayfield-Johnson S, De Zapien JG. Community health workers then and now: an overview of national studies aimed at defining the field. J Ambul Care Manage. 2011;34(3):247–259. http://dx.doi.org/10.1097/JAC.0b013e31821c64d7
15. Pan American Health Organization and World Health Organization. Final report. Empowering local communities to improve children's health in ten Latin American countries [report on the Internet]. 2007 [cited 2012 April 17]. Available from. http://www.paho.org/us/index.php?option=com_content&view=frontpage&lang=en&limitstart=30

16. Alfaro-Trujillo B, Valles-Medina AM, Vargas-Ojeda AC. Profiles, perceptions and mo tivations of community health workers of NGOs in a border city of US-Mexico. J Commun Health. 2012;37:583–590. http://dx.doi.org/10.1007/s10900-011-9486-z

17. Mannan I, Rahman SM, Sania, A. Can early postpartum home visits by trained community health workers improve breastfeeding of newborns? J Perinatol. 2008;28(9):632–640. http://dx.doi.org/10.1038/jp.2008.64

18. Ghimire M, Pradhan YV, Maskey MK. Community-based interventions for diarrhoeal diseases and acute respiratory infections in Nepal. Bull World Health Organ. 2010;88(3):216–221. http://dx.doi.org/10.2471/BLT.09.065649

19. Provincial Government of the Western Cape, Department of Health. Community based services delivery framework. 7th draft. Cape Town: District Health Services & Health Programmes; 2010.

20 Statistics South Africa. Mortality and causes of death in South Africa, 2011. Findings from death notification. Pretoria: Statistics South Africa; 2014. Statistical release P0305.

21. Burns NB, Grove SK. The practice of nursing research: appraisal, synthesis and generation of evidence. 6th ed. St Louis: Saunders; 2009.

22. Kramer MS, Kakuma R. The optimal duration of exclusive breastfeeding: a systematic review. 2002 [cited 2015 November 18]. Available from http://www.who.int/maternal_child_adolescent/documents/nhd_01_08/en/.

23. Pérez-Escamilla R. Evidence-based breast-feeding promotion: the Baby-friendly Hospital Initiative. J Nutr. 2007;137:484–487.

24. World Health Organization. Diarrhoeal disease. Fact sheet N°330. April 2013 [document on the Internet]. c2015 [cited 2015 May 27]. Available from http://www.who.int/mediacentre/factsheets/fs330/en/.

25. World Health Organization, UNICEF. Handbook: IMCI integrated management of childhood illness. Geneva: World Health Organization; 2005. Available from http://apps.who.int/iris/bitstream/10665/42939/1/9241546441.pdf.

26. Western Cape Department of Health 2014 Road to Health Card. Available from https://www.westerncape.gov.za/general-publication/road-health-card.

27. Lehmann U, Sanders D.. Community health workers: what do we know about them? The state of the evidence on programmes, activities, costs and impact on health outcomes of using community health workers. Geneva: World Health Organization; 2007. Available from http://www.who.int/hrh/documents/community_health_workers.pdf.

28. South Africa. Department of Health and Department of Social Development. Community care worker policy management framework. Draft version 6 [report on the Internet]. 2009 [cited 2012 August 20]. Available from http://www.cabsa.org.za/sites/default/files/2009%20-%20Community%20Care%20Worker%20Management%20Policy%20Framework.pdf.

29. Redick C, Faich HSD, Long L. The current state of CHW training programs in sub-Saharan Africa and South Asia: What we know, what we don't know, and what we need to do. 2014 [cited 2015 November 18]. Available from http://1millionhealthworkers.org/files/2013/01/1mCHW_mPowering_LitReview_Formatted.compressed.pdf

36

Exploring the meaning of caring amongst student midwives, professional midwives and educators in Tshwane, South Africa

Authors:
Mmajapi E.T. Masala-Chokwe[1]
Tendani S. Ramukumba[1]

Affiliations:
[1]Adelaide Tambo School of Nursing Science, Tshwane University of Technology, South Africa

Correspondence to:
Mmajapi Masala-Chokwe

Email:
chokweme@tut.ac.za

Postal address:
PO Box 911-1569, Rosslyn 0200, South Africa

Background: In spite of caring being the core of midwifery and nursing, there is a constant public outcry about uncaring behaviours of midwives towards clients. Local media reports and recent discussion in the health system have highlighted the concerns regarding caring behaviours of midwives. Thus, there is a need to compare the meaning of caring from the perspectives of student midwives, midwives and educators.

Aims: The aim of this article was to determine the meaning of caring from the perspectives of the undergraduate student midwives, the professional midwives, and the educators teaching midwifery in Tshwane.

Setting: The study was conducted at healthcare institutions which the undergraduate student midwives attended for work integrated learning and at nursing education institutions in Tshwane, South Africa.

Methods: The strategy was qualitative and exploratory in nature. The population comprised student midwives, professional midwives and educators. Purposive sampling was done. Focus group discussions were held with student midwives and professional midwives, whilst the naïve sketch form was used as data-collection instrument for educators. Content data analysis was done. The total sample realised was 38.

Results: The findings revealed that 'caring' was taken to mean being well conversant, up-to-date and proficient in the field of work as well as considerate and respectful to others. The professional midwives indicated that they have seen colleagues demonstrate uncaring behaviour whilst educators emphasised respect as caring.

Conclusion: The student midwives, professional midwives and educators described caring as being a competent nurse with compassion and respect for others.

Examen de la signification du concept de "soins" chez les étudiantes sages-femmes, les sages-femmes professionnelles et les éducateurs à Tshwane, en Afrique du Sud

Contexte : Bien que les soins soient au cœur de la profession de sage-femme et d'infirmière, le public se plaint constamment du comportement sans compassion des sages-femmes envers leurs clients. Les déclarations dans les médias locaux et les récentes discussions dans le système de santé ont souligné les inquiétudes au sujet du comportement sans compassion des sages-femmes. Ainsi, il faut comparer la signification du concept de soins du point de vue des élèves sages-femmes, des sages-femmes et des éducateurs.

Objectifs : Le but de cet article était de déterminer la signification du concept de soins du point de vue des étudiantes sages-femmes de premier cycle, des sages-femmes professionnelles et des éducateurs formant les sages-femmes à Tshwane.

Lieu : L'étude a été faite dans les établissements de santé où vont les étudiantes sages-femmes pour leurs cours pratiques et aux collèges d'infirmières à Tshwane, en Afrique du Sud.

Méthodes : La stratégie était de nature qualitative et exploratoire. La population comprenait des étudiantes sages-femmes, des sages-femmes professionnelles et des éducateurs. On a procédé à un échantillonnage dirigé. On a organisé des discussions de groupes témoins avec des étudiantes sages-femmes et des sages-femmes professionnelles, et on a utilisé des sketchs naïfs comme instrument de collecte de données pour les éducateurs. On a fait une analyse des données relatives au contenu. On a obtenu un total de 38 échantillons.

Résultats : Les résultats ont montré que « soins » signifiait bien au courant, à jour et compétent dans le domaine du travail ainsi que attentionné et respectueux envers les autres. Les sages-femmes professionnelles ont indiqué qu'elles avaient vu des collègues qui n'étaient pas attentionnées alors que les éducateurs soulignaient que le respect était une forme de soins.

Conclusion : Les étudiantes sages-femmes, les sages-femmes professionnelles et les éducateurs ont décrit l'infirmière attentionnée comme une infirmière compétente qui traite les autres avec compassion et respect.

Introduction

No-one exists in isolation because humans are connected to one another by caring, an aspect which is important for human existence.[1] When people are in vulnerable situations, such as being ill or pregnant, they express a strong need for care and caring.[1] Nursing, which includes midwifery, is a profession of relationships. Therefore, the profession has the obligation to revisit the value central to the profession, namely caring.[1]

Caring is primary to nursing and midwifery. According to Fahrenwald et al.[2] caring is demonstrated in nursing when the nurse or midwife expresses the five core values of the profession: human dignity, integrity, autonomy, altruism and social justice. Student midwives should observe caring behaviours by the educators and professional midwives as the custodians of and role models for caring. Furthermore, in order to build a strong caring profession, caring should be interlaced through the curriculum of nursing and midwifery training.

Teaching caring should include both the emotional and the physical aspects, so that all nursing and midwifery actions provided to patients are accompanied by empathy, respect, compassion.[2] To effectively teach caring, educators and midwives should model the attributes of caring, value the students and believe in the students' potential for growth.[2] In addition, the professionals must feel good about themselves and confident in their roles; educators should excel in their subjects and midwives should be willing to become involved with the students.[3]

Nursing and midwifery do not always show outcomes of care in the same way as doctors' curative acts of care do. Nursing outcomes are mostly based on the caring attributes experienced by those who are cared for. The attributes which help to identify specific caring behaviours during nursing and midwifery care are competence, conscience, confidence, commitment, comportment and creativity.[3] Therefore, it is important for the nursing and midwifery professions to model caring so that the intended outcomes of interconnectedness are realised.[1]

Although caring is the core of midwifery, there is a constant public outcry about uncaring behaviours of midwives towards clients.[4] Local media reports and recent discussion in the health system have highlighted the concerns regarding caring behaviours of midwives.[5,6] In the past many institutions and literature raised awareness of and enormous concern about the negative midwife-client relationship; nonetheless the problem still exists in South Africa and internationally.[7] Miller and Keane[8] define caring as an emotional commitment to and willingness to act on behalf of persons with whom one has a special relationship. These include family members, relatives, friends and patients. In that relationship there is love, trust, compassion, sympathy and empathy.[7]

Flyn[9] states that caring is unique to each individual and therefore the definition of caring will be dependent on the needs of the individual. One therefore cannot assume that caring will be defined the same by health professionals, student midwives, educators and patients.[10] Perhaps the starting point therefore is to establish the meaning of caring as described by student midwives, professional midwives and educators.

Like other professions, midwifery in South Africa has experienced changes as a result of political, technological, health and disease specialisations.[11] In addition, overexpansion of services is complicated by staff shortages, resulting in decreased contact time with patients whilst pressure regarding patient throughput increases.[11,12] According to Watson,[13] nursing in general has lost its humanness and caring; these have been replaced by machines, technology and the medicalisation of childbirth. Some authors[11,12,14] claim that caring is further affected by the worsening conditions under which nurses and midwives work. Griffiths[14] agrees with Corbin[15] about the changing environment of nursing and how caring has been affected by staff shortage staff and the use of technology[16]; however, Griffiths suggests that in order to counteract these conditions, caring must constantly be nurtured in each individual on a continuous basis.

Many theorists have defined caring. Leininger[17] defines professional caring as knowledge acquired through institutions used to assist, support and enable another individual to improve a health condition. Furthermore, caring behaviours can be categorised as belonging to the emotional or cognitive aspect or the instrumental or physical aspect of caring.[18] The cognitive type of caring is based on assisting the recipient of caring in coping with the situation, whereas the instrumental type of caring focuses on the actions of alleviating suffering, for example giving analgesia to a patient.[18]

Notwithstanding the efforts by stakeholders to improve caring in the midwifery and nursing profession, there is still lack of caring in midwifery practice.[19,20,21] The purpose of this study was to determine the meaning of caring from the perspectives of undergraduate student midwives, professional midwives working at hospitals and clinics, and educators teaching midwifery. The objectives of the study were to explore and describe the meaning of caring from the perspectives of student midwives, professional midwives and educators in midwifery clinical practice.

Problem statement

The science of caring is changing and developing continuously. In addition, individuals' views are altered by cultural change, diversity of philosophies and legal and political milieus. From the introduction it is clear that much has been written about nurses and caring but practically, caring seems to be lacking. Unpublished information gathered during debriefing sessions in class with student midwives revealed that they experienced uncaring behaviours from the educators and the professional midwives in clinical practice.[22] In addition, they had different experiences and definitions of caring, although they belonged to the same institution and were at the same level of study.[23] If educators instruct student midwives about caring, why do student midwives seem to lose their caring attributes when they start practising midwifery and nursing? In addition, how do educators define and express caring to student midwives? The uncaring behaviour of professional midwives observed in clinical practice is also a matter for concern.

Therefore, there is a need to explore the perception of caring amongst the three groups of participants in order to find a starting point for improving caring behaviours in midwifery clinical practice. As a result of the inconsistent caring experienced by student midwives, and the general public outcry regarding uncaring behaviours of professional midwives in clinical practice, the researcher identified a need to explore the meaning of caring from the perspective of student midwives, professional midwives and educators.

Research question

The research question therefore is: what does caring mean from the perspective of the student midwives, professional midwives and educators?

Significance of the study

Caring is the basis of the nursing and midwifery professions, therefore misconceptions regarding care or a lack thereof may affect patient care negatively. We intend to show that student midwives, professional midwives and educators ascribe different meanings to the concept of caring. If the meaning of caring is described as an activity and not as an emotional encounter, then the recipients of caring might not experience it as expected. Furthermore, the difference in meaning may have an impact on the type of care and caring imparted to patients, colleagues and the community. If caring is defined based on the cognitive aspect only, excluding the emotional and expressive aspect which is the core of caring, the profession might be missing an important aspect of caring as an affective skill. The importance of the affective, emotional aspect of caring cannot be underestimated as it is what the recipients of care expect when they encounter nursing and midwifery services.[23,24]

Research methods and design

Design

The study was qualitative and exploratory in nature.[18]

Population and sampling

The study population consisted of level III student midwives at university, professional midwives at state and private hospitals and educators employed at a university and a college. The study was conducted at the university in Tshwane where the level III student midwives were registered for an undergraduate nursing programme. The target group of participants for level III student midwives was all the undergraduate full-time students who were registered for third-year Midwifery theoretical and practical subjects in 2007 – a total of 31.[4] The second group of participants was the professional midwives who were employed by state and private health institutions in Tshwane where the undergraduate nursing students were placed for work integrated learning (WIL). The third group of participants was the educators teaching Midwifery in nursing colleges and universities in Tshwane.[25]

The sampling method for the level III student midwives and the professional midwives was convenient and purposive. The level III students were sampled as they were more informed about the topic under study as they had been instructed about the concept of caring, had passed midwifery II and were placed for WIL in the maternity sections of clinics and hospitals in Tshwane.

All the professional midwives who had been permanently employed for five years or more in clinics and hospitals in Tshwane were invited to participate in the study as they are expected to practice and have an in-depth knowledge of caring. A census sampling method was used for the educators as all those who were invited to take part agreed to participate in the study.

Data-collection instruments

Self-report was the main data-collection method for all three groups of participants. Focus group sessions and focus group schedules were the method and instrument used for the student midwives and professional midwives, whilst narratives and the naive sketch form were used as method and instrument for educators.

The focus group schedule and the naive sketch form comprised two sections. Section A was dedicated to the demographic profile of the participants, such as age and years of work experience. Section B of the focus group schedule posed a central question, namely:

> 'From your own perspective, please tell me the meaning of caring in midwifery clinical practice.'

Section B of the naive sketch form asked the educators to narrate the meaning of caring:

> 'As a midwifery educator, please tell me the meaning of caring in midwifery clinical practice.'

Pretesting of the instruments

Pretesting of the focus group interview was conducted with a group of six level III student midwives who were not included in the study. It was confirmed that the interview lasted 45 to 60 minutes and the central question was rephrased. The instrument for the professional midwives was pretested on four professional midwives working at a hospital which was not included in the study, and there was no need to adjust any part of the instrument. The naïve sketch was pretested at a university not included in the study; years of experience as an educator was added to the tool.

Data collection

The data were collected by the first author, who used English as language of communication. The study purpose and data collection process were explained to the student midwives in a class-room at the university where they were registered in the undergraduate programme. Those who agreed to participate signed a consent form. Arrangements were made with the Head of the Nursing Department of the university to access the student midwives. Appointments were made with them a week before the focus group session took place. Two focus groups were conducted with the level III student midwives. A third focus group was conducted but no new information emerged.

The focus group was conducted in the skills laboratory, with the assistance of the moderator, a psychiatric nurse who had interviewing skills. Three focus group interviews comprising six to seven student midwives were planned for data collection purposes. The seating arrangement was in the form of a circle in order to facilitate eye contact in the focus group. A tape recorder was used to record the interviews after the student midwives granted permission to record the interview. The researcher was the student midwives' lecturer hence the student midwives were called by their names during the interview; however, pseudonyms were used during transcription of the data.

The Department of Health, managers of the hospitals, clinics, and the University Ethics committee were consulted and permission to interview the professional midwives and the educators respectively was obtained. Prior arrangement was made with the professional midwives to conduct the focus group and a briefing about the nature of the study was made. Professional midwives were reminded of the focus group on the morning of the interview. On the day of the interview, the professional midwives were informed of the nature of the study and that a tape recorder was to be used. They were requested to sign a consent form to indicate their willingness to participate. Seventeen professional midwives were interviewed in two focus groups. The researcher conducted the focus group, whilst the moderator operated the tape recorder and took field notes. The focus group took place in the duty room, away from the rest of the personnel, in order to minimise disturbances. The process took about an hour.

Permission to conduct the study at the university and college to access the educators was granted. Also, arrangements were made with the Heads of Department at the college and university. Email addresses of the educators were obtained and the naïve sketch forms were dispatched to them; they were given a week to complete the form. Ten naïve sketch forms were sent to the educators; nine were completed and returned. Table 1 indicates the number of participants, data-collection methods, and the instruments used.

The total sample realised for the study was 38: two focus groups of student midwives with six participants each, eight and nine participants in the first and second group of professional midwives respectively, and nine educators.

TABLE 1: Population, data-collection methods and instruments.

Population	Sample size	Data-collection method	Instrument
Students midwives	12	Two focus groups	Focus group schedule
Midwives	17	Two focus groups	Focus group schedule
Educators	9	Narratives	Naïve sketch form

Data analysis

Data analysis commenced as soon as the first interview was conducted and the first naïve sketch was received. The content analysis approach was taken using open coding according to Tesch's approach.[26] Responses from the interviews were transcribed verbatim and later categorised into themes and subcategories. The findings from each of the three groups of participants were classified into themes, categories and subcategories.

Trustworthiness

The principles of trustworthiness proposed by Lincoln and Guba[27] were considered.

Credibility was ensured by the fact that the researcher had 10 years' experience as a researcher, educator and midwife. As a result, she had a relationship of trust with the student midwives, educators in the midwifery field and midwives in the clinical areas. The researcher conducted the focus group amongst all three groups of participants in order to promote consistency using the designed tool. Furthermore, the researcher and the moderator each analysed the data separately, compared their findings, and reached an agreement regarding the meaning the participants ascribed to caring. This was done to increase the credibility of the findings.

Confirmability was ensured by conducting a member checking to confirm with the participants that the data recorded were the true reflection of the focus group session and the narratives.

Dependability was ensured by following the scientific process of conducting a research.

Transferability was ensured by clearly describing the context of the study so that the findings could be applied in similar settings.

Ethical considerations

Approval to conduct the study was granted by the Research and Ethics Committee of the University (2006/10/025), the Gauteng Department of Health Research Unit, the heads of the institutions of learning and the managers of the different hospitals identified.[15] Respect for persons, autonomy, beneficence, justice, confidentiality and anonymity principles were adhered to.[18] In addition, the participants completed a written informed consent form to indicate their voluntary participation in the study. The participants were further informed that they were allowed to terminate their participation without facing any penalty.

Findings of the study

Demographic profile of the participants

Table 2 shows the demographic profile of the three groups of participants.

The 12 undergraduate student midwives' ages ranged from 18 to 30 years; 7 of the 12 were in the age group 18 to 21 years. There is an age gap of more than 10 years between the youngest student midwife and the youngest educator, and a further age gap of 10 years between the youngest educator and the youngest midwife. Eleven out of 12 student midwives spoke 1 of the 11 South African official languages; two of this group were Afrikaans speaking whilst one spoke a foreign language.

Eleven of the 17 professional midwives were between 31 and 50 years old whilst 4 of the 9 educators were between 41 and 50 years old. Seven educators had 16 to 20 years' of work experience. Sixteen midwives stated that they enjoyed working in midwifery clinical practice.

Themes

Three themes emerged from the data (Table 3). Both negative and positive sentiments were expressed; examples of these are provided under each theme.

Caring and competence as the basis of nursing

According to the some participants, preparing the favourable conducive environment for care is perceived as caring. The student midwives expressed caring as when one gives the best care to patients using expert knowledge. They described the confidence the professional midwives had when assisting them during a delivery and how they felt comfortable during a birth as competence and caring. The educators expressed that rendering service based on individual needs, respect, affection, and dignity reflect caring whilst the midwives perceived dedication to one's work as competency and caring. In addition, the midwives ascribed caring to instances where there was integration of cultural beliefs, practices and values in the scientific assessment and care of their patients.

Realities related to caring and competence as the basis of nursing

The realities of this category are both positive and negative as experienced by the student midwives, professional midwives and educators. Students observed behaviour that demonstrated competency as well as a lack of competency. The student midwives expressed that they were supported and mentored during their WIL experience whilst some of them experienced negative realities.

The midwives stated that there was uncooperativeness and unfriendliness amongst some of their colleagues

TABLE 2: Demographic profile of the participants (n = 38).

Criteria	Student midwives	n	Professional midwives	n	Educators	n
Age	18–21	7	21–30	3	31–40	3
	22–30	5	31–50	11	41–50	4
	> 30	0	> 50	3	> 50	2
South African languages†	Afrikaans	2	Afrikaans	4	Setswana	6
	Sesotho	1	Sesotho	4	Sesotho	2
	TshiVenda	3	TshiVenda	3	isiTsonga	1
	isiTsonga isiNdebele		isiTsonga isiNdebele			
	isiXhosa isiSwati English	3	isiXhosa isiSwati English	3	-	0
	Sepedi Setswana	2	Setswana Sepedi isiZulu	3	-	0
Foreign languages	Foreign	11	-	0	-	0
Gender	Female	10	Female	17	Female	9
	Male	2	Male	0	Male	0
Years of work experience	Not applicable to student midwives		≤ 5	5	5–10	0
			6–10	3	11–15	1
			11–20	6	16–20	7
			> 21	3	> 21	1
Total	**12**		**17**		**9**	

†, South African languages: Sepedi, TshiVenda, Sesotho, Tsonga, Setswana, isiZulu, isiXhosa, isiNdebele, English, isiSwati and Afrikaans.

TABLE 3: Findings of the study.

Theme	Student midwives	Professional midwives	Educators
Caring and competence as the basis of nursing	Realising the basic needs of the patient	Being dedicated to the work	Ensuring that one remains competent
Compassion and support	Being there for somebody when the need arises	Assisting the person to maintain his physical, mental and emotional aspect of health	Identifying and attending to student midwives' or patients' needs
Respect for humankind	Showing respect	Giving respect to the patients	Respecting individuality

which resulted in uncaring and incompetent behaviour. Furthermore, midwives expressed lack of trust and confidence as a result of criticism from colleagues. As a result, there were no role models for newly qualified and student midwives. The educators stated that the ability to make accurate assessments and make good decisions to meet the students' needs demonstrate caring and competence.

Participants expressed the following positive realities:

> 'The midwife at the clinic was professional and passionate about her work. Sister made me and the patient ... comfortable.' (S5, 21 years)

> 'A positive welcome of the patients and family in the unit and exercising patience demonstrate caring. Being knowledgeable about the work.' (P2, 30 years)

> 'Ensuring that one remains competent with the profession's current body of knowledge.' (E1, 40 years)

However, negative realities were also expressed:

> 'No orientation to the unit or supervision of the students was done. This resulted in me becoming frustrated and wishing to take my bag and going home on that day.' (S1, 19 years)

> 'Patients suffer because of lack of teamwork. Some of the midwives refuse to give patients attention and treatments.' (P4, 23 years)

> 'Providing the student midwives with physical, psychological and social support. Caring means allowing the students to reflect on their learning and facilitation.' (E6, 47 years)

Compassion and support to others in need

According to some participants, caring means giving people comfort. Caring was perceived as understanding someone's difficult situation. According to the student midwives, caring means to 'be there' for somebody when the need arises, and nurturing is a positive way of helping someone. The professional midwives described caring as unconditional support of the woman and her family. The educators referred to caring as assisting the student midwives who are not performing well in class, following up with them and providing remedial action. The educators expressed that attending to student midwives' or patients' needs demonstrate caring.

Realities related to compassion and support to others in need

Student midwives experienced mostly negative realities related to compassion and support to others in need. Student midwives observed that the behaviours of some of the professional midwives were disturbing, citing some incidents that occurred in their presence as uncaring. In one incident, the student midwives work schedule was amended without informing them of it. When student midwives came to work the following day, they were sent back home as they were not supposed to be on duty according to the changed duty list. The student midwives regarded that as insensitivity and lack of positive regard.

The midwives also reported that they observed uncaring behaviours amongst their own colleagues. From the professional midwives' perspectives, their colleagues did not care for one another as colleagues; the outcome is an environment which is demotivating, resulting in the deterioration of work quality. The educators expressed 'academic' and physical definitions of the reality of caring. They demonstrated that they have been taught the meaning of caring. The following definitions of caring were expressed:

> 'Caring means assisting someone without expecting reward. A partner or a family member was allowed into the delivery room to provide support to the woman. This I think was real caring.' (S11, 30 years)

> 'Administration of analgesia to ensure comfort when someone is in pain, means caring.' (P3, 51 years)

> 'Giving your time, service and holistic attention to others, being interested in the wellbeing of others, being empathetic, means caring.' (E9, 31 years)

The participants also experienced negative realities:

> 'A patient who had miscarriage earlier in the year was scolded for being pregnant twice in one year. The patient was so embarrassed.' (S10, 25 years)

> 'As a result of an uncaring environment, the turnover of the midwives is high and some of the midwives engage in overtime encounters in an attempt to acquire financial and job satisfaction elsewhere.' (P3, 49 years)

Respect for humankind

According to the participants' perceptions, caring is demonstrated when individuals, their families and their beliefs are respected. The student midwives and professional midwives stated that one should show respect or give respect to others whilst the educators mentioned that respecting the other person's individuality, norms, values and cultural practices demonstrates caring. Some of the student midwives observed disrespectful behaviour towards patients and other professionals by professional midwives, whilst the midwives articulated that respect shown to patients and other professionals was inconsistent.

Realities related to respect for humankind

The student midwives stated that some of the professional midwives were seen mishandling patients without talking to them. Some professional midwives claimed that respect by some of their colleagues is inconsistent. According to them, there often was infighting about allocation of work, which indicates disrespect of authority. The professional midwives mentioned that some of their colleagues undermined the decisions taken by others. This state of affairs negatively affected the quality of patient care. The educators' view was that respecting the patient's decision-making abilities and individuality means caring:

> 'Showing respect and unconditional focus directed at the person means caring.' (S7, 25 years)

> 'Respect to the patients' wishes in the management and care shows caring. Treating the patient as unique individual whilst providing privacy and exercising confidentiality.' (P3, 37 years)

> 'Providing respectful treatments, being gentle, nurturing, respecting the family and their beliefs.' (E8, 33 years)

Discussion

From the findings about the meaning of caring in midwifery practice, it is apparent that the student midwives, professional midwives and educators have almost the same interpretation and understanding of caring at a cognitive level. The student midwives, however, emphasised emotional presence and showing respect as expressions of caring. These two aspects denote that the student midwives knew that caring is both instrumental and expressive, as postulated by Woodward[29] and Mulaudzi[30] et al. A study by Murphy[31] et al. in the United Kingdom found that because of an uncaring clinical environment, the expressive caring value of student nurses were gradually lost over the period of training. In the current study, however, the student midwives were not discouraged or preoccupied by an uncaring midwifery clinical environment.

Smith et al.[32] stated in their study about caring in nursing that no other profession is as totally concerned with caring behaviours, caring processes and caring relationship as nursing and midwifery. In the current study, the professional midwives and educators indicated the same – that caring, competence and compassion constitute caring in midwifery clinical practice. Roach[10] asserts that compassion without competence in nursing and midwifery is meaningless.

The professional midwives stated that teamwork is poor and some professional midwives have no respect for authority. Disconcertingly, poor teamwork has a negative influence on quality of care and patient outcomes.[33] In a study by Smith et al.[32] the registered nurses were asked to rank several meanings of caring in order of importance. Some of the meanings were attentive listening, comforting, honesty, patience, responsibility, providing information for decision making, touch, sensitivity, respect, and individuality. The participants in the current study referred to a few of these, namely respect, individuality and comforting. Once again, this agrees with Roach's definition of caring, which is being compassionate.[10]

Caring is unique to each individual and it the right of everyone to define this concept according to psychological, cultural, social and spiritual needs.[9] In the current study, all the participants defined caring as being compassionate and showing respect; however, it seems the educators put more emphasis on the instrumental role of caring. The educators referred to 'identifying' and attending to the needs of patients or students and 'respecting individuality' as the meaning of caring. Therefore, they were emphasising the physical aspect of caring more than the emotional. The definition is related to Watson's clinical caritas of caring, which states that caring is being considerate and assisting someone with basic needs.[13] It seems teaching caring has also been affected by the political, social and technological changes in the profession, which resulted in the profession losing its humanness, as stated by Watson.[13] There seems to be a gap in the process of professional growth on caring which shows a difference between cognitive assertions of the concept, the psychomotor and the affective behaviour.

Some participants mentioned that respecting patients' privacy, individuality and wishes in their management and care constitute caring.[4] This is an important aspect in the management of women in labour, as failure to involve women in their management could increase catecholamine in the body as a response to anxiety, pain and fear.[34] Indeed, this will result in prolonged labour and hampers the woman's coping mechanism regarding the pain of labour.[34] Watson supports this aspect and mentions that caring includes promotion of sensitivity to oneself and going beyond your ego self.[13,31,32] With this study, the researchers aimed to emphasise that humanness is the foundation of midwifery and to encourage the interconnectedness of the one providing care and the one being cared for.

Limitations

Data were collected from student midwives, professional midwives and educators only; a possible limitation of the study is that patients were not asked to define caring. This might have enriched the data.

Recommendations

The midwifery and nursing professions should have frequent in-service training on caring and include caring processes and relationships during clinical practice and at training institutions. The caring curriculum should run through the undergraduate nursing programme, the attributes of caring highlighted throughout and emphasised more as students become more senior.

Conclusion

In this study, student midwives', professional midwives' and educators' meaning of caring were explored. The participants described caring as respect, compassion and competence – the basis for nursing. The training of students should expose them to authentic learning opportunities about caring. Furthermore, novice midwives should be exposed to positive caring role models.

Acknowledgements

The authors acknowledge the authorities who granted the permission to conduct the study and the participants for taking part in the study.

Competing interests

The authors declare that they have no financial or personal relationship(s) that may have inappropriately influenced them in writing this article.

Authors' contributions

M.E. (Tshwane University of Technology) was the project leader and compiled the manuscript. T.S. (Tshwane University of Technology) came up with the concept under study.

References

1. Miyawaki M. Reconsidering the value of caring in nursing practice. J Philos Eth Health Care Med. 2010;4:5–17.
2. Fahrenwald NL, Bassett SD, Tschetter L, Carson PP, White L, Winterboer VJ. Teaching core nursing values. J Prof Nurs. 2005;21(1):46–51. PMID: 15682160.
3. Bauer JA. Caring as the central focus in nursing curriculum development. NLN Publ. 1990;41:255–266. PMID: 2308805.
4. Chokwe ME, Wright SCD, Erasmus DGJ. Perceptions and experiences of caring in midwifery [unpublished M Tech Nursing Science dissertation]. Pretoria: Tshwane University of Technology; 2010.
5. Borland S. If you don't hurry up, I'll cut you: What one mother was told by midwife at NHS Trust where five died during labour. MailOnline [newspaper online]. 2011 Nov 11 [cited 2015 May 2]. Available from: http://www.dailymail.co.uk/health/article-2054171/NHS-maternity-care-Midwife-tells-mother-dont-hurry-Ill-cut-you.html
6. Department of Health. Towards quality care for patients: National core standards for health establishments in South Africa [8–45]. 2011 [cited 2015 May 28]. Available from: http://www.rhap.org.za/wp-content/uploads/2014/05/National-Core-Standards-2011-1.pdf
7. Lourens G. The National Core Standards and evidenced-based nursing. Prof Nurs Today [serial online]. 2012 [cited 2015 Apr 12]; 16(1):3. Available from: http://www.rmchsa.org/wp-content/uploads/2014/04/NCS_Clinical-Audits.pdf
8. Miller BF, Keane CB. Encyclopedia and dictionary of medicine, nursing, and allied health. 7th ed. Philadelphia: Elsevier; 2003.
9. Flynn S. Who cares? A critical discussion of the value of caring from a patient and healthcare professional perspective. Int J Orthop Trauma Nurs. 2015. http://dx.doi.org/10.1016/j.ijotn.2015.06.001
10. Roach SM. A foundation for nursing ethics. In: Carmi A, Schneider S, editors. Nursing law and ethics. Berlin: Springer Verlag, 1985; p. 170–177.
11. Maben J, Cornwell J, Sweeney K. In praise of compassion. J Res Nurs. 2010;15(1):9–13. http://dx.doi.org/10.1177/1744987109353689
12. Costello J, Haggart CJ. The nature of nursing: Can we teach students how to care? CARE [serial online]. 2008 [cited 2014 Feb 29]; 2(2):41–55. Available from: http://www.gcu.ac.uk/care/issuesarchive/issue2volume2/vol2iss2.the-nature-of-nursing.can-we-teach-students-how-to-care.-8310.pdf
13. Watson J. Caring science as sacred science. Philadelphia: FA Davis; 2005.
14. Griffiths J, Speed S, Horne M, Keeley PA. Caring professional attitude: What service users and carers seek in graduate nurses and the challenge for educators. Nurse Educ Today. 2012;32:121–127. PMID: 21737189, http://dx.doi.org/10.1016/j.nedt.2011.06.005
15. Cobin J. Is caring a lost art in nursing? Int J Nurs Stud. 2008;45(2):163–165. PMID: 18031746.
16. Kitson AL. A comparative analysis of lay-caring and professional (nursing) caring relationships. Int J Nurs Stud. 2003;40:503–510. PMID: 12828972.
17. Leininger M. Culture care theory: A major contribution to advance transcultural nursing knowledge and practices. J Transcult Nurs. 2002;13(3):189–192. PMID: 12113148, http://dx.doi.org/10.1177/10459602013003005
18. Moroney R. Caring and competent caregivers. Athens, GA: University of Georgia Press; 1998.
19. Elliasson M, Kainz G, Von Post I. Uncaring midwives. Nurs Ethics. 2008;15(4):500–511. PMID: 18515439, http://dx.doi.org/10.1177/0969733008090521
20. Olayinka O, Mombel MO, Achi OT, Azibaben I. Perceived effects of midwives attitudes toward women in labour in Bayelsa State. Arch Appl Sci Res [serial online]. 2012 [cited 2015 Apr 22]; 4(2):960–964. Available from: http://scholarsresearchlibrary.com/aasr-vol4-iss2.html
21. Korsah KA. Nurses' stories about their interactions with patients at the Holy Family Hospital, Techiman, Ghana. Open J Nurs. 2011;1(1):1–9. http://dx.doi.org/10.4236/ojn.2011.11001
22. Ramukumba TS, Wright SCD, Chokwe ME. Caring behaviour displayed by health professionals in the clinical institutions of learning as experienced by students of nursing. Paper presented at the International Conference on Global Public Health; 2005 Nov 2–4; Gaborone, Botswana.
23. Davison N, Williams K. Compassion in nursing. 2: Factors that influence compassionate care in clinical practice. Nurs Times. 2009;105(37):18–19. PMID: 19882850.
24. Pearcey P, Draper P. Exploring nursing experiences: Listening to student nurses. Nurse Educ Today. 2008;28(5):595–601. PMID: 17950499, http://dx.doi.org/10.1016/j.nedt.2007.09.007
25. Chokwe ME, Wright SCD. Caring as a core concept in educating midwifery learners: A qualitative study. Health SA Gesondheid. 2012;17(1):7. http://dx.doi.org/10.4102/hsag.v17i1.653
26. Creswell JW. Research design: Qualitative, quantitative and mixed methods. Thousand Oaks: Sage; 2003.
27. Lincoln YS, Guba EG. Naturalistic inquiry. Thousand Oaks: Sage; 1995.
28. Speziale HJS, Carpenter DR. Qualitative research in nursing: Advancing the humanistic imperative. 4th ed. Philadelphia: Lippincott; 2007.
29. Woodward V. Caring for women: The potential contribution of formal theory to midwifery practice. Midwifery. 2000;16(1):68–75. PMID: 11139863.
30. Mulaudzi FM, Mokoena JD, Troskie R. Basics in nursing ethics. Sandown: Heinemann; 2001.
31. Murphy F, Jones S, Edwards M, James J, Mayer A. The impact of nurse education on the caring behaviours of nursing students. Nurse Educ Today. 2009;29:254–264. PMID: 18945526, http://dx.doi.org/10.1016/j.nedt.2008.08.016
32. Smith MC, Turkel MC, Wolf ZR. Caring in nursing classics: An essential resource. New York: Springer; 2013.
33. Purdy NM, Laschinger HKS. Effects of work environments on nursing and patient outcomes [dissertation online]. London (ON): University of Western Ontario; 2011 [cited 2015 Aug 4]. Available from: http://ir.lib.uwo.ca/etd/92/
34. Fraser DM, Cooper MA, Nolte AGW. Myles textbook for midwives – African edition. Philadelphia: Elsevier; 2006.

Two-year longitudinal health-related fitness, anthropometry and body composition status amongst adolescents in Tlokwe Municipality: The PAHL Study

Authors:
Oluwatoyi O. Toriola[1]
Makama A. Monyeki[1]
Abel L. Toriola[2]

Affiliations:
[1]Physical Activity, Sport and Recreation Focus Area, North-West University, Potchefstroom Campus, South Africa

[2]Department of Sport, Rehabilitation and Dental Sciences, Tshwane University of Technology, South Africa

Correspondence to:
Makama Monyeki

Email:
andries.monyeki@nwu.ac.za

Postal address:
Private Bag X6001, Potchefstroom 2520, South Africa

Aim: To evaluate a two-year longitudinal development of health-related fitness, anthropometry and body composition status amongst adolescents in Tlokwe Municipality, Potchefstroom, South Africa.

Setting: A total of 283 high-school learners (111 boys and 172 girls) of ages 14 and 15 years who were part of the ongoing Physical Activity and Health Longitudinal Study (PAHLS) participated in the study. For the purpose of the present study, data collected for 2011 and 2012 for anthropometric, body composition and health-related physical fitness were used.

Results: Body mass index (BMI) classification of boys and girls for 2011 and 2012 showed that 24.3% of them were underweight compared with 21% in 2012. In 2011, 50% of boys and girls had normal body weight compared with 52% in 2012, whilst 25.5% of the total group of participants were overweight compared with 27% in 2012. Both boys and girls showed significant increases of 5.9% in body fat (BF) and 3.2 kg in body weight over two years' measurements, respectively. Regarding health-related fitness (i.e BAH), boys showed an increase of 14.8 seconds whilst girls gained 9.6 seconds. Significant decreases were found for sit-ups in both boys and girls. A significant VO_2max increase of 2.9 mL/kg/min. was found in boys over the time period. A non-significant decrease of -0.5 mL/kg/min. was observed in girls. Regression coefficients showed that changes in BMI were inversely associated with those in health-related physical fitness. The changes in percentage BF were negatively associated with standing broad jump (SBJ), bent arm hang (BAH) and VO_2 max in both boys and girls. A low significant positive association was found between changes in waist-to-height ratio (WHtR) and SBJ in both genders, whilst inverse low associations were found between WHtR and BAH in girls and for VO_2max in both genders.

Conclusion: Changes in BMI, %BF and WHtR were negatively associated with strength and running performances in the participating children. The relative increase in overweight, especially in girls, negatively affected their endurance running and static strength performances. The health implications of the observed findings are discussed and recommendations offered for physical activity intervention in school physical education (PE) programmes.

Etude longitudinale de deux ans de la condition physique liée à la santé, de l'anthropométrie et de l'état de la composition corporelle chez des adolescents de la municipalité de Tlokwe: Etude ELAPS.

Objectifs: Evaluer pendant deux ans le développement longitudinal de la condition physique liée à la santé, de l'anthropométrie et de l'état de la composition corporelle chez les adolescents de la municipalité de Tlokwe, à Potchefstroom, en Afrique du Sud.

Lieu: 283 élèves du secondaire (111 garçons et 172 filles) de 14-15 ans faisant partie de l'Etude longitudinale de l'Activité physique et de la Santé (ELAPS) ont participé à l'étude. Pour cette étude on a utilisé les données collectées en 2011 et 2012 pour l'anthropométrie, la composition corporelle et la condition physique liée à la santé.

Résultats: La classification de l'index de masse corporelle (IMC) des garçons et des filles en 2011 et 2012 a montré que 24.3% d'entre eux avaient un poids insuffisant comparé à 21% en 2012. En 2011, 50% des garçons et des filles avaient un poids normal comparé à 52% en 2012, alors que 25.5% du groupe participant étaient en surpoids comparé à 27% en 2012. Les garçons tout comme les filles montraient une augmentation significative de 5.9% de graisse corporelle (GC) et 3.2 kg de masse corporelle sur deux ans, respectivement. En ce qui concerne la condition physique liée à la santé (i.e. BAH), les garçons avaient gagné 14.8 secondes et les filles 9.6 secondes. On a trouvé une diminution significative pour les redressements assis chez les garçons comme chez les filles. On a remarqué une augmentation VO_2max de 2.9 mL/kg/min. chez les garçons pendant cette période. On a noté une diminution peu importante de -0.5 mL/kg/min. chez les filles. Les coefficients de régression ont montré que les changements en IMC étaient inversement associés à ceux de la condition physique liée à la santé. Les changements dans le pourcentage de GC étaient liés négativement avec le saut en longueur sans élan (SLSE), la suspension à bras pliés (SBP) et le VO_2max chez les garçons et les filles. On a trouvé un rapport significatif entre les changements du rapport Tour de taille sur Taille (RTtT) et le SLSE chez les deux sexes, alors qu'il y avait un faible rapport inverse entre le RTtT et la SBP chez les filles et pour le VO_2max chez les deux sexes.

Conclusion: Les changements dans l'IMC, le %GC et le RTtT étaient associés négativement avec la force et la performance à la course des enfants participants. L'augmentation relative de poids, surtout chez les filles, a affecté leur endurance à la course et leurs performances de force statique. Les implications pour la santé des résultats observés sont discutées et des recommandations sont proposées de plans d'activités physiques dans les programmes d'Education physique (EP) des écoles.

Introduction

Childhood obesity has become a major public health concern in the new millennium[1] and is one of the most important risk factors of non-communicable diseases in both developed and developing countries.[2] The prevalence of underweight, overweight and obesity in youth has resulted in an increased mortality rate worldwide.[3,4] Therefore, it is of vital importance to understand trends in the development of body weight disorders in the youth and the negative effect thereof on overall health.[5]

According to the World Health Organization (WHO), physical inactivity is one of the fastest growing risk factors of non-communicable diseases.[6] For instance, the WHO reported that the number of children below the age of 5 who were overweight was estimated to be at least 42 million worldwide.[7] Furthermore, obesity and overweight have been found to be major contributors to the risk factors of cardiovascular disease amongst children and adolescents.[8,9] Measured in terms of body mass index (BMI) and percentage body fat (%BF), obesity has been found to be negatively associated with performance tasks in which the body is raised off the ground, such as standing broad jump (SBJ), and the tasks for which the body has to be lifted in space, such as bent arm hang (BAH) and sit-ups.[10]

From early childhood, a sedentary lifestyle and poor health-related fitness lead to undesirable health consequences,[11] including imbalances in body composition. The increasing prevalence of childhood overweight and obesity over the past decades therefore raises concern.[11] Amongst the detrimental consequences of childhood overweight on current and future health are that children and adolescents who are overweight have very low levels of fitness compared with those who are slimmer.[12,13] Furthermore, overweight is found to be a leading factor associated with inactivity amongst children.[14]

Excessive consumption of food high in kilojoules, and physical inactivity, worsened by prolonged TV viewing, the use of social media and playing computer video games, have also been identified as major contributory factors to the high incidence of overweight and obesity amongst children and adolescents.[8] Wiecha et al.[15] reported that the prevalence of overweight children and adolescents has increased between 1976 and 1994 to 13%, is continuously increasing, and reached about 15.5% in 2000. Furthermore, it was revealed that most of the youths affected lived in developing nations. The rate at which children in this domain consume fatty food is alarming.[1] The WHO stated that the excessive consumption of processed food leads to accumulation of body fat (BF) and a high BMI, causing overweight and finally leading to obesity.[16]

From an epidemiological standpoint, obesity is associated with physical inactivity and is assumed to be the outcome of several health risk factors during childhood and adolescence[17]; hence, the need for strategic interventions to stem the menace of overweight and physical inactivity in children is imperative.[5]

In view of the link between physical activity, physical fitness and body composition in children, it is important to have a comprehensive understanding of the relationship, using prospective research design in order to implement appropriate intervention strategies. However, very little epidemiological research exists that examines such longitudinal trends.[18,19] Furthermore, few studies on the longitudinal relationship between health-related physical fitness, physical activity and body composition amongst South African children have been conducted.[20,21,22] Therefore, the purpose of the present study was to evaluate the two-year longitudinal development of health-related fitness, anthropometry and body composition status amongst adolescents in Tlokwe Municipality, South Africa.

Methods

Design

The present research was part of the ongoing Physical Activity and Health Longitudinal Study (PAHLS),[5] which commenced in 2010 following a mixed longitudinal survey designed to evaluate the development of physical activity (PA), determinants of health risk, and factors affecting participation in sport and recreational activities amongst 14-year-old high school learners in Tlokwe Municipality, an area within Dr Kenneth Kaunda District Municipality which is located near Potchefstroom, the capital city of North-West Province, South Africa. For the purpose of the present study, analyses of findings from the cross-sectional measurements of 2011 and measurements of 2012 are presented.

Participants

A total of 283 high school learners (111 boys and 172 girls), aged 14 and 15 years, who were purposefully drawn from six secondary schools in Tlokwe Municipality, which granted permission to carry out the research, participated in the study. The participants provided demographic information regarding gender, race and school locale (i.e. town or township). The school-based locales comprised four schools from the town and four others in economically deprived township areas. The former group of schools (Potchefstroom town) thus comprised learners predominantly of high socioeconomic background, and the latter group of schools (Ikageng township) comprised learners predominantly of low socioeconomic background. The South African Department of Education categorises schools in quintiles (1 to 5) according to physical condition, facilities and crowding, and the relative poverty of the community around the schools.[23] Of the 8 schools initially selected, 2 urban schools declined to participate in the study, without giving any reasons. Detailed information regarding the participants[5] and methods of data collection have been published elsewhere.[8]

Anthropometric measurements

The participants' height, body weight, skinfold thickness (triceps and subscapular skinfolds), and waist circumference (WC) respectively were measured using the protocol of the International Society for the Advancement of Kinanthropometry (ISAK).[24] Waist-to-height ratio (WHtR) and BMI were calculated as waist (cm)/height (cm) and mass/stature^2 (kg.m^{-2}), respectively. Subsequently, age-specific BMI for children was used to determine the following categories: overweight, normal weight and underweight/thinness.[25] Percentage body fat (%BF) for boys was: 2 = very low; 6–12 = low; 13–18 = optimal range; 19–25 moderately high; 26–31 = high; ≥ 32 very high; and %BF for girls was: 4–10 = very low; 11–15 = low; 15–24 = optimal range; 26–30 = moderately high; 31–35.5 = high; ≥ 35.5 = very high). % BF was calculated from skinfold measurements using Slaughter et al.'s[26] equation which is internationally accepted for use in children and adolescents from different ethnic groups.

Health-related physical fitness measurements

The participants' health-related physical fitness status was determined by assessing their cardiorespiratory endurance, muscle strength and endurance, and flexibility, using standardised techniques.[27,28] Cardiovascular endurance was assessed with the 20-metre multistage shuttle run test which is a valid measure of aerobic capacity in adolescents.[29] The following health-related fitness test items were measured according to the EUROFIT[28] test protocol: sit-and-reach (SAR) (a test of hamstring flexibility, expressed in centimetres); sit-up (SU) (a measure of abdominal strength and endurance, determined by the number of correctly performed SUs in 30 seconds); SBJ (a test of explosive strength of leg extensors measured in centimetres), and BAH (which measures functional arm and shoulder muscular endurance to exhaustion in seconds).

Measurement procedures

Before data collection, permission to conduct the measurements was granted by the District Manager of the Department of Basic Education in Potchefstroom, North-West Province. Clearance was also received from the Ethics Committee of North-West University, Potchefstroom Campus (Ethics no: NWU-0058-01-A1). The participating schools were briefed about the purpose of the study, and informed consent forms were signed by the school authorities as well as the learners and their parents. To minimise loss of interest and fatigue amongst the participants and prevent disruption of teaching and learning activities at the schools, data were collected on days agreed to by the participating schools. Only the data of learners who were 14 and 15 years old at the time of testing were analysed.[5]

Before the anthropometric and health-related fitness measurements were carried out, a demographic questionnaire, under the supervision of the principal investigator, was completed. The physical and physiological variables were measured in the following order: anthropometry, health-related fitness, and gross and fine motor fitness. All anthropometric sites were measured twice by Level 2 ISAK-certified anthropometrists according to standardised procedures.

Data analyses

The cross-sectional data on the high school learners' health-related fitness, body composition and PA were analysed using descriptive statistics, such as means and standard deviations. Independent *t*-tests were computed to determine age and sex differences in the variables amongst the high school learners. A non-parametric paired *t*-test was used to examine significant differences between two outcome variables, and a chi-square test to evaluate significant differences. The effect size statistics reported as Cohen's d (standardised mean differences) and 95% confidence interval (CI) were calculated. Values of Cohen's d = 0.2, 0.5 and 0.8 were regarded as small, medium and large effects, respectively. To study the development over time of the body composition indicators and health-related physical fitness, Pearson's product moment correlation coefficients were calculated for the first and second measurements for all outcome variables. To further examine the relationships between the independent and dependent measures, linear regression analyses corrected for gender, race and locality were computed. If a significant interaction with gender was established, separate coefficients were reported for boys and girls separately. All data analyses were performed with the Statistical Package for the Social Sciences (SPSS), Version 20.0 2011. A probability level ≤ 0.05 was taken to indicate significance.

Results

Table 1 presents the percentage distribution of the learners' BMI categories by year of study (i.e. for both 2011 and 2012). Based on BMI classifications of boys and girls over the 2-year period, 24.3% of them were underweight, with a decrease of 3.3 (21%) in 2012. For 2011, 50% of the boys and girls were in the normal weight category, with an increase of 2% (52%) in 2012, whilst 25.5% of the total group of participants was overweight in 2011, thus yielding an overall increase of 1.5% (27%) in 2012.

Table 2 comprises data on the percentage distribution of BMI by gender for the learners in 2011 and 2012. In the measurements for 2011, 23% of the boys were in the underweight category; a decrease of 3.5% in the incidence of underweight was found amongst them in the second measurement session in 2012. For girls, 25% were underweight in 2011, and in 2012 a decrease of 3.1% was found. Amongst

TABLE 1: Percentage distribution of BMI categories for total group of participants by year of study.

BMI classification	2011 (boys and girls)		2012 (boys and girls)	
	Frequency	%	Frequency	%
Underweight (BMI between 17 and 18.5)	60	24.3	52	21
Normal weight (BMI between 18.5 and 25)	124	50.2	128	52
Overweight (BMI > 22.62 for boys and > 23.34 for girls)	63	25.5	66	27
Total	**247**	**100.0**	**246**	**100**

BMI, body mass index.

TABLE 2: Percentage distribution of BMI of participants by gender for 2011 and 2012.

BMI classification	2011				2012			
	Boys		Girls		Boys		Girls	
	Frequency	%	Frequency	%	Frequency	%	Frequency	%
Underweight (BMI between 17 and 18.5)	20	23.0	40	25.0	17	19.5	35	21.9
Normal weight (BMI between 18.5 and25)	49	56.3	75	46.9	42	48.3	86	53.8
Overweight (BMI > 22.62 for boys and > 23.34 for girls)	18	20.7	45	28.1	28	32.2	38	23.8
Total	**87**	**100.0**	**160**	**100**	**87**	**100.0**	**159**	**99.4**

BMI, body mass index.

TABLE 3: Gender differences in the high school learners' anthropometric and body composition characteristics.

Variables	Boys			Girls				Cohen's *d*
	2011 (*n* = 87)	2012 (*n* = 86)		2011 (*n* = 159)		2012 (*n* = 158)		
	Mean ± SD	Mean ± SD	Average mean change over time and confidence intervals	Cohen's *d*	Mean ± SD	Mean ± SD	Mean differences	
Stature (cm)	160.7 ± 10.0	162.6 ± 9.4	1.9 (-7.42 to -1.06)†	0.65	157.8 ± 7.09	163.0 ± 9.43	5.2 (-7.16 to -3.39)†	0.67
Body mass (kg)	57.1 ± 14.17	57.0 ± 13.4	-0.1 (-4.10 to 4.25)	0.02	54.1 ± 13.15	57.3 ± 14.0	3.2 (-6.23 to -0.21)†	0.25
BMI ($kg.m^{-2}$)	20.5 ± 3.81	21.7 ± 4.56	1.2 (-2.48 to 0.04)	0.69	21.6 ± 4.45	21.4 ± 4.30	-0.2 (-0.52 to 1.17)	0.03
%BF	14.44 ± 9.09	20.3 ± 9.36	5.9 (-8.41 to -3.11)†	0.89	26.4 ± 8.61	19.4 ± 9.68	-7 (4.87 to 9.10)†	0.89
WHtR (mm)	0.42 ± 0.04	0.43 ± 0.05	0.01(-0.02 to 0.01)	0.33	0.43 ± 0.05	0.42 ± 0.51	-0.01 (-0.00 to 0.02)†	0.47
SBJ (cm)	156.4 ± 26.2	162.5 ± 86.7	6.1 (-26.11 to 13.82)	0.48	165.7 ± 30.8	159.8 ± 54.7	-5.9 (-3.77 to 15.59)	0.09
BAH (x/sec.)	8.0 ± 9.38	22.8 ± 12.4	14.8 (-18.43 to -11.15)†	0.88	10.8 ± 12.1	20.4 ± 14.2	9.6 (-12.50 to -6.71)†	0.87
SU (x/sec.)	29.3 ± 10.7	13.9 ± 15.36	-15.4 (11.32 to 19.42)†	0.92	28.0 ± 10.46	17.0 ± 14.3	-11 (8.43 to 13.66)†	0.84
VO_2max (mL/kg/min)	31.2 ± 7.75	34.2 ± 7.96	3 (-5.58 to -0.36)†	0.56	34.6 ± 8.33	34.1 ± 8.56	-0.5 (-1.58 to 2.61)	0.15
SAR (cm)	44.7 ± 8.64	45.8 ± 8.42	1.1 (-3.55 to 1.25)	0.10	45.6 ± 8.55	46.1 ± 8.76	0.5 (-2.33 to 1.38)	0.02

†, A significant change over time with $p < 0.05$.
SD, standard deviation; BMI, body mass index; %BF, percentage body fat; WHtR, waist-to-height ratio; SBJ, standing broad jump; BAH, bent arm hang; SU, sit-up; VO_2max, maximal oxygen uptake; SAR, sit-and-reach.

the boys, those overweight showed an increase in incidence of 11.5%, whilst a decrease in incidence of 4.3% was found amongst the girls.

Descriptive data by gender differences in the anthropometric and body composition characteristics (boys and girls in 2011 and 2012) are shown in Table 3. In 2011, the boys' mean height was 160.7 ± 9.1 cm ($n = 87$) which reveals that they were not significantly taller than the mean height of 162.6 ± 9.4 cm ($n = 87$) ($p > 0.117$) noted in 2012. For the girls in 2012, results showed that they were taller (163.0 ± 9.43 cm; $n = 159$) than they were (157.8 ± 7.09 cm; $n = 159$) in 2011, but the difference was not significant ($p > 0.608$). Boys were slightly heavier (57.09 ± 14.17 kg; $n = 87$) in the first year than in the second year (57.02 ± 13.4 kg; $n = 87$), but the difference was also not statistically significant ($p > 0.959$). However, in the second year, girls were heavier (57.33 ± 14.0 kg; $n = 159$) than they were in the first year (54.11 ± 13.15 kg; $n = 159$), similarly yielding a non-significant difference ($p > 0.992$).

Both series of measurements for boys showed a significant increase of 1.9 cm (95% CI -7.42 to -1.06 and Cohen's $d = 0.63$) in height, and 5.9% BF (95% CI -8.41 to -3.11 and Cohen's $d = 0.89$), over 2 years. Amongst the girls, a significant increase of 5.2 cm (95% CI -7.16 to -3.39 and Cohen's $d = 0.67$) in height and 3.2 kg (95% CI -6.23 to -0.21 and Cohen's $d = 0.25$) in body weight were found. Regarding health-related physical fitness, boys showed a significant increase of 14.8 seconds (95% CI -18.43 to -11.15 and Cohen's $d = 0.88$) in BAH and 3 mL/kg/min. (95% CI -5.58 to -0.36 and Cohen's $d = 0.56$) in VO_2max. A significant decrease of 15.4 counts per second (95% CI 11.32 to 19.42 and Cohen's $d = 0.88$) was found in SUs in boys. For girls, a significant increase of 9.6 seconds (95% CI -12.50 to -6.71 and Cohen's $d = 0.87$) in BAH was found. Additionally, a significant decrease of 11 counts (95% CI 8.43 to 13.66 and Cohen's $d = 0.85$) was found for SUs in girls. A non-significant decrease of 5.9 cm (95% CI -3.77 to 15.59 and Cohen's $d = 0.09$) in SBJ and 0.5 mL/kg/min (95% CI -1.58 to 2.61 and Cohen's $d = 0.15$) in VO_2max were observed (Table 4).

Significantly high correlation coefficients were found for BMI and %BF, sum of skinfolds and WHtR at all measurements points for all participants (Table 5).

TABLE 4: Correlation coefficients for body composition variables over two annual measurements.

Variables	%BF2	Body mass2	BMI2	%BF2	ΣSKF2	WHtR2
% BF1	-	0.02	-0.02	-0.06	-0.06	-0.07
Body mass1	.02	-	0.86†	0.44†	0.55†	0.70†
BMI1	-.02	0.86†	-	0.72†	0.81†	0.88†
% BF1	-.06	0.44†	0.72†	-	0.96†	0.65†
ΣSKF1	-.06	0.55†	0.81†	0.96†	-	0.75†
WHtR1	-.07	0.70†	0.88†	0.65†	0.75†	-

†, Correlation is significant at the 0.01 level (2-tailed).
%BF, percentage body fat; BMI, body mass index; ΣSKF, sum of skinfolds; WHtR, waist-to-height ratio.

TABLE 5: Correlation coefficients for health-related fitness over two annual measurements.

Variables	SBJ2	SUP2	BAH2	SAR2	VO_2max2
SBJ1	-0.02	0.07	0.02	0.001	0.02
BAH1	-0.03	0.11	-0.01	0.04	0.02
SUP1	0.04	0.09	0.10	-0.002	0.05
VO_2max1	-0.05	0.10	-0.02	0.002	0.02
SAR1	-0.01	-0.06	0.04	0.13†	0.09

†, correlation is significant at the 0.05 level (2-tailed).

TABLE 6: Age- and race-adjusted regression coefficients (ß) and p-values for the relationship of changes in body composition and changes in health-related fitness parameters.

Variable	Gender	Parameter	SBJ (cm)		BAH (sec.)		SAR (cm)		SUP		VO_2max	
			ß	p	ß	p	ß	p	ß	p	ß	p
BMI	Boys	Crude	-0.011	0.057	-0.037	0.38	-0.09	0.138	-0.04	0.198	-0.229	0.001
		Adjusted	-0.012	0.56	-0.03	0.51	-0.10	0.155	-0.049	0.163	-0.226	0.002
	Girls	Crude	-0.012	0.05	-0.075	0.002	-0.015	0.72	-0.01	0.696	-0.19	0.000
		Adjusted	-0.12	0.068	-0.08	0.001	-0.008	0.84	-0.01	0.694	-0.197	0.000
%BF	Boys	Crude	-0.03	0.007	-0.229	0.006	0.15	0.566	-0.31	0.000	-.081	0.000
		Adjusted	-0.03	0.01	-0.227	0.01	0.13	0.34	-0.32	0.000	-0.82	0.000
	Girls	Crude	-0.056	0.000	-0.335	0.000	0.03	0.756	-0.22	0.000	-0.899	0.000
		Adjusted	-0.058	0.000	-0.334	0.000	0.03	0.71	-0.23	0.000	-0.88	0.000
WHtR	Boys	Crude	0.00	0.009	0.00	0.34	-0.070	0.589	-0.001	0.067	-0.02	0.00
		Adjusted	0.00	0.008	0.00	0.47	-0.071	0.602	-0.001	0.05	-0.003	0.001
	Girls	Crude	0.00	0.02	-0.001	0.00	-0.070	0.41	0.000	0.44	-0.002	0.00
		Adjusted	0.00	0.028	-0.001	0.00	-0.056	0.52	0.000	0.49	-0.002	0.00

BMI, body mass index; %BF, percentage body fat; WHtR, waist-to-height ratio; SBJ, standing broad jump; BAH, bent arm hang; SAR, sit-and-reach; SU, sit-up; VO_2max, maximal oxygen uptake.

The results also showed low non-significant correlation coefficients between health-related physical fitness in the first and second measurements, except for a significant correlation found between SAR at first and second measurements.

Table 6 presents the age-adjusted regression coefficients for the relationship of changes in body composition and the health-related fitness parameters. The changes in BMI were inversely associated with health-related physical fitness. The changes in %BF were negatively associated with SBJ, BAH and VO_2max in both boys and girls. A low significant positive association was found between changes in WHtR and SBJ in both genders, whilst low inverse associations were found between WHtR and BAH in girls and for VO_2max amongst both genders.

Discussion

The present study was carried out to examine a two-year longitudinal development in health-related physical fitness, PA and body composition in randomly selected South African schoolchildren. In general, the results showed a steady decrease in underweight on the one hand, whilst on the other hand a relative increase in overweight amongst the boys and girls was observed. In a study on health-related fitness and weight status in Hong Kong adolescents, Mak et al.[30] reported higher body weight characteristics and comparatively poorer age- and gender-specific performance measures than amongst the South African children in the present study. However, our study showed an increasing tendency to be fatter and overweight, as indicated by BMI scores of the South African boys and girls over the 2-year period. As many factors affect body composition, it is important that those factors be identified so that preventative measures can be put in place to address them. The outcome of the negative health effects of underweight and obesity is likely to be the development of diseases that emanate from a sedentary lifestyle such as hypertension, cancer and Type II diabetes[5,31,32,33] which can considerably reduce children's health-related physical fitness.[34]

In the present study, significantly high inter-correlations were found for BMI and %BF, sum of skinfolds and WHtR over the two testing sessions. This finding is not surprising as studies have consistently shown that, because these variables are all indicators of fatness, positive associations amongst them are to be expected.[35]

It was of particular interest in the present study to examine the longitudinal relationship between body composition and fitness performance measures amongst the South African learners; the results showed that changes in BMI and %BF were inversely associated with health-related physical fitness amongst the boys and girls. Furthermore, significant positive relationships were found between changes in WHtR and SBJ in both genders, with correspondingly low inverse correlations noted between WHtR and BAH in girls, and VO_2max in both genders. These results are probably linked to the decrease in physical activity/exercise and work capacity amongst the children, which consequently reduced their health-related physical fitness performances.[4] Furthermore, Shang et al.[36] reported that overweight and obese youth do not perform well, as was shown by their poor performance in SBJ, and in the 50 m sprint and shuttle run, compared with youths of normal weight. These observations show that explosive strength, cardiorespiratory fitness, speed, agility and muscular capability of the youths are progressively reduced owing to excess fat accumulated in the body,[36] which becomes an extra load for them to carry in weight-bearing tasks or whilst performing gross motor skills.

Research has shown that physical fitness is another important issue from a public health perspective.[13,37] According to Brunet et al.[38] and Artero et al.[4] who examined whether there is a relationship between weight status and health-related physical fitness in youth, there was a decrease in physical fitness with increasing BMI amongst children. Although the major influence of fat mass and fat-free mass is still not clear,[4] it should be noted that body composition constitutes an important element of health-related physical fitness and is a powerful factor in providing specific information on wellness.[5]

One influence that could account for the tendency for South African children to develop excess BF and weight is the fact that they have limited exposure to PA in school. For instance, it was reported in the study conducted by Reddy et al.[39] that, amongst South African adolescents, more than 54.3% have physical education (PE) classes as part of their school curriculum, and more than 52.8% engage in vigorous physical activity (PA) during school hours. Despite this shortcoming (i.e. excessive BF amongst learners), attention is not paid to PE in the public school system, and many schools are constructed without playgrounds.[39] To stem the rising trend of obesity and physical inactivity in South African high school learners, it is of vital importance that the school system provides children and adolescents ample opportunity to be physically active. The need to design PA intervention programmes, even in the temporary absence of PE, is therefore urgent and imperative.

Limitations of the study

The findings of the present study should be interpreted in the light of the following limitations. In view of the longitudinal nature of the study, only a small sample of schoolchildren was involved. It was also not feasible to involve more children as the sample was based on the permission granted by the authorities of the schools where the study was conducted, and care was taken not to disrupt the learners' classes as a result of their participation in the research. The results might have been different if a larger sample size had been used. As the study was undertaken in 6 public high schools in the Tlokwe Municipality area of the Dr Kenneth Kaunda District Municipality, the findings should not be generalised as reflecting the status of PA, physical fitness and body composition amongst schoolchildren in Tlokwe Municipality and North-West Province as a whole. Such a generalisation would require much larger samples that would be representative of schools in the province.

Conclusion and recommendations

Based on the findings, it is concluded that changes in BMI, %BF and WHtR are negatively associated with strength and running performances in children. The relative increase in overweight, especially in girls, negatively affected their endurance running and static strength performances. Based on these findings, we therefore recommend the need for PA interventions in school PE programmes. In addition, future studies that will cover larger samples of South African learners are required.

Acknowledgements

The co-operation of the District Office of the Department of Basic Education, school authorities, teachers, parents and children in Tlokwe Municipality is greatly appreciated. We thank the fourth-year students in the School of Biokinetics, Recreation and Sport Science and the PAHLS research team for their valuable support in the study. The material is based upon work supported financially by the National Research Foundation (NRF) and the Medical Research Council of South Africa (MRC).

Competing interests

The authors declare that they have no financial or personal relationship(s) that may have inappropriately influenced them in writing this article.

Authors' contributions

O.T. (North-West University), a PhD student, is responsible for the development of the objectives, data arrangements, interpretation and write-up of the article. M.M. (North-West University) is the principal investigator in the PAHL study, and was responsible for the total design, planning, logistics and funding application of the entire study. Furthermore, M.M. contributed to the data analyses and write-up of the article, and commented on the final article. A.T. (Tshwane University of Technology) contributed to the write-up and commented on the final version.

References

1. Ademola OA, Monday OM. Aerobic and progressive resistance exercise effects on body composition of primary school children in Ibadan, Nigeria. Br J Educ Soc Behav Sci. 2013;3:163–173.
2. Bishwalata R, Brogen SA, Joy-Singh A, Usharani L. Assessment of body composition and body mass index of adolescent school children in Imphal-West district, Manipur. J Med Sociol. 2012;26:184–188.
3. Hands B, Larkin D, Parker, H, Straker L, Perry M. The relationship among physical activity, motor competence and health-related fitness in 14-year-old adolescents. Scand J Med Sci Sports. 2009;19:655–663. PMID: 18694431, http://dx.doi.org/10.1111/j.1600-0838.2008.00847.x
4. Artero EG, España-Romero V, Ortega FB, et al. Health-related fitness in adolescents: Underweight, and not only overweight, as an influencing factor. The AVENA Study. Scand J Med Sci Sports. 2010;20:418–427. PMID: 19558383, http://dx.doi.org/10.1111/j.1600-0838.2009.00959.x
5. Monyeki MA, Neetens R, Moss SJ, Twisk J. The relationship between body composition and physical fitness in 14 year old adolescents residing within the Tlokwe local municipality, South Africa: The PAHL study. BMC Public Health. 2012;12:374. PMID: 22626033, http://dx.doi.org/10.1186/1471-2458-12-374
6. World Health Organization. Global health risks. Mortality and burden of disease attributable to selected major risks. c2009 [cited 2011 October 2]. Available from: www.who.int/healthinfo/global _burden_disease/ GlobalHealthRisks _report_ full.pdf
7. World Health Organization. Global strategy on diet, physical activity and health: Childhood overweight and obesity. c2011 [cited 2012 February 8]. Available from: www.who.int/dietphysicalactivity/childhood/en/
8. Toriola OM, Monyeki MA. Health-related fitness, body composition and physical activity status among adolescent learners: The PAHL study. Afr J Phys Health Educ Recreat Dance. 2012;18:795–811.
9. Tremblay MS, Williams JD. Is the Canadian childhood obesity epidemic related to physical inactivity? Int J Obes Relat Metab Disord. 2003;27:1100–1105. PMID: 12917717, http://dx.doi.org/10.1038/sj.ijo.0802376
10. Monyeki MA, Koppes LLJ, Kemper HCG, et al. Body composition and physical fitness of undernourished South African rural primary school children. Eur J Clin Nutr. 2005;59:877–883. PMID: 15915157, http://dx.doi.org/10.1038/sj.ejcn.1602153
11. Pahkala K, Hernelahti M, Heinonen OJ, et al. Body mass index, fitness and physical activity from childhood through adolescence. Br J Sports Med. 2013;47:71–77. PMID: 22809525, http://dx.doi.org/10.1136/bjsports-2011-090704
12. Kriemler S, Manser-Wenger S, Zahner L, Braun-Fahrländer C, Schindler C, Puder JJ. Reduced cardiorespiratory fitness, low physical activity and an urban environment are independently associated with increased cardiovascular risk in children. Diabetologia. 2008;51:1408–1415. PMID: 18560801, http://dx.doi.org/10.1007/s00125-008-1067-z
13. Ortega FB, Ruiz JR, Castillo MJ, Sjöström M. Physical fitness in childhood and adolescence: A powerful marker of health. Int J Obes. 2008;32:1–11. PMID: 18043605, http://dx.doi.org/10.1038/sj.ijo.0803774
14. Metcalf BS, Hosking J, Jeffery AN, Voss LD, Henley W, Wilkin TJ. Fatness leads to inactivity, but inactivity does not lead to fatness: A longitudinal study in children (EarlyBird 45). Arch Dis Child. 2011;96:942–947. PMID: 20573741, http://dx.doi.org/10.1136/adc.2009.175927

15. Wiecha JL, El Ayadi AM, Fuemmeler BF, et al. Diffusion of an integrated health education programme in an urban school system: Planet health. J Paediatr Psychol. 2004;29:467–474. PMID: 15277589, http://dx.doi.org/10.1093/jpepsy/jsh050

16. World Health Organization. Media centre: Obesity and overweight. c2011 [cited 2012 February 8]. Available from: http:// www.who.int/mediacentre/factsheets/fs311/en/

17. Kovacs VA, Fajcsak Z, Gabor A, Martos E. School-based exercise program improves fitness, body composition and cardiovascular risk profile in overweight/obese children. Acta Physiol Hung. 2009;96:337–347. PMID: 19706375, http://dx.doi.org/10.1556/APhysiol.96.2009.3.7

18. Kristensen PL, Møller NC, Korsholm L, Wedderkopp N, Andersen LB, Froberg K. Tracking of objectively measured physical activity from childhood to adolescence: The European youth heart study. Scand J Med Sci Sports. 2008;18:171–178. PMID: 17555542, http://dx.doi.org/10.1111/j.1600-0838.2006.00622.x

19. Nelson MC, Neumark-Stzainer D, Hannan PJ, Sirard JR, Story M. Longitudinal and secular trends in physical activity and sedentary behaviour during adolescence. Pediatrics. 2006;118:e1267–e1634. PMID: 17142492, http://dx.doi.org/10.1542/peds.2006-0926

20. Kruger R, Kruger HS, Macintyre UE. The determinants of overweight and obesity among 10- to 15-year-old schoolchildren in the North West Province, South Africa – the THUSA BANA (Transition and Health during Urbanisation of South Africans; BANA, children) study. Public Health Nutr. 2006;9:351–358. PMID: 16684387, http://dx.doi.org/10.1079/PHN2005849

21. Amusa LO, Goon DT, Amey AK, Toriola AL. Health-related physical fitness among rural primary school children in Tshannda, South Africa. Sci Res Essay. 2011;6:4665–4680. http://dx.doi.org/10.5897/SRE10.522

22. Monyeki MA, Koppes LLJ, Monyeki KD, Kemper HCG, Twisk JWR. Longitudinal relationships between nutritional status, body composition, and physical fitness in rural children of South Africa: The Ellisras longitudinal study. Am J Hum Biol. 2007;19:551–558. PMID: 17546607, http://dx.doi.org/10.1002/ajhb.20616

23. Department of Education. National norms and standards for school funding. Government notice 20. Pretoria: Department of Education; 2003.

24. Marfell-Jones M, Old T, Steward A, et al. International standards for anthropometric assessment. Auckland: ISAK; 2006.

25. Cole TJ, Flegal KM, Nicholls D, Jackson AA. Body mass index cut offs to define thinness in children and adolescents: International survey. BMJ. 2007;335(7612):194. PMID: 17591624 http://dx.doi.org/10.1136/bmj.39238.399444.55

26. Slaughter MH, Lohman TG, Boileau RA, et al. Skinfold equations for estimation of body fatness in children and youth. Hum Biol. 1988;60:709–723. PMID: 3224965.

27. Australian Sports Commission. 20m shuttle run test: A progressive shuttle run test for measuring aerobic fitness. Belconnen: Australian Coaching Council; 1999.

28. EUROFIT. Handbook for the EUROFIT test of physical fitness. Strasbourg: Council of Europe Committee for the development of sport, Committee of experts on sport research; 1988.

29. Davis JA. Direct determination of aerobic power. In: Maud PJ, Foster C, editors. Physiological assessment of human fitness. 2nd ed. Champaign, IL: Human Kinetics; 2006; p. 9–18.

30. Mak K, Ho S, Lo W, et al. Health-related physical fitness and weight status in Hong Kong adolescents. BMC Public Health. 2010;10:88. PMID: 20178615, http://dx.doi.org/10.1186/1471-2458-10-88

31. Bovet P, Shamlaye C, Gabriel A, Riesen W, Paccaud F. Prevalence of cardiovascular risk factors in a middle-income country and estimated cost of a treatment strategy. BMC Public Health. 2006;6:9. PMID: 16423280, http://dx.doi.org/10.1186/1471-2458-6-9

32. Rivera IR, Mendoca-Da Silva MA, Almeida-Silva RDT, et al. Physical inactivity, TV-watching hours and body composition in children and adolescents. Socieda de Brasileira De Cardiologia. 2009;67:278–295.

33. Lubans DR, Boreham CA, Kelly P, Foster CE. The relationship between active travel to school and health-related fitness in children and adolescents: A systematic review. Int J Behav Nutr Phys Act. 2011;8:5. PMID: 21269514, http://dx.doi.org/10.1186/1479-5868-8-5

34. Rey-Lopez JP, Vincent-Rodriguez G, Biosca M, Moreno LA. Sedentary behaviour and obesity development in children and adolescents. Nutr Metab Cardiovasc Dis. 2008;18:242–251. PMID: 18083016, http://dx.doi.org/10.1016/j.numecd.2007.07.008

35. Katzmarzyk PT, Barreira TV, Broyles ST, et al. The international study of childhood obesity, lifestyle and the environment (ISCOLE): Design and methods. BMC Public Health. 2013;13:900. PMID: 24079373, http://dx.doi.org/10.1186/1471-2458-13-900

36. Shang X, Liu A, Li Y, et al. The association of weight status with physical fitness among Chinese children. Int J Pediatr. 2010;2010: 6. PMID: 20652083, http://dx.doi.org/10.1155/2010/515414

37. Myers J, Kaykha A, George S, et al. Fitness versus physical activity patterns in predicting mortality in men. Am J Med. 2004;117:912–918. PMID: 15629729, http://dx.doi.org/10.1016/j.amjmed.2004.06.047

38. Brunet M, Chaput JP, Tremblay A. The association between low physical fitness and high body mass index or waist circumference is increasing with age in children: The 'Quebec en Forme' Project. Int J Obes. 2007;31:637–643. PMID: 17006443, http://dx.doi.org/10.1038/sj.ijo.0803448

39. Reddy SP, Panday S, Swart D, et al. Umthente Uhlaba Usamila – The South African Youth Risk Behaviour Survey. Cape Town: South African Medical Research Council; 2002 [cited 2009 October 18]. Available from: www.mrc.ac.za/ health promotion/reports.htm

Understanding the organisational culture of district health services: Mahalapye and Ngamiland health districts of Botswana

Authors:
Oathokwa Nkomazana[1]
Robert Mash[2]
Nthabiseng Phaladze[3]

Affiliations:
[1]Faculty of Medicine, University of Botswana, Botswana

[2]Division of Family Medicine and Primary Care, Stellenbosch University, South Africa

[3]School of Nursing, University of Botswana, South Africa

Correspondence to:
Oathokwa Nkomazana

Email:
nkomazanao@mopipi.ub.bw

Postal address:
Private Bag 00713, Gaborone, Botswana

Background: Botswana has a shortage of health care workers, especially in primary health care. Retention and high performance of employees are closely linked to job satisfaction and motivation, which are both highest where employees' personal values and goals are realised.

Aim: The aim of the study was to evaluate employees' personal values, and the current and desired organisational culture of the district health services as experienced by the primary health care workers.

Setting: The study was conducted in the Ngamiland and Mahalapye health districts.

Method: This was a cross sectional survey. The participants were asked to select 10 values that best described their personal, current organisational and desired organisational values from a predetermined list.

Results: Sixty and 67 health care workers completed the survey in Mahalapye and Ngamiland districts, respectively. The top 10 prevalent organisational values experienced in both districts were: teamwork, patient satisfaction, blame, confusion, job insecurity, not sharing information and manipulation. When all the current values were assessed, 32% (Mahalapye) and 36% (Ngamiland) selected by health care workers were potentially limiting organisational effectiveness. The organisational values desired by health care workers in both districts were: transparency, professional growth, staff recognition, shared decision-making, accountability, productivity, leadership development and teamwork.

Conclusions: The experience of the primary health care workers in the two health districts were overwhelmingly negative, which is likely to contribute to low levels of motivation, job satisfaction, productivity and high attrition rates. There is therefore urgent need for organisational transformation with a focus on staff experience and leadership development.

Comprendre la culture organisationnelle des services de santé de district: les districts de santé de Mahalapye et Ngamiland au Botswana.

Contexte: Le Botswana a une pénurie de personnel de santé, surtout dans les soins de santé primaire. La fidélisation et la bonne performance des employés sont étroitement liées à la satisfaction et à la motivation au travail, qui sont le plus élevées quand les valeurs personnelles et les objectifs des employés sont atteints.

Objectif: Le but de l'étude était d'évaluer les valeurs personnelles des employés, ainsi que la culture organisationnelle actuelle et voulue des services de santé de district vécue par le personnel de santé primaire.

Lieu: L'étude a été menée dans les districts de santé de Ngamiland et Mahalapye.

Méthode: C'était une étude transversale. On a demandé aux participants de choisir dix valeurs qui décrivent le mieux leurs valeurs organisationnelles personnelles actuelles et désirées à partir d'une liste prédéterminée.

Résultats: Soixante des 67 membres du personnel de santé ont complété le sondage dans les districts de Mahalapye et Ngamiland, respectivement. Les dix valeurs organisationnelles les plus importantes dans les deux districts étaient : le travail d'équipe, la satisfaction des patients, les reproches, la confusion, l'insécurité professionnelle, la non communication des informations et la manipulation. Quand toutes les valeurs actuelles ont été évaluées, on a noté que 32% (Mahalapye) et 36% (Ngamiland) des valeurs sélectionnées par le personnel de santé pouvait limiter l'efficacité organisationnelle. Les valeurs organisationnelles désirées par le personnel de santé des deux districts étaient: la transparence, le développement professionnel, la reconnaissance du mérite des employés, le partage des prises de décision, la responsabilité, la productivité, le développement du leadership et du travail d'équipe.

Conclusions: L'expérience des travailleurs de santé primaire dans les deux districts sanitaires était largement négative, ce qui probablement contribue aux faibles niveaux de motivation, de satisfaction professionnelle, de productivité et aux taux d'attrition élevés. Il est donc urgent de faire des transformations organisationnelles en mettant l'accent sur l'expérience du personnel et le développement du leadership.

Introduction

Primary health care has been identified as an essential part of the health system when countries strive to provide universal access to quality cost effective health services.[1] Effective primary health care services in many low-to-middle-income countries are, however, limited by high disease burdens, dysfunctional health systems and shortage of appropriately skilled and sufficiently motivated healthcare workers.[2,3,4,5,6]

Job satisfaction and motivation are strongly associated with retention and high performance of health care workers.[5,7,8] Motivation, however, is complex as it is influenced by multiple intrinsic and extrinsic factors.[5,7,8,9] Nevertheless, employees are known to have higher levels of productivity, commitment and creativity in organisations where their personal values and goals can be expressed or realised. These workers are said to have a kind of 'psychological contract' with the organisation.[10,11] Successful organisations therefore will highly value their employee's satisfaction and experience in order to enhance their engagement, retention and the organisation's performance.[10,11,12]

Botswana's national health policy (2010) and the 10 year Integrated Health Services Plan (2010–2020) seek to ensure that there is 'an appropriately skilled, motivated, well distributed and productive workforce for the provision of quality health services effectively and efficiently, to all the people living in Botswana.'[13,14] The two policies subscribe to the following core values: 'ethics, equity, ownership, evidence base, innovation, gender equity, client satisfaction, skilled staff retention and circulation and partnership'. The national Ministry of Health, which is the custodian and driver of policy and strategic planning, has the following core values: 'customer focus (consistently meeting customer expectations), *botho* [providing service with respect, kindness in a friendly manner], timeliness (always delivering services on time to clients), equity (equal service delivery to all regardless of religion, social status or geographical location), teamwork (working together for a common goal) and accountability (responsible, liable and answerable for one's actions)'.[13] All the district health management teams (DHMTs) espouse the values of the Ministry of Health. It is notable that the Ministry of Health, and hence the DHMTs, place no value on staff experience or satisfaction despite the plan to have a motivated and productive health workforce.

Shortage of health care workers and their inequitable distribution were identified as major bottlenecks to the delivery of quality health services in Botswana.[6,14] The health workers, especially doctors, are also more concentrated in urban areas and hospital services compared to rural areas and primary care clinics.[2,6,14] The government has used training (both in and outside the country), recruitment of expatriate workers as well as bilateral agreements with China and Cuba to address the shortage of health professionals in the public health system. Conversely, many Batswana (citizens of Botswana) health professionals trained in other countries have remained in the host countries on completion of their training.[2,6,14] In addition, a significant number of those who returned, and a number of those trained locally have migrated from the public to the private or non-governmental sectors or have left the country.[6] (Thupayagale-Tshweneagae G. Migration of Nurses in Botswana. Botswana Nursing Council. Gaborone 2009, personal communication).

Administratively, Botswana is divided into 28 health districts, and primary health care is provided through a network of 265 primary care clinics (101 with maternity beds), 343 health posts and 861 mobile clinic sites.[2] The health facilities have been grouped into functional clusters centred around a larger clinic with maternity beds. Clinical services in the clusters are coordinated by cluster heads who are senior nursing officers. Management of all health services, including recruitment and deployment of health care workers (HCWs), procurement and distribution of equipment and drugs, is centralised at the national Ministry of Health headquarters. DHMTs were created in 2010 to administer healthcare services in their respective districts. Being a relatively recent structure many of the managers at the health districts are still being appointed and there is uncertainty about their roles.

Ineffective human resources and health care management systems, and inadequate supportive supervision that does not focus on improving staff satisfaction and experience have been identified as important determinants of low health worker motivation and retention in Botswana's public health service.[6] This manuscript reports on the findings of a survey to evaluate the HCWs experience of the primary care organisation within Ngamiland and Mahalapye districts. The survey evaluated the organisational culture and was also intended to inform the work of a cooperative inquiry group that was initiated in the Ngamiland district. The last-mentioned group had been established to improve supportive supervision by the DHMT and cluster heads and to evaluate if this would increase staff motivation, experience and retention. The cooperative inquiry group was seen as the intervention in a quasi-experimental study and its findings will be presented later in separate articles.

Methods

Study design

A cross sectional survey of personal values, current organisational culture and desired future organisational culture, from the health workers' perspective, was conducted in Ngamiland and Mahalapye health districts.

The values assessment was based on a conceptual framework that recognised the interrelation between the individual personality and character on the one hand and the organisational culture and structures or systems on the other (Table 1).[11] At the individual level, one's internal values drive one's personality and are expressed through actions and behaviours as one's character. At the collective level the

TABLE 1: Four quadrants of human systems (Adapted from R Barrett).[12]

Variables	Individual	Collective
Objective (External)	Character: Individual actions and behaviours	Structures and procedures: Collective actions, behaviours and processes
Subjective (Internal)	Personality: Individual values and beliefs	Culture: Guiding values, attitudes that limit, shared strategic vision

TABLE 2: Seven levels of organisational consciousness (adapted from R Barrett).[12]

Consciousness level	Example of collective values
7. Service to humanity and social contribution	Social responsibility, long-term perspective, future generations, ethics, compassion, humility
6. Making a difference to the local community or health district	Environmental awareness, community involvement, strategic partnerships, employee fulfilment, coaching, mentoring and leadership development
5. Sense of purpose and strong internal cohesion	Shared vision and values, commitment, creativity, enthusiasm, integrity, generosity, fairness, honesty, openness, transparency and trust
4. On-going improvement and employee participation	Adaptability, accountability, empowerment, teamwork, goals orientation and continuous improvement
3. High performance and quality of care	Reliability, quality, efficiency, productivity, excellence, best practice, systems and processes. Bureaucracy†, hierarchy†, confusion†, arrogance†, hoarding information† and complacency†
2. Relationship with colleagues and patients	Loyalty, open communication, patient experience and friendship. Blame†, internal competition†, rivalry†, favouritism† and manipulation†
1. Survival: Resources and safety	Sufficient budget, equipment, employee health and safety. Control†, greed†, chaos†, caution†, job insecurity†, exploitation† and micromanagement†

†, Limiting values.

organisation's values drive its culture and are expressed in its collective actions, structures, procedures and processes.

Organisations therefore, like individuals, are living systems which possess internal values and external behaviours.[11,12] The survey tools supplied by the Barrett's Value Centre make the internal individual and collective values visible and allow an assessment of the alignment between the four quadrants shown in Table 1.[11,12] Highly functioning organisations have greater alignment or congruence between the four quadrants of this model. Personal alignment refers to the degree of congruence between one's individual values and behaviour, whilst structural alignment refers to the alignment between organisational values and structures or procedures. Values alignment refers to the extent to which individual values are congruent with organisational values and mission alignment refers to how well individual behaviour is congruent with organisational behaviour and procedures.[10] A system that is well aligned across the quadrants will have employees that are more engaged and motivated, with high organisational performance.[12] This model implies that a system or organisation that wants to improve its performance must work on alignment in and between all four quadrants simultaneously as they are interdependent.[11] At the organisational level, the leadership has the greatest influence over creating and maintaining the prevailing culture and therefore transformation almost always involved leadership transformation.[15]

In the model developed by Richard Barrett the values selected in the survey can also be assigned to seven different levels of organisational consciousness (Table 2). The seven levels of consciousness were originally developed from Maslow's hierarchy of needs, and the distribution of values provides insight into what the organisation currently needs from its employees and what the employees need the organisation to focus on in the future. A well-functioning organisation will have positive values across all the levels.[11,12,15] In the bottom three levels there can be both limiting as well as positive values. Limiting values are values which are usually detrimental to the functioning of the organisation and limit the organisation's performance. In the model the total percentage of all values chosen that are potentially limiting values corresponds to the organisational entropy, which is a measure of the amount of dysfunction and wasted energy in the system.[12,15]

Setting

The research was performed in the health districts of Ngamiland (population: 96 356) and Mahalapye (population: 117 492), which are serviced by 29 and 40 primary care facilities (clinics and health posts) respectively. According to the 2011 National Health Policy, 80% of the Botswana population use public health services.[13]

The DHMT is led by a head, who is usually a doctor with public health training, with heads of preventive, curative and corporate services reporting to him or her, whilst he or she reports to the Deputy permanent secretary, clinical services. The clinic clusters are managed by cluster heads who are nursing officers based at the larger clinics. Each clinic in turn is managed by a nursing sister-in-charge, who reports to the cluster heads. The majority of the HCWs employed at these clinics and health posts are nurses and midwives with small numbers of pharmacy technicians, social workers, health education assistants and medical officers (generalist doctors). The doctors are based at the larger clinics and support the smaller facilities through regular outreach.

Study population

All the primary HCWs in Ngamiland and Mahalapye health districts were eligible to participate in the survey, whereas support staff, such as drivers and cleaners and HCWs based in hospitals, were excluded. The research teams visited most primary care facilities to deliver the survey forms and for those facilities that were not visited the forms were given to the cluster heads. The plan was to recruit all consenting health workers on duty in the facilities during the two weeks of data collection. All the HCWs on duty during the two weeks of data collection were invited to complete the survey. Cluster heads were also invited to complete the survey as they are also based in the primary health care facilities.

Data collection

The questionnaire was a standardised and validated tool developed by the Barrett Value Centre.[16] The participants were asked to select 10 values, from a predetermined list, that best described their personal values, the organisational culture as they currently experienced it and the culture they desired in the district health service. The researchers also collected demographic data which included, gender, age, name of health facility, length of stay at the facility and job title. The anonymous questionnaire was administered in English, which is the normal language of communication in the organisation. The tool was piloted for understanding amongst HCWs working at the University of Botswana clinic who were considered to be of the same level of training and experience as the study population. The hardcopy survey was self-administered by the participants, and trained research assistants provided clarification as required. The collated questionnaires were then captured in the password controlled Barrett Value Centre website by one of the research assistants.

Data analysis

The Barrett's Value Centre analysed the data and provided the study team with the results and a report. The results were descriptive and provided the numbers and frequencies for the selected values. The results were presented in figures and words and mapped to the seven levels of organisational consciousness.

The results were presented to the HCWs in each district in order to explore the meanings of the selected values. They were also presented to the Ngamiland District Health Management Team and cluster heads as part of the input into the cooperative inquiry process.

Ethical consideration

Approval to conduct the study was given by the University of Botswana Institutional Review Board, the Ngamiland District Ethics Committee, the Stellenbosch University Health Research Ethics Committee (Protocol Number: S13/03/051) and the Botswana Ministry of Health, Health Research Development Committee (Reference No: PPME 13/18/1 V11 (368)). Written consent was obtained from each study participant.

Results

Demographical data

In Mahalapye, 60 primary HCWs on duty during the data collection period completed the survey compared to 67 in Ngamiland (Table 3). All those on duty during the data collection period agreed to participate in the survey, although one form from Mahalapye and five from Ngamiland were incomplete and therefore excluded from the data analysis. The health workers were recruited from 25 of Mahalapye's 40 (63%) clinics and health posts and 19 of Ngamiland's 29 (66%) primary care facilities. The majority of participants were female in Ngamiland (64%) and Mahalapye (66%).

TABLE 3: Age, length of service in the district and the different staff categories.

Variables	Mahalapye $N = 60$ *n* (%)	Maun $N = 67$ *n* (%)
Staff categories		***n* (%)**
Doctors	1 (1.7)	1 (1.7)
Nurses	55 (91.7)	60 (89.5)
Others	4 (6.8)	3 (4.5)
Unknown	0	3 (4.5)
Mean age (range) years	35.7 (23–51)	35.4 (23–60)
Mean length of service in district (range) years	5.6 (1–20)	4.9 (1–21)

Most of the HCWs in primary care in these districts were nurses (Table 3). The staff category labelled 'others' included social workers, pharmacists and health education assistants. Health education assistants are specifically trained for 18 months to be a link between primary care facilities and the community.

Ngamiland health district values

Table 4 shows the top 10 values in rank order for the Ngamiland respondents' personal values, current experience of the organisation and desired future experience of the organisation. The values in italics are personal values that were also desired organisational values and those in bold were current organisational values that health workers wanted to continue to experience in the future. None of the personal values were currently experienced in the organisation.

Seven of the top 10 current organisational values were potentially limiting (marked with L) and only three were positive (Table 4). When all the limiting values were analysed there was a cultural entropy rate of 36%, which is a high level of entropy 'requiring cultural and structural transformation, and leadership development'.[10]

There were no limiting values amongst the top 10 desired organisational values. These include only one currently experienced organisational value, teamwork, and one personal value, accountability (Table 4).

Mahalapye health district values

Table 5 shows the top 10 values in rank order for the Mahalapye respondents' personal values, current organisational and desired future organisational values. The values in italics were personal values that were also desired organisational values and those in bold were current

TABLE 4: Top 10 personal, current organisational and desired future organisational values for Ngamiland health district.

Personal values	N = 62 n	Current organisational values	N = 62 n	Desired organisational values	N = 62 n
Accountability§	40	Working in isolation†	22	Transparency	26
Caring	30	Confusion†	21	Leadership development	20
Trust	24	Job Insecurity†	20	Teamwork‡	20
Respect	23	Information sharing	20	Staff recognition	17
Honesty	22	Working strictly by the rules†	19	Accountability§	16
Cooperation	20	Blame†	18	Productivity	16
Commitment	19	Not sharing information†	18	Shared decision making	15
Openness	18	Teamwork‡	18	Professional growth	14
Compassion	16	Patient satisfaction	17	Staff engagement	13
Responsibility	16	Manipulation†	16	Staff health	12

†, limiting value; ‡, values that are both current organisational values and desired organisational values; §§§, values that a both personal values and desired organisational values.

TABLE 5: Top 10 personal, current organisational and desired organisational values: Mahalapye health district.

Personal values	N = 59 n	Current organisational values	N = 59 n	Desired organisational values	N = 59 n
Accountability§	37	Teamwork‡	22	Transparency	24
Caring	24	Blame†	18	Professional growth	18
Respect	20	Community involvement	17	Staff recognition	18
Commitment	19	Confusion†	17	Shared decision making	15
Compassion	19	Job insecurity†	15	Accountability§	14
Honesty	19	Patient satisfaction	15	Productivity	14
Cooperation	17	Not sharing information†	14	Organisational growth	12
Responsibility	17	Long hours†	13	Staff fulfilment	12
Trust	15	Control†	12	Empowerment	11
Fairness§	14	Manipulation†	12	Fairness§	11
		Professionalism	12	Leadership development	11
		Shared vision	12	Mission focus	11
		Working strictly by the rules†	12	Teamwork‡	11

†, limiting value; ‡, values that are both current and desired organisational values; §, values that a both personal values and desired organisational values.

TABLE 6: The top 10 common personal current and future organisational values for Mahalapye and Ngamiland.

Personal values	Current organisational values	Desired organisational values
Accountability	Teamwork	Transparency‡
Caring	Patient satisfaction	Professional growth‡
Respect	Blame†	Staff recognition‡
Commitment	Confusion†	Shared decision-making‡
Compassion	Job insecurity†	Accountability‡
Honesty	Not sharing information†	Productivity‡
Cooperation	Manipulation†	Leadership development‡
Responsibility	Working strictly by the rules†	Teamwork
Trust	-	-

†, Limiting values; ‡, Desired values that are not part of the prevalent organisational culture.

organisational values that health workers wanted to continue to experience in the future. None of the personal values were currently experienced in the organisation.

Eight of the current organisational values were potentially limiting (marked with L) and five were positive. When all the limiting values are analysed there was a high cultural entropy rate of 32%.

None of the top 10 desired organisational values were potentially limiting. Teamwork was the only desired value currently experienced in the organisation. Two of the top 10 personal values, accountability and fairness, were desired for the future organisation (Table 5).

Comparison of Mahalapye and Ngamiland health district values

Primary HCWs in Mahalapye and Ngamiland share nine common personal values (Table 6) and two dissimilar values, namely, fairness (Mahalapye) and openness (Ngamiland).

Eight of the top 10 values in the current culture were also shared by the two districts. These included two positive values and six limiting values, as shown in Table 6. Working in isolation was another potentially limiting value currently experienced in Ngamiland whilst long hours and control were experienced in Mahalapye. Furthermore, Mahalapye had the following positive values: community involvement, shared vision and professionalism compared with

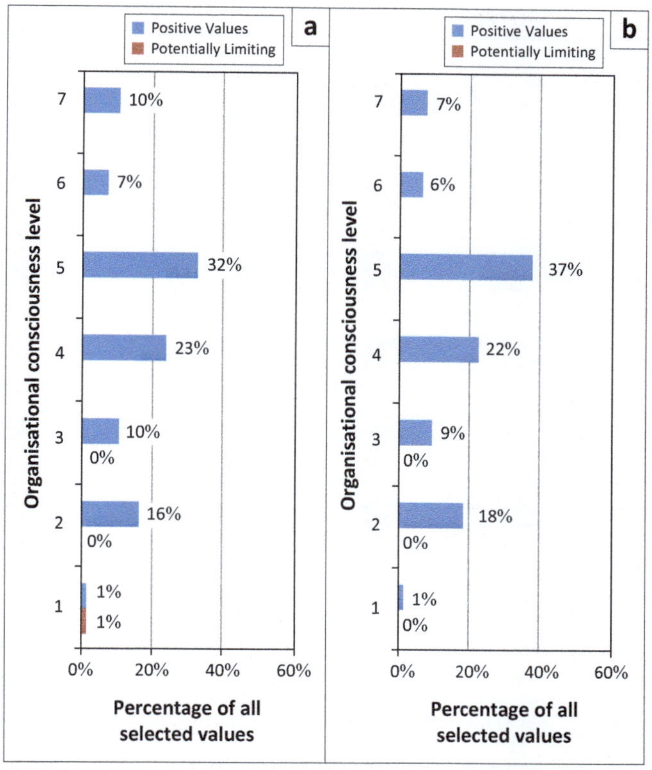

FIGURE 1: (a) Personal values of Mahalapye HCWs mapped to organisational consciousness level. (b) Personal values of Ngamiland HCWs mapped to organisational consciousness level.

information sharing for Ngamiland. None of the personal values of the health workers were experienced in either district.

The primary HCWs in Ngamiland and Mahalapye also shared 8 of the top 10 desired organisational values (Table 6). These included seven new (bold) values and one that is currently experienced in both districts. Moreover, Mahalapye health workers also selected the following desired values: organisational growth, staff fulfilment, empowerment, fairness and mission focus, whilst those in Ngamiland chose staff health and staff engagement.

Figure 1 shows the percentages of all personal values of HCWs in Mahalapye and Ngamiland according to the level of organisational consciousness. HCWs in the two districts had almost identical distributions of personal values that were concentrated at Level 5 followed by Levels 4 and 2.

The distribution of current organisational values for the two districts was concentrated at Level 3 (Figure 2). The employees' experience of the organisations at this level was largely negative. The organisations were experienced as bureaucratic and people felt confused, isolated and needed more information. This was followed by Level 4 with an organisational emphasis on teamwork and Level 2 with a positive focus on relationships with patients, but a negative experience of relationships in the organisation due to a sense of being both blamed and manipulated. At Level 1 there was also a concern about job security.

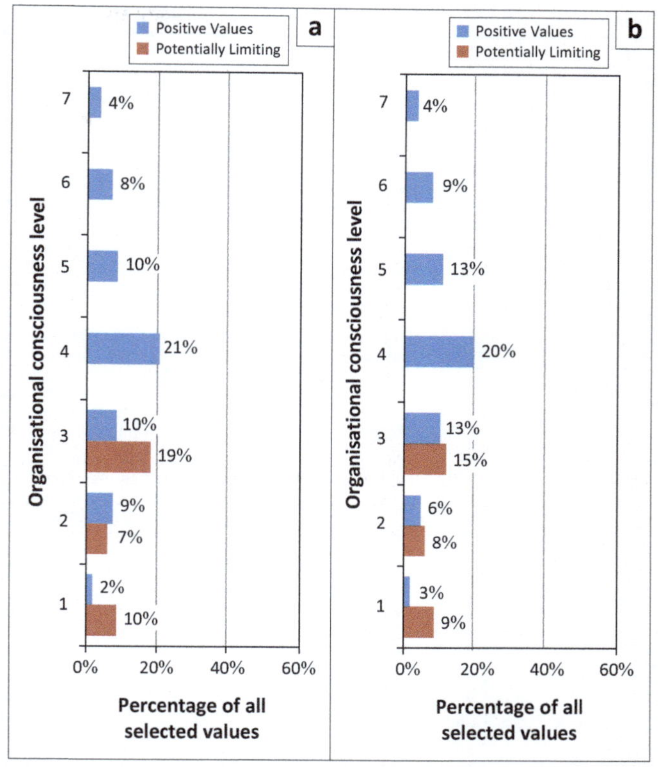

FIGURE 2: (a) Current organisational values Mahalapye health districts mapped to organisational consciousness level. (b) Current organisational values Ngamiland health districts mapped to organisational consciousness level.

The distribution of the desired values for the two districts was similarly concentrated at Level 4 with a need for more accountability and shared decision-making, followed by

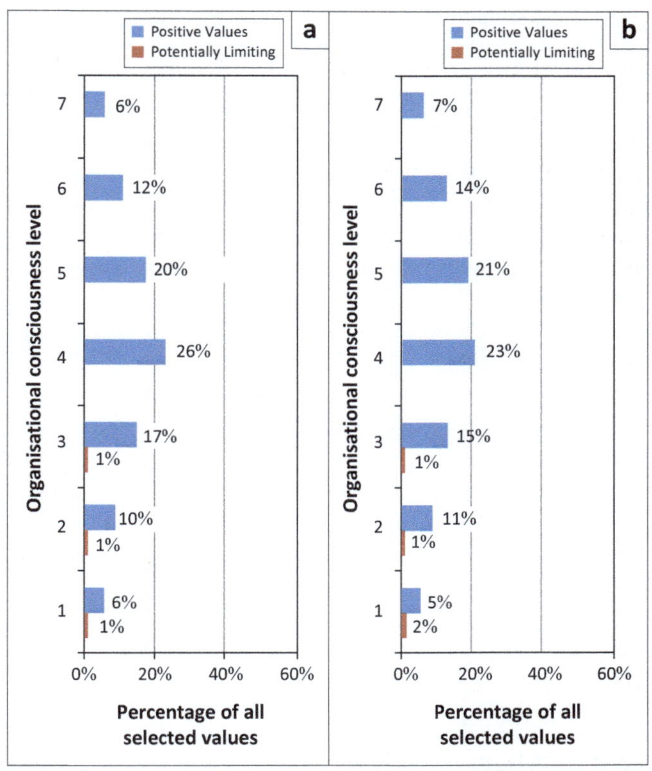

FIGURE 3: (a) Desired organisational values for Mahalapye health districts mapped to organisational consciousness level. (b) Desired organisational values for Ngamiland health districts mapped to organisational consciousness level.

TABLE 7: Implications of the top current organisational values for Mahalapye and Ngamiland health districts as interpreted by healthcare workers.

Value	Implication
Teamwork	People in the two districts were aware that they could accomplish more together than alone. The continued appeal for teamwork in the future was a call to build a complete team. The people believed the team was incomplete and as such ineffective as some critical health care cadres were either missing or in short supply. The people also wanted their contribution to the team effort to be recognised and rewarded (*staff recognition*).
Blame	Some people in both organisations were being mistreated by being held accountable for the misdeeds of others. Poor communication in a bureaucratic environment had led to employees also blaming management for problems and vice versa. The call for *accountability* implied that employees wanted to be acknowledged and rewarded for good performance and made to account for poor performance. They also placed a very high value on *transparency* and *honesty* to facilitate accountability.
Community involvement	The clinics are embedded in the community and in Mahalapye the respondents saw the district health services as engaged in local issues and working closely with the community. The interaction with the community though was not always perceived as positive by health workers, who often felt unfairly criticised by the community for things they had no control over. Unrealistic expectations and interference by some community and political leaders was also disruptive to efficient running of the clinics.
Confusion	The DHMTs were a fairly recent invention whose implementation was not properly communicated to the health workers, who were still unsure of the district health system governance structure. Moreover the people in both districts experienced a lack of clarity as well as mixed messages from the national Ministry of Health and DHMT, which left them unsure of motives and directives. This confusion was compounded by poor communication. The request for *leadership development* implied they saw the need for learning opportunities that would help their leaders in uniting and guiding the employee population. The people were also calling for clear transparent communication and staff engagement to bring about common understanding, especially in issues that affected the way they work.
Job insecurity	There was fear and uncertainty in both districts about the people's ability to keep their jobs. As such, people tended not to question the status quo, but worked strictly by the rules. An environment of blame, poor information sharing, control and manipulation all heightened this insecurity. Some human resources management policies were construed as unclear and unfairly applied. There was a call for *professional growth* as employees sought learning and career opportunities in their organisations. The people also sought transparency and fairness in implementation of human resources policies.
Patient satisfaction	Each of the districts emphasised the fact that they existed to meet the needs of their patients.
Not sharing information	The people in the two districts did not have access to the truths that would provide clarity and understanding about what was going on in the organisation. Information flow was often just from top to bottom and not vice versa. Even the information from the top often did not trickle down to all the health facilities and especially not to all employees. These employees called for *transparency* and *openness* and that those giving directives should actively provide clarity around their motives and orders in order to promote shared understanding.
Long hours	In Mahalapye people were overworked. They acknowledged that some clinics had few patients, but these sought health care around the clock leaving very little time for nurses working alone in the clinic to rest. Increased numbers of programmes without increase in staff had also stretched this limited resource with minimal reward and recognition. They were therefore burnt out and demoralised. Employees were therefore calling for an organisational focus on *staff fulfilment* and *staff recognition*.
Control	In Mahalapye the people were not empowered to do their work, but were rather micromanaged. The employees sought to be empowered to utilise and develop their skills and be held accountable for their actions. They also wanted to share in decision making. Leadership development at all levels was also wanted to create a more open and supportive management style.
Manipulation	Nurses in both districts felt exploited as they were expected to do tasks traditionally done by doctors, pharmacists and laboratory technicians without any extra reward. The clear call for *shared decision making*, *staff recognition* and *staff fulfilment* was intended to address this.
Professionalism	Mahalapye had a focus on high standards of care and conduct.
Shared vision	Mahalapye health district also recognised the importance of a sense of purpose and direction that united and inspired their efforts.
Working strictly by the rules	In both districts bureaucracy and the status quo hampered the employees efforts who tended to keep quiet and adhere to the business norms of the health districts. The call for *empowerment* (Mahalapye) and *staff engagement* (Ngamiland), *professional* and *leadership development* were made in order to free the innovation and creativity of the staff.
Information sharing	Those from Ngamiland were focused on exchanging knowledge and resources across the business in order to help empower employees' efforts. Despite this, a similar number of respondents experience lack of information sharing as the predominant culture.
Working in isolation	Ngamiland is a large remote and rural district where many health workers work alone. These health workers felt detached from the rest and unsupported. Consequently, depression and loneliness were experienced by many. The employees, therefore, sought support for their basic well-being (*staff health*). They also want to be involved in decisions about their deployment as well as opportunities (*staff engagement*) to fully utilise their talents and skills.

Level 5 with a call for more transparency to build alignment and internal cohesion (Figure 3). Level 3 represented a positive commitment to improved productivity and professional growth. The other levels suggested a need for more attention to staff welfare and more recognition of the work they were doing as well as a call for development of the leadership within the organisation.

Table 7 summarises the feedback from the health workers in both districts on their interpretation of the values seen in the current organisational culture. 'The current organisational values reflect the employees' perceptions of what their organisation focuses on and how it behaves. These attributes provide a picture of the working environment, the positive aspects of the business, and its potential problem areas. These are a description of what the situation is between these groups at this point in time'.[11,12]

Discussion

This study has investigated the personal values of the HCWs in the Mahalapye and Ngamiland health districts as well as the perceived current and desired organisational culture of the health districts. Organisational culture has been strongly linked to employee satisfaction and organisational commitment and hence their retention.[17] An understanding of the prevailing organisational culture in the Botswana district health system and how this is likely to affect retention of primary HCWs is critical to guide organisational transformation.

The results of this study showed that the HCWs' personal values were focused on demonstrating ownership for their actions, being truthful and trustworthy. They also placed emphasis on fostering kind and supportive interactions with the people around them. The prevailing culture in the districts, on the other hand, was predominantly perceived as potentially limiting and likely to cause frustration amongst employees and hinder organisational performance. None of the personal values of the HCWs were currently experienced in either district where a culture of blame, control, manipulation, poor communication and working strictly by the rules dominated. HCWs in both districts additionally experienced high levels of job insecurity. It is also notable that more than a third of the current organisational values were perceived as constraining organisational performance. The incongruence between personal and organisational values is likely to negatively affect job satisfaction, performance and organisational commitment.[12,17]

The personal values of the primary HCWs in the two health districts in Botswana were almost identical to their counterparts in the Cape Town primary care services where the primary health care services were also equally experienced as negative with levels of entropy above 30%.[18] Similar organisational dysfunction has also been reported by Kenyan HCWs in Kenya's district hospitals.[19]

With the exception of teamwork and customer focus (patient satisfaction), the current organisational values were not aligned to the espoused values of the national Ministry of Health and district health services of *botho* [kindness, compassion, respect], integrity, timeliness and accountability.[14] These espoused values, however, are similar to the actual personal values of the employees, implying that the staff have the potential to manifest the espoused values of the Ministry if given a chance to do so. Interestingly, the Western Cape government embraces similar core values of caring, competence, accountability, integrity, responsiveness and respect, despite its mostly negative employee experiences.[20] This incongruity between personal and organisational values as well as espoused and actual values is very likely to result in low health worker motivation, high attrition and poor patient outcome.[8,10,11,12]

Primary care workers in the two districts desire organisational transformation that concentrates on building a sense of shared purpose, internal community and employee participation. They were in agreement that a more supportive and innovative culture with a focus on transparency, professional growth, staff recognition, shared decision-making, accountability, productivity and leadership development should replace the current largely limiting culture. The HCWs also wanted to see teamwork continue as part of the future culture of the district health services. A more supportive and innovative culture together with considerate supportive supervisors has been associated with increased job satisfaction and organisational commitment.[17] Organisational culture and leadership styles determine the work environment, which can be either helpful or detrimental to organisational effectiveness and job satisfaction.[21] Furthermore, the perception of a limiting work environment and paucity of supportive supervision is strongly correlated with low job satisfaction and intention to migrate.[22] Alignment of the distribution of the desired organisational culture and personal values denotes that the health workers are capable of affecting the change they want to see.[18]

Botswana's human resources for health are heavily skewed towards cities and hospital care, displaying an 'inverse care law,'[23,24] despite the national Ministry of Health and the district health systems espoused value of equity.[14] Attraction and retention of motivated and committed health workers to primary health care services, especially in rural areas, should therefore be prioritised. This mandates a new emphasis on employee experience with a focus on professional development, shared decision-making and staff engagement in the district health system.

The response rates were relatively low, but the study captured the views of all the different health care cadres working in two thirds of the health facilities of each district. The study was conducted in two of the 27 health districts in the country, which means the findings may not be applicable to the rest of the health system. The concordance in the personal and perceived organisational values in these two dissimilar districts, however, suggests that similar findings may be elicited in other health districts. The very strong similarity and distribution of the values and culture with Cape Town primary care services also suggests that this state of affairs may be prevalent in the region.

Conclusion

The primary HCWs in Mahalapye and Ngamiland health districts perceive the organisational culture of the health districts to be mostly limiting organisational effectiveness. The health workers personal attributes were strongly correlated with the transformed culture they desired to see in their health districts, reflecting personal capacity to effect the changes. The employees' personal attributes and those they want to see in the future transformed organisation are in keeping with what is known about organisational cultures and leadership styles that create employee satisfaction, organisational commitment and retention. Transformation of the leadership from a bureaucratic controlling style focused on keeping the status quo to a more supportive type is urgent in order to restore employee trust and retain them in primary care.

There is an urgent need for organisational transformation of the health care services at the district and national levels to translate the espoused organisational values to the felt culture. This transformation should accentuate employee experience with an emphasis on accountability, transparency, professional growth, staff recognition and shared decision making. Opportunities for professional growth as well as employee recognition are well known to improve health care worker motivation and retention.

Leadership have the greatest influence in creating and sustaining the prevailing organisational culture. Leadership development is therefore imperative at all levels of the health system for organisational transformation to succeed.

Implementation research to explore whether developing more supportive leaders will improve employee motivation and retention is required. Additionally, investigation of aspects of organisational transformation that will significantly impact staff motivation and retention in the Botswana primary health care services will need to accompany the transformation.

Acknowledgements

This work is part of the Human Resources for African Primary Care and is supported through the European Union's FP7 programme, grant agreement no. 265727: http://www.huraprim-project.eu. The researchers acknowledge the facilitation of the research from the Ministry of Health, Ngamiland and Mahalapye DHMTs. The team want to thank Mr Pilatwe Pilatwe, Mrs Tlotlo Thutoemang and Miss Seonyatseng Moseki for collecting the data for this study.

Competing interests

The authors declare that they have no financial or personal relationship(s) that may have inappropriately influenced them in writing this article.

Authors' contributions

O.N. (University of Botswana, School of Medicine) conceptualised the project, collected and drafted the manuscript. R.M. (Stellenbosch University) guided the conceptualisation of the project, facilitated the data analysis, reviewed the draft manuscript and approved the final version. N.P. (University of Botswana, School of Nursing) reviewed the manuscript and approved the final version.

References

1. World Health Organization. Primary care: Now more than ever, 2008 World Health Report. Geneva: World Health Organization Press; 2008.
2. Nkomazana O, Peersman W, Willcox M, Mash R, Phaladze N. Human resources for health in Botswana: The results of in-country database and reports analysis. Afr J Prim Health Care Fam Med [serial on the Internet]. 2014;6(1):E1–E8. PMID: 26245420, http://dx.doi.org/10.4102/phcfm.v6i1.716
3. World Health Organization. The world health report 2006 - Working together for health. Geneva: World Health Organization Press; 2006.
4. World Health Organization. World health statistics. Geneva: World Health Organization Press; 2012.
5. Bonenberger M, Aikins M, Akweongo P, Wyss K. The effects of health worker motivation and job satisfaction on turnover intention in Ghana: A cross-sectional study. Hum Resour Health [serial on the Internet]. 2014;12:43. PMID: 25106497, http://dx.doi.org /10.1186/1478-4491-12-43
6. Nkomazana O, Mash R, Shaibu S, Phaladze N. Stakeholders' perceptions on shortage of healthcare workers in primary healthcare in Botswana: Focus group discussions. PLoS One. 2015;10(8):e0135846. PMID: 26284617, http://dx.doi.org/10.1371/journal.pone.0135846
7. Manafa O, McAuliffe E, Maseko F, Bowie C, MacLachlan M, Normand C. Retention of health workers in Malawi: Perspectives of health workers and district management. Hum Resour Health [serial on the Internet]. 2009;7:65. PMID: 19638222, http://dx.doi.org/10.1186/1478-4491-7-65
8. Rowe AK, de Savigny D, Lanata CF, Victora CG. How can we achieve and maintain high-quality performance of health workers in low-resource settings? Lancet. 2005;366:1026–1035. PMID: 16168785, http://dx.doi.org/10.1016/S0140-6736(05)67028-6
9. Willis-Shattuck M, Bidwell P, Thomas S, Wyness L, Blaauw D, Ditlopo P. Motivation and retention of health workers in developing countries: A systematic review [homepage on the Internet]. BMC Health Serv Res. 2008;8:247. PMID: 19055827, http://dx.doi.org/10.1186/1472-6963-8-247
10. Barrett R. Liberating the corporate soul: Building visionary organizations. Oxford: Butterworth-Heinemann; 1998.
11. Eneroth T, van Meer P, Jiang N, Clothier P, Infer H. Get connected: A practical guide to grow a desired team culture [homepage on the Internet]. 2013 [cited 2015 Feb 18]. Available from: http://www.valuescentre.com/sites/default/files/uploads/2013-05-13/Get%20Connected_2013.pdf
12. Barrett R. Building a values-driven organization: A whole system approach to cultural transformation. Oxford: Butterworth-Heinemann; 2006.
13. Ministry of Health. National health policy: Towards a healthier Botswana [homepage on the Internet]. 2011 [cited 2015 Mar 19]. Available from: http://www.moh.gov.bw/Publications/policies/revised_national_health_policy.pdf
14. Ministry of Health. Integrated health services plan: A strategy for changing the health sector for a healthy Botswana 2010-2020 [homepage on the Internet]. 2010 [cited 2015 Mar 12) Available from: http://www.moh.gov.bw/Publications/policies/Botswana%20IHSP%20Final%20HLSP.pdf
15. Cultural capital: The new frontier of competitive advantage [homepage on the Internet]. [cited 2013 Jun 20]. Available from: http://www.valuescentre.com/
16. Barrett's Value Centre [homepage on the Internet]. [cited 2013 Jun 20]. Available from: http://www.valuescentre.com/
17. Lok P, Crawford J. The effect of organisational culture and leadership style on job satisfaction and organisational commitment: A cross-national comparison. JMD [serial on the Internet]. 2004;23:321–338. http://dx.doi.org/10.1108/02621710410529785
18. Mash RJ, Govender S, Isaacs AA, De Sa A, Schlemmer A. An assessment of organisational values, culture and performance in Cape Town's primary healthcare services. S Afr Fam Pract. 2013;55:459–466. http://dx.doi.org/10.1080/20786204.2013.10874396
19. Mbindyo P, Gilson L, Blaauw D, English M. Contextual influences on health worker motivation in district hospitals in Kenya. Implement Sci [serial on the Internet]. 2009;4:43. PMID: 19627590, http://dx.doi.org/10.1186/1748-5908-4-43
20. Western Cape. Department of Health. Vision 2020 [homepage on the Internet]. Cape Town: Department of Health; 2011 [cited 2015 Apr 1]. Available from: https://www.westerncape.gov.za/other/2011/12/healthcare_2020_-_9_december_2020.pdf
21. Krogstad U, Hofoss D, Veenstra M, Hjortdahl P. Predictors of job satisfaction among doctors, nurses and auxiliaries in Norwegian hospitals: Relevance for micro unit culture. Hum Resour Health [serial on the Internet]. 2006;4:3. PMID: 16483384, http://dx.doi.org/10.1186/1478-4491-4-3
22. McAuliffe E, Bowie C, Manafa O, *et al.* Measuring and managing the work environment of the mid-level provider – The neglected human resource. Hum Resour Health [serial on the Internet]. 2009;7:13.PMID: 19228391, http://dx.doi.org/10.1186/1478-4491-7-13
23. Moosa S, Wojczewski S, Hoffmann K, *et al.* The inverse primary care law in sub-Saharan Africa: A qualitative study of the views of migrant health workers. Br J Gen Pract. 2014;64(623):e321–e328. PMID: 24868069, http://dx.doi.org/10.3399/bjgp14X680089
24. Hart JT. The inverse care law. Lancet. 1971;1:405–412. PMID: 4100731, http://dx.doi.org/10.1016/S0140-6736(71)92410-X

Intestinal helminth infections amongst HIV-infected adults in Mthatha General Hospital, South Africa

Authors:
Olukayode A. Adeleke[1]
Parimalaranie Yogeswaran[2]
Graham Wright[3]

Affiliations:
[1]Department of Family Medicine, Walter Sisulu University, Mthatha, South Africa

[2]Department of Family Medicine and Rural Health, Walter Sisulu University, Mthatha, South Africa

[3]Centre for Health Informatics Research and Development, University of Fort Hare, South Africa

Correspondence to:
Olukayode Adeleke

Email:
kay2kay001@gmail.com

Postal address:
Private Bag X1007, Grahamstown 6140, South Africa

Background: In South Africa, studies on the prevalence of intestinal helminth co-infection amongst HIV-infected patients as well as possible interactions between these two infections are limited.

Aim: To investigate the prevalence of intestinal helminth infestation amongst adults living with HIV or AIDS at Mthatha General Hospital.

Setting: Study participants were recruited at the outpatient department of Mthatha General Hospital, Mthatha, South Africa.

Methods: This cross-sectional study was conducted between October and December 2013 amongst consecutive consenting HIV-positive adult patients. Socio-demographic and clinical information were obtained using data collection forms and structured interviews. Stool samples were collected to investigate the presence of helminths whilst blood samples were obtained for the measurement of CD4+ T-cell count and viral load.

Results: Data were obtained on 231 participants, with a mean age of 34.9 years, a mean CD4 count of 348 cells/µL and a mean viral load of 4.8 $\log_{10}$ copies/mL. Intestinal helminth prevalence was 24.7%, with *Ascaris Lumbricoides* (42.1%) the most prevalent identified species. Statistically significant association was found between CD4 count of less than 200 cells/µL and helminth infection ($p = 0.05$). No statistically significant association was found between intestinal helminth infection and the mean CD4 count ($p = 0.79$) or the mean viral load ($p = 0.98$).

Conclusion: A high prevalence of intestinal helminth infections was observed amongst the study population. Therefore, screening and treatment of helminths should be considered as part of the management of HIV and AIDS in primary health care.

Les infections par les helminthes intestinaux chez les adultes séropositifs à l'Hôpital Général de Mthatha, en Afrique du Sud.

Contexte: Peu d'études ont été faites en Afrique du Sud sur la prévalence de la coïnfection par les helminthes intestinaux chez les patients séropositifs ainsi que les interactions possibles entre ces deux infections.

Objectif: Etudier la prévalence d'infection par les helminthes intestinaux chez les adultes séropositifs avec le VIH ou le SIDA à l'Hôpital Général de Mthatha.

Lieu: Les participants à l'étude ont été recrutés au service de consultations externes de l'Hôpital Général de Mthatha, à Mthatha en Afrique du Sud.

Méthodes: Cette étude transversale a été faite d'octobre à décembre 2013 chez des patients séropositifs consécutifs, adultes et consentants. On a obtenu les informations sociodémographiques et cliniques au moyen de formulaires de collecte de données et d'entretiens structurés. Des échantillons de selles ont été prélevés pour déterminer la présence d'helminthes et des échantillons sanguins ont été obtenus pour mesurer le nombre de cellules T CD4+ et la charge virale.

Résultats: On a obtenu des données de 231 participants, avec un âge moyen de 34.9 ans, une moyenne de cellules CD4 de 348 cellules/µL et une charge virale moyenne de 4.8 log10 copies/mL. La prévalence d'helminthes intestinaux était de 24.7%, avec les *Ascaris Lumbricoides* (42.1%) qui étaient les espèces les plus fréquentes. On a trouvé un lien important du point de vue statistique entre le nombre de CD4 de moins de 200 cellules/µL et l'infection par les helminthes ($p = 0.05$). Aucune corrélation importante du point de vue statistique n'a été trouvée entre l'infection par les helminthes intestinaux et le nombre moyen de CD4 ($p = 0.79$) ou la charge virale moyenne ($p = 0.98$).

Conclusion: On a remarqué une forte prévalence d'infections par les helminthes intestinaux chez les sujets à l'étude. Ainsi, le dépistage et le traitement des helminthes devrait faire partie de la gestion du VIH et du SIDA dans les soins de santé primaire.

Introduction

Helminths are the most common parasitic agents of humans in Africa and other developing countries, producing a burden of disease that exceeds better-known conditions, including malaria and tuberculosis.[1] Sub-Saharan Africa bears an inordinate proportion of the global HIV pandemic, being home to more than two-thirds of the estimated 35.3 million people worldwide living with HIV in 2012.[2] There is significant overlaps in the geographical distribution of HIV and helminthiasis, and co-infection is highly endemic in this region.[3]

South Africa has the highest HIV epidemic in the world,[2] with an estimated 10% of the total population, approximately 5.2 million people, living with HIV or AIDS in 2013.[4] A significant proportion of South Africans live in areas characterised by poverty and under-development,[5] conditions that have been shown to fuel the continuing spread of HIV and helminthic infections.[6] Although the national estimates of helminth prevalence are not known, data from surveys in various parts of South Africa reveal infestation levels that range between 70% and 100% in school-age children and pre-schoolers.[5] For example, the prevalence of intestinal parasites amongst school children in four schools in Mthatha is reported to be 64.8%.[7] In addition, helminths were identified in 21.7% of stool specimen from adults obtained from some public hospital laboratories in Kwazulu-Natal Province.[8] However, data on the prevalence of intestinal parasites in the country's adult population are insufficient.

Despite the high prevalence of these two infections in Sub-Saharan Africa, the effect of intestinal helminths on the epidemiology of HIV infection, including the risk of HIV transmission and disease progression and management, remains uncertain.[9] Studies have shown that infestation by intestinal worms adversely affects the immune response, causing immune dysfunction and diminishing the host's capacity to mount appropriate defence against infections such as tuberculosis and HIV infection.[10,11] Although they vary in their biology, route of infection and developmental stages in which they exist in the human host, most helminth parasites evoke a similar immune response in the host. This entails a polarisation of CD4+ T-cells towards a Th2 phenotype, with reduced Th1-type responses, as well as immunosuppression of both worm-specific and generalised immune responses.[12] Th1 cells are important in eliminating intracellular pathogens, and inflammatory responses. Th2 cells, on the other hand, target extracellular pathogens and produce cytokines, which enhance antibody production. The profound Th2 and diminished Th1 responses as well as the chronic immune activation found in patients with intestinal helminth infection have been hypothesised to lead to an increased susceptibility to HIV infection and enhanced HIV replication in helminth-infected individuals.[12,13]

Intestinal helminthic infection has been shown to be common amongst people living with HIV or AIDS in Africa, with prevalence ranging from 17% to 66% depending on the methods used to identify the helminths.[5,9,14] However, studies conducted in several African countries have produced conflicting results regarding the impact of intestinal helminthic infection on the epidemiology of HIV. Though most authors agree on the potential theoretical deleterious immunological consequences of HIV and helminthic infection co-existing in an individual, the results from various studies evaluating the practical implication of treating intestinal helminthic infection in HIV disease progression are inconclusive.[15] Whilst some studies found no effect of treatment of intestinal helminth infections on HIV disease progression,[9,16,17] other authors have reported a beneficial effect, with a reduction in HIV viral load, including reduction in the risk of HIV transmission following treatment of intestinal helminthic infection.[18,19,20]

This study sought to explore the extent of the problem of intestinal infestation in HIV-positive adults at the Mthatha General Hospital, a district hospital located in the OR Tambo district of the Eastern Cape Province, South Africa. About 12.6% of the South African population lives in the province, the third largest and one of the poorest in the country, with the highest percentage of households living without toilet facilities.[21] Although there is a paucity of data on the prevalence of HIV-helminth co-infection in the province, the endemic poverty, lack of access to clean water and poor sanitation makes it highly probable that HIV-helminth co-infection will be common in this area.

Research methods and design

Study design, setting and sampling strategy

This cross-sectional study was conducted within the outpatient department of Mthatha General Hospital, Mthatha, Eastern Cape Province of South Africa. This is a district hospital that is a part of the Mthatha Academic Hospital Complex, one of the teaching complexes of the Faculty of Health Sciences, Walter Sisulu University. Consecutive patients aged 18 years and above, confirmed to be HIV-positive and HAART (Highly active antiretroviral therapy)-naïve, were enrolled between October and December 2013. They were provided with written and verbal information about the study and were required to provide written informed consent. Exclusion criteria were the presence of acute severe illnesses like pneumonia, tuberculosis or meningitis. Over a three-month period, the population of HAART-naïve HIV-positive adults attending the outpatient department was estimated at 720. As the prevalence of helminth infection amongst the population was unknown, this was computed as 50%. Using a confidence level of 95% and a design effect of 1.0, a sample size of 251 was calculated using OpenEpi software.[22] None of the eligible participants declined to participate in the study.

Collection, transport and processing of specimens

Stool samples were collected according to World Health Organization (WHO) standard procedure.[23] Submitted stool specimens were transported in a cooler box to the department of Medical Microbiology at Walter Sisulu University within an hour of collection for microscopy. About 5 mL of venous blood specimen was collected in ethylenediaminetetraacetic acid (EDTA) and plasma preparation tubes, for estimation of CD4 count and plasma HIV-RNA level, immediately after collection. A pilot study was conducted amongst 20 participants who were not included in the main study. Necessary adjustments were made to the interview guide and specimen collection technique. For example, all 20 participants strongly objected to the application of transparent adhesive tape to skin around the anus to obtain ova of *Enterobius vermicularis* (the scotch-tape technique). The technique was omitted in the main study.

Stool specimens were processed using the formalin-ethyl acetate concentration method. An experienced medical technologist performed microscopy of the concentrated specimen, and a consultant medical microbiologist examined a random selection of the microscope slides for the purpose of quality control. Parasites were quantified based on the number of parasites seen per high microscopic power field (hpf). CD4 count was determined at the National Health Laboratory Service in Mthatha from venous blood using the Panleucogating (PLG) methodology, whilst HIV viral load was determined using COBAS® AmpliPrep/COBAS® TaqMan® HIV-1 Test, version 2.0.

Participants identified as having intestinal helminth infection were treated with anti-helminthic drugs according to standard practice. Participants who were eligible for antiretroviral therapy based on CD4 count were contacted and appropriately referred for treatment initiation.

Statistical analysis

Data analysis was performed using the Statistical Package for the Social Sciences (SPSS) version 21.0 (SPSS Inc., Chicago, IL, USA). Data were expressed as means ± standard error (s.e.) of the mean or as means ± standard deviation (s.d.) for the continuous variables and proportions (percentages) for the categorical variables. The chi-square test or Fischer's exact test was used to test the degree of association of categorical variables. Student's *t*-test was performed to assess differences between two means and analysis of variance (ANOVA) between groups. All tests were two-sided and a *p*-value of ≤ 0.05 was considered significant.

Ethical considerations

Ethical approval was obtained from the Human Research Committee of Walter Sisulu University (Protocol number: 005/2013). Institutional approval to conduct the research was obtained from the Eastern Cape Department of Health, Bisho.

Results

A total of 252 HIV seropositive adults were enrolled in the study. Twenty-one of these (6 male, 15 female) were excluded from the analysis because of incomplete data. The excluded participants were not different from the remaining participants in terms of age, gender, level of education, income, employment status, CD4 count or viral load. Of the remaining 231 HIV seropositive patients with complete data, 72 (31%) were male and 231 (69%) female. The mean age of the study participants was 34.9 years (s.d. = 10.6 years), ranging from 18 years to 64 years. Other social, demographic and clinical characteristics of the participants are presented in Table 1.

Of the 231 participants, 132 (57.1%) were unemployed, the majority of whom were dependent on various forms of social grants. The average monthly income of 53.7% of these patients was less than R1000. There was no statistically significant association between participants' age, gender, level of education or average monthly income and intestinal helminth infection. Helminth-infected participants reported

TABLE 1: Socio-demographic characteristics of the study population (n = 231).

Characteristics	Total participants (n = 231) n (%)		Helminth-infected (n = 57) n (%)		Helminth-uninfected (n = 174) n (%)		ANOVA (p-value)
Age (years), mean ± s.d.	34.7 ± 10.6		35.4 ± 9.7		34.7 ± 10.9		0.66
Gender							**0.36**
Male	72	31.2	15	26.3	57	32.8	0.41
Female	159	68.8	42	73.7	117	67.2	0.40
Number of household members, mean ± s.d.	5 ± 4		6 ± 7		5 ± 3		0.05
Employment							**0.09**
Yes	99	42.9	31	54.4	68	39.1	0.09
No	132	57.1	26	45.6	106	60.9	0.09
Level of education							**0.5**
None	4	1.7	2	3.5	2	1.2	0.23*
Primary	43	18.6	10	17.5	33	18.9	0.81*
Secondary	146	63.2	38	66.7	108	62.4	0.53*
Tertiary	38	16.5	7	12.3	31	17.9	0.32*
Average monthly income (Rand)							**0.51**
< 1000	125	53.7	27	47.4	98	56.3	0.27*
1000 to 5000	86	37.5	25	43.8	61	35.1	0.26*
> 5000	20	8.7	5	8.8	15	8.6	0.96*

ANOVA, analysis of variance (calculated with Asymp. Sig 2-sided or Exact Sig 2-sided ANOVA); s.d., standard deviation; *, 2-tailed Z -score test

a higher number of household members (mean = 6) than their helminth-uninfected counterpart (mean = 5) ($p = 0.05$).

As shown in Table 2, 163 (70.6%) participants had access to tap water, whilst 178 (77.1%) used pit latrines, mostly shared with other families. There was no statistically significant association between source of water or toilet type and helminth infection. Only 6.1% of the participants indicated that they clean their hands with soap and water after defecation, and 93.1% indicated that they wash their hands with water only. No statistically significant association was found between hand-washing practices and intestinal helminthic infection ($p = 0.076$).

Of the 231 participants whose stools were examined for intestinal parasites, helminth infection was detected in 57, representing 24.7% of the study population. Seven species of helminths were identified: *Ascaris Lumbricoides* (42.1%), *Trichuris trichura* (5.26%), *Strongyloides stercoralis* (5.26%), Hookworm species (5.26%) (*Necator americanus, Ancylostoma duodenale*), Hymenolepis *nana* (5.26%), *Diphylobothrium latum* (28.07%) and *Fasciolopsis buski* (8.8%) (Figure 1).

TABLE 2: Sanitation-related characteristics of the study population (n = 231).

Characteristics	Total participants (n = 231) n (%)		Helminth-infected (n = 57) n (%)		Helminth-uninfected (n = 174) n (%)		ANOVA (p-value)
Water source							**0.37**
Tap	163	70.6	39	68.4	124	71.3	0.68*
River	48	20.8	12	21.1	36	20.7	0.95*
Tank	20	8.7	6	10.6	14	8	0.56*
Toilet type							**0.45**
Pit	178	77.1	46	80.7	132	75.9	0.59
Flush	53	22.9	11	19.3	42	24.1	0.59
Bucket	0	0	0	0	0	0	
Refuse disposal							**0.76**
Burning	172	74.5	44	77.2	128	73.6	0.58*
Municipal collection	58	25.1	13	22.8	45	25.8	0.64*
Others	1	0.4	0	0	1	0.6	0.56*
Hand care							**0.20**
None	2	0.9	0	0	2	1.1	0.41*
Water and soap	14	6.1	1	1.8	13	7.5	0.11*
Water only	215	93.1	56	98.2	159	91.4	0.11*

ANOVA, analysis of variance (calculated with Asymp. Sig 2-sided or Exact Sig 2-sided ANOVA); *, 2-tailed Z-score test

The CD4+ cell count of the study participants ranged widely from 3 to 1283 cells/µL, with a mean of 348 cells cells/µL. Sixty-nine participants (29.9%) were severely immunosuppressed with a CD4+ cell count of less than 200 cells/µL, of whom 37 (16%) had a CD4 count of less than 100. A total of 105 (45.4%) patients had a CD4+ count of more than 350 cells/µL. The mean plasma viral load for the study participants was 4.8 $\log_{10}$ copies/mL (Table 3). Although the participants with helminth infection had a slightly lower mean CD4 count and a slightly higher mean viral load than those with no infection, there was no statistically significant differences in the mean viral load ($p = 0.98$) or mean CD4+ cell count ($p = 0.79$) in both groups. However, low CD4 count (< 200 cells/µL) was associated with intestinal helminthic infection. This was statistically significant ($p = 0.05$).

Apart from the seven species of intestinal helminth identified during the study, *Entamoeba histolytica*, a protozoan, was identified in two of the participants (0.9% prevalence) whilst the bacterium *Escherica coli* was found in 35 patients (15.2% prevalence). Thirteen (5.5%) of the participants had mixed infection (Table 4).

Discussion

Nearly 70% of participants in the study were female (Table 1), which might be an indication of low attendance of men at the outpatient department of the hospital. It has been noted that in most part of Africa, men in general seek treatment for all ailments (HIV/AIDS-related or otherwise) less often than

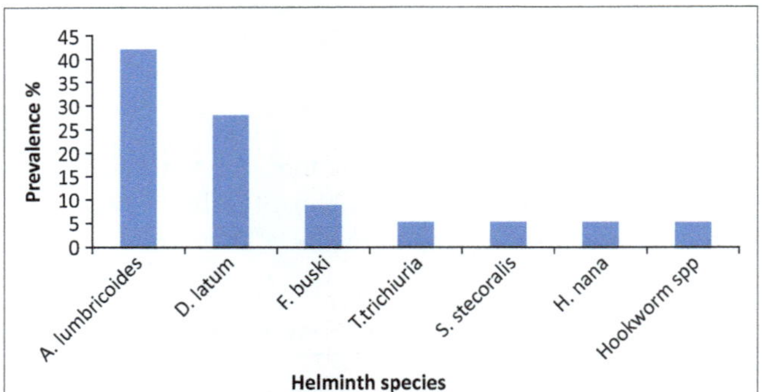

FIGURE 1: Prevalence of helminth species amongst helminth-infected participants (n = 57).

TABLE 3: CD4+ T-cell count and HIV viral load of the study population.

CD4+ cell count and viral load	Total participants (n = 231) n (%)		Helminth-infected (n = 57) n (%)		Helminth-uninfected (n = 174) n (%)		ANOVA (p-value)
CD4+ cell count category							**0.14**
< 200 cells/µL	69	29.9	23	40.4	46	26.4	0.05*
200–350 cells/µL	57	24.7	12	21.0	45	25.9	0.47*
350 cells/µL	105	45.4	22	38.6	83	47.7	0.23*
Log10 HIV-RNA category (copies/mL)							**0.35**
≤ 3 log10	11	4.8	1	1.8	10	5.7	-
3–5 log10	120	51.9	33	57.9	87	50	-
5 log10	100	43.3	23	40.4	77	44.3	-
CD4+ cell count, mean (±s.d.) cells/µL	348 ± 239		340 ± 264		350 ± 232		0.79
Log10 HIV-RNA, mean (±SEM) copies/mL	4.8 ± 0.06		4.8 ± 0.08		4.7 ± 0.11		0.98

ANOVA, analysis of variance (calculated with Asymp. Sig 2-sided or Exact Sig 2-sided ANOVA).
*, 2-tailed Z-score test; s.d., standard deviation; SEM, standard error of the mean; log, logarithm.

TABLE 4: Multiple infections amongst the study participants (n = 231).

Parasites	Prevalence (n)	Prevalence (%)
A. lumbricoides and *E. coli*	4	1.73
A. lumbricoides and *F. buski*	1	0.43
A. lumbricoides and *E. histolytica*	1	0.43
E. coli and *H. nana*	5	2.2
E. coli and *D. latum*	1	0.43
E. coli and *F. buski*	1	0.43

women. This has been attributed to the culture of 'tough' masculinity which assumes that men are more powerful and less vulnerable than women.[24] It has also been shown that more women than men accessed HIV and/or AIDS care and treatment[25] and were more than twice as likely to be on antiretroviral therapy (ART) than men.[26]

The study found that 178 (77.1%) of the participants use pit latrines. This is similar to findings from a community-based survey conducted in 2008 by Mfenyana et al.[27] in which only 17.9% of the households had access to a flush toilet. The low socio-economic status noted amongst the participants in this study could be because of the setting of the study. As noted by Nattrass,[24] people of higher socio-economic status are less likely to use public health facilities than those of lower socio-economic status. Consistent with the findings of Modjarrad et al.[28] as well as Mwambete et al.[29] the participants' age, gender, income, level of education or occupation were not predictive of helminth status in the present study.

A statistically significant association was found between a large number of household members and helminthic infection amongst the participants. This was similar to the findings of the report by Anuar et al.[30] in which increased number of household members was associated with a higher frequency of intestinal parasitic infections. Crowded living conditions in developing countries have been shown to be one of the factors that increase susceptibility to soil-transmitted helminth infection.[31]

Although no statistically significant association was found between hand washing and helminthic infection, the proportion of participants with helminth infection who used soap and water was smaller than those without intestinal helminth infection (1.8% vs. 7.5%; p = 0.11). The lack of a statistically significant association in this study could be as a result of the small sample size. A review by Strunz et al.[32] shows that hand washing with soap after defecation significantly reduces the risk of helminth infection. Primary care physicians and indeed all health care workers practising in this community should therefore opportunistically provide patients with information on hand-washing practices and motivate a behavioural change during every consultation.

The species of intestinal helminths detected in this study and their prevalence were similar to the findings of some of the previously published reports of helminth infection amongst adults living with HIV and AIDS in Africa.[8,28,33] However, the 24.7% prevalence found in the present study was significantly lower than those from several other studies, which range from 48.7% to 66%.[5,34] This difference in prevalence reported in the various studies could be because of the differences in sample sizes, setting of the studies, inclusion and exclusion criteria used in participant selection as well as the difference in the methods used in the identification of the parasites (stool microscopy with or without serology)[5].

The Mthatha region of the Eastern Cape Province of South Africa has one of the highest prevalences of *Taenia solium* neurocysticercosis in the country.[35] The absence of the eggs of tapeworms in any of the stool specimens examined is therefore noteworthy, considering the high prevalence of neurocysticercosis in the community. The absence could be attributed to the small sample size or could be a result of HIV enteropathy, which affects the colonisation of the intestinal tract by parasites.[36] Larger studies should be conducted to explore the relationship between the prevalence of *T. solium* and HIV infection in this community.

The mean CD4 count of the study population was 348 cells/µL. The relatively lower CD4 count of the participants in this study could be attributed to the fact that this was a facility-based study, involving individuals who are more immunosuppressed than those found in the community. In this study, 69 (29.9%) of the participants were considerably immunosuppressed with a CD4 count of less than 200.

Consistent with the findings of Mwambete et al.[29] a statistically significant association was observed in the present study between a CD4 count less than 200 cells/µL and helminth infection (Table 3). This is in contrast to the report by Walson et al.[14] who noted an increased prevalence of intestinal helminth infection amongst patients with higher CD4 counts. The correlation of helminth infection with higher CD4 count found by Walson et al.[14] could be attributed to the inclusion in the study of only individuals with CD4 counts greater than 250 cells/µL and without WHO Stage 3 or 4 disease. This represents patients with less severe immune suppression than those in the present study.

No statistically significant difference was found between the mean CD4+ cell count (p = 0.79) of the helminth co-infected participants compared to the helminth-uninfected. This is similar to findings from similar studies conducted in Uganda,[17] South Africa[5] and Ethiopia.[37] In addition, no statistically significant association was observed between intestinal helminth infection and viral load in this study (p = 0.98), similar to the findings of Modjarrad et al.[38] and Hosseinipour et al.[9] but contrary to the findings of others.[5,37]

The lack of association between CD4 count, viral load and intestinal helminth infection in the present study could be attributed to the small sample size as well as possible under-estimation of the presence of intestinal helminth because stool microscopy was used as the sole method of diagnosing helminthiasis. It could also be attributed to the difference in the prevalence of the various helminth species identified in this study compared to those identified in studies where association has been found between CD4 count or viral load and helminthic infection. As Mkhize-Kwitshana et al.[5] have argued, diagnosis of helminthiasis based on stool microscopy alone could lead to a wrong classification of infection or non-infection and could affect the evaluation of the immunological effect of helminth co-infection on HIV and AIDS. Further studies that incorporate monitoring of markers of immune activation are necessary in order to provide a better understanding of the HIV-helminth relationship.

Limitations

As a cross-sectional survey, this study is useful in generating hypothesis but cannot show any causal or risk relationships. The use of a hospital-based population in this study was not representative of the adult population in Mthatha. Moreover, the study population may not be representative of all patients at the outpatient department because of the use of convenient sampling.

HIV-negative individuals were not included in this study to serve as a comparison group. As a result of this, comparative inferences cannot be made on the prevalence of helminth infections across populations of differing HIV status. Only one stool specimen was collected from each participant and helminth detection was based only on the use of light microscopy. These could have led to an under-estimation of the prevalence of helminthiasis.

Recommendation

It is recommended that larger community-based studies be conducted to determine the extent of intestinal helminth co-infection amongst people living with HIV or AIDS. Future studies should include HIV-negative comparison groups and be appropriately designed to explore several aspects of HIV-helminth interactions, including the effect of the various helminth species as well as multiple infections on HIV disease. Diagnosis of intestinal helminth infections in such studies should include, in addition to microscopy, parasite serology and molecular diagnostic techniques.

Conclusion

The study revealed that intestinal helminth infection was relatively common amongst the study population, with 24.7% prevalence. Helminthiasis was diagnosed in this study using a simple and cost-effective technique of stool microscopy, but the prevalence of intestinal helminth could actually be higher if other methods of identification (such as serology) were combined with microscopy.

Intestinal helminthic infections are known to be associated with high morbidity, adversely affecting the host's general health and nutritional status.[39] In HIV-positive patients, this represents an additional burden on already compromised hosts. In this study, no statistically significant association was found between intestinal helminth infection and markers of HIV disease progression; however, intestinal helminth infection was found to be significantly associated with lower CD4 count (< 200 cells/µL). Routine anti-helminth treatment should therefore be included as part of patients' comprehensive care, at least amongst this group of patients.

Acknowledgements

The authors thank Mr Eric Nombekela, Dr T. Apalata and Prof. S. Vasaikar of the Microbiology Department, Water Sisulu University for their assistance in the identification of intestinal parasites in stool specimens.

Competing interests

The authors declare that they have no financial or personal relationship(s) that may have inappropriately influenced them in writing this article.

Authors' contributions

O.A.A. (Walter Sisulu University) was the primary researcher. He designed the study, collected the specimen and analyse the data to fulfil the requirements for the degree of Master of Medicine (MMed) in Family Medicine at Walter Sisulu University. He wrote the article in a publishable format. P.Y. (Walter Sisulu University) was the study leader. She took part in conceptualising and designing the study. She provided appropriate and invaluable contributions towards the completion of the project and the final draft of the manuscript. G.W. (University of Fort Hare) was a co-supervisor and contributed to the study design and sampling procedure. He provided guidance towards the completion of the project and documentation.

References

1. Hotez PJ, Brindley PJ, Bethony JM, King CH, Pearc EJ, Jacobson J. Helminth infections: The great neglected tropical diseases. J Clin Invest. 2008;118(4):1311–1321. PMID: 18382743, http://dx.doi.org/10.1172/JCI34261
2. Joint United Nations Programme on HIV/AIDS (UNAIDS). Global report: UNAIDS report on the global AIDS epidemic 2013 [page on the Internet]. Geneva: UNAIDS; 2013 [cited 2014 Jan 3]. Available from: http://www.unaids.org/en/resources/campaigns/globalreport2013/globalreport
3. Webb EL, Ekii AO, Pala P. Epidemiology and immunology of helminth–HIV interactions. Curr Opin HIV AIDS. 2012;7(3):245–253. PMID: 22411451, http://dx.doi.org/10.1097/COH.0b013e32835210cd
4. Statistics South Africa. Mid-year population estimates, 2013 [page on the Internet]. Pretoria: Statistics South Africa; 2013 [cited 2013 Dec 28]. Available from: http://beta2.statssa.gov.za/publications/P0302/P03022013.pdf
5. Mkhize-Kwitshana ZL, Taylor M, Jooste P, Mabaso ML, Walzl G. The influence of different helminth infection phenotypes on immune responses against HIV in co-infected adults in South Africa. BMC Infect Dis. 2011;11(1):273. PMID: 21999928, http://dx.doi.org/10.1186/1471-2334-11-273
6. Fincham JE, Markus MB, Adams VJ. Could control of soil-transmitted helminthic infection influence the HIV/AIDS pandemic. Acta Trop. 2003;86(2):315–333. PMID: 12745148, http://dx.doi.org/10.1016/S0001-706X(03)00063-9
7. Nxasana N, Baba K, Bhat V, Vasaikar S. Prevalence of intestinal parasites in primary school children of Mthatha, Eastern Cape Province, South Africa. Ann Med Health Sci Res. 2014;13(3):511–516. PMID: 24380000, http://dx.doi.org/10.4103/2141-9248.122064
8. Kwitshana ZL, Tsoka JM, Mabaso ML. Intestinal parasitic infections in adult patients in KwaZulu-Natal. S Afri Med J. 2008;98(9):709. PMID: 19113052.
9. Hosseinipour MC, Napravnik S, Joaki G, et al. HIV and parasitic infection and the effect of treatment among adult outpatients in Malawi. J Infect Dis. 2007;195(9):1278–1282. PMID: 17396996, http://dx.doi.org/10.1086/513274
10. Bentwich Z, Teicher CL, Borkow G. The helminth HIV connection: Time to act. AIDS. 2008;22(13):1611–1614. PMID: 18670220, http://dx.doi.org/10.1097/QAD.0b013e32830a506e
11. Da'dara AA, Harn DA. Elimination of helminth infection restores HIV-1C vaccine-specific T cell responses independent of helminth-induced IL-10. Vaccine. 2010;28(5):1310–1317. PMID: 19941988, http://dx.doi.org/10.1016/j.vaccine.2009.11.019

12. Bourke CD, Maizels RM, Mutapi F. Acquired immune heterogeneity and its sources in human helminth infection. Parasitology. 2011;138(2):139–159. PMID: 20946693, http://dx.doi.org/10.1017/S0031182010001216

13. Borkow G, Bentwich Z. Chronic immune activation associated with chronic helminthic and human immunodeficiency virus infections: Role of hyporesponsiveness and anergy. Clin Microbiol Rev. 2004;17(4):1012–1030. PMID: 15489359, http://dx.doi.org/10.1128/CMR.17.4.1012-1030.2004

14. Walson JL, Stewart BT, Sangaré L, et al. Prevalence and correlates of helminth co-infection in Kenyan HIV-1 infected adults. PLoS Negl Trop Dis. 2010;4(3):e644. PMID: 20361031, http://dx.doi.org/10.1371/journal.pntd.0000644

15. Sangaré LR, Herrin BR, John-Stewart G, Walson JL. Species-specific treatment effects of helminth/HIV-1 co-infection: A systematic review and meta-analysis. Parasitology. 2011;138(Special Issue 12):1546–1558. PMID: 21729353, http://dx.doi.org/10.1017/S0031182011000357

16. Elliott AM, Mawa PA, Joseph S, et al. Associations between helminth infection and CD4+ T cell count, viral load and cytokine responses in HIV-1-infected Ugandan adults. Trans R Soc Trop Med Hyg. 2003;97(1):103–108. PMID: 12886815, http://dx.doi.org/10.1016/S0035-9203(03)90040-X

17. Brown M, Kizza M, Watera C, et al. Helminth infection is not associated with faster progression of HIV disease in coinfected adults in Uganda. J Infect Dis. 2004;190(10):1869–1879. PMID: 15499545.

18. Walson JL, Herrin BR, John-Stewart G. Deworming helminth co-infected individuals for delaying HIV disease progression. Cochrane Database Syst Rev. 2009;3(3). PMID: 19588389, http://dx.doi.org/10.1002/14651858.CD006419.pub3

19. Modjarrad K, Vermund SH. Effect of treating co-infections on HIV-1 viral load: A systematic review. Lancet Infect Dis. 2010;10(7):455–463. PMID: 20610327, http://dx.doi.org/10.1016/S1473-3099(10)70093-1

20. Gallagher M, Malhotra I, Mungai PL, et al. The effects of maternal helminth and malaria infections on mother-to-child HIV transmission. AIDS. 2005;19(16):1849–1855. PMID: 16227793, http://dx.doi.org/10.1097/01.aids.0000189846.90946.5d

21. Statistics South Africa. General household survey, 2012 [page on the Internet]. Pretoria: Statistics South Africa; 2013 [cited 2013 Dec 29]. Available from: http://www.statssa.gov.za/publications/P0318/P0318August2012.pdf

22. Open Source Epidemiologic Statistics for Public Health (OpenEpi). Sample size for frequency in a population [page on the Internet]. 2013 [cited 2013 Feb 10]; Available from: http://www.openepi.com/SampleSize/SSPropor.htm

23. World Health Organization (WHO). Basic laboratory methods in medical parasitology [page on the Internet]. Geneva: WHO; 1991 [cited 2011 Aug 20]; Available from: http://whqlibdoc.who.int/publications/9241544104_(part1).pdf

24. Nattrass N. Gender and access to antiretroviral treatment in South Africa. Fem Econ. 2008;14(4):19–36. http://dx.doi.org/10.1080/13545700802266452

25. Coetzee D, Hildebrand K, Boulle A, et al. Outcomes after two years of providing antiretroviral treatment in Khayelitsha, South Africa. AIDS. 2004;18(6):887–895. PMID: 15060436.

26. Bärnighausen T, Tanser F, Herbst K, Mutevedzi T, Mossong J, Newell ML. Structural barriers to antiretroviral treatment: A study using population-based CD4 cell count and linked antiretroviral treatment programme data. Lancet. 2013;382:S5. http://dx.doi.org/10.1016/S0140-6736(13)62253-9

27. Mfenyana K, Griffin M, Yogeswaran P, et al. Socio-economic inequalities as a predictor of health in South Africa: The Yenza cross-sectional study. S Afr Med J. 2008;96(4):323–330. PMID: 16670806.

28. Modjarrad K, Zulu I, Redden DT, Njobvu L, Freedman DO, Vermund SH. Prevalence and predictors of intestinal helminth infections among human immunodeficiency virus type 1–infected adults in an urban African setting. Am J Trop Med Hyg. 2005;73(4):777–782. PMID: 16222025.

29. Mwambete KD, Justin-Temu M, Peter S. Prevalence and management of intestinal helminthiasis among HIV-infected patients at Muhimbili National Hospital. J Int Assoc Physicians AIDS Care 2010;9(3):150–156. PMID: 20530468, http://dx.doi.org/10.1177/1545109710368138

30. Anuar TS, Salleh FM, Moktar N. Soil-transmitted helminth infections and associated risk factors in three Orang Asli tribes in peninsular Malaysia. Sci Rep. 2014;4:1–7. PMID: 24525479, http://dx.doi.org/10.1038/srep04101

31. De Silva NR, Brooker S, Hotez PJ, Montresor A, Engels D, Savioli L. Soil-transmitted helminth infections: Updating the global picture. Trends Parasitol. 2003;19(12):547–551. PMID: 14642761, http://dx.doi.org/10.1016/j.pt.2003.10.002

32. Strunz EC, Addiss DG, Stocks ME, Ogden S, Utzinger J, Freeman MC. Water, sanitation, hygiene, and soil-transmitted helminth infection: A systematic review and meta-analysis. PLoS Med. 2014;11(3):e1001620. PMID: 24667810, http://dx.doi.org/10.1371/journal.pmed.1001620

33. Idindili B. Challenges of continuum of HIV/AIDS care and treatment in Tanzania: The effects of parasites co-infections, HIV clinical manifestations, and adherence to antiretroviral therapy [doctoral dissertation] Basel: University of Basel; 2012 [cited 2014 Apr 26]. Available from: http://edoc.unibas.ch/22092/1/PhD_dissertation_Boniphace_Idindili.pdf

34. Hailemariam G, Kassu A, Abebe G, et al. Intestinal parasitic infections in HIV/AIDS and HIV seronegative individuals in a teaching hospital, Ethiopia. Jpn J Infect Dis. 2004;57(2):41–43. PMID: 15118206.

35. Foyaca-Sibat H, Del Rio-Romero I. Prevalence of epilepsy in an endemic area for neurocysticercosis in South Africa. Internet J Neurol. 2008;9(1):8–18.

36. Babatunde SK, Salami AK, Fabiyi JP, Agbede OO, Desalu OO. Prevalence of intestinal parasitic infestation in HIV seropositive and seronegative patients in Ilorin, Nigeria. Ann Afr Med. 2010;9(3). 123–128. PMID: 20710101, http://dx.doi.org/10.4103/1596-3519.68356

37. Mulu A, Maier M, Liebert UG. Deworming of intestinal helminths reduces HIV-1 subtype C viremia in chronically co-infected individuals. Int J Infect Dis. 2013;17(10):e897–e901. PMID: 23688549, http://dx.doi.org/10.1016/j.ijid.2013.03.022

38. Modjarrad K, Zulu I, Redden DT, et al. Treatment of intestinal helminths does not reduce plasma concentrations of HIV-1 RNA in coinfected Zambian adults. J Infect Dis. 2005b;192(7):1277–1283. PMID: 16136473, http://dx.doi.org/10.1086/444543

39. Hotez PJ, Bundy D, Beegle K, et al. Helminth infections: Soil-transmitted helminth infections and schistosomiasis [chapter on the Internet]. In: Jamison DT, Breman JG, Measham AR, et al., editors. Disease control priorities in developing countries. New York: Oxford University Press; 2006 [cited 2012 Nov 21]; p. 467–82. Available from: http://www.dcp-3.org/sites/default/files/dcp2/DCP24.pdf

The expected and actual communication of health care workers during the management of intrapartum: An interpretive multiple case study

Authors:
Doreen K.M. M'Rithaa[1,2]
Sue Fawcus[3,4]
Mikko Korpela[1,5]
Retha De la Harpe[1]

Affiliations:
[1]Information Technology, Cape Peninsula University of Technology, South Africa

[2]Department of Interdisciplinary Health Sciences, Stellenbosch University, South Africa

[3]Mowbray Maternity Hospital, South Africa

[4]Obstetrics and Gynaecology, University of Cape Town, South Africa

[5]School of Computing, University of Eastern Finland, Finland

Correspondence to:
Doreen M'Rithaa

Email:
doreen.mugendi@gmail.com

Postal address:
PO Box 1634, Milnerton, Cape Town 7435, South Africa

Background: Daily activities within a health care organisation are mediated by information communication processes (ICP) involving multiple health care professionals at different levels of care. Effective perinatal management requires critical information to be accurately communicated. If there is a breakdown in this communication patient safety is at risk for various reasons such as: inadequate critical information, misconception of information and uninformed decisions being made. The purpose of this study was to interpret the complexities around ICP in order to contribute to the effective management of the intrapartum period.

Methods: Multi method, multiple case study approach was used to understand the ICP during the management of the intrapartum period. During the study, the expected ICP, the actual ICP, the challenges involved and the desired ICP were analysed. Twenty-four in-depth interviews with skilled birth attendants (SBAs) employing observer-as-participant roles, field notes, and document review methods were utilised to gather the data. Thematic analysis was utilised to analyse the data using Atlas TI software.

Results: The study revealed three subthemes which emerged from the expected ICP, whilst three others that emerged formed the theme actual ICP. The subthemes from the expected ICP included: accessibility of obstetric services, expected referral, recommended tools, expected communication and expected documentation. The theme actual ICP held three emerging subthemes: the handover processes, collaborative information seeking, information communicated and referral processes.

Conclusion: This study showed that what was expected was not what was actually happening. The requirements of the policies and protocols need to be effectively implemented to improve practice building these into current biomedical guidelines.

La communication attendue et effective entre les travailleurs de santé pendant la gestion des soins périnatals: une étude interprétative de cas multiples.

Contexte: Les activités journalières au sein d'un établissement de santé sont influencées par le processus de communication des informations (PCI) impliquant de nombreux professionnels de la santé aux différents niveaux de soins. La prise en charge périnatale efficace exige une communication précise des informations essentielles. S'il y a un manque de communication la sécurité des patients est en danger pour plusieurs raisons: des informations essentielles inadéquates, des malentendus sur les informations et des décisions malavisées peuvent être prises. Le but de cette étude était de relever les complexités du PCI afin de contribuer à la prise en charge efficace de la période périnatale.

Méthodes: On a utilisé une étude multi-méthode de plusieurs cas pour comprendre le PCI pendant la prise en charge de la période périnatale. Au cours de l'étude, le PCI attendu, le PCI effectif, l'enjeu et le PCI désiré ont été analysés. Pour collecter les données on a eu vingt-quatre entrevues en profondeur avec des sages-femmes qualifiées (SFQ) au moyen de rôles d'observateur participant, des notes de terrain, et des méthodes de revue des documents. On s'est servi de l'analyse thématique pour analyser les données au moyen du logiciel Atlas Ti.

Résultats: L'étude a mis en évidence trois sous-thèmes qui sont ressortis du PCI attendu, alors que les trois autres qui sont apparus forment le thème du PCI effectif. Les sous-thèmes du PCI attendu sont: l'accessibilité des services obstétriques, l'orientation attendue, les outils recommandés, la communication attendue et la documentation attendue. Le thème effectif du PCI contenait trois sous-thèmes émergeants: les processus de transfert, la recherche d'informations collaborative, les informations communiquées et les processus de recommandation.

Conclusion: Cette étude a montré que ce qu'on attendait n'était pas ce qui se passait réellement. Les exigences des politiques et des protocoles devaient être mises en œuvre efficacement pour améliorer les pratiques et les intégrer dans les directives biomédicales actuelles.

Background

Maternal mortality is referred to as death caused by complications from pregnancy or childbirth. According to the current report by the WHO, there is a decline in the Maternal Mortality Rate (MMR) from 1990 to 2013 by 45% – from 380 deaths to 210 deaths per 100 000 live births. The decline does not necessarily meet the 5.5% rate required for the three quarters reduction targeted in the MDG goal 5 by 2015.[1] Although all regions have shown significant advancement, the levels of maternal mortality in sub-Saharan Africa remain unacceptably high.[1] In South Africa, the average MMR of 140 with a lower rate of 85 and 210 on the higher side indicates the need to implement further measures to reduce the lifetime risk of maternal death. Currently, the industrialized countries have a lifetime risk of maternal death of 1 in 4000, versus 1 in 51 in countries classified as 'least developed'.[1] Effective information communication during the management of labour and birth is an effective strategy to reduce maternal morbidity and mortality through identification of risks and abnormalities and promptly attending to them.[2]

Within the perinatal environment, interdisciplinary teams collaborate in providing quality care to women and the new-born during pregnancy, birth and the postpartum period with the ultimate goal of delivering a healthy mother and baby.[2] The collaboration during perinatal care in addition to the management of obstetric emergencies allows the skilled birth attendants (SBAs) to intercept errors before they happen.[2]

The coordination of these collaborative activities requires information communication to be clear, timely, accurate, comprehensive and respectful in order to achieve cohesiveness within the perinatal setting.[3,4] Fragmented activities, failure in systems and breakdown in communication contributes to a chain of actions that cause unexpected fatal outcomes.[5]

Improving maternal health requires health systems that function as an entity rather than silos with single interventions or actions by individual actors that form part of the activities of a team of actors.[6] The complexity of management of perinatal care requires a variety of complex, yet comprehensive, interventions in order to reduce maternal mortality.[7] The fact that complications can arise at any time and place requires single interventions which are comprehensive yet achievable. These interventions may be networked by several activities which require specific means of coordination. This, therefore, requires maternal health care which is dependent on appropriate health systems to have policies whose objective is dependent on each intervention to be achieved, whilst managing the complex interventions.[8]

Various factors were attributed to the expected information communication processes (ICP) within the obstetric units and between the referring facilities in the Cape Town Metro. The policies, protocols and guidelines are used as a means of coordination of activities in the management of the perinatal period. The definition of a protocol according to[9] is all steps in the management of a clinical condition which could cover the steps to develop a diagnosis or treat an illness. The protocols used in the study were used to describe the steps in diagnosis and management whilst describing the required processes to be followed in case of further management.

Guidelines are synonymously used with the term protocol emphasising guidance in the clinical management rather than ordering the course of action required. The practitioners are expected to use judgment in the care of patients. In an attempt to describe evidence-based health policy,[8] it is important to know what is needed and to facilitate those needs, although that does not necessarily mean that the health is improved. Conducting studies on health policy process in especially low and middle-income settings, whilst focusing on the current activities, will allow for better identification of the content needed for the health policies.[8]

Regardless of whether the content of a guideline or a protocol reflects best practice, the usefulness and the impact is reflected by the adoption rate. Consequently, there is need for the developers of the policies, guidelines and protocols to contemplate the best representation or the guidelines for dissemination.[9] Policies have to be contextualised in both context and place,[10] meaning that the environment requiring policies is influenced by inter-organisational and network relationships. The purpose of the study was to understand the complexities involved during the ICP in the management of the intrapartum period. The review of what is expected in this study is based on the domestic policies, protocols and guidelines which guide the daily practices that determine what is actually happening within, and between, the health facilities.

Methods

Setting

The study was carried out in the Western Cape Province of South Africa. The province has two tertiary hospitals for obstetric referrals. Cape Town Metro has four intermediate level referral hospitals with 11 Midwifery Obstetric Units (MOUs) within the Metro District Health Services (DHS) managing low-risk women. The MOUs have the highest number of births, approximately 300 births per month, and are managed exclusively by midwives. The obstetric specialists are situated in the secondary and tertiary level hospitals managing intermediate and high-risk women. A multi-method qualitative case study approach with multiple units of analysis was utilised. Two case studies were purposefully selected from the Cape Metro from the MOUs with the highest number of deliveries per month. All the MOUs have specific referral criteria and management protocols for either intermediate or high-risk women when complications arise during labour and birth. The two selected MOUs in the study (referred to as MOU A and MOU B) were selected with the consecutive referring intermediate level hospitals (referred to as RH A and RH B).

Data collection

Data were collected through conducting 24 interviews with the skilled birth attendants (SBAs) (doctors and midwives); eight midwives from MOU A, and six from MOU B; three doctors from RH A, one midwife, four doctors from referral hospital B and three midwives. These interviews explored activities influencing the ICP during the management of the intrapartum period. They were conducted in English lasting between 30 to 60 min as this was the medium of communication amongst other languages utilised, such as Afrikaans and Xhosa. All interviews were tape recorded with the permission of the participants and later transcribed and analysed thematically. The interviews were conducted in the health facilities at the convenience of the participants in a quiet room.

The document review of protocols, guidelines and policies was done in order to understand the expected ICP. These documents included: national maternal guidelines, provincial maternal guidelines, specific hospital protocols and the maternal case records (MCRs). The last-mentioned records include labour plans and partograms by identifying trends and patterns of the expected ICP. The partograms reviewed were those that were completed by the SBAs during the study observation period. During observation, the researcher assumed the role of the observer–as-participant, which involved observing and conducting short interviews regarding the observation. The researcher's role was overt, and the rapport created allowed the participants to freely speak about their experiences.

Analysis

The researcher transcribed all interviews and analysed data using Atlas TI software 7. Furthermore, all documents were uploaded onto the Atlas TI and data coding was done. The thematic analysis was used to organise the emergent codes and categories in order to ensure rigorous analysis. The coded transcripts were read and reread whilst listening to the recorded tapes to identify emerging themes. Data were analysed according to each unit of analysis (MOU A, MOU B, RH A, and RH B). A report was created for the cases that considered the similarities and differences within, and between, the cases. Themes were created in consultation with the fellow researchers through discussion and amendment after the feedback.

Ethical considerations

The research was approved by the review board and the ethics committee of the University Higher Degrees Committee (HDC) and the Western Cape Province, Department of Health, (RP052/2013) and the health facilities where the research was carried out. An informed consent was obtained from each interview participant. Ethical procedures were followed according to the ethics committee recommendations.

Results

The main themes, expected ICP and the Actual ICP, were deduced from the objectives of the study, whilst the subthemes emerged inductively from the data coding and categorizing process.

Theme expected information communication processes: Means of coordination

The policies, protocols and the maternal guidelines, which included SA national maternity guidelines and Western Cape guidelines, were reviewed. These included: the Western Cape level of care document, Metro West and Metro East protocols and referral criteria, neonatal protocols and referral criteria for the Cape Metro. The review revealed the expectations for the SBAs to ensure accurate and appropriate ICP whilst managing the women in the perinatal period. The subthemes that emerged from the data included accessibility, recommended tools for communication, the expected documentation, expected communication and referral criteria.

Expected accessibility of obstetric services

The need for accessibility of obstetric services was described as being able to provide women with 24 hour care during pregnancy, birth and motherhood. Appropriate ICP ensures a swift reliable access to care especially during referrals:

> Ensure 24-hour access to functioning emergency obstetric care (both basic and comprehensive).[1]

This accessibility to care was required from management at low-risk levels with the expectation that there are policies and protocols to ensure appropriate support between referring units.

The expected documentation

The expected documentation included the data which was expected to be collected and the tools that were required to be used in the documentation. The early warning chart (EWC) was one of the tools required for use to recognise abnormalities and refer the woman:

> Poor response to abnormal observations prompts an urgent need for the routine use of a national obstetric early warning chart used for all obstetric women ...[11]

Situation, Background, Assessment and Recommendation (SBAR), which is a structured document, was also recommended to prompt an urgent need for referral and should also be used for consultation with referral hospital doctors, followed by appropriate training on the use of the tool:

> ... the SBAR communication format refers to the Situation, Background, Assessment and Recommendation format. It is

> important that the health care workers formulate an appropriate request and clearly document the response … Ensure training in the early warning charts and SBAR referral system is provided.[11]

The structured communication format is expected to increase the effectiveness of communication whilst formulating an appropriate request and documenting the response. Although most individuals used the SOAP (Subjective, Objective, Assessment, and Plan) criteria to hand over information, the recommended SBAR and the EWC have not been implemented and are in the process of implementation.

Expected communication

Communication was expected to be effective, with tools such as radio, telephone and SBAR charts available between referring sites. Advice calls were recommended to be taken by doctors:

> Effective communication system (radio or telephone) and reliable 24 hour transport service for emergency transfer to hospital … Ensure dedicated telephonic linkages for consultation for emergencies between referring and referral site are available. (SBAR charts).[12]

The expected communication requires intercollegial interactions to always be conducted in a respectful and professional manner. The communicator is required to be clear and upfront regarding the reason for calling the senior practitioner:

> Intercollegial interactions should always be conducted in a respectful and professional manner.[13]

All data regarding the management of the intrapartum period was expected to be entered into the partogram with specific description of the required entry of information for progress of labour, condition of the mother and the condition of the foetus:

> All observations pertinent to the progress of labour and the condition of the mother and the foetus during labour must be recorded on the partogram in the prescribed manner and intervals.[14]

Although the ISBAR was recommended for use during the referral of the woman, the partogram was also expected to be used for communication, and all information regarding the communication clearly written up on the reverse side of the partogram:

> The professional taking action or phoning the next level of health management, must clearly document the actions on the reverse side of the observation chart …[12]

The expected communication required professionals to use precise, accurate and appropriate documentation in order to communicate effectively.

Expected referral

The expected referral required a reliable mode of transport referral routes and appropriate communication processes. Protocols were required to streamline the routes whilst monitoring the referral processes:

> A well-coordinated referral system, with access to transport and facilities, is essential for the provision of optimal care to all pregnant women in the district; it is essential to have in place a referral system with clear protocols of management, referral, transport and responsibility.[13]

An expected solution for mistakes during referrals was also suggested as the responsibility of the doctor at the referring level of care. It is her or his responsibility to contact the next level of care and communicate that information with the referring midwife. It was also recommended that the consultant in the higher level of care should resolve any disputes that arise during the referrals.

Theme Actual information communication processes: Activities involved in the information communication processes

All SBAs viewed communication as essential for the coordination of work activities within each unit and had developed a culture that was understood by the other members. The handover process, collaborative information seeking, information communicated and referral processes were the categories emerging under this theme.

Actual handover process in the midwifery obstetric units

The critical role of the handover process in the management of women during the intrapartum period was, by and large, the first statement expressed by midwives when asked about a day whilst on duty. The handover process involved the entry point for information exchange between shifts that enabled midwives to gain insight to the women already in the labour ward:

> 'We go from bed to bed we discuss in detail if it's a post-partum woman, what has happened from when she came in through the labour, if there were any difficulties, focus on that, and when they leave you take over the woman and you go on.' (P1:3)

All midwives and students are usually present during the handover process, as they are required to have information about each woman as they work through the day. The verbal handover is required to be documented in the maternal case record by the midwives handing over and those receiving the information:

> '… Ok in the mornings I take over with the rest of the staff so everybody, irrespective of whether you are working in the ante-natal clinic, we all take over in the labour ward. The reason why I do that is because I always feel that everybody should know what is going on you see because it might just happen that I need to call somebody for them to help me in the labour ward then they know what is going on in the labour ward.' (P2:10)

The information exchange also referred to by midwives as 'takeover' also took place as the women arrived and progressed through the stages of labour. Being a midwifery-led unit that managed low-risk women, the midwives relied on phone calls for consultation, because there were no doctors in the MOU to consult when the midwives were unsure of how to proceed. The referral hospital was about 10 km away and, in case of a need for consultation, they would use telephones to call the hospital where the obstetric and paediatric specialists were located:

> '... No we don't have doctors in the MOU, we phone according to, say we have our whole criteria on where the woman needs to go, depending on the problem. Say if we find that the woman needs to go to RH A – which is mostly for the high-risk people. I consider level I as an intermediate that means the woman can be seen there and here.' (P1:9)

Apart from the handover process, collaborative information seeking was noted during the management of the intrapartum period.

Actual collaborative information seeking

The midwives cross-checked information that was given to be sure of the accuracy. Even though there was no specific allocation of a midwife per woman, the midwives worked as a team and kept each other informed of any new information regarding the women, including a particular woman's progress. This took place between the breaks for tea and lunches and also as they managed the women:

> '... Well I go and see and I check because there are times when the FHR is there and the progress is going slowly. The membranes are still intact and we need to see in 2 hours if this woman is dilated further or she stayed like that ...' (P8:23)

Using colleagues to record information when the midwife was busy allowed the midwife to write up information immediately, thus preventing loss of the required data. The use of non-medical personnel, such as the general assistants (GA), who were able to write down data was raised by the midwives. However, the question of whether or not the GAs wrote the correct information was not considered. GAs are unskilled staff who include cleaners or administrative assistants. The GAs would document the data on a piece of paper, which the midwife would later transfer to the maternal case record. The midwives also relied on memory to transcribe the notes:

> 'But when we don't have students, we call out "weight" and someone will write it down but maybe she is busy while you are doing that and you ask her please to write it down on a piece of paper and will write 39, 47, blah blah blah.' (P3:8)

In describing their day whilst working with women in labour, it emerged that the information collected by the midwives was part of the management of the intrapartum. The collection of information began with the assessment of the woman to determine when she was in labour:

> 'Ok every admission that walks in here, we have got an admission bed and we do tests and urine, it's a routine we do for blood pressure, pulse, temperature and the h/b on admission. Then we do palpations and stretching of the abdomen, we palpate, we monitor the contractions, whether she is having contractions or not, as long as there no history of spontaneous rupture of membranes or if it's just a history of pains, even if you can't feel those pains we do the vaginal examinations so as to know where we stand.' (P2:26)

The women were kept in the antenatal ward for four hours and, if diagnosed in labour, they would be admitted and managed in the antenatal ward during the latent phase of labour. During this time, the progress of labour was recorded in the maternal case record on the partogram. Those women who progressed to active phase > 4 cm dilated would be transferred to a labour bed and allowed to be mobile until delivery. All information collected during the management of labour was documented:

> 'And when they are in active phase we prefer our women to walk around in the ante natal ward until they have the urge to bear down and when they reach the stage that they can't take the pain then we transfer them to the labour ward and then our trays are prepared in advance so that even if we don't have women that are in labour, whoever comes in with their head on the perineum, we have got a tray ready.' (P3:24)

The midwives indicated that they worked as a team within the MOU. Even though the ward was busy, everyone was aware of what was happening in the ward as they would inform each other, or the midwife would examine the women to evaluate how far they were in labour. Sharing tasks was also common amongst the midwives in order to deal with the busy wards.

Actual information communicated

The information communicated in the referral hospital is usually performed quickly, especially during emergency situations. The midwives from the MOU A would give the information to the doctors in order for them to decide whether to refer a woman to an intermediate risk or a high-risk hospital. The midwives would immediately explain the history of the woman as well as any concerns they had about her:

> 'Sisters give me the whole information and what is the history of the woman?' (P8:59).

> 'Give us the meaty information so we can decide whether they need to come in or go there, can they stay there or do they need to go to RH B.' (P10:10)

Disparities on which information was given, and prioritizing the information differed between the expectations of the doctors and what the midwives would give.

The specific information that is required to be communicated is important to prevent wasting of time and giving inappropriate information. The age, gravidity, the parity, and the reason for calling the referral hospital was deemed as important. The order in which the information was given differed from one midwife to another, and the doctors preferred the reason for calling as the most important information:

> 'You need to say the background history of the woman, but they are very good at that – they will tell you the age, the gravidity/ parity and how far the woman is, they are very good at that presentation but the important part is why you're phoning!

[*Laughs*].' (P10:36)

The age, gravidity, parity, investigations and the reason for calling, especially the current history, was information required to be communicated to the doctors by the midwives.

Actual referral process

The referral process was emphasised as it was understood by both midwives and the doctors in the referral hospital. If a woman changes condition whilst in labour and becomes either a high risk or intermediate risk, they are expected to refer her in labour. Protocols for the Metro East are used to determine the types of women and where they are expected to be referred. When the midwives in MOU A phone the referral hospital they use the required criteria (in the protocol) to determine where they will send the woman. The protocols are adjusted according to the hospital capacity to accommodate the woman in labour:

> '... we phone according to, say we have our whole criteria on where the woman needs to go, depending on the problem ... Then we discuss it with the doctor but we know already what kind of problem goes where ...' (P1:9)

When the MOU's call the referral hospital there are four MOU's that refer to RH A. The phone calls go through the switchboard and the doctors are contacted via intercom; they then contact the MOU. The doctors do not wait for the phone calls from the MOU as they have other tasks elsewhere in the hospital. The doctors prefer a hot line as the MOUs contact the hospital directly:

> 'You can put it down to switchboard and say they can broadcast the call but they will put it through to their cell phone if it's after hours because after 10 pm there is no broadcasting of calls.' (P11:32)

The consultation process requires the midwife in MOU A to give enough information for the doctor to make an informed decision. This happens when midwives encounter problems they are unsure of how to manage:

> '... I prefer them phoning if they need advice than sitting at that side not knowing what to do without a doctor that side, so I don't mind them doing that but not all doctors feel the same way.' (P10:19)

The doctors' work load in the referral hospital influences the ICP. There is no specific doctor allocated to answer the phone calls in the MOU. There are mainly two doctors on call who will answer calls and deal with the consultations and referrals as they come in. This means that the MOU A has to wait for the referral hospital to contact the doctors, whether in an emergency or merely for consultation purposes:

> 'Yes there are two people ... We are two of us on call and we will be taking calls and we will be seeing all the gynae women and all the obstetrics women, doing all the surgery as well. So there isn't a way for them to communicate with us other than the way that it is because as I said, it's not always us sitting in one place.' (P10:64)

The fact that doctors can be anywhere in the hospital influences the flow of phone calls. The calls are directed to the area where the doctor is busy at that particular time. If the doctor is in theatre and scrubbed up the anaesthetist may receive calls and pass the information verbally to the doctor ... However, the anaesthetist might not be conversant with obstetrics terminology, so that she or he will be unable to communicate the message from the midwives to the doctors properly:

> 'If we are operating, scrubbed up or the anaesthetist needs to be our receptionist to convey the message, I think it's very frustrating for them as they mention it multiple times.' (P10:5)

The doctors indicated that they mostly used the protocols to decide on women management and referral. Although there are protocols in place for the management of the intrapartum women, different doctors seemed to have different ways of managing the referrals and the consultations of the women.

Discussion

Means of coordination

The need to have policies, protocols and guidelines that can be easily adopted within a clinical setting is recommended.[8] In the study, although most policies were made at the national level, the context within which they were applied required more specific approaches. The means of coordination should be specific to the interventions required, especially in the maternal health setting.[7] As mentioned in the findings, the requirement for primary health care facilities to be accessible 24 hours allows low-risk women to have available services. The availability of the services is also linked to acceptability by the community and availability to the community.[10] For accessibility to really have an impact on maternal heath, there is a need for a well-functioning system for accessing comprehensive emergency obstetric services.[10] The accessibility of obstetric services emerged as the 'umbrella' of the other interventions such as expected documentation, recommended tools for documentation communication and the expected referral.

The recommended tools for communication had duplication of requirements where the information documented on the partogram was also required to be documented on the ISBAR and the EWC for every woman during the management of the intrapartum period. This tool required all information regarding the condition of the foetus, the progress of labour maternal condition and the management to be recorded. The effectiveness of use of the partogram evaluated in systematic reviews by[15] reports low and middle-income settings recommendation for use of partograms.

Furthermore, the EWC was also recommended for use in detecting deviations from the normal during the management of the intrapartum period. This chart was also needed for communication. The tool SBAR was recommended for use during communication within and between referring centres. Although the structured communication document is recommended in literature for its effectiveness in communication,[16] inappropriate use can lead to adverse outcomes. The duplication of information required in the three tools for documentation would increase the work of the SBAs in documenting information. Although telephones and radios were recommended for communication, the precise flow of information was not described in any of the guidelines. Specific guidelines are required in order to improve on all paper and electronic information tools to improve ICP

The expected communication was linked to the structure in the tools for communication. However, the need for specific protocols or communication guidelines is required to be drafted as context-specific, and training of the practitioners actualised during the implementation. The communication recommendations were mainly linked to referral requirements. The influence of documentation was not linked to communication processes but was seen as a separate entity.

Understanding the actual information communication processes

The handover process within this study played the role of passing information regarding the management of perinatal women between SBA within and between shifts, which could be verbal and written summary notes.[17] The communication was a culture that was considered important for transferring information between the team members, but the sufficiency of the information transferred was subjective to the receiver and sender. There was no structured communication between the SBAs. The use of nursing handover minimum data set and nursing notes for the specific context is recommended.[17] There is a need to develop intrapartum midwifery-specific handover minimum data set and transcribed notes.[17]

The existence of finding, using and communicating the information in the study was complex-emphasised by the SBAs' need to obtain information regarding the women in labour. The search for information was either between the experienced birth attendants, from protocols which they are familiar with, or other sources such as books and cell phones in the case of students. Information seekers, according to[18] decide to seek information from a number of sources to choose from. The credibility, which refers to perceived trustworthiness, and utility described as usefulness, relevance, timeliness, accessibility and ease of use of the sources are characteristics described by[19] as being relative to the perceptions and environments of the different users.

Although the SBAR tool was recommended for communication according to the means of communication, most of the SBAs were not aware of the existence of the SBAR, nor were they using the EWC. The partogram was heavily relied on for communication, and past history documented on the maternal case record. This is a very important tool for ICP, provided it is comprehensively completed and accompanies the woman in referral.

Protocols should be designed according to best evidence and, most importantly, should consider the context that includes the patient, treatment goals, local resources, staff and the local processes.[8] The study highlighted the need for information communication protocols that are usable and understood by the intended users. Understanding work activities of the actors would enable development of appropriate means of coordination.

Conclusion

What is expected by the means of coordination is not what is actually happening. The expected information communication is not the actual information communication. Context-specific culture for information collection, documentation and communication has allowed practitioners to use preferred processes in communicating amongst themselves. The ICP requires a structured process to be implemented with accurate monitoring and evaluation of the activities involved in the ICP. The author urges that the framework should provide a basis for the evaluation of the effectiveness involved in the ICP for the effective management of the intrapartum period.

Acknowledgements

This study was partly supported by the ISD4D project funded by the Academy of Finland, grant no. 253275.

Competing interests

The authors declare that they have no financial or personal relationship(s) that may have inappropriately influenced them in writing this article.

Authors' contributions

D.K.M.M. was the researcher and main author of the article. S.F. was co-researcher and second author of the article sections of the article. M.K. was co-researcher and third author contributed sections of the article. R.D. was co-researcher and edited the article.

References

1. WHO, UNICEF, UNFPA, World Bank, United Nations Population Division. Trends in maternal mortality: 1990 to 2013. Estimates by WHO, UNICEF, UNFPA, The World Bank and the United Nations Population Division. Geneva: World Health Organization; 2014.
2. Gephart SM, Cholette M. Pure communication: A strategy to improve care coordination for high-risk birth. Newborn Infant Nurs Rev. 2012;12(2):109–114. PMID: 22773922, http://dx.doi.org/10.1053/j.nainr.2012.03.007
3. Gephart SM, McGrath JM, Effken JA. Failure to rescue in neonatal care. J Perinat Neonatal Nurs. 2011;25:275–282. PMID: 21825918, http://dx.doi.org/10.1097/JPN.0b013e318227cc03
4. Lyndon A, Kennedy HP. Perinatal safety: From concept to nursing practice. J Perinat Neonatal Nurs. 2010;24(1):22–31. PMID: 20147827, http://dx.doi.org/10.1097/JPN.0b013e3181cb9351
5. Nyamtema AS, Urassa DP, van Roosmalen J. Maternal health interventions in resource limited countries: A systematic review of packages, impacts and factors for change. BMC Pregnancy Childbirth. 2011;11(1):30. PMID: 21496315, http://dx.doi.org/10.1186/1471-2393-11-30

6. Campbell OMR, Graham WJ. Strategies for reducing maternal mortality: Getting on with what works. Lancet. 2006;368(9543):1284–1299. PMID: 17027735, http://dx.doi.org/10.1016/S0140-6736(06)69381-1

7. Sanneving L, Kulane A, Iyer A, Ahgren B. Health system capacity: Maternal health policy implementation in the state of Gujarat, India. Glob Health Action.2013;6:1–8. PMID: 23522352, http://dx.doi.org/10.3402/gha.v6i0.19629

8. Coiera E. Guide to health informatics. 2nd ed. Boca Raton: CRC Press; 2003.

9. Walt G, Shiffman J, Schneider H, Murray SF, Brugha R, Gilson L. 'Doing' health policy analysis: Methodological and conceptual reflections and challenges. Health Policy Plan. 2008; 23(5):308–317. PMID: 18701552, http://dx.doi.org/10.1093/heapol/czn024

10. Silal SP, Penn-Kekana L, Harris B, Birch S, McIntyre D. Exploring inequalities in access to and use of maternal health services in South Africa. BMC Health Serv Res. 2012;12(1):120. PMID: 22613037, http://dx.doi.org/10.1186/1472-6963-12-120

11. Pattinson R, Fawcus S, Moodley J. Tenth interim report on confidential enquiries into maternal deaths in South Africa 2011 and 2012. National Committee for Confidential Enquiries into Maternal Deaths; 2013.

12. National Committee on Confidential Enquiries into Maternal Deaths. Saving mothers: Fifth report on confidential enquiries into maternal deaths in South Africa 2008–2010. Pretoria: Department of Health; 2011.

13. Department of Health. Guidelines for maternity care in South Africa. 3rd ed. Pretoria: Department of Health; 2007.

14. Department of Health. Metro east protocols for basic antenatal care. Cape Town: Western Cape Department of Health; 2012.

15. Lavender T, Hart A, Smyth RMD. Effect of partogram use on outcomes for women in spontaneous labour at term. Cochrane Database Systc Rev [serial online]. 2012;8:CD005461. PMID: 23843091, http://dx.doi.org/10.1002/14651858.CD005461.pub4

16. Woodhall LJ, Vertacnik L, McLaughlin M. Implementation of the SBAR communication technique in a tertiary center. J Emerg Nurs. 2008;34(4):314–317. PMID: 18640411, http://dx.doi.org/10.1016/j.jen.2007.07.007

17. Johnson M, Sanchez P, Suominen H, et al. Comparing nursing handover and documentation: forming one set of patient information. Int Nurs Rev. 2014;61(1):73–81. PMID: 24308444, http://dx.doi.org/10.1111/inr.12072

18. Johnson M, Jefferies D, Nicholls D. Developing a minimum data set for electronic nursing handover. J Clin Nurs. 2012;21(3–4):331–343. PMID: 22082347, http://dx.doi.org/10.1111/j.1365-2702.2011.03891.x

19. Robson A, Robinson L. Building on models of information behaviour: Linking information seeking and communication. J Doc. 2013;69(2):169–193. http://dx.doi.org/10.1108/00220411311300039

Permissions

All chapters in this book were first published in PHCFM, by AOSIS Publishing; hereby published with permission under the Creative Commons Attribution License or equivalent. Every chapter published in this book has been scrutinized by our experts. Their significance has been extensively debated. The topics covered herein carry significant findings which will fuel the growth of the discipline. They may even be implemented as practical applications or may be referred to as a beginning point for another development.

The contributors of this book come from diverse backgrounds, making this book a truly international effort. This book will bring forth new frontiers with its revolutionizing research information and detailed analysis of the nascent developments around the world.

We would like to thank all the contributing authors for lending their expertise to make the book truly unique. They have played a crucial role in the development of this book. Without their invaluable contributions this book wouldn't have been possible. They have made vital efforts to compile up to date information on the varied aspects of this subject to make this book a valuable addition to the collection of many professionals and students.

This book was conceptualized with the vision of imparting up-to-date information and advanced data in this field. To ensure the same, a matchless editorial board was set up. Every individual on the board went through rigorous rounds of assessment to prove their worth. After which they invested a large part of their time researching and compiling the most relevant data for our readers.

The editorial board has been involved in producing this book since its inception. They have spent rigorous hours researching and exploring the diverse topics which have resulted in the successful publishing of this book. They have passed on their knowledge of decades through this book. To expedite this challenging task, the publisher supported the team at every step. A small team of assistant editors was also appointed to further simplify the editing procedure and attain best results for the readers.

Apart from the editorial board, the designing team has also invested a significant amount of their time in understanding the subject and creating the most relevant covers. They scrutinized every image to scout for the most suitable representation of the subject and create an appropriate cover for the book.

The publishing team has been an ardent support to the editorial, designing and production team. Their endless efforts to recruit the best for this project, has resulted in the accomplishment of this book. They are a veteran in the field of academics and their pool of knowledge is as vast as their experience in printing. Their expertise and guidance has proved useful at every step. Their uncompromising quality standards have made this book an exceptional effort. Their encouragement from time to time has been an inspiration for everyone.

The publisher and the editorial board hope that this book will prove to be a valuable piece of knowledge for researchers, students, practitioners and scholars across the globe.

List of Contributors

Nicodemus O. Owusu
Faculty of Human and Social Sciences, University of Southampton, United Kingdom

Wendwosen T. Nibabe
Ethiopian Society of Obstetricians and Gynaecologists, Addis Ababa

Tennyson Mgutshini
College of Human Sciences, University of South Africa, South Africa

Kabiru K. Salami
Department of Sociology, University of Ibadan, Nigeria

William R. Brieger
Department of International Health, Bloomberg School of Public Health, Johns Hopkins University, USA

Linda Jonker and Ethelwynn L. Stellenberg
Faculty of Health Sciences, Department of Nursing, Stellenbosch University, South Africa

Sumaya Mall and Leslie Swartz
Alan J Flisher Centre for Public Mental Health, Department of Psychology, Stellenbosch University, South Africa

Leticia Fernandez, Theresa Rossouw, Tessa Marcus, Angelika Reinbrech-Schutte and Nicoleen Smit
Department of Family Medicine, University of Pretoria, South Africa

Hans F. Kinkel and Shehla Memon
Department of Family Medicine, University of Pretoria, South Africa
Foundation for Professional Development, South Africa

Takalani G. Tshitangano
Department of Public Health, University of Venda, South Africa

Kristopher Hartwig and Paul Z. Mmbando
Evangelical Lutheran Church in Tanzania, Tanzania

Mervyn Dean
Consulting Palliative Care Physician, Tanzania

Kari Hartwig
College of Health Sciences, Walden University, United States

Abduraoof Sayed
Department of Community Health, University of Cape Town, South Africa

Elma de Vries
Division of Family Medicine, University of Cape Town, South Africa

Soornarain S. Naidoo
Department of Family Medicine, University of KwaZulu-Natal, South Africa

Lourens Schlebusch
Department of Behavioural Medicine, University of KwaZulu-Natal, South Africa

Surona Visagie
Centre for Rehabilitation Studies, University of Stellenbosch, South Africa

Marguerite Schneider
Department of Psychology, Stellenbosch University, South Africa

Alphonsus U. Idung and Sunday B. Udoh
Faculty of Clinical Sciences, Department of Family Medicine, College of Health Sciences, University of Uyo, Nigeria

Festus Abasiubong
Faculty of Clinical Sciences, Department of Psychiatry, College of Health Sciences, University of Uyo, Nigeria

Uwemedimbuk S. Ekanem
Department of Community Health, Faculty of Clinical Sciences, College of Health Sciences, University of Uyo, Nigeria

Indiran Govender, Honey L. Mabuza and Gboyega A. Ogunbanjo
Department of Family Medicine & PHC, Sefako Makgatho Health Sciences (formerly known as the University of Limpopo, Medunsa Campus), South Africa

Sam T. Ntuli
Department of Public Health Medicine, University of Limpopo, Polokwane Campus, South Africa

Gboyega A. Ogunbanjo
Department of Family and Primary Health Care, University of Limpopo, Medunsa Campus, South Africa

Folafolu A. Adebolu and Mergan Naidoo
Department of Family Medicine, University of Kwazulu-Natal, South Africa

Douglas Newman-Valentine and Sinegugu Duma
Division of Nursing and Midwifery, University of Cape Town, South Africa

Lauren M. Terblanche and Ethelwynn L. Stellenberg
Division of Nursing, Department of Interdisciplinary Health Sciences, Faculty of Medicine and Health Sciences, Stellenbosch University, South Africa

Louis S. Jenkins and Colette Gunst
Division of Family Medicine and Primary Care, Faculty of Medicine and Health Sciences, Stellenbosch University, South Africa
Western Cape Department of Health, South Africa

Julia Blitz and Johan F. Coetzee
Division of Family Medicine and Primary Care, Faculty of Medicine and Health Sciences, Stellenbosch University, South Africa

Samuel A. Ajayi, Lawrence A. Adebusoye and Adetola M. Ogunbode
Family Medicine Department, University College Hospital, Ibadan, Nigeria

Joshua O. Akinyemi
Department of Epidemiology and Medical Statistics, College of Medicine, University of Ibadan, Nigeria

Ayodeji M. Adebayo
Department of Preventive Medicine and Primary Care, College of Medicine, University of Ibadan, Nigeria

Adeleye M. Awolola, Laura Campbell and Andrew Ross
Department of Family Medicine, University of KwaZulu-Natal, South Africa

Kholiwe Shabangu
Discipline of Pharmaceutical Sciences, School of Health Sciences, University of KwaZulu-Natal, Durban, South Africa

Fatima Suleman
Discipline of Pharmaceutical Sciences, School of Health Sciences, Westville Campus, University of KwaZulu-Natal, South Africa

Nkhensani Mogale
Department of Anatomy, Sefako Makgatho Health Sciences University, South Africa
Department of Anatomy, University of Pretoria, South Africa

Albert-Neels van Schoor and Marius C. Bosman
Department of Anatomy, University of Pretoria, South Africa

Rachel Wood, Vanessa Viljoen, Lisa Van Der Merwe and Robert Mash
Family Medicine and Primary Care, Stellenbosch University, South Africa

Johnface F. Mdala and Robert Mash
Division of Family Medicine and Primary Care, Stellenbosch University, South Africa

Jeannie van der Linde
Department of Speech- Language Pathology and Audiology, University of Pretoria, South Africa

De Wet Swanepoel
Department of Speech- Language Pathology and Audiology, University of Pretoria, South Africa
Ear Sciences Centre, School of Surgery, University of Western Australia, Nedlands, Australia
Ear Science Institute Australia, Subiaco, Australia

Frances P. Glascoe
Department of Pediatrics, Vanderbilt University, United States

E.M. Louw
Department of Statistics, University of Pretoria, South Africa

Jannie F.M. Hugo
Department of Family Medicine, University of Pretoria, South Africa

Bart Vinck
Department of Speech- Language Pathology and Audiology, University of Pretoria, South Africa
Department of Speech- Language Pathology and Audiology, Ghent University, Belgium

Augustin R.M. Amboko and Petra Brysiewicz
School of Nursing and Public Health, University of KwaZulu-Natal, South Africa

Sam T. Ntuli
Research Development and Administration, University of Limpopo, Polokwane Campus, South Africa Department of Public Health, University of Limpopo, Polokwane Campus, South Africa

Eric Maimela
Epidemiology Services, Limpopo Department of Health, South Africa

Mariannes Alberts, Solly Choma and Sekgothe Dikotope
Medical Science Department, University of Limpopo, Turfloop Campus, South Africa

Ethelwynn L. Stellenberg and Johanna M. Abrahams
Division of Nursing, Stellenbosch University, South Africa

Mary I. Ofili
Department of Nursing Science, Delta State University, Nigeria

Busisiwe P. Ncama and Benn Sartorius
School of Nursing and Public Health, University of KwaZulu-Natal, South Africa

Benjamin Mills and Indiran Govender
Department of Family Medicine, Sefako Makgatho Health Sciences University, South Africa

Jannie Hugo
Department of Family Medicine, University of Pretoria, South Africa

Talitha Crowley
Department of Interdisciplinary Health Sciences, Stellenbosch University, South Africa

Pat Mayers
Department of Health and Rehabilitation Sciences, University of Cape Town, South Africa

Adeyinka A. Alabi and Don O'Mahony
Department of Family Medicine, Faculty of Health Sciences, Walter Sisulu University, South Africa

Graham Wright
School of Health Sciences, University of Fort Hare, East London, South Africa

Mohlomi J. Ntsaba
Department of Nursing, Faculty of Health Sciences, Walter Sisulu University, South Africa

N.K. Mgori
Division of Family Medicine and Primary Care, Stellenbosch University, South Africa
Oshakati Intermediate Hospital, Namibia

Robert Mash
Division of Family Medicine and Primary Care, Stellenbosch University, South Africa

Doudou Nzaumvila and Indiran Govender
Department of Family Medicine, Sefako Makgatho Health Sciences University, South Africa

Efraim B. Kramer
Division of Emergency Medicine, School of Medicine, University of the Witwatersrand, South Africa

Sam Surka, Krisela Steyn and Katherine Everett-Murphy
Chronic Disease Initiative for Africa, Cape Town, South Africa

Thomas A. Gaziano
Brigham and Women's Hospital, Harvard University, United States

Naomi Levitt
Chronic Disease Initiative for Africa, Cape Town, South Africa
Department of Medicine, University of Cape Town, South Africa

Ethelwynn Stellenberg, Marjorie van Zyl and Johanna Eygelaar
Division of Nursing, Stellenbosch University, South Africa

Mmajapi E.T. Masala-Chokwe and Tendani S. Ramukumba
Adelaide Tambo School of Nursing Science, Tshwane University of Technology, South Africa

Oluwatoyi O. Toriola and Makama A. Monyeki
Physical Activity, Sport and Recreation Focus Area, North-West University, Potchefstroom Campus, South Africa

Abel L. Toriola
Department of Sport, Rehabilitation and Dental Sciences, Tshwane University of Technology, South Africa

Oathokwa Nkomazana
Faculty of Medicine, University of Botswana, Botswana

Robert Mash
Division of Family Medicine and Primary Care, Stellenbosch University, South Africa

Nthabiseng Phaladze
School of Nursing, University of Botswana, South Africa

Olukayode A. Adeleke
Department of Family Medicine, Walter Sisulu University, Mthatha, South Africa

Parimalaranie Yogeswaran
Department of Family Medicine and Rural Health, Walter Sisulu University, Mthatha, South Africa

Graham Wright
Centre for Health Informatics Research and Development, University of Fort Hare, South Africa

Doreen K.M. M'Rithaa
Information Technology, Cape Peninsula University of Technology, South Africa
Department of Interdisciplinary Health Sciences, Stellenbosch University, South Africa

Sue Fawcus
Mowbray Maternity Hospital, South Africa
Obstetrics and Gynaecology, University of Cape Town, South Africa

Mikko Korpela
Information Technology, Cape Peninsula University of Technology, South Africa
School of Computing, University of Eastern Finland, Finland

Retha De la Harpe
Information Technology, Cape Peninsula University of Technology, South Africa